FOURTH EDITION

ADMINISTRATIVE PROCEDURES

for Medical Assisting

Kathryn A. Booth, RN, RMA (AMT), RPT, CPhT, MS
Total Care Programming, Inc.
Palm Coast, Florida

Leesa G. Whicker, BA, CMA (AAMA)
Central Piedmont Community College
Charlotte, North Carolina

Terri D. Wyman, CPC, CMRS
Wing Memorial Hospital
Palmer, Massachusetts

Sandra Moaney Wright, BS, M.Ed., RMA (AMT)
Moaney Wright & Associates Consulting Group
Palmetto, Georgia

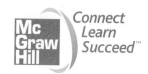

Connect
Learn
Succeed™

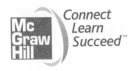

ADMINISTRATIVE PROCEDURES FOR MEDICAL ASSISTING

Published by McGraw-Hill, a business unit of The McGraw-Hill Companies, Inc., 1221 Avenue of the Americas, New York, NY, 10020. Copyright © 2011 by The McGraw-Hill Companies, Inc. All rights reserved. Previous editions © 1999, 2005, and 2009.

Some ancillaries, including electronic and print components, may not be available to customers outside the United States.

This book is printed on acid-free paper.

1 2 3 4 5 6 7 8 9 0 WDQ/WDQ 1 0 9 8 7 6 5 4 3 2 1 0

ISBN   978-0-07-734007-0
MHID   0-07-734007-8

Vice president/Editor in chief: *Elizabeth Haefele*
Vice president/Director of marketing: *John E. Biernat*
Publisher: *Kenneth S. Kasee Jr.*
Senior sponsoring editor: *Debbie Fitzgerald*
Director of development, Allied Health: *Patricia Hesse*
Developmental editor: *Connie Kuhl*
Editorial coordinator: *Parissa DJangi*
Marketing manager: *Mary B. Haran*
Lead digital product manager: *Damian Moshak*
Media development editor: *Marc Mattson*
Director, Editing/Design/Production: *Jess Ann Kosic*
Lead project manager: *Susan Trentacosti*

Senior production supervisor: *Janean A. Utley*
Senior designer: *Srdjan Savanovic*
Lead photo research coordinator: *Carrie K. Burger*
Photo researcher: *Pam Carley*
Media project manager: *Brent dela Cruz*
Outside development house: *Triple SSS Press—Alexis Ferraro*
Typeface: *10/12 Slimbach*
Compositor: *MPS Limited, A Macmillan Company*
Printer: *Worldcolor*
Cover credit: *Tablet: ©Getty Images/Comstock Images*
Credits: The credits section for this book begins on page 473 and is considered an extension of the copyright page.

Library of Congress Cataloging-in-Publication Data

Administrative procedures for medical assisting / Kathryn A. Booth ... [et al.]. — 4th ed.
    p. ; cm.
Includes bibliographical references and index.
ISBN-13: 978-0-07-734007-0 (alk. paper)
ISBN-10: 0-07-734007-8 (alk. paper)
1. Medical assistants. I. Booth, Kathryn A., 1957-
    [DNLM: 1. Allied Health Personnel. 2. Practice Management, Medical—organization & administration. 3. Medical Records. W 21.5 A238 2011]
R728.8.A28 2011
610.73'72069—dc22

2009048194

WARNING NOTICE: The procedures and other matters described in this publication are based upon research of current literature and consultation with knowledgeable persons in the field. The procedures and matters described in this text reflect currently accepted administrative medical practice. However, this information cannot and should not be relied upon as necessarily applicable to a given individual's case. Accordingly, each person must be treated as an individual to discern the patient's unique circumstances. Publisher disclaims all liability for any inaccuracies, omissions, misuse, or misunderstanding of the information contained in this publication. Publisher cautions that this publication is not intended as a substitute for the professional judgment of trained medical personnel.

The Internet addresses listed in the text were accurate at the time of publication. The inclusion of a Web site does not indicate an endorsement by the authors or McGraw-Hill, and McGraw-Hill does not guarantee the accuracy of the information presented at these sites.

www.mhhe.com

Brief Contents

PART ONE

Introduction to Medical Assisting 2

SECTION 1
Foundations and Principles 4

Chapter 1   The Profession of Medical Assisting   5
Chapter 2   Types of Medical Practice   24
Chapter 3   Legal and Ethical Issues in Medical Practice, Including HIPAA   42
Chapter 4   Communication with Patients, Families, and Coworkers   71

PART TWO

Administrative Medical Assisting 98

SECTION 1
Office Work 100

Chapter 5   Using and Maintaining Office Equipment   101
Chapter 6   Using Computers in the Office   123
Chapter 7   Managing Correspondence and Mail   145
Chapter 8   Managing Office Supplies   171
Chapter 9   Maintaining Patient Records   189
Chapter 10   Managing the Office Medical Records   216

SECTION 2
Interacting with Patients 239

Chapter 11   Telephone Techniques   240
Chapter 12   Scheduling Appointments and Maintaining the Physician's Schedule   258
Chapter 13   Patient Reception   278
Chapter 14   Patient Education   295

SECTION 3
Financial Responsibilities 314

Chapter 15   Health Insurance Billing Procedures   315
Chapter 16   Medical Coding   342
Chapter 17   Patient Billing and Collections   361
Chapter 18   Accounting for the Medical Office   384

APPENDIXES

Appendix I   Prefixes, Suffixes, and Word Roots in Commonly Used Medical Terms   420
Appendix II   Abbreviations and Symbols Commonly Used in Medical Notations   423

Glossary 425

Credits 473

Index 474

Contents

PART ONE

Introduction to Medical Assisting 2

SECTION 1
Foundations and Principles 4

Chapter 1 The Profession of Medical Assisting 5

Your Success as a Student 8
Growth of the Medical Assisting Profession 8
Medical Assistant Credentials 10
Membership in a Medical Assisting Association 11
Training Programs and Other Learning Opportunities 12
Accreditation 12
Daily Duties of Medical Assistants 15
Career Opportunities/Certified Office Laboratory Technician 16
Personal Qualifications of Medical Assistants 17
Points on Practice/Recycling in the Medical Office, Hospital, Laboratory, or Clinic 18
The AAMA Occupational Analysis 21

Chapter 2 Types of Medical Practice 24

Medical Specialties 26
Working with Other Allied Health Professionals 30
Career Opportunities/Medical Office Administrator or Manager 32
Specialty Career Options 36
Professional Associations 38

Chapter 3 Legal and Ethical Issues in Medical Practice, Including HIPAA 42

Medical Law and Ethics 45
The Patient-Physician Contract 46
Special Circumstances for Physician Practices 48
Preventing Lawsuits 49
Federal Legislation Affecting Health Care 56

OSHA Regulations 57
Laws That Protect the Employee 57
HIPAA 57
Risk Management 62
Confidentiality Issues and Mandatory Disclosure 63
Caution: Handle with Care/Notifying Those at Risk for Sexually Transmitted Disease 63
Code of Ethics 64
Points on Practice/AAMA Code of Ethics 66
Labor and Employment Laws 66
Legal Medical Practice Models 67

Chapter 4 Communication with Patients, Families, and Coworkers 71

Communicating with Patients and Families 73
The Communication Circle 74
Understanding Human Behavior and How It Relates to the Provider-Patient Relationship 75
Types of Communication 77
Improving Your Communication Skills 78
Communicating in Special Circumstances 82
PROCEDURE 4-1 Communicating with the Anxious Patient 83
Reflecting On . . . Cultural Issues/Multicultural Attitudes About Modern Medicine 84
Points on Practice/Talking with the Geriatric Patients 87
Communicating with Coworkers 88
Written Communication Tools and Community Resources 90
PROCEDURE 4-2 Identifying Community Resources 92
Personnel Management 92
Managing Stress 92
Preventing Burnout 93
Points on Practice/Potential Causes of Stress 93
Points on Practice/Tips for Reducing Stress 94
Reflecting On . . . Communication Issues/Scope of Practice 95

PART TWO

Administrative Medical Assisting 98

SECTION 1
Office Work 100

Chapter 5 Using and Maintaining Office Equipment 101

Office Communication Equipment 103

Reflecting On . . . HIPAA/Avoiding Abuse of Patient Confidentiality 105

Points on Practice/Routing Calls Through an Automated Menu 106

Reflecting On . . . HIPAA/HIPAA and Faxing 107

PROCEDURE 5-1 Using a Facsimile (Fax) Machine 108

Office Automation Equipment 110

PROCEDURE 5-2 Using a Photocopier Machine 111

PROCEDURE 5-3 Using a Postage Meter 113

PROCEDURE 5-4 Using a Dictation-Transcription Machine 115

PROCEDURE 5-5 Using a Check-Writing Machine 115

Purchasing Decisions 116

Reflecting On . . . HIPAA/HIPAA and Shredding 116

Reflecting On . . . HIPAA/HIPAA and Electronic Media 117

Maintaining Office Equipment 119

Points on Practice/Equipment Manual Tips 119

Chapter 6 Using Computers in the Office 123

The Computer Revolution 125

Types of Computers 125

Components of the Computer 127

Caution: Handle with Care/Carpal Tunnel Syndrome 129

Using Application Software 133

PROCEDURE 6-1 Creating a Form Letter 135

Reflecting On . . . HIPAA/HIPAA and E-mail 135

Points on Practice/Working Efficiently Online 137

Selecting Computer Equipment 138

Medical Practice Websites 139

Security in the Computerized Office 139

Reflecting On . . . HIPAA/Guidelines for HIPAA Privacy Compliance and the Computer 140

Computer System Care and Maintenance 140

Computers of the Future 142

Chapter 7 Managing Correspondence and Mail 145

Correspondence and Professionalism 147

Choosing Correspondence Supplies 147

Written Correspondence 148

Effective Writing 152

Interoffice Memorandums (Memos) 154

Editing and Proofreading 154

PROCEDURE 7-1 Creating a Letter 159

Preparing Outgoing Mail 160

Mailing Equipment and Supplies 163

U.S. Postal Service Delivery 163

Other Delivery Services 164

Processing Incoming Mail 166

PROCEDURE 7-2 Sorting and Opening Mail 167

Points on Practice/How to Spot Urgent Incoming Mail 168

Chapter 8 Managing Office Supplies 171

Organizing Medical Office Supplies 173

Taking Inventory of Medical Office Supplies 176

PROCEDURE 8-1 Step-by-Step Overview of Inventory Procedures 176

Ordering Supplies 180

Points on Practice/Ordering by Telephone or Fax or Online 183

Chapter 9 Maintaining Patient Records 189

Importance of Patient Records 191

Contents of Patient Charts 192

Reflecting On . . . HIPAA/Guidelines for Handling Protected Health Information within the Medical Record 198

Initiating and Maintaining Patient Records 199

The Six Cs of Charting 200

PROCEDURE 9-1 Preparing a Patient Medical Record/Chart 200

Types of Medical Records 202

Appearance, Timeliness, and Accuracy of Records 203

Electronic Health Records 204

Medical Transcription 205

Points on Practice/Working with Electronic Health Records 206

PROCEDURE 9-2 Transcribing Letters, Reports, and Notes 207

Career Opportunities/Medical Transcriptionist 207

Correcting and Updating Patient Records 208

PROCEDURE 9-3   Correcting Medical Records   209
Release of Records   209
PROCEDURE 9-4   Maintaining Medical
    Records   210

Chapter 10   Managing the Office Medical Records   216

The Importance of Records Management   218
Filing Equipment   218
Reflecting On . . . HIPAA/Safeguarding Protected
    Health Information   220
Filing Supplies   221
Filing Systems   222
Points on Practice/Indexing Rules   224
PROCEDURE 10-1   Creating a Filing System for
    Patient Records   226
PROCEDURE 10-2   Setting Up an Office Tickler
    File   227
The Filing Process   228
Points on Practice/Evaluating Your Office Filing
    System   231
Inactive and Closed File Storage   231
PROCEDURE 10-3   Developing a Records Retention
    Program   234
Career Opportunities/Registered Health Information
    Technician   235

SECTION 2
Interacting with Patients   239

Chapter 11   Telephone Techniques   240

Using the Telephone Effectively   242
Communication Skills   242
Managing Incoming Calls   242
Points on Practice/Screening Incoming Calls   245
Types of Incoming Calls   245
PROCEDURE 11-1   Performing Telephone
    Screening   246
PROCEDURE 11-2   Handling Emergency
    Calls   249
Using Proper Telephone Etiquette   250
Taking Messages   251
PROCEDURE 11-3   Retrieving Messages from an
    Answering Service   253
Telephone Answering Systems   253
Placing Outgoing Calls   253
Telephone Triage   254
Telephone Slamming and Cramming   255
Pagers and Cell Phones   255
Facsimile (Fax) Machines   255

Chapter 12   Scheduling Appointments and Maintaining the Physician's Schedule   258

The Appointment Book   260
Appointment Scheduling Systems   262
PROCEDURE 12-1   Creating a Cluster
    Schedule   266
Online Scheduling   266
Arranging Appointments   266
Special Scheduling Situations   268
Points on Practice/Scheduling Emergency
    Appointments   269
Scheduling Outside Appointments   270
PROCEDURE 12-2   Scheduling and Confirming
    Surgery at a Hospital   271
Maintaining the Physician's Schedule   273

Chapter 13   Patient Reception   278

First Impressions   280
Career Opportunities/Medical Receptionist   281
The Importance of Cleanliness   284
Caution: Handle with Care/Maintaining Cleanliness
    Standards in the Reception Area   285
The Physical Components   286
Keeping Patients Occupied and Informed   287
Points on Practice/Tailoring Office Magazines to
    Patient Interests   288
PROCEDURE 13-1   Creating a Pediatric
    Playroom   290
Patients with Special Needs   290
PROCEDURE 13-2   Creating a Reception Area
    Accessible to Patients with Special Needs   292

Chapter 14   Patient Education   295

The Educated Patient   297
Types of Patient Education   297
PROCEDURE 14-1   Developing a Patient Education
    Plan   298
Promoting Health and Wellness Through
    Education   299
The Patient Information Packet   301
Educating Patients with Special Needs   304
Reflecting On . . . Cultural Issues/Respecting Patients'
    Cultural Beliefs   305
Educating the Patient/Instructing Patients with
    Hearing Impairments   305
Patient Education Prior to Surgery   306
PROCEDURE 14-2   Informing the Patient of
    Guidelines for Surgery   308
Additional Educational Resources   309
Career Opportunities/Occupational Therapy
    Assistant   311

SECTION 3
Financial Responsibilities 314

Chapter 15   Health Insurance Billing Procedures 315
Basic Insurance Terminology 317
Types of Health Plans 318
Government Plans 319
PROCEDURE 15-1   Verifying Workers' Compensation Coverage 324
The Claims Process: An Overview 325
Fee Schedules and Charges 328
Preparing and Transmitting Health-Care Claims 333
PROCEDURE 15-2   Completing the CMS-1500 Claim Form 335
Points on Practice/Data Elements for HIPAA Electronic Claims 339

Chapter 16   Medical Coding 342
Diagnosis Codes: The ICD-9-CM 344
PROCEDURE 16-1   Locating an ICD-9-CM Code 349
Procedure Codes: The CPT 351
HCPCS 354
PROCEDURE 16-2   Locating a HCPCS Code 355
PROCEDURE 16-3   Locating a CPT Code 356
Avoiding Fraud: Coding Compliance 356
Career Opportunities/Medical Coder, Physician Practice 358

Chapter 17   Patient Billing and Collections 361
Basic Accounting 363
Standard Payment Procedures 363
Standard Billing Procedures 367
PROCEDURE 17-1   Processing a Credit Balance 368
PROCEDURE 17-2   Processing Refunds to Patients 368
Standard Collection Procedures 370
PROCEDURE 17-3   How to Bill with the Superbill 372
PROCEDURE 17-4   Preparing an Age Analysis 375
Points on Practice/Choosing a Collection Agency 377
Credit Arrangements 378
Common Collection Problems 380
Career Opportunities/Coding, Billing, and Insurance Specialist 381

Chapter 18   Accounting for the Medical Office 384
The Business Side of a Medical Practice 386
Patient Accounting Methods 386
PROCEDURE 18-1   Posting Entries, Adjustments, and Collection Payments 392
Banking for the Medical Office 393
PROCEDURE 18-2   Posting a Nonsufficient Funds (NSF) Check 394
PROCEDURE 18-3   Making a Bank Deposit 397
PROCEDURE 18-4   Reconciling a Bank Statement 400
Points on Practice/Telephone Banking 401
PROCEDURE 18-5   Setting Up the Accounts Payable System 402
Managing Accounts Payable 402
Managing Disbursements 402
Handling Payroll 405
Points on Practice/Handling Payroll Through Electronic Banking 408
PROCEDURE 18-6   Generating Payroll 409
Calculating and Filing Taxes 411

APPENDIXES

Appendix I   Prefixes, Suffixes, and Word Roots in Commonly Used Medical Terms 420

Appendix II   Abbreviations and Symbols Commonly Used in Medical Notations 423

Glossary 425

Credits 473

Index 474

Procedures

PROCEDURE 4-1   Communicating with the Anxious Patient   83

PROCEDURE 4-2   Identifying Community Resources   92

PROCEDURE 5-1   Using a Facsimile (Fax) Machine   108

PROCEDURE 5-2   Using a Photocopier Machine   111

PROCEDURE 5-3   Using a Postage Meter   113

PROCEDURE 5-4   Using a Dictation-Transcription Machine   115

PROCEDURE 5-5   Using a Check-Writing Machine   115

PROCEDURE 6-1   Creating a Form Letter   135

PROCEDURE 7-1   Creating a Letter   159

PROCEDURE 7-2   Sorting and Opening Mail   167

 PROCEDURE 8-1   Step-by-Step Overview of Inventory Procedures   176

PROCEDURE 9-1   Preparing a Patient Medical Record/Chart   200

PROCEDURE 9-2   Transcribing Letters, Reports, and Notes   207

PROCEDURE 9-3   Correcting Medical Records   209

PROCEDURE 9-4   Maintaining Medical Records   210

PROCEDURE 10-1   Creating a Filing System for Patient Records   226

PROCEDURE 10-2   Setting Up an Office Tickler File   227

PROCEDURE 10-3   Developing a Records Retention Program   234

PROCEDURE 11-1   Performing Telephone Screening   246

PROCEDURE 11-2   Handling Emergency Calls   249

PROCEDURE 11-3   Retrieving Messages from an Answering Service   253

WORK // PRODUCT   PROCEDURE 12-1   Creating a Cluster Schedule   266

PROCEDURE 12-2   Scheduling and Confirming Surgery at a Hospital   271

PROCEDURE 13-1   Creating a Pediatric Playroom   290

PROCEDURE 13-2   Creating a Reception Area Accessible to Patients with Special Needs   292

PROCEDURE 14-1   Developing a Patient Education Plan   298

PROCEDURE 14-2   Informing the Patient of Guidelines for Surgery   308

WORK // PRODUCT   PROCEDURE 15-1   Verifying Workers' Compensation Coverage   324

WORK // PRODUCT   PROCEDURE 15-2   Completing the CMS-1500 Claim Form   335

PROCEDURE 16-1   Locating an ICD-9-CM Code   349

PROCEDURE 16-2   Locating a HCPCS Code   355

PROCEDURE 16-3   Locating a CPT Code   356

PROCEDURE 17-1   Processing a Credit Balance   368

PROCEDURE 17-2   Processing Refunds to Patients   368

WORK // PRODUCT   PROCEDURE 17-3   How to Bill with the Superbill   372

WORK // PRODUCT   PROCEDURE 17-4   Preparing an Age Analysis   375

PROCEDURE 18-1   Posting Entries, Adjustments, and Collection Payments   392

PROCEDURE 18-2   Posting a Nonsufficient Funds (NSF) Check   394

WORK // PRODUCT   PROCEDURE 18-3   Making a Bank Deposit   397

WORK // PRODUCT   PROCEDURE 18-4   Reconciling a Bank Statement   400

PROCEDURE 18-5   Setting Up the Accounts Payable System   402

PROCEDURE 18-6   Generating Payroll   409

Preface

Administrative Procedures for Medical Assisting, fourth edition, is a comprehensive textbook for the administrative medical assisting student. It provides the student with information about all aspects of the administrative medical assisting profession, from the general to the specific, it covers the key concepts, skills, and tasks that administrative medical assistants need to know. The book speaks directly to the student, and its chapter introductions, case studies, procedures, chapter summaries, and chapter reviews are written to engage the students attention and build a sense of positive anticipation about joining the profession of medical assisting.

When referring to patients in the third person, we have alternated between passages that describe a male patient and passages that describe a female patient. Thus, the patient will be referred to as he half the time and as she half the time. The same convention is used to refer to the physician. The medical assistant is consistently addressed as you.

New to This Edition

- 2010 ABHES standards now open each chapter, thus providing the student and instructor with the most current standards of any medical assisting textbook currently in print.
- 2008 CAAHEP standards now open each chapter, providing the student and instructor with the most current standards.
- Media boxes appear at the beginning of each chapter and list all of the media supplements available to support the content presented in the chapter.
- Preparation for Certification Boxes outline the content on the CMA (AAMA), RMA (AMT), and CMAS certification examinations.
- ACTIVSim™ Medical Assisting is an entirely Web-based patient simulator that provides real world cases and a variety of virtual patients. It gives extensive, individualized feedback, providing students with a realistic clinical experience.
- 30+ Electronic Health Record (E.H.R) activities using SpringCharts® from Spring Medical Systems, Inc. are housed in ConnectPlus+ and provide students with activities that simulate real patient encounters.

- LearnSmart™ Medical Assisting aids the student in focusing on the information required to successfully pass certification exams. This diagnostic tool assesses each student's responses to establish a clearly defined learning path that instructors can measure.
- Connect Plus+™ allows students and instructors to access all their course materials including the media-rich textbook in one place. With its unique integrated learning system, Connect Plus™ combines market-leading content, a proven course architecture, and unmatched flexibility to help students apply the principles in the textbook.
- Competency work products, including sample forms for student practice, are now found in the completely revised workbook.
- Practice Exam Questions now end each chapter of the textbook. New to this edition are multiple-choice questions, which appear at the close of each chapter.
- The coverage in the Administrative section has been vastly improved based on extensive user and reviewer feedback.

Content Correlations

Administrative Procedures for Medical Assisting provides new features that will enhance its usefulness to both students and instructors. We have been careful to ensure that the text and supplements provide ample coverage of topics used to construct all of the following:

- CAAHEP (Commission on Accreditation of Allied Health Education Programs) Standards and Guidelines for Medical Assisting Education Programs
- ABHES (Accrediting Bureau of Health Education Schools) Competencies and Curriculum
- AAMA (American Association of Medical Assistants) CMA (Certified Medical Assistant) Occupational Analysis
- AMT (American Medical Technologists) RMA (Registered Medical Assistant) Task List
- AMT CMAS (Certified Medical Assistant Specialist) Competencies and Examination Specifications
- NHA (National Healthcareer Association) Medical Assisting Duty/Task List
- CMA (AAMA) Certification Examination Content Outline

CAAHEP requires that all medical assistants be proficient in the 71 entry-level areas of competence when they begin medical assisting work. ABHES requires proficiency in the competences and curriculum content at a minimum. The opening page of each chapter provides a list of the areas of competence that are covered within the chapter. A complete correlation to both the ABHES Competencies and Curriculum and the CAAHEP Standards and Guidelines appears on pages xi–xx. In addition, you will find that each procedure is correlated to the ABHES and CAAHEP competencies within the workbook on the procedure sheets. These sheets can be easily pulled out of the workbook and placed in the student file to document the proficiency.

Complete content correlations to the NHA Medical Assisting Duty/Task List, the AAMA (CMA) Occupational Analysis, the AMT (RMA) Task List, and the AMT Certified Medical Administrative Specialists (CMAS) Competencies and Examination Specifications can be found on pages xxi–xxxii. To ensure complete coverage as well as ease in use of the *Medical Assisting,* fourth edition, text and supplements package, a new feature titled "Preparation for Certification" has been added to the beginning of each chapter. This feature includes as list of the content that is covered in the chapter from the AMT (RMA) Task List, AMT (CMAS) Competencies and Exam, and the AAMA (CMA) Certification/Recertification Content Outline.

Correlation of Text to CAAHEP Core Curriculum for Medical Assistants

APPLIED COMMUNICATIONS	CHAPTER #
IV. C. Cognitive (Knowledge Base)	
IV. Concepts of Effective Communication	
1. Identify styles and types of verbal communication	4
2. Identify nonverbal communication	4
3. Recognize communication barriers	4
4. Identify techniques for overcoming communication barriers	4
5. Recognize the elements of oral communication using a sender–receiver process	4
6. Differentiate between subjective and objective information	9
7. Identify resources and adaptations that are required based on individual needs, i.e., culture and environment, developmental life stage, language, and physical threats to communication	4, 14
8. Recognize elements of fundamental writing skills	7
9. Discuss applications of electronic technology in effective communication	4, 6
10. Diagram medical terms, labeling the word parts	Appendix I
13. Identify the role of self boundaries in the health care environment	4
14. Recognize the role of patient advocacy in the practice of medical assisting	4, 13, 14
15. Discuss the role of assertiveness ineffective professional communication	4
16. Differentiate between adaptive and non–adaptive coping mechanisms	4
IV. P Psychomotor Skills	
IV. Concepts of Effective Communication	
1. Use reflection, restatement and clarification techniques to obtain a patient history	4, 9
2. Report relevant information to others succinctly and accurately	4
3. Use medical terminology, pronouncing medical terms correctly, to communicate information, patient history, data and observations	4
4. Explain general office policies	4
5. Instruct patients according to their needs to promote health maintenance and disease prevention	14
6. Prepare a patient for procedures and/or treatments	14
7. Demonstrate telephone techniques	11
8. Document patient care	9
9. Document patient education	9, 14
10. Compose professional/business letters	7
11. Respond to nonverbal communication	4
12. Develop and maintain a current list of community resources related to patients' healthcare needs	4, 14
13. Advocate on behalf of patients	4, 13

(*continued*)

APPLIED COMMUNICATIONS (*continued*)	CHAPTER #
IV. A Affective (Behavior)	
IV. Concepts of Effective Communication	
1. Demonstrate empathy in communicating with patients, family and staff	4
2. Apply active listening skills	4
3. Use appropriate body language and other nonverbal skills in communicating with patients, family and staff	4
4. Demonstrate awareness of the territorial boundaries of the person with whom communicating	4
5. Demonstrate sensitivity appropriate to the message being delivered	4
6. Demonstrate awareness of how an individual's personal appearance affects anticipated responses	4
7. Demonstrate recognition of the patient's level of understanding in communications	4
8. Analyze communications in providing appropriate responses/feedback	4
9. Recognize and protect personal boundaries in communicating with others	4
10. Demonstrate respect for individual diversity, incorporating awareness of one's own biases in areas including gender, race, religion, age and economic status	4
MEDICAL BUSINESS PRACTICES	CHAPTER #
V. C Cognitive (Knowledge Base)	
V. Administrative Functions	
1. Discuss pros and cons of various types of appointment management systems	12
2. Describe scheduling guidelines	12
3. Recognize office policies and protocols for handling appointments	12
4. Identify critical information required for scheduling patient admissions and/or procedures	12
5. Identify systems for organizing medical records	10
6. Describe various types of content maintained in a patient's medical record	9, 10
7. Discuss pros and cons of various filing methods	10
8. Identify both equipment and supplies needed for filing medical records	10
9. Describe indexing rules	10
10. Discuss filing procedures	10
11. Discuss principles of using Electronic Medical Records (EMR)	9
12. Identify types of records common to the healthcare setting	9
13. Identify time management principles	9
14. Discuss the importance of routine maintenance of office equipment	5
V. P Psychomotor (Skills)	
V. Administrative Functions	
1. Manage appointment schedule, using established priorities	12
2. Schedule patient admissions and/or procedures	12
3. Organize a patient's medical record	9, 10
4. File medical records	10

MEDICAL BUSINESS PRACTICES (*continued*)	CHAPTER #
5. Execute data management using electronic healthcare records such as the EMR	9
6. Use office hardware and software to maintain office systems	6
7. Use Internet to access information related to the medical office	6, 9
8. Maintain organization by filing	10
9. Perform routine maintenance of office equipment with documentation	5
10. Perform an office inventory	5
V. A Affective (Behavior)	
V. Administrative Functions	
1. Consider staff needs and limitations in establishment of a filing system	10
2. Implement time management principles to maintain effective office function	1
VI. C Cognitive (Knowledge Base)	
VI. Basic Practice Finances	
1. Explain basic bookkeeping computations	18
2. Differentiate between bookkeeping and accounting	18
3. Describe banking procedures	12, 18
4. Discuss precautions for accepting checks	18
5. Compare types of endorsement	18
6. Differentiate between accounts payable and accounts receivable	18
7. Compare manual and computerized bookkeeping systems used in ambulatory healthcare	18
8. Describe common periodic financially reports	18
9. Explain both billing and payment options	17, 18
10. Identify procedure for preparing patient accounts	18
11. Discuss procedures for collecting outstanding accounts	18
12. Describe the impact of both the Fair Debt Collection Act and the Federal Truth in Lending Act of 1968 as they apply to collections	18
13. Discuss types of adjustments that may be made to a patient's account	17, 18
VI. P Psychomotor (Skills)	
VI. Basic Practice Finances	
1. Prepare a bank deposit	18
2. Perform accounts receivable procedures, including: a. Post entries on a dayshee b. Perform billing procedures c. Perform collection procedures d. Post adjustments e. Process a credit balance f. Process refunds g. Post non–sufficient funds (NSF) checks h. Post collection agency payments	18
3. Utilize computerized office billing systems	18

(*continued*)

MEDICAL BUSINESS PRACTICES (*continued*)	CHAPTER #
VI. A Affective (Behavior)	
VI. Basic Practice Finances	
1. Demonstrate sensitivity and professionalism in handling accounts receivable activities with clients	18
VII. C Cognitive (Knowledge Base)	
VII. Managed Care/Insurance	
1. Identify types of insurance plans	15
2. Identify models of managed care	15
3. Discuss workers' compensation as it applies to patients	15
4. Describe procedures for implementing both managed care and insurance plans	15
5. Discuss utilization review principles	15
6. Discuss referral process for patients in a managed care program	15
7. Describe how guidelines are used in processing an insurance claims	10, 15
8. Compare processes for filing insurance claims both manually and electronically	17
9. Describe guidelines for third–party claims	17
10. Discuss types of physician fee schedules	17
11. Describe the concept of RBRVS	15
12. Define Diagnosis–Related Groups (DRGs)	15
VII. P Psychomotor (Skills)	
VII. Managed Care/Insurance	
1. Apply both managed care policies and procedures	15
2. Apply third party guidelines	17
3. Complete insurance claim forms	15
4. Obtain precertification, including documentation	15
5. Obtain preauthorization, including documentation	15
6. Verify eligibility for managed care services	15
VII. A Affective (Behavior)	
VII. Managed Care/Insurance	
1. Demonstrate assertive communication with managed care and/or insurance providers	15, 17
2. Demonstrate sensitivity in communicating with both providers and patients	4, 11, 17
3. Communicate in language the patient can understand regarding managed care and insurance plans	4, 11
VII. C Cognitive (Knowledge Base)	
VII. Procedural and Diagnostic Coding	
1. Describe how to use the most current procedural coding system	16
2. Define upcoding and why it should be avoided	16
3. Describe how to use the most current diagnostic coding classification system	16
4. Describe how to use the most current HCPCS coding	16

MEDICAL BUSINESS PRACTICES (*continued*) | CHAPTER

	CHAPTER #
VII. P Psychomotor (Skills)	
VIII. Procedural and Diagnostic Coding	
1. Perform procedural coding	16
2. Perform diagnostic coding	16
VIII. P. Psychomotor (Skills)	
VIII. Procedural and Diagnostic Coding	
1. Work with physician to achieve the maximum reimbursement	15, 16

MEDICAL LAW AND ETHICS | CHAPTER

	CHAPTER #
IX. Cognitive (Knowledge Base)	
IX. Legal Implications	
1. Discuss legal scope of practice for medical assistants	3
2. Explore issue of confidentiality as it applies to the medical assistant	3
3. Describe the implications of HIPAA for the medical assistant in various medical settings	3
4. Summarize the Patient Bill of Rights	3
5. Discuss licensure and certification as it applies to healthcare providers	1, 2
6. Describe liability, professional, personal injury, and third party insurance	3, 17
7. Compare and contrast physician and medical assistant roles in terms of standard of care	2
8. Compare criminal and civil law as it applies to the practicing medical assistant	3
9. Provide an example of tort law as it would apply to a medical assistant	3
10. Explain how the following impact the medical assistant's practice and give examples: a. Negligence b. Malpractice c. Statute of Limitations d. Good Samaritan Act(s) e. Uniform Anatomical Gift Act f. Living will/Advanced directives g. Medical durable power of attorney	3
11. Identify how the Americans with Disabilities Act (ADA) applies to the medical assisting profession	3, 13
13. Discuss all levels of governmental legislation and regulation as they apply to medical assisting practice, including FDA and DEA regulations	3
14. Describe the process to follow if an error is made in patient care	3, 9
IX. P Psychomotor (Skills)	
IX. Legal Implications	
1. Respond to issues of confidentiality	3
2. Perform within scope of practice	1, 2, 3
3. Apply HIPAA rules in regard to privacy/release of information	3
4. Practice within the standard of care for a medical assistant	1
5. Incorporate the Patient's Bill of Rights into personal practices and medical office policies and procedures	3

(*continued*)

MEDICAL LAW AND ETHICS (*continued*)	CHAPTER #
6. Complete an incident report	9
7. Document accurately in the patient record	9
8. Apply local, state, and federal health care legislation and regulation appropriate to the medical assisting practice setting	1, 3

IX. A Affective (Behavior)
IX. Legal Implications

1. Demonstrate sensitivity to patient rights	4
2. Demonstrate awareness of the consequences of not working within the legal scope of practice	3
3. Recognize the importance of local, state and federal legislation and regulations in the practice setting	3

X. C Cognitive (Knowledge Base)
X. Ethical Considerations

1. Differentiate between legal, ethical, and moral issues affecting healthcare	3
2. Compare personal, professional and organizational ethics	3
3. Discuss the role of cultural, social and ethnic diversity in ethical performance of medical assisting practice	3
4. Identify where to report illegal and/or unsafe activities and behaviors that affect health, safety and welfare of others	3
5. Identify the effect personal ethics may have on professional performance	3

X. P. Psychomotor (Skills)
X. Ethical Considerations

1. Report illegal and/or unsafe activities and behaviors that affect health, safety and welfare of others to proper authorities	3
2. Develop a plan for separation of personal and professional ethics	3

X. A. Affective (Behavior)
X. Ethical Considerations

1. Apply ethical behaviors, including honesty/integrity in performance of medical assisting practice	3
2. Examine the impact personal ethics and morals may have on the individual's practice	3
3. Demonstrate awareness of diversity in providing patient care	3

SAFETY AND EMERGENCY PRACTICES	CHAPTER #

X. C. Cognitive (Knowledge Base)
XI. Protective Practices

1. Describe personal protective equipment	3
2. Identify safety techniques that can be used to prevent accidents and maintain a safe work environment	3
3. Describe the importance of Materials Safety Data Sheets (MSDS) in a healthcare setting	3
7. Describe fundamental principles for evacuation of a healthcare setting	13
9. Discuss requirements for responding to hazardous material disposal	3
10. Identify principles of body mechanics and ergonomics.	10

SAFETY AND EMERGENCY PRACTICES (*continued*)	CHAPTER #
X. P Psychomotor (Skills)	
XI. Protective Practices	
7. Explain an evacuation plan for a physician's office	13
8. Demonstrate methods of fire prevention in the healthcare setting	13
12. Maintain a current list of community resources for emergency preparedness	14
X. A Affective (Behavior)	
XI. Protective Practices	
1. Recognize the effects of stress on all persons involved in emergency situations	4
2. Demonstrate self awareness in responding to emergency situations	4

Correlation of Text to ABHES Competencies

1. GENERAL ORIENTATION	CHAPTER #
a. Comprehend the current employment outlook for the medical assistant	1
b. Compare and contrast the allied health professions and understand their relation to medical assisting	1, 2
c. Understand medical assistant credentialing requirements and the process to obtain the credential. Comprehend the importance of credentialing	1
d. Have knowledge of the general responsibilities of the medical assistant	1, 2
e. Define scope of practice for the medical assistant, and comprehend the conditions for practice within the state that the medical assistant is employed	1, 2

2. ANATOMY AND PHYSIOLOGY	CHAPTER #
a. Comprehend and explain to the patient the importance of diet and nutrition. Effectively convey and educate patients regarding the proper diet and nutrition guidelines. Identify categories of patients that require special diets or diet modifications.	14

3. MEDICAL TERMINOLOGY	CHAPTER #
a. Define and use entire basic structure of medical words and be able to accurately identify in the correct context, i.e., root, prefix, suffix, combinations, spelling and definitions	Appendix I
b. Build and dissect medical terms from roots/suffixes to understand the word element combinations that create medical terminology	Appendix I
d. Recognize and identify acceptable medical abbreviations	16, Appendix II

4. MEDICAL LAW AND ETHICS	CHAPTER #
a. Document accurately	3, 15, 16
b. Institute federal and state guidelines when releasing medical records or information	3, 9
c. Follow established policies when initiating or terminating medical treatment	
d. Understand the importance of maintaining liability coverage once employed in the industry	3
e. Perform risk management procedures	3
f. Comply with federal, state, and local health laws and regulations	3, 15, 16, 18

5. PSYCHOLOGY OF HUMAN RELATIONS	CHAPTER #
a. Define and understand abnormal behavior patterns	4
b. Identify and respond appropriately when working/caring for patients with special needs	4
c. Use empathy when treating terminally ill patients. Identify common stages that terminally ill patients go through and list organizations/support groups that can assist patients and family members of patients struggling with terminal illness	4
d. Identify common stages that terminally ill patients go through and list organizations/support groups that can assist patients and family members of patients struggling with terminal illness	4
e. Advocate on behalf of family/patients, having ability to deal and communicate with family	4
f. Identify and discuss developmental stages of life	4
g. Analyze the effect of hereditary, cultural, and environmental influences	4

6. PHARMACOLOGY

	CHAPTER #
d. Understand legal aspects of writing prescriptions, including federal and state laws.	3
e. Comply with federal, state, and local health laws and regulations	

7. BASIC KEYBOARDING/COMPUTER CONCEPTS

	CHAPTER #

a. Perform basic keyboarding skills including:
  1. Locating the keys on a keyboard
  2. Typing medical correspondence and basic reports
	7, 9

b. Identify and properly utilize office machines, computerized systems and medical software such as:
  1. Efficiently maintain and understand different types of medical correspondence and medical reports
  2. Apply computer application skills using variety of different electronic programs including both practice management software and EMR software
	6, 7, 9, 10

8. MEDICAL OFFICE BUSINESS PROCEDURES MANAGEMENT

	CHAPTER #
a. Perform basic clerical functions	7
b. Prepare and maintain medical records	9, 10
c. Schedule and manage appointments	12
d. Apply concepts for office procedures	7, 8, 9, 10
e. Locate resources and information for patients and employers	13
f. Schedule in patient and outpatient admissions	12
g. Prepare and reconcile a bank statement and deposit record	18
h. Post entries on a day sheet	18
i. Perform billing and collection procedures	17
j. Perform accounts payable procedures	18
k. Perform accounts receivable procedures	18
l. Establish and maintain a petty cash fund	18
m. Post adjustments	18
n. Process credit balance	17
o. Profess refunds	18
p. Post non–sufficient funds (NSF)	18
q. Post collection agency payments	18
r. Apply third party guidelines	17, 18
s. Obtain managed care referrals and pre–certification	15
t. Perform diagnostic and procedural coding	16
u. Prepare and submit insurance claims	15
v. Use physician fee schedule	15
w. Use manual or computerized bookkeeping systems	18
x. Maintain medical facility	13
y. Perform routine maintenance of administrative and clinical equipment	5, 7
z. Maintain inventory equipment and supplies	8
aa. [Graduates] Are attentive, listen and learn	4
cc. Communicate on the recipient's level of comprehension	1, 4
dd. Serve as liaison between physician and others	4, 12, 14
ee. Use proper telephone techniques	11, 15, 17

(continued)

8. MEDICAL OFFICE BUSINESS PROCEDURES MANAGEMENT (*continued*)

	CHAPTER #
gg. Use pertinent medical terminology	9
hh. Receive, organize, prioritize, and transmit information expediently	11, 13, 14, 15, 16, 17, 18
ii. Recognize and respond to verbal and non–verbal communication	4
jj. Perform fundamental writing skills including correct grammar, spelling, and formatting techniques when writing prescriptions, documenting medical records, etc.	7
kk. Adapt to individualized needs	6
ll. Apply electronic technology	6

9. MEDICAL OFFICE CLINICAL PROCEDURES

	CHAPTER #
p. Advise patients of office policies and procedures	4
q. Instruct patients with special needs	14
r. Teach patients methods of health promotion and disease prevention	14

10. CAREER DEVELOPMENT

	CHAPTER #
Demonstrate professionalism by: 1. Exhibiting dependability, punctuality, and a positive work ethic 2. Exhibiting a positive attitude and a sense of responsibility 3. Maintaining confidentiality at all times 4. Being cognizant of ethical boundaries 5. Exhibiting initiative 6. Adapting to change 7. Expressing a responsible attitude 8. Being courteous and diplomatic 9. Conducting work within scope of education, training, and ability	1–18

Correlation of Text to National Healthcareer Association (NHA) Medical Assisting Duty/Task List

DUTY A: DISPLAY PROFESSIONALISM	CHAPTER #
A. 01 Project a Positive Attitude	1, 4
A. 02 Demonstrate Ethical Behavior	1, 4
A. 03 Practice Within the Scope of Education, Training and Personal Capabilitie	4
A. 04 Maintain Confidentiality	4, 15
A. 05 Work as a Team Member	4
A. 06 Conduct Oneself in a Courteous and Diplomatic Manner	4
A. 07 Adapt to Change	4
A. 08 Show Initiative and Responsibility	4
A. 09 Promote the Profession	4
A. 10 Apply Critical Thinking Skills to Workplace Situations	4
A. 11 Manage Stress	4

DUTY B: APPLY COMMUNICATION SKILLS	CHAPTER #
B. 01 Listen and Observe	4
B. 02 Treat all Patients with Empathy and Impartiality	4
B. 03 Adapt Communication to Individual's Abilities to Understand	4
B. 04 Recognize and Respond to Verbal and Nonverbal Communication	4, 11
B. 05 Serve as Liaison Between Physicians and Others	4, 11, 14
B. 06 Evaluate Understanding of Communication	4
B. 07 Receive, Organize, Prioritize and Transmit Information	4
B. 08 Use Proper Telephone Technique	11
B. 09 Interview Effectively	4, 9, 11
B. 10 Use Medical Terminology Appropriately	7
B. 11 Compose Written Communication Using Correct Grammar, Spelling and Format	7

DUTY C: DEMONSTRATE KEYBOARDING SKILL AND COMPUTER AWARENESS	CHAPTER #
C. 01 Perform Keyboarding by Touch on a Microcomputer	6
C. 02 Use Basic Terminology Common in the Computer Industry	6
C. 03 Demonstrate Care and Routine Maintenance of Computer Systems	6
C. 04 Identify the Types and Functions of Hardware and Peripheral Components	6
C. 05 Identify the Types of Operating Systems	6
C. 06 Define Differences in the Application of Microcomputer Software	6

DUTY D: PERFORM BUSINESS SOFTWARE APPLICATIONS	CHAPTER #
D. 01 Explain the Characteristics and Components of Word Processing	6
D. 02 Start Up Word Processing Software	6
D. 03 Produce and Format Common Business Documents Such as Letters, Memos, and Reports	6, 7
D. 04 Edit a Document	7

(continued)

DUTY D: PERFORM BUSINESS SOFTWARE APPLICATIONS (continued)

	CHAPTER #
D. 05 Print a Document	7
D. 06 Retrieve a Document	7
D. 07 Enhance a Document	7
D. 08 Utilize Software Reference/ Documentation	6
D. 09 Explain the Use of Database Management Concepts and Applications	6

DUTY F: PERFORM ADMINISTRATIVE DUTIES

	CHAPTER #
F. 01 Perform Records Management	3, 10
F. 02 Use and Maintain Office Equipment	5
F. 03 Handle Incoming Mail	7
F. 04 Schedule and Monitor Appointments	12
F. 05 Prepare and Maintain Medical Records	9, 10
F. 08 Information for Patients and Employers	15
F. 09 Manage Calendar/Itineraries	13, 14
F. 10 Organize Meetings and Presentations	12

DUTY G: PERFORM CLINICAL DUTIES

	CHAPTER #
G. 07 Interview and Take Patient History	4
G. 08 Prepare Patients for Procedures	4, 14
G. 21 Utilize Proper Body Mechanics	6

DUTY H: APPLY LEGAL, ETHICAL, AND CONFIDENTIALITY CONCEPTS

	CHAPTER #
H. 01 Document Accurately	3, 9
H. 04 Follow Established Policy in Initiating, Withdrawing, Withholding, or Terminating Medical Treatment	3
H. 05 Dispose of Controlled Substances in Compliance with Government Regulations	3
H. 06 Maintain Licenses and Certification	1
H. 07 Monitor Legislation Related to Current Health Care and Practice	3
H. 08 Perform Within Ethical Boundaries	3

DUTY I: MANAGE THE OFFICE

	CHAPTER #
I. 01 Maintain the Physical Plant	13
I. 02 Operate and Maintain Facilities and Equipment Safely	13
I. 03 Maintain and Operate Medical Equipment	5, 6
I. 04 Observe Safety Precautions in the Office	3
I. 05 Inventory Equipment and Supplies	5
I. 06 Identify Supply Resources	5
I. 07 Evaluate and Recommend Equipment and Supplies	5
I. 08 Maintain Liability Coverage	4
I. 09 Maintain Documentation of Continuing Education	1
I. 10 Exercise Efficient Time Management	4

DUTY J: PROVIDE PATIENT INSTRUCTION

	CHAPTER #
J. 01 Orient Patients to Office Policies and Procedures	13, 14
J. 02 Instruct Patients With Special Needs	4, 14

DUTY J: PROVIDE PATIENT INSTRUCTION (*continued*)	CHAPTER #
J. 03 Teach Patients Methods of Health Promotion and Disease Prevention	14
J. 04 Provide Verbal and Written Information	4
J. 05 Orient and Train Personnel	4

DUTY K: MANAGE PRACTICE FINANCES	CHAPTER #
K. 01 Use Bookkeeping Systems	18
K. 02 Implement Current Diagnostic/Procedural Coding Systems (CPT and ICD–9–CM coding)	16
K. 03 Analyze and Use Current Third–Party Guidelines for Reimbursement	17
K. 04 Manage Accounts Receivables	18
K. 05 Manage Accounts Payable	18
K. 06 Maintain Records for Accounting and Banking Purposes	18

Correlation of Text to Occupational Analysis of the CMA (AAMA)

GENERAL SKILLS	CHAPTER #
Communication	
• Recognize and respect cultural diversity	4, 14
• Adapt communication to individual's understanding	4
• Employ professional telephone and interpersonal techniques	11
• Recognize and respond effectively to verbal, nonverbal, and written communications	1, 4, 11
• Receive, organize, prioritize, store and maintain transmittable information utilizing electronic technology	6
• Serve as "communication liaison" between the physician and patient	1, 4
• Serve as patient advocate professional and health coach in a team approach in health care	13, 14
• Identify basics of office emergency preparedness	11
Legal Concepts	
• Perform within legal (including federal and state statutes, regulations, opinions, and rulings) and ethical boundaries	3, 15, 16, 17, 18
• Document patient communication and clinical treatments accurately and appropriately	3, 9
• Maintain medical records	9, 10
• Follow employer's established policies dealing with the health care contract	3
• Comply with established risk management and safety procedures	3
• Recognize professional credentialing criteria	1, 2
• Identify and respond to issues of confidentiality	3
Instruction	
• Function as a health care advocate to meet individual's needs	4, 14
• Education individuals in office policies and procedures	4, 10
• Educate the patient within the scope of practice and as directed by supervising physician in health maintenance, disease prevention, and compliance with patient's treatment plan	4, 14
• Identify community resources for health maintenance and disease prevention to meet individual patient needs	4, 14
• Maintain current list of community resources, including those for emergency preparedness and other patient care needs	4, 14
• Collaborate with local community resources for emergency preparedness	14
• Educate patients in their responsibilities relating to third-party reimbursement	15, 17
Operational Functions	
• Perform inventory of supplies and equipment	5, 7
• Perform routine maintenance of administrative and clinical equipment	5, 8
• Apply computer and other electronic equipment techniques to support office operations	5, 6
• Perform methods of quality control	3

CLINICAL SKILLS	CHAPTER #
Fundamental Principles	
• Identify the roles and responsibilities of other team members in the medical office	2
Patient Care	
• Perform initial-response screening following protocols approved by supervising physician	12
• Obtain, evaluate, and record patient history employing critical thinking skills	4, 9, 10
ADMINISTRATIVE SKILLS	**CHAPTER #**
• Schedule, coordinate, and monitor appointments	12
• Schedule inpatient/outpatient admissions and procedures	12
• Apply third-party and managed care policies, procedures and guidelines	15
• Establish, organize, and maintain patient medical record	9, 10
• File medical records appropriately	10
PRACTICE FINANCES	**CHAPTER #**
• Perform procedural and diagnostic coding for reimbursement	16
• Perform billing and collection procedures	17
• Perform administrative functions, including book-keeping and financial procedures	18
• Prepare submittable ("clean") insurance forms	15

Correlation of Text to RMA (AMT) Task List

I. GENERAL MEDICAL ASSISTING KNOWLEDGE	CHAPTER #
B. Medical Terminology	
1. Identify word parts	Appendix I
2. Define medical terms	Appendix I
3. Identify common abbreviations and symbols	Appendix II
4. Accurately spell medical terms	Appendix I
C. Medical Law	
1. Identify and understand the application of medical law	3
2. Identify licensure, certification, and registration regulations	3
D. Medical Ethics	
1. Identify and employ principles of medical ethics	2, 3, 9
2. Recognize and apply ethical conduct	2, 3, 9
3. Recognize and apply professional development	1, 2, 3, 9
E. Human Relations	
1. Understand and employ group specific responses in patient relations	2, 4, 9
2. Employ appropriate interpersonal skills	4, 5, 9
3. Observe and respect cultural diversity	4
F. Patient Education	
1. Identify and apply proper communication methods in patient instruction	4
2. Develop, assemble, and maintain patient resource materials	4, 14

II. ADMINISTRATIVE MEDICAL ASSISTING	CHAPTER #
A. Insurance	
1. Identify and apply insurance related terminology	15, 16, 17
2. Identify and understand application of various insurance plans	15, 16, 17
3. Complete and file claim forms	15
4. Understand and perform electronic insurance claims	15, 16, 17
5. ICD–9/CPT Coding applications	16, 17
6. Identify and apply HIPAA mandated coding systems	16
7. Understand proper financial applications of medical insurance	18
B. Financial Bookkeeping	
1. Understand terminology associated with medical financial book keeping	18
2. Maintain and employ proper patient billing procedures	17, 18
3. Understand and perform proper collection procedures	18
4. Perform appropriate fundamental medical office accounting procedures	18
5. Understand and perform office banking duties	18
6. Understand and prepare employee payroll	18
7. Apply appropriate financial calculations and accounting procedures	18

II. ADMINISTRATIVE MEDICAL ASSISTING (*continued*)   CHAPTER

C. Medical Secretarial-Receptionist

	CHAPTER #
1. Understand and correctly apply terminology associated with receptionist duties	9, 10, 11, 12
2. Understand and perform general reception of patients and visitors	9, 10, 11, 12
3. Employ appointment scheduling system	12
4. Understand and employ appropriate oral and written communication	4, 7, 9
5. Understand and perform appropriate medical records management	9, 10
6. Understand and apply appropriate charting guidelines and regulations	9
7. Protect, store, and retain medical records according to HIPAA regulations	3, 9, 10
8. Understand and perform electronic insurance claims	15, 16
9. Understand preparation and release of protected health information adhering to HIPAA regulations	3, 6, 9, 10
10. Perform accurate transcription of dictation	5, 9
11. Employ supplies and equipment management	8
12. Identify and understand medical office computer applications	6
13. Employ procedures in compliance with OSHA guidelines and regulations of office safety	10, 13, 14

III. CLINICAL MEDICAL ASSISTING   CHAPTER

B. Sterilization

	CHAPTER #
5. Identify and employ proper record keeping procedures	9

E. Physical Examinations

1. Obtain patient history information, employing proper charting procedures	9

F. Clinical Pharmacology

6. Understand Drug Enforcement Agency regulations for ordering, dispensing, storage, and documentation of medication use	3

I. Laboratory Procedures

8. Maintain laboratory records according to state and federal guidelines	9

American Medical Technologists Certified Medical Administrative Specialists (CMAS) Competencies and Examination Specifications

I. MEDICAL ASSISTING FOUNDATIONS (13% OF EXAMINATION)	CHAPTER #
A. Medical Terminology	
• Identify root words, prefixes, and suffixes	Appendix I
C. Legal and Ethical Considerations	
• Apply principles of medical law and ethics to the heath care setting	3
• Recognize legal responsibilities of, and know scope of practice for the medical administrative specialist	3
• Know basic laws pertaining to medical practice	3
• Know and observe disclosure laws (patient privacy, minors, confidentiality)	3
• Know the principles of medical ethics established by the AMA	3
• Recognize unethical practices and identify ethical responses for situations in the medical office	3
D. Professionalism	
• Employ human relations skills appropriate to health care setting	4, 12, 13, 14
• Display behaviors of a professional medical administrative specialist	1, 2
• Participate in appropriate continuing education	1, 2
II. BASIC CLINICAL MEDICAL OFFICE ASSISTING (8% OF EXAMINATION)	CHAPTER #
A. Basic Health History Interview	
• Obtain preliminary health histories from patients	4
B. Basic Charting	
• Chart patient information	4, 9
D. Asepsis in the Medical Office	
• Observe Standard Precautions	3, 4
III. MEDICAL OFFICE CLERICAL ASSISTING (10% OF EXAMINATION)	CHAPTER #
A. Appointment Management and Scheduling	
• Schedule and monitor patient and visitor appointments	12
• Address cancellations and missed appointments	12
• Prepare information for referrals and preauthorizations	12
• Arrange hospital admissions and surgery, and schedule patients for out-patient diagnostic tests	12
• Manage recall system and file	10, 12

III. MEDICAL OFFICE CLERICAL ASSISTING (10% OF EXAMINATION) *(continued)*

	CHAPTER #
B. Reception	
• Receive and process patients and visitors	4, 13, 14
• Screen visitors and vendors requesting to see physician	4
• Coordinate patient flow into examining rooms	4, 12
C. Communication	
• Employ effective written and oral communication	7
• Address and process incoming telephone calls form outside providers, pharmacies, and vendors	11
• Employ appropriate telephone etiquette when screening patient calls and addressing office business	11
• Recognize and employ proper protocols for telephone emergencies	11
• Format business documents and correspondence appropriately	7
• Process incoming and outgoing mail	7
D. Patient Information and Community Resources	
• Order and organize patient informational materials	14
• Maintain list of community referral resources	14

IV. MEDICAL RECORDS MANAGEMENT (14% OF EXAMINATION)

	CHAPTER #
A. Systems	
• Demonstrate knowledge of, and manage patient medical records systems	9, 10
• Manage documents and patient charts using paper methods	9
• Manage documents and patient charts using computerized methods	9
B. Procedures	
• File records alphabetically, numerically, by subject, and by color	10
• Employ rules of indexing	10
• Arrange contents of patient charts in appropriate order	10
• Document and file laboratory results and patient communication in charts	10
• Perform corrections and additions to records	9
• Store, protect, retain, and destroy records appropriately	10
• Transfer files	10
• Perform daily chart management	9
• Prepare charts for external review and audits	9
C. Confidentiality	
• Observe and maintain confidentiality of records, charts, and test results	4, 5, 9, 10
• Observe special regulations regarding the confidentiality of protected information	3, 5, 6, 9, 10, 15

V. HEALTH CARE INSURANCE PROCESSING, CODING, AND BILLING (17% OF EXAMINATION)

	CHAPTER #
A. Insurance Processing	
• Understand private/commercial health care insurance plans (PPO, HMO, traditional indemnity)	15

(continued)

V. HEALTH CARE INSURANCE PROCESSING, CODING, AND BILLING (17% OF EXAMINATION) *(continued)*	CHAPTER #
• Understand government health care insurance plans (Medicare, Medicaid, Veteran's Administration, CHAMPUS, Tricare, use of Advance Beneficiary Notices)	15
• Process patient claims using appropriate forms (including superbills) and time frames	17
• Process Workers' Compensation/disability reports and forms	17
• Submit claims for third-party reimbursements including the use of electronic transmission methods	17
B. Coding	
• Understand procedure and diagnosis coding	16
• Employ Current Procedural Terminology (CPT) and Evaluation and Management codes appropriately	16
• Employ International Classification of Diseases 9 (ICD9) codes appropriately	16
• Employ Health Care Financing Administration Common Procedure coding System (HCPCS) codes appropriately	16
C. Insurance Billing and Finances	
• Understand health care insurance terminology (deductible, copayment, preauthroizations, capitation, coinsurance)	15, 16, 17
• Understand billing requirements for health care insurance plans	15, 17
• Process insurance payments	15, 17
• Track unpaid claims, and file and track appeals	17
• Understand fraud and abuse regulations	17

VI. MEDICAL OFFICE FINANCIAL MANAGEMENT (17% OF EXAMINATION)	CHAPTER #
A. Fundamental Financial Management	
• Understand basic principles of accounting	18
• Perform bookkeeping procedures including balancing accounts	18
• Perform financial computations	18
• Manage accounts payable	18
• Manage accounts receivable	18
• Prepare monthly trial balance (reports)	18
• Understand basic audit controls	18
• Understand professional fee structures	15, 18
• Understand physician/practice owner compensation provisions	18
• Understand credit arrangements	17, 18
• Manage other financial aspects of office management	18
B. Patient Accounts	
• Manage patient accounts/ledgers	17, 18
• Manage patient billing (methods, cycle billing procedures)	17, 18
• Manage collections in compliance with state and federal regulations	17
C. Banking	
• Understand banking services and procedures (accounts, lines of credit, checking endorsements, deposits, reconciliations, and statements)	17
• Manage petty cash	18

VI. MEDICAL OFFICE FINANCIAL MANAGEMENT (17% OF EXAMINATION) (continued)

	CHAPTER #
D. Payroll	
• Prepare employee payroll and reports	18
• Maintain payroll tax deduction procedures and records	18

VII. MEDICAL OFFICE INFORMATION PROCESSING (7% OF EXAMINATION)

	CHAPTER #
A. Fundamentals of Computing	
• Possess fundamental knowledge of computing in the medical office including keyboarding, data entry, and retrieval	5, 6, 7
• Possess fundamental knowledge of PC-based environment	6
• Possess fundamental knowledge of word processing, spreadsheet, database, and presentation graphics applications	7
• Employ procedures for ensuring the integrity and confidentiality of computer-stored information	6, 7, 9, 10
B. Medical Office Computer Applications	
• Employ medical office software applications	6, 7
• Use computer for billing and financial transactions	17
• Employ e-mail applications	6

VIII. MEDICAL OFFICE MANAGEMENT* (14% OF EXAMINATION)

	CHAPTER #
A. Office Communications*	
• Facilitate staff meetings and in-service, and ensure communication of essential information to staff	10
B. Business Organization Management*	
• Manage medical office business functions	10
• Manage office mailing and shipping services	10
• Manage outside vendors and supplies	10, 11
• Manage contracts and relationships with associated health care providers	10
• Comply with licensure and accreditation requirements	1
C. Human Resources*	
• Manage/supervise medical office staff	10
• Conduct performance reviews and disciplinary action	10
• Maintain office policy manual	10
• Mange staff payroll and scheduling	18
• Mange staff recruiting in compliance with state and federal laws	10
• Orient and train new staff	10
• Manage employee benefits	10
D. Safety	
• Maintain office safety, maintain office safety manual, and post emergency instructions	10, 13
• Observe emergency safety requirements	3, 13
• Maintain records of biohazardous waste, hazardous chemicals, (Material Safety Data Sheets), and safety conditions	3
• Comply with Occupational Safety and Health Act (OSHA) guidelines and regulations	3

(continued)

VIII. MEDICAL OFFICE MANAGEMENT* (14% OF EXAMINATION) (*continued*)

	CHAPTER #
E. Supplies and Equipment	
• Manage medical and office supply inventories and order supplies	8
• Maintain office equipment and arrange for (and maintain records of) equipment maintenance and repair	8
F. Physical Office Plant	
• Maintain office facilities and environment	13
G. Risk Management and Quality Assurance	
• Understand and employ risk management and quality assurance concepts	3

Note: Asterisked areas addressed by the Medical Office Management job function may or may not be performed by the Certified Medical Administrative Specialist at entry-level practice. Nevertheless, the competent Specialist should have sound knowledge of these management functions at certification level.

Content Highlights

In this book we focus particularly on patient education and on the role of the medical assistant in encouraging patients to be active participants in their own health care. It is always desirable for patients to be as knowledgeable as possible about their health. Patients who do not understand what is expected of them may become confused, frightened, angry, and uncooperative; educated patients are better able to understand why compliance is important.

Chapter 14 is devoted entirely to patient education. Other chapters cover various aspects of patient interaction such as Chapter 4, on communicating with the patient, and Chapter 11, on Telephone Techniques. Throughout the book, we provide the medical assistant with the information needed to educate patients so that they can participate fully in their health care.

We have also made a consistent effort to discuss patients with special needs. Several chapters contain special sections of text devoted to the particular concerns of certain patient groups. These groups include the following:

- **Elderly patients.** Special care is often required with elderly patients. The body undergoes many changes with age, and patients may have difficulty adjusting to their changing physical needs. Several chapters deal with the special needs of elderly patients, such as Chapter 4 which includes a Points on Practice feature on Talking with the Geriatric Patient.

- **Children.** The special needs of children are complex, because not only their bodies but also their minds and social situations are very different from those of adults. Dealing with children usually means dealing with their parents as well, and medical assistants must hone their communication skills to meet the needs of both patient and parent when working with children. One chapter that focuses on children is Chapter 13, which includes a special text section and a procedure for designing a patient reception area to accommodate children.

- **Patients with disabilities.** Many different diseases and disabilities require extra effort or consideration on the part of the medical assistant. Patients in wheelchairs and patients with diabetes, hemophilia, or visual or hearing impairments all require specific accommodations. For example, Chapter 13 addresses the needs of such patients; including a section that discusses the Americans With Disabilities Act. This chapter also explains how be assure that patients with special needs, such as those utilizing a wheelchair or walker, can easily access not only the parking lot and building entrance, but can also maneuver easily within the office itself.

- **Patients from other cultures.** Communicating with patients from other cultures, especially when language barriers are involved, poses a special challenge for the medical assistant. In addition, patients from other cultures may have attitudes about medicine or about social interaction that differ sharply from those of the medical assistants culture. Chapter 4 is one chapter that deals in depth with patients from other cultures. It contains a text section and a Reflecting On . . . Cultural Issues feature about different cultures attitudes toward medicine.

Because safety is a primary concern for both the patient and the administrative medical assistant, we have emphasized this aspect of medical assisting work. Safety and legal guidelines and administrations such as OSHA and HIPAA are introduced in Chapter 3 and are a recurring theme throughout the rest of the text.

Organization of the Text

Administrative Procedures for Medical Assisting, fourth edition, is divided into two distinct sections.

Part One provides a basic explanation of the role of the medical assistant in a medical practice. It includes an overview of the profession and covers the different types of medical practices, legal, and ethical issues including important information on HIPAA (Health Information Portability and Accountability Act) regulations and communication with patients, their families, and coworkers.

Part Two explores the administrative duties of the medical assistant, including basic office work, patient interaction, and the financial responsibilities including claims processing of a medical practice. Chapter 19 provides the medical assisting student with information about the externship process and how to prepare to find a position as a medical assistant.

The ordering of chapters within each part allows the student and the instructor to build a knowledge base starting with the fundamentals and working toward an understanding of highly specialized tasks. Part Two introduces the basics of working with office equipment before covering the details of maintaining patient records, scheduling appointments, and processing insurance.

Chapters are also grouped into sections when their subjects relate to a broader topic or area of skills. Each section is set apart and the section opener includes the list of chapters within that section.

Each chapter opens with a page of material that includes the ABHES and CAAHEP medical assisting competencies covered in the chapter, a list of key terms, a list of media supplements available to support the content of the chapter, the chapter outline, the preparation for certification feature, and the learning outcomes the student can expect to achieve after completing the chapter. The main text of each chapter begins with an overview of chapter content and includes a case study for students to consider as they read the chapter. Chapters are organized into topics that move from the general to the specific. Updated color photographs, anatomic and technical drawings, tables, charts, and text features help educate the student about various aspects of medical assisting. The text features, set off in boxes within the text, include the following:

- **Case Studies** are provided at the beginning of all chapters. They represent situations similar to those that the medical assistant may encounter in daily practice. Students are encouraged to consider the case study as they read each chapter. Case Study Questions in the end-of-chapter review check students' understanding and application of chapter content.
- **Procedures** give step-by-step instructions on how to perform specific administrative tasks that an administrative medical assistant will be required to perform. A list of the procedures, which follows the Contents, details the procedures found in each chapter.
- **Points on Practice** boxes provide guidelines on keeping the medical office running smoothly and efficiently.
- **Educating the Patient** boxes focus on ways to instruct patients about caring for themselves outside the medical office.
- **Reflecting On . . .** boxes provide specialized information about legal and ethical issues, communication issues, cultural issues, professionalism, age considerations, and HIPAA.
- **Caution:** *Handle with Care* boxes cover the precautions to be taken in certain situations or when performing certain tasks.
- **Career Opportunities** boxes provide the student with information on various specialized medical professions or duties related to the medical assistant's role within the health-care team.

Each chapter closes with a summary of the chapter material that focuses on the role of the administrative medical assistant. The summary is followed by an end-of-chapter review that consists of the following elements:

- Case Study Questions
- Multiple-Choice Questions
- Discussion Questions
- Critical Thinking Questions
- Application Activities
- Virtual Fieldtrip

A list of further readings, including related books and journal articles, will be provided for each chapter within the Instructor's Manual and on McGraw-Hill's *Medical Assisting* Online Learning Center. The end-of-chapter questions and activities, as well as the additional online resources, provide supplementary information about the subjects presented in the chapter and allow students to practice specific skills.

The book also includes a glossary and two appendixes for use as reference tools. The glossary lists all the words presented as key terms in each chapter along with a pronunciation guide and the definition of each term. The appendixes include a list of common medical terminology including prefixes, root words, and suffixes as well as medical abbreviations and symbols.

Digital Supplements

Student CD-ROM. The Student CD-ROM provides a comprehensive learning program that is correlated to each chapter of the text and reinforces competencies required to become a medical assistant. Short video clips and pictures introduce skills and case studies for application. In addition, numerous interactive exercises and applications are provided for every chapter in the text. The Student CD, included with each student textbook and updated to include new administrative practice activities, provides the following menu choices:

- 1 Day in the Life Critical Thinking
- Administrative Practice Activities
- Anatomy and Physiology Review
- Games: Spin the Wheel, Key Term Concentration, and Medical Assisting Challenge
- Interactive Review
- Audio Glossary
- Progress Report (can be saved, printed, and e-mailed to the instructor)
- Online Learning Center

Online Learning Center. The Online Learning Center (OLC) is a text-specific website that offers an extensive array of learning and teaching tools, including chapter quizzes with immediate feedback, news-feeds, links to relevant websites, and many more study resources. Log on at www.mhhe.com/medicalassisting4e.

Instructor Productivity CD-ROM. The Instructor Productivity CD-ROM provides easy-to-use resources for class preparation. The Instructor Productivity CD-ROM includes the following:

- EZTest test generator with over 5,000 questions and answer rationales and correlations to AAMA competencies PowerPointfi Presentations
- Correlations to AAMA-CMA, AMT-RMA, NHA, CAAHEP, ABHES, and AMT-CMAS Standards
- Course syllabi
- Figure browser
- Video clip library
- Lesson plans
- Course management allows you to monitor and record student progress on the student CD activities
- Ability to modify the interactive questions on the CD

Print Supplements

The *Student Workbook* provides an opportunity for the student to review and practice the material and skills presented in the textbook. Divided into parts and presented by chapter, Part One provides:

- Vocabulary review exercises, which test knowledge of key terms in the chapter

- Content review exercises, which test the students knowledge of key concepts in the chapter
- Critical thinking exercises, which test the students understanding of key concepts in the chapter
- Application exercises, which include figures and practice forms and test mastery of specific skills
- Case studies, which apply the chapter material to real-life situations or problems

Part Two includes procedure checklists, presented in the order in which they are presented in the student textbook. These checklists have been revised for each of use, and include correlations to the ABHES and CAAHEP competencies mastered with the successful completion of each procedure.

Part Three, Work Product Documentation, provides blank charting forms for many of the procedures that include a work product. These forms can be used to practice and test the procedure competencies.

The *Instructor's Resource Binder* provides the instructor with materials to help organize lessons and classroom interactions. It includes:

- A list of learning outcomes, the chapter outline, a complete lesson plan for each chapter, including an introduction to the lesson, teaching strategies, alternate teaching strategies, case studies, assessment, chapter close, resources, and an answer key to the student textbook
- An answer key to the *Student Workbook*
- Charts that show the location in the student textbook, the *Student Workbook*, and the *Instructor's Resource Binder* of material that correlates with the following:
  - The 2008 American Association of Medical Assistants (AAMA) Occupational Analysis
  - The Association of Medical Technologists (AMT) Registered Medical Assistant (RMA) Certified Exam Topics
  - The National Healthcareer Association (NHA) Medical Assisting Duty/Task List
  - The National Occupational Competency Testing Institute (NOCTI) Job Ready Sample Assessment competencies and skills
  - The Commission on Accreditation of Allied Health Education Programs (CAAHEP) Standards and Guidelines for Medical Assisting Education Programs competencies
  - The Secretarys Commission on Achieving Necessary Skills (SCANS) areas of competence
  - The Accrediting Bureau of Health Education Schools (ABHES) Medical Assisting competencies and curriculum
- PowerPoint Presentations on the Instructor Productivity CD-ROM
- The EZ Test generator with over 5,000 questions to use or modify to meet your course needs
- Computer software for the student and instructor is also available. The Student CD-ROM is packaged with.

The *Pocket Guide to Accompany Medical Assisting, 4e* is a quick and handy reference to use while working as a medical assistant or during training. It includes critical procedure steps, bulleted lists, and brief information all medical assistants should know. Information is sorted by Administrative, Clinical, and General content.

Together, the Student Edition, the *Student Workbook*, and the *Instructor's Resource Binder* form a complete teaching and learning package. The *Administrative Procedures for Medical Assisting* course will prepare students to enter the medical assisting field with all the knowledge and skills needed to be a useful resource to patients, a valued asset to employers, and a credit to the medical assisting profession.

Acknowledgments

The publisher and authors would like to thank the reviewers and contributors for their assistance in shaping this revision. We appreciate their suggestions, insights, and commitment to providing information that is relevant and valuable to medical assisting students.

In addition, many people and organizations provided invaluable assistance in the process of illustrating the highly technical and detailed topics covered in the text. Their contributions helped ensure the accuracy, timelines, and authenticity of the illustrations in the book.

We would like to thank the following organizations for providing source materials and technical advice: the American Association of Medical Assistants, Chicago, Illinois; Becton Dickinson Microbiology Systems, Sparks, Maryland; Becton Dickinson VACUTAINER Systems, Franklin Lakes, New Jersey; Bibbero Systems, Petaluma, California; Burdick, Schaumberg, Illinois; the Corel Corporation, Ottawa, Ontario, Canada; Hamilton Media, Hamilton, New Jersey; Nassau Ear, Nose, and Throat, Princeton, New Jersey; Princeton Allergy and Asthma Associates, Princeton, New Jersey; Richmond International, Boca Raton, Florida; and Winfield Medical, San Diego, California.

We would like to express our appreciation to the following New Jersey physicians and medical facilities for allowing us to photograph a variety of procedures and procedural settings at their facilities: the Eric B. Chandler Medical Center, New Brunswick; Helene Fuld School of Nursing of New Jersey, Trenton; Mercer Medical Center, Trenton; Mercer County Vocational-Technical Health Occupations Center, Trenton; Plainfield Health Center, Plainfield; Princeton Allergy and Asthma Associates, Princeton; the Princeton Medical Group, Princeton; Robert Wood Johnson University Hospital, New Brunswick; Robert Wood Johnson University Hospital at Hamilton, Hamilton; St. Francis Medical Center, Trenton; St. Peters Medical Center, New Brunswick; Dr. Edward von der Schmidt, neurosurgeon, Princeton; Wound Care Center/Curative Network, New Brunswick.

We would also like to thank the following facilities and educational institutions for graciously allowing us to photograph procedures and other technical aspects related to the profession of medical assisting: Total Care Programming, Henrico, North Carolina; Wildwood Medical Clinic, Henrico, North Carolina; Central Piedmont Community College, Charlotte, North Carolina; Daytona Beach Community College, Daytona Beach, Florida; Roanoke Rapids Clinic, Roanoke Rapids, Virginia; and Everest University, Jacksonville, Florida.

Thanks also to Lynn Egler and Susan Findley for their assistance with various aspects of the project. A special thank you to Tiffany Heath for her content review.

Reviewers

Every area of the text was reviewed by practitioners and educators in the field. Their insights helped shape the direction of the book.

Medical Advisory Board

Gerry A. Brasin, AS, CMA (AAMA), CPC
Premier Education Group

Dr. Marina Klebanov, BDS, MSPH
Mandl College of Allied Health

Tabitha L. Lyons, NCMA, AS
Corporate Program Manager-Medical Assisting
Anthem Education Group

Barry Newman, MD
Lincoln Educational Services

Diane Peavy
Fortis Colleges

Adrienne Predko, M.A. Ed.
National Director of Education
MedVance Institute

Dr. Gary Zuckerman
Washington University School of Medicine

CONNECT Contributors

Dolly R. Horton, CMA(AAMA), BS, M.Ed.
Asheville Buncombe Technical Community College

Sepanta Jalali, M.D.
Columbus State

Merideth Sellars, M.S.
Columbus State Community College

Sherry Stanfield, RN, BSN, MSHPE
Miller-Motte Technical College

Nerissa Tucker, MHA, CPC
Kaplan University School of Health Sciences

Dr. Wendy Vermillion DVM
Columbus State Community College

Mindy Wray, BS, CMA (AAMA), RMA
ECPI College of Technology

Byron Hamilton, BA, MA
Australian College of Advanced Education

Digital Symposium Attendees

Courtney M. Conrad, MBA, MPH, CMA
Robert Morris University Illinois

Bonnie J. Crist, BS, CMA, AAS, (AAMA)
Harrison College

Patrick J. Debold, Vice President of Academic Affairs
Concorde Career Colleges, Inc.

Robert Delaney
Chair, Allied Health
Brookline College

Alice Macomber, RN, RMA, AHI, RPT, CPI, BXO
Keiser University, Port Saint Lucie Campus

Barry Newman, MD
Kathleen Olewinski, MS, RHIA, NHA, FACHE
Medical Assisting Program Director
Bryant & Stratton College—Milwaukee Market

Mickie Roy, LPN, CCMA
Delta College of Arts & Technology

Lisa M. Smith, B.S., RMA(AMT), BXMO
Medical Assisting Program & Externship Coordinator
Keiser University

Michael Weinand
Kaplan Higher Education

Dr. Barbara Worley, DPM, BS, RMA
Program Manager, Medical Assisting
King's College

Patti Zint, M.A., N.C.H.I.
Apollo College

Reviewers

Hooshiyar Ahmadi, MD, DC
Remington College

Diana Alagna, RN, RMA (AMT)
Branford Hall Career Institute

Yvonne Beth Alles, MBA
Davenport University

Ramona Atiles, LPN
Allied Health Program Chair
Career Institute of Health and Technology

Vanessa J. Austin, RMA (AMT), CAHI, BS
Clarian Health Sciences Education Center

Dr. Joseph H. Balatbat, MD
Sanford-Brown Institute

Katie Barton, BA, LPN
Savannah River College

Suzanne Bitters, RMA (AMT)-NCPT/NCICS
Harris Business School

Alecia C. Blake, MD
Medical Careers Institute at ECPI College of Technology

Kathleen Bode, MS
Flint Hills Technical College

Cynthia Boles, CMA (AAMA)
Bradford School

Cindi Brassington, MS, CMA (AAMA)
Quinebaug Valley Community College

Robin K. Choate, LPN, CHI
Pennsylvania Institute of Technology

Stephen M. Coleman, NCMA
    Central Florida Institute

Sheronda Cooper, BSD, BSN, MSFN, RMA (AMT),
    NRCPT(NAHP)
    Director of Medical Assisting
    Bradford School of Business

Janet H. Davis, BSN, MS, MBA, PhD
    Robert Morris College

Linda Demain, LPN, BS, MS
    Wichita Technical Institute

Carol Dew, MAT, CMA-AC (AAMA)
    Baker College

James R. Dickerson, AAS
    Remington College

Cheryl Lacey Donovan, CMA (AAMA)
    Academy of Health Care Professions

Patricia Dudek, RN
    McCann School of Business and Technology

Jane W. Dumas, MSN
    Remington College

Tamara Epperson Mottler, BA, CMA (AAMA)
    Daytona Beach College

Rhonda K. Epps, AS
    National College of Business and Technology

Dr. Herbert J. Feitelberg, D.P.M.
    King's College

Suzanne S. Fielding, BS
    Daytona Beach College

Walter E. Flowers
    Medical Director
    Lamson Institute

Martina T. Forte Brown, CCMA (AAMA),
    CPT, CET
    Brookstone College of Business

Janette Gallegos, RMA (AMT)
    ECPI College of Technology

Christine Goldwater, NCMOA, AA
    Campus Director
    Ross Medical Education Center

Darlene S. Grayson Harmon, BS
    Remington College

Gay Grubbs, MEd
    Griffin Technical College

Tiffany Heath, CMA (AAMA)
    Porter and Chester Institute

Lisa M. Herrera
    Concorde Career College

Claudia N. Hewlett, AS
    Remington College

Elizabeth Hoffman, MA Ed., CMA,
    (AAMA), CPT (ASPT)
    Baker College

Adriane Holliman
    Westwood College ATM

Joanna L. Holly, MS, RN, CMA (AAMA)
    Midstate College

Deborah Honstad, MA, RHIA
    San Juan College

Susan Horn, AAS CMA (AAMA)
    Indiana Business College

Janet Hunter, Ph.D.
    Northland Pioneer College

Dara A. Indish, CMA (AAMA), EMT
    Alpena Community College

Carol Lee Jarrell, MLT, AHI
    Brown Mackie College

Shara-Leigh Kauffman, RN
    University of Northwestern Ohio

Jody Kirk
    Cambria-Rowe Business College

Doris Klein, BA
    Concorde Career College

Pam Kowalski, MA
    Ross Medical Education Center

Linda E. LaGrange, NCMA
    Remington College

Amy L. Lake, RMA (AMT)
    Wright Career College

Paul Lucas, CMA (AAMA), CPbt, PN, AS
    Brown Mackie College

Alice Macomber, RN, RMA (AMT)
    Keiser University

Gregory Martinez, BS, MS
    Wichita Technical Institute

Wilsetta McClain, MBA, ABD
    Baker College of Auburn Hills

Diana K. McWilliams
    Remington College

Nancy Measell, BS, CMA (AAMA)
    IVY Tech Community College

Maureen Messier, AS, BA
    Branford Hall Career Institute

Helen Mills, RN
    MA Instructor
    Keiser University

Edward Moreno
    STVT

Diane Morlock, BA, CMA (AAMA)
    Owens Community College

Roger K. Oatman, DC
    Logan Chiropractic College

Thomas O'Brien, AS CCT CST
    Central Florida Institute

Londa L. Ogden, RN, BSN
    Keiser University E-Campus

Everlee O'Nan, RMA (AMT)
    National College

Janet S. Pandzik, BA, CMT, RMA (AMT)
   Hallmark College of Technology

June M. Petillo
   Capital Community College

Alisa J. Petree, MHSM, MT (ASCP)
   McLennan Community College

Robert Plick, BA, BS
   Alta/Westwood College

Angela N. Resnick, RMA (AMT)
   School of Health Careers

Diane Roche Benson, CMA (AAMA), MSA, BS
   Wake Technical Community College,
   University of Phoenix

Rebecca Rodenbaugh, CMA (AAMA)
   Baker College of Cadillac

Janette Rodriguez, RN
   Wood Tobe Coburn

Pratima Sampat-Mar, M. Ed.
   Pima Medical Institute

Judy Scire, BS
   Stone Academy

Noreen T. Semanski, AS, LPN
   McCann School of Business

Lynn G. Slack, BS CMA (AAMA)
   Kaplan Career Institute

Robin Snider-Flohr, EdD, RN, CMA (AAMA)
   Jefferson Community College

Sherry A. Stanfield, RN, BSN, MSHPE
   Miller-Motte Tech College

Judith D. Symons
   McCann School of Business

Tricia Taylor
   Kaplan College

Catherine A. Teel, AST, RMA (AMT), CMA (AAMA)
   McCann School of Business and Technology

Lynne A. Thomas, BS
   Clarita Career College

Cindy Thompson, RN, RMA (AMT), MA, BS
   Davenport University

Carlota Zuniga Tienda, AS
   San Joaquin Valley College

Drew D. Totten, CLT, NRCMA
   Charter College

Nerissa C. Tucker, BS, MHA
   ECPI College of Technology

Marilyn M. Turner, R.N., C.M.A. (AAMA)
   Ogeechee Technical College

Sally Vrooman, MA Ed.
   Career Quest Learning Centers, Inc.

Judy K. Ward, BS
   Ivy Tech Community College

Marsha Lynn Wilson, MA, BS, MS (ABT)
   Clarian Health Sciences Education Center

Stacey F. Wilson, BS, MHA
   Cabarrus College of Health Sciences

Constance M. Winter, MPH, RN
   Bossier Parish Community College

Dr. Barbara Worley
   Program Manager,
   Medical Assisting Program
   King's College

Mindy Wray, BS, CMA (AAMA), RMA (AMT)
   ECPI College of Technology

Will L. Wright, BS
   Atlanta Medical Academy

Carole A. Zeglin, MS, BS, RMA (AMT)
   Westmoreland County Community College

Susan K. Zolvinski, BS, MBA
   Brown Mackie College

Previous Edition Reviewers

Roxane M. Abbott, MBA
   Sarasota County Technical Institute

Dr. Linda G. Alford, Ed.D.
   Reid State Technical College

Suzzanne S. Allen
   Sanford Brown Institute

Ann L. Aron, Ed.D.
   Aims Community College

Emil Asdurian, MD
   Bramson ORT College

Rhonda Asher, MT, ASCP, CMA
   Pitt Community College

Adelina H. Azfar, DPM
   Total Technical Institute

Joseph H. Balatbat, MD, RMA, RPT, CPT
   Sanford Brown Institute

Mary Barko, CMA, MA Ed
   Ohio Institute of Health Careers

Katie Barton, LPN, BA
   Savannah River College

Kelli C. Batten, NCMA, LMT
   Medical Assisting Department Chair
   Career Technical College

Nina Beaman, MS, RNC, CMA
   Bryant and Stratton College

Kay E. Biggs, BS, CMA
   Columbus State Community College

Norma Bird, M.Ed., BS, CMA
   Medical Assisting Program Director/
   Master Instructor

Kathleen Bode, RN, MS
   Flint Hills Technical College

Natasha Bratton, BSN
   Beta Tech

Karen Brown, RN, BC, Ed.D.
   Kirtland Community College

Kimberly D. Brown, BSHS, CHES, CMA
  Swainsboro Technical College

Nancy A. Browne, MS, BS
  Washington High School

Teresa A. Bruno, BA
  EduTek College

Marion I. Bucci, BA
  Delaware Technical and Community College

Michelle Buchman, BSN, RNC
  Springfield College

Michelle L. Carfagna, RMA, ST, BMO, RHE
  Brevard Community College

Carmen Carpenter, RN, MS, CMA
  South University

Pamela C. Chapman, RN, MSN
  Caldwell Community College and Technical Institute

Patricia A. Chappell, MA, BS
  Director, Clinical Laboratory Science
  Camden County College

Phyllis Cox, MA Ed, BS, MT(ASCP)
  Arkansas Tech University

Stephanie Cox, BS, LPN
  York Technical Institute

Christine Cusano, CMA, CPhT
  Clark University CCI

Glynna Day, M.Ed
  Dean of Education
  Academy of Professional Careers

Anita Denson, BS
  National College of Business and Technology

Leon Deutsch, RMA, BA, MA Ed
  Keiser College

Walter R. English, MA, MT(AAB)
  Akron Institute

Dennis J. Ernst, MT(ASCP)
  Center for Phlebotomy Education

C.S. Farabee, MBA, MSISE
  High-Tech Institute Inc.

Deborah Fazio, CMAS, RMA
  Sanford Brown Institute Cleveland

William C. Fiala, BS, MA
  University of Akron

Cathy Flores, BHS
  Central Piedmont Community College

Brenda K. Frerichs, MS, MA, BS
  Colorado Technical University

Michael Gallucci, PT, MS
  Assistant Professor of Practice,
  Program in Physical Therapy,
  School of Public Health,
  New York Medical College

Susan C. Gessner, RN, BSN, M Ed
  Laurel Business Institute

Bonnie J. Ginman, CMA
  Branford Hall Career Institute

Robyn Gohsman, RMA, CMAS
  Medical Career Institute

Cheri Goretti, MA, MT(ASCP), CMA
  Quinebaug Valley Community College

Marilyn Graham, LPN
  Moore Norman Technology Center

Jodee Gratiot, CCA
  Rocky Mountain Business Academy

Donna E. Guisado, AA
  North-West College

Debra K. Hadfield, BSN, MSN
  Baker College of Jackson

Carrie A. Hammond, CMA, LPRT
  Utah Career College

Kris A. Hardy, CMA, RHE, CDF
  Brevard Community College

Toni R. Hartley, BS
  Laurel Business Institute

Brenda K. Hartson, MS, MA, BS
  Colorado Technical University

Marsha Perkins Hemby, BA, RN, CMA
  Pitt Community College

Linda Henningsen, RN, MS, BSN
  Brown Mackie College

Carol Hinricher, MA
  University of Montana College
  of Technology

Elizabeth A. Hoffman, MA Ed., CMA
  Baker College of Clinton Township

Gwen C. Hornsey, BS
  Medical Assistant Instructor
  Tulsa Technology Center, Lemley Campus

Helen J. Houser, MSHA, RN, RMA
  Phoenix College

Melody S. Irvine, CCS-P, CPC, CMBS
  Institute of Business and Medical Careers

Kathie Ivester, MPA, CMA(AAMA), CLS(NCA)
  North Georgia Technical College

Josephine Jackyra, CMA
  The Technical Institute of Camden County

Deborah Jones, BS, MA
  High-Tech Institute

Karl A. Kahley, CHE, BS
  Instructor, Medical Assisting
  Ogeechee Technical College

Barbara Kalfin Kalish
  City College, Palm Beach Community College

Cheri D. Keenan, MA Instructor, EMT-B
  Remington College

Barbara E. Kennedy, RN, CPhT
  Blair College

Tammy C. Killough, RN, BSN
Texas Careers Vocational Nursing
Program Director

Jimmy Kinney, AAS
Virginia College at Huntsville

Karen A. Kittle, CMA, CPT, CHUC
Oakland Community College

Diane M. Klieger, RN, MBA, CMA
Pinellas Technical Education Centers

Mary E. Larsen, CMT, RMA
Academy of Professional Careers

Nancy L. Last, RN
Eagle Gate College

Holly Roth Levine, NCICS, NCRMA, BA, BSN, RN
Keiser College

Christine Malone, BS
Everett Community College

Janice Manning
Baker College

Loretta Mattio-Hamilton, AS, CMA, RPT, CCA, NCICS
Herzing College

Gayle Mazzocco, BSN, RN, CMA
Oakland Community College

Patti McCormick, RN, PHD
President, Institute of Holistic Leadership

Stephanie R. McGahee, AATH
Augusta Technical College

Heidi M. McLean, CMA, RMA, BS, RPT, CAHI
Anne Arundel Community College

Tanya Mercer, BS, RN, RMA
KAPLAN Higher Education Corporation

Sandra J. Metzger, RN, BSN, MS. Ed
Red Rocks Community College

Joyce A. Minton, BS, CMA, RMA
Wilkes Community College

Grace Moodt, RN, BSN
Wallace Community College

Sherry L. Mulhollen, BS, CMA
Elmira Business Institute

Deborah M. Mullen, CPC, NCMA
Sanford Brown Institute

Michael Murphy, CMA
Berdan Institute @ The Summit
Medical Group

Lisa S. Nagle, CMA, BS.Ed
Augusta Technicial College

Peggy Newton, BSN, RN
Galen Health Institute

Brigitte Niedzwiecki, RN, MSN
Chippewa Valley Technical College

Thomas E. O Brien, MBA, BBA, AS, CCT
Central Florida Institute

Linda Oliver, MA
Vista Adult School

Linda L. Oprean, BSN
ACT College

Holly J. Paul, MSN, FNP
Baker College of Jackson

Shirley Perkins, MD, BSE
Everest College

Kristina Perry, BPA
Heritage College

James H. Phillips, BS, CMA, RMA
Central Florida College

Carol Putkamer, RHIA, MS
Alpena Community College

Mary Rahr, MS, RN, CMA-C
Northeast Wisconsin Technical College

David Rice, AA, BA, MA
Career College of Northern Nevada

Dana M. Roessler, RN, BSN
Southeastern Technical College

Cindy Rosburg, MA
Wisconsin Indian Technical College

Deborah D. Rossi, MA, CMA
Community College of Philadelphia

Donna Rust, BA
American Commercial College

Ona Schulz, CMA
Lake Washington Technical College

Amy E. Semenchuk, RN, BSN
Rockford Business College

David Lee Sessoms, Jr., M.Ed., CMA
Miller-Motte Technical College

Susan Shorey, BA, MA
Valley Career College

Lynn G. Slack, BS
ICM School of Business and Medical Careers

Patricia L. Slusher, MT(ASCP), CMA
Ivy Tech State College

Deborah H. Smith, RN, CNOR
Southeastern Technical College

Kristi Sopp, AA
MTI College

Nona K. Stinemetz, Practical Nurse
Vatterott College

Patricia Ann Stoddard, MS, RT(R), MT, CMA
Western Business College

Sylvia Taylor, BS, CMA, CPC-A
Cleveland State Community College

Cynthia H. Thompson, RN, MA
Davenport University

Geiselle Thompson, M. Div.
The Learning Curve Plus NC

Barbara Tietsort, M. Ed.
   University of Cincinnati, Raymond Walters

Karen A. Trompke, RN
   Virginia College at Pensacola

Marilyn M. Turner, RN, CMA
   Ogeechee Technical College

L. Joleen VanBibber, AS
   Davis Applied Technology College

Lynette M. Veach, AAS
   Columbus State Community College

Antonio C. Wallace, BS
   Sanford Brown Institute

Jim Wallace, MHSA
   Maric College

Denise Wallen, CPC
   Academy of Professional Careers

Mary Jo Whitacre, MSN, RN
   Lord Fairfax Community College

Donna R. Williams, LPN, RMA
   Tennessee Technology Center

Marsha Lynn Wilson, BS, MS (ABT)
   Clarian Health Sciences Education Center

Linda V. Wirt, CMA
   Cecil Community College

Dr. MaryAnn Woods, PhD, RN
   Prof. Emeritus,
   Fresno City College

Bettie Wright, MBA, CMA
   Umpqua Community College

Mark D. Young, DMD, BS
   West Kentucky Community and
   Technical College

Cynthia M. Zumbrun, MEd, RHIT, CCS-P
   Allegany College of Maryland

Guided Tour

Case Studies

represent situations similar to those that the medical assistant may encounter in daily practice.

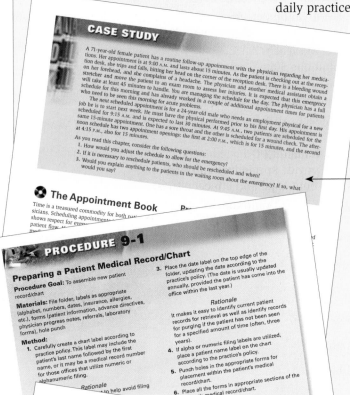

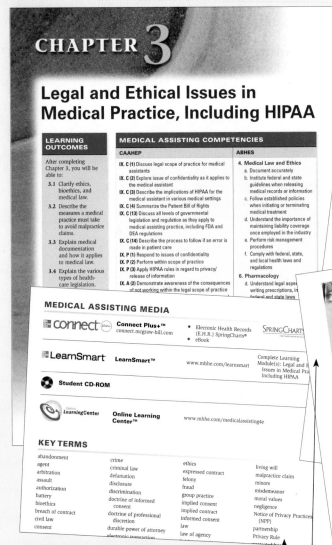

Chapter Openers include the CAAHEP and ABHES competencies covered in the chapter, a list of learning outcomes, a list of the media supplements available to accompany the chapter, a list of key terms, the chapter outline, and the new Preparation for Certification feature boxes.

Procedure boxes Specific administrative or clinical tasks are illustrated in a step-by-step format. A new work product icon denotes the need for documentation to successfully complete the procedure, which can be found and completed in the Student Workbook.

CAUTION *Handle with Care* boxes cover precautions to be taken when performing certain tasks.

Points on Practice boxes
provide guidelines on keeping the medical office running smoothly and efficiently.

Educating the Patient boxes
Patient instruction on self-care outside the medical office is the focus.

Reflecting On . . . boxes
provide specialized information about legal and ethical issues, communication issues, cultural issues, professionalism, age considerations, and HIPAA.

Career Opportunities boxes
provide information on professions and duties related to medical assisting.

Summary and Review
A summary of the chapter material and an end-of-chapter review close out each chapter. New to this edition are multiple-choice questions that also appear here.

Points on Practice

Working with Electronic Health Records

Electronic health records (EHRs) are essentially a computer-based or a digital recording of patient information. They are also called computer records, electronic medical records (EMRs), electronic charts, and computer health records. Paper records can be lost and information is not consistent. In addition, hand-writing is often illegible. EHRs provide a multitude of advantages, including the following:

- Access. Electronic records _____
by health-care _____
includ_____

be performed. More sophisticated programs can document health trends, provide _____ recognition, and convert _____ sentences.

As a m_____

Respecting Patients' Cultural Beliefs

Patients come from many diverse cultures and often have different beliefs about the causes and treatments of illness. These differences may affect their treatment expectations, as well as their willingness to follow medical directions. When talking with patients, it is important to understand and respect their cultural beliefs. Patients may not be willing to accept instructions or consent to treatment based on their cultural background. Consider these simple steps when giving instructions to patients of diverse cultures:

1. Speak slowly and clearly.
2. Request or provide a translator as needed.

3. Ask for and look for feedback from the patient, indicating that she understands and intends to follow the patient instructions.
4. Ask the patient if there is any reason that she will not be able to follow the instructions.
5. Address any concerns addressed by the patient, notifying the doctor if the concerns will mean that patient is not likely to follow instructions.
6. Provide educational resources in the patient's primary language, if available.

Educating the Patient

Instructing Patients with Hearing Impairments

Educating patients who have hearing impairments need not be difficult if you pay a little extra attention in the following areas.

- Try to eliminate all background noise. Talk in a quiet room, if possible.
- Make sure the room is well lit.
- _____ the patient, and make sure the patient can _____ Having the patient watch your _____ help him understand

would like you to go over any particular part of the explanation or instructions again.

Loss of hearing can cause people to withdraw and feel isolated. Being empathic and patient greatly enhances the educational process.

Elderly Patients with Hearing Loss
Most people experience a gradual loss of hearing as they get older. In addition to the preceding suggestions, try to talk in a lower pitch whenever possible. As people get older, they often lose the ability to hear higher tones first.

_____ Wear Hearing Aids
_____ who wears a hearing aid, it _____ Many hearing aids _____ and noises.

Reflecting On . . . HIPAA

Avoiding Abuse of Patient Confidentiality

HIPAA law describes **abuse** as a practice or behavior that is not indicative of sound medical or fiscal activity. Improper or careless use of a patient's answering system or fax machine can be viewed as abusive behavior in the eyes of the law. It is imperative that the

patient's right to privacy be carefully _____ times. If in doubt that the patien_____ violated by leaving it _____ machine, it is b_____

Leaving a Message on an An_____ or Fax Machine. On _____
leave a message on _____
send a m_____

PROCEDURE 10-3

Developing a Records Retention Program (concluded)

retrieving these files from storage, circulate a notice to the office staff stating which records will be destroyed. Indicate that the staff must let you know by a specific date if any of the files should be saved. You may want to keep a separate file with these notices.

10. After the deadline has passed, retrieve the files from storage. Review each file before it is destroyed. Make sure the staff members who will destroy the files are trained to use the equipment properly. Develop a sheet of instructions for destroying files. Post it prominently with the retention schedule, near the machinery used to destroy the files.

Rationale
To guard patient confidentiality and follow all HIPAA laws governing the protection of patient information.

11. Update the index card, giving the date the file was destroyed and by whom.
12. Periodically review the retention schedule. Update it with the most current legal and governmental requirements. With the staff, evaluate whether the current schedule is meeting the needs of your office or whether files are being kept too long or destroyed prematurely. With the doctor's approval, change the schedule as necessary.

Career Opportunities

Registered Health Information Technician

To gain medical assistant credentials, you must fulfill the requirements of either the American Association of Medical Assistants (for a Certified Medical Assistant) or the American Medical Technologists (for a Registered Medical Assistant). After obtaining your medical assistant certification or registration, you may wish to acquire additional skills in specialty areas through course work or on-the-job training. Although this course work or training may not lead to an additional certification or degree, it will enable you to expand your role in the medical office and advance your career as the demand for skilled health professionals increases. Should you wish to add an additional certification, the opportunity, with further training in health information technology, does exist through the American Health Information Management Association (AHIMA).

Skills and Duties
Sometimes called a medical record technician or a medical chart specialist, a Registered Health Information Technician (RHIT) maintains patient records for a physician or group of physicians. The RHIT is responsible for ensuring that all medical information is accurate and complete. In a hospital, a RHIT deals strictly with health information and has no patient contact. In a small office, however, the RHIT may

have additional clerical duties such as answering the telephone.

A patient's medical record includes a medical history and statement of symptoms as well as the results of exams, laboratory tests, and x-rays. The physician's diagnoses and treatment plans are also included. The information in the patient's record may be needed for insurance purposes or to aid in further diagnosis and treatment. In addition, it may be used for research purposes.

continued →

---

procedures, equipment, and supplies either not listed in CPT or containing more detail than CPT.

16.6 In locating a procedure code, you first become familiar with the format and guidelines. First look up the procedure description in the alphabetic listing in the back of the CPT manual. Then verify the correct code, codes, or code range in the numeric index. For detailed information in completing this process, see Procedure 16-3.

16.7 Medical codes must be correctly linked (one diagnosis for each procedure) when reporting them for reimbursement because payers analyze this connection to determine the medical necessity for the charge.

16.8 Insurance fraud is an act of deception used to take advantage of another entity. An example of billing and coding fraud is when a physician reports services that were not performed.

REVIEW

CHAPTER 16

CASE STUDY QUESTIONS

Now that you have completed this chapter, review the case study at the beginning of the chapter and answer the following questions:

1. How would you select the ICD-9 and CPT codes for a health-care claim for this visit?
2. What diagnosis and procedure codes will result in the correct payment for these services?
3. How should the claim show the medical necessity of the procedures?
4. Locate the ICD-9 code for the patient's asthma. How many digits are required? What code did you assign?
5. Locate the CPT code for the cardiovascular stress test. What information did you use to select it from the list of related codes?

Multiple-Choice Questions

1. The Alphabetic Index for ICD-9-CM is organized by
   a. the part of the body involved.
   b. symptoms the patient displays.
   c. codes found in the Tabular List.
   d. the condition.
2. The Tabular List of ICD-9-CM is organized by
   a. the condition of the patient.
   b. the codes found in the Alphabetic Index.
   c. the symptoms of the patient.
   d. the part of the body involved.
3. The _____ codes are considered to be the most important of the CPT codes.
   a. modifier   c. add-on
   b. E/M   d. unlisted procedure

4. For reporting purposes, CPT considers a patient "new" if he or she has not received professional services within the past _____ year(s).
   a. one   c. three
   b. two   d. five
5. The Health Care Common Procedure Coding System (HCPCS) was developed for use in coding services for
   a. Blue Cross.
   b. HMOs.
   c. Medicare patients.
   d. Managed care organizations.

Discussion Questions

1. What are the differences among the three code sets discussed in the chapter?
2. Are see cross-references in the Alphabetic Index of the ICD-9 followed by codes? Why?
3. Would you expect to locate codes for the following services or procedures in CPT? What range or series of codes would you investigate?
   a. Routine obstetric care including antepartum care, cesarean delivery, and postpartum care
   b. Echocardiography (cardiac)
   c. Radiologic examination, nasal bones, complete
   d. Home visit for evaluation and management of an established patient
   e. Drug test for amphetamines
   f. Anesthesia for cardiac catheterization
4. Why are both the ICD-9 and CPT codes updated each year?
5. What three main changes in coding are included in the ICD-10-CM revision?
6. What is the value of modifiers in coding?

FOURTH EDITION

ADMINISTRATIVE PROCEDURES

for Medical Assisting

Introduction to Medical Assisting

"The medical assisting profession is filled with challenges and rewards every day. Everything is important when you are assisting a patient. You should get to know your patient and his family, if possible, in order to understand the patient's specific needs. This is especially true with an elderly patient. Treat your patient like you would want to be treated. Be considerate and concerned, and always maintain a pleasant attitude.

"It is also essential to know your physician well, and how he or she likes to work. Let the physician know all the information the patient has shared with you, to help him or her make a better diagnosis. Keep informed about what the physician has recommended for treatment. The patient will have questions along the way. It's good medicine to be able to give him solid information about his condition and reinforce the doctor's orders when necessary. A skilled physician and an organized, cooperative, receptive medical assistant promote and maintain exceptional patient care."

Sue Haines
Medical Assistant, Princeton, New Jersey

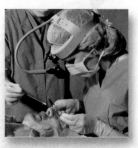

SECTION ONE
Foundations and Principles

Chapter 1   The Profession of Medical Assisting

Chapter 2   Types of Medical Practice

Chapter 3   Legal and Ethical Issues in Medical Practice, Including HIPAA

Chapter 4   Communication with Patients, Families, and Coworkers

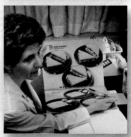

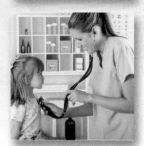

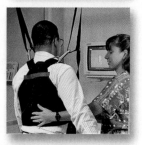

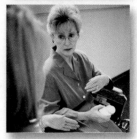

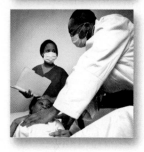

SECTION 1

FOUNDATIONS AND PRINCIPLES

CHAPTER 1

The Profession of Medical Assisting

CHAPTER 2

Types of Medical Practice

CHAPTER 3

Legal and Ethical Issues in Medical Practice, Including HIPAA

CHAPTER 4

Communication with Patients, Families, and Coworkers

The Profession of Medical Assisting

MEDICAL ASSISTING COMPETENCIES

CAAHEP

IX.C (5) Discuss licensure and certification as it applies to health-care providers

IX.P (2) Perform within scope of practice

IX.P (4) Practice within the standard of care for a medical assistant

ABHES

1. General Orientation
- a. Comprehend the current employment outlook for the medical assistant
- b. Compare and contrast the allied health professions and understand their relation to medical assisting
- c. Understand medical assistant credentialing requirements and the process to obtain the credential; comprehend the importance of credentialing.
- d. Have knowledge of the general responsibilities of the medical assistant
- e. Define scope of practice for the medical assistant, and comprehend the conditions for practice within the state that the medical assistant is employed

11. Career Development

Demonstrate professionalism by:
- 1) Exhibiting dependability, punctuality, and a positive attitude and a sense of responsibility
- 4) Being cognizant of ethical boundaries
- 9) Conducting work with in scope of education, training, and ability

LEARNING OUTCOMES

After completing Chapter 1, you will be able to:

1.1 Identify the job responsibilities of a medical assistant.

1.2 Describe the professional training of a medical assistant.

1.3 Model personal characteristics a medical assistant needs.

1.4 Describe a multi-skilled health professional.

1.5 Explain the importance of continuing education for a medical assistant.

1.6 Explain the process and benefits of certification and registration.

1.7 Distinguish the benefits of becoming a member of a professional association.

MEDICAL ASSISTING MEDIA

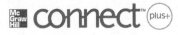 **Connect Plus+™**
connect.mcgraw-hill.com

- Electronic Health Records (E.H.R.) SpringCharts®
- eBook

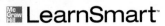 **LearnSmart™**   www.mhhe.com/learnsmart

Complete Learning Module: The Profession of Medical Assisting

 Student CD-ROM

 Online Learning Center™   www.mhhe.com/medicalassisting4e

KEY TERMS

accreditation

American Association of Medical Assistants (AAMA)

American Medical Technologists (AMT)

Certified Medical Assistant (CMA)

Clinical Laboratory Improvement Amendments of 1988 (CLIA '88)

contaminated

cross-training

externship

Health Insurance Portability and Accountability Act (HIPAA)

managed care organization (MCO)

Occupational Safety and Health Administration (OSHA)

practitioner

Registered Medical Assistant (RMA)

résumé

CHAPTER OUTLINE

- Growth of the Medical Assisting Profession
- Medical Assistant Credentials
- Membership in a Medical Assisting Association
- Training Programs and Other Learning Opportunities
- Accreditation
- Daily Duties of Medical Assistants
- Personal Qualifications of Medical Assistants
- The AAMA Occupational Analysis

Introduction

Medical assisting is one of the fastest-growing occupations in allied health care today. Health care is changing at a rapid rate, from advanced technology to implementing cost-effective medicine while maintaining quality patient care. The medical assistant is the perfect complement to this changing industry. Employers are looking for health care professionals who are "generalists." A generalist is someone who is trained in all departments in the facility in which he or she is employed. Medical assistants who graduate from an accredited institution will gain the skills that enable them to multitask. A multitasking professional is someone who is able to work in the administrative areas, the clinical areas, and the financial areas. Employers are seeking credentialed health-care professionals who are dedicated to the profession and the patient.

This chapter will introduce the professional standards that are required in medical assisting.

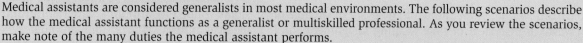

CASE STUDY

Medical assistants are considered generalists in most medical environments. The following scenarios describe how the medical assistant functions as a generalist or multiskilled professional. As you review the scenarios, make note of the many duties the medical assistant performs.

Scenario 1 Debbie is 23 years old. She has been working as a medical assistant for 2 years. She is currently working in a family practice office with two doctors, two other medical assistants, and a medical records clerk. Her role is primarily administrative; she is mainly responsible for phone reception and patient check-in and check-out.

A 29-year-old female patient calls complaining of lower back pain. As Debbie listens to the patient describe her condition, she determines the severity of the patient's discomfort and schedules a same-day appointment. When the patient arrives at the office, Debbie greets her at the front desk, verifies her address and insurance information, and escorts her to an exam room. After the physician completes the exam, the patient is instructed to see Debbie on the way out. Debbie reviews the patient's prescriptions and schedules a diagnostic test and laboratory work for the patient at another facility. Debbie then collects the patient co-pay and gives the patient a receipt. After the patient leaves, Debbie prepares the insurance forms for reimbursement and files the patient's chart.

Scenario 2 Tom is 30 years old. He has been working as a medical assistant for 7 years. He currently works as a clinical medical assistant in an urgent care center that specializes in occupational medicine and basic emergency medicine. He is flexible and works a combination of days, afternoons, and weekends. He normally works with two doctors, two nurses, and four other medical assistants during his shift. The center's patients usually arrive on a walk-in basis.

A 40-year-old man signs in with the receptionist. She helps the patient complete the necessary forms for the medical chart. After the chart is completed, she places the chart at the clinical station. Tom reviews the medical chart and makes note that the patient, a truck driver, is here for an occupational physical. He obtains the protocol from the trucking company file and verifies the testing requested by the company. He then escorts the patient to an exam room and interviews the patient regarding his medical history. He explains all the testing that will be completed and escorts the patient to the laboratory. Tom collects a urine drug screen, following precise directions, and collects a blood specimen. Tom then performs an auditory and visual screening and escorts the patient back to the exam room. The patient is given a gown with instructions on how to put it on. After a few minutes, Tom obtains an EKG on the patient. The patient is now ready for the physical part of the exam, which is performed by the doctor. Tom verifies the information again and gives the chart to the doctor. After the doctor is finished with the exam, Tom returns to the patient, explains how the physical is reported to his employer, and escorts him to the x-ray technician for a chest x-ray. After the patient leaves, Tom completes the paperwork, submits the laboratory work to an outside reference lab, and submits the x-ray to be read by a radiologist.

Scenario 3 Patty begins her day at 5:00 A.M. Her first stop is the reference laboratory, where she collects all the necessary phlebotomy equipment needed to complete the daily visits. She then drives to the first nursing facility on her route, where she is scheduled to collect blood specimens from 10 patients. She returns to the lab to drop off the specimens and paperwork, and heads out to her second nursing facility to collect blood specimens. She continues to collect specimens throughout the day and returns to the laboratory at 1:30 P.M. She is given her schedule for the following day.

As you read this chapter, consider the following questions:

1. How are the three jobs different?
2. How are the three jobs the same?
3. How do these three medical assistants function as multiskilled health-care professionals?

Your Success as a Student

The world of medical assisting is an exciting and rewarding career path. Your success is determined by the path that you take toward your goal of becoming a medical assistant. As a new student in this field, there are several key factors that will assist you while embarking on this great career.

Key Factors for Success

There are several factors that will impact your success as a student.

1. *Organizational skills.* Students who are disorganized waste a great deal of time locating assignments and other materials before they get started on their work. Organizational skills are crucial to your success. Prepare in advance. Make sure you purchase a binder, notebook, or folders that have your homework assignments in them, reminders about upcoming tests, your course syllabus, and other pertinent information such as your instructor's office hours and phone and classmates' information for study sessions.

2. *Study habits.* Study habits will assist you with concentration and retention of the materials. Make sure you study in a quiet area away from distractions; find a study "buddy" who is just as committed and focused on success as you are; and prepare flashcards to assist you with independent studying.

3. *Set goals.* By setting goals for yourself, you can take responsibility for the results of your efforts. You must take ownership toward your success as a student. You can generate on the computer or manually a goal-setting sheet such as the one in Table 1-1.

Growth of the Medical Assisting Profession

As a medical assistant, you will be an allied health professional trained to work in a variety of health-care settings: medical offices, clinics, and ambulatory care facilities. Your role, with varied and challenging administrative and clinical duties, will be integral to creating a health-care facility that operates smoothly and provides a patient-centered approach to quality health care. Your specific responsibilities will likely depend on the location and size of the facility as well as its medical specialties.

Medical assisting is now one of the fastest-growing occupations. As the health services industry expands, the U.S. Department of Labor projects that medical assisting will be the fastest-growing occupation between 2006 and 2016. The growth in the number of physicians' group practices and other health-care practices that use support personnel will in turn continue to drive up demand for medical assistants.

TABLE 1-1 Sample Goal-Setting Sheet				
Goal(s)	Study Strategies	Who? (persons involved in carrying out your strategies)	Specific Concerns?	Completion Date?
To make an "A" in my Medical Terminology class.	1. Flashcards and note cards 2. Study with Andrea (my study buddy) on Thursday nights before each test.	1. Shania (myself) 2. Shania and Andrea	1. I can't remember the prefixes and suffixes of medical terms 2. Finishing my presentation on time 3. I feel I am lacking the typing skills to finish presentation	June 28, 2010 (the day before final exam)

According to the U.S. Department of Labor Bureau of Statistics, by 2016 it is expected that medical assistants will hold 565,000 jobs. This is up 35% from the 417,000 jobs that were held in 2006. Of these, 60% were in physicians' offices and approximately 14% were in hospitals, including outpatient and inpatient facilities. Almost 10% were in nursing homes and the offices of other health **practitioners** (those who practice a profession), such as chiropractors, optometrists, and podiatrists. The rest worked mostly in outpatient care centers, public and private educational services, other ambulatory health-care services, state and local government agencies, medical and diagnostic laboratories, nursing care facilities, and employment services. Modern health insurance, Medicare, and Medicaid now make medical care available to more people, and the number of physicians is increasing. Thus, more medical assistants will be needed to run these physicians' offices.

The following factors will also increase job opportunities for medical assistants: growth of outpatient clinics and health maintenance organizations (HMOs), and the population increase. Specifically, greater numbers of older people now require a relatively higher level of medical care. Today, the elderly are the fastest-growing segment of the U.S. population, bringing an increase in demand for health-care services.

History of the Medical Assisting Profession

With the emergence of formal training programs for medical assistants and the continuous changes in health care today, the role of the medical assistant has become dynamic and wide ranging. These changes have raised the expectations for medical assistants. The knowledge base of the modern medical assistant includes:

- Administrative and clinical skills
- Patient insurance product knowledge (specific to the workers' geographical locations)
- Compliance, especially of OSHA and HIPAA guidelines
- Exceptional customer service
- Practice management
- Current patient treatments and education

The medical assisting profession today requires a commitment to self-directed, lifelong learning. Health care is changing rapidly because of new technology, new health-care delivery systems, and new approaches to facilitating cost-efficient, high-quality health care. A medical assistant who can adapt to change and is continually learning will be in high demand.

Creating the American Association of Medical Assistants

The seed of the idea for a national association of medical assistants—to be called the **American Association of Medical Assistants (AAMA)**—was planted at the 1955 annual

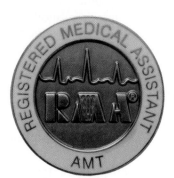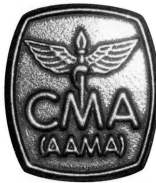

Figure 1-1. The pin on the left is worn by medical assistants registered by the American Medical Technologists. The pin on the right is worn by members of the American Association of Medical Assistants.

state convention of the Kansas Medical Assistants Society. The next year, at an American Medical Association (AMA) meeting, the AAMA was officially created. In 1978 the U.S. Department of Health, Education, and Welfare declared medical assisting an allied health profession. In the early 1970s the American Medical Technologists (which has been a national certifying body for laboratory personnel since 1939) began a program to register medical assistants at accredited schools. You will read more about the benefits of joining one of these organizations later in the chapter. Figure 1-1 shows the pins worn by medical assistants who are certified by the AAMA and by those registered by the American Medical Technologists.

The AAMA's Purpose. The AAMA works to raise standards of medical assisting to a more professional level. It is the only professional association devoted exclusively to the medical assisting profession. Its creator and first president, Maxine Williams, had extensive experience in orchestrating medical assisting projects for the Kansas Medical Assistants Society. She also served as co-chair of the planning committee that formed the AAMA.

The AAMA Creed. To maintain the professional standards of the medical assisting profession, the AAMA has developed the following creed, which is reprinted here with the permission of the organization:

> I believe in the principles and purposes of the profession of medical assisting.
> I endeavor to be more effective.
> I aspire to render greater service.
> I protect the confidence entrusted to me.
> I am dedicated to the care and well-being of all people.
> I am loyal to my employer.
> I am true to the ethics of my profession.
> I am strengthened by compassion, courage, and faith.

AAMA Code of Ethics. The AAMA has also established a code of ethics, which is reprinted here with the permission of the organization:

The Code of Ethics of AAMA shall set forth principles of ethical and moral conduct as they relate to the medical profession and the particular practice of Medical Assisting.

Members of AAMA dedicated to the conscientious pur-suit of their profession, and thus desiring to merit the high regard of the entire medical profession and the respect of the general public which they serve, do pledge themselves to strive always to:

A. render service with full respect for the dignity of humanity;
B. respect confidential information obtained through employment unless legally authorized or required by responsible performance of duty to divulge such information;
C. uphold the honor and high principles of the profession and accept its disciplines;
D. seek to continually improve the knowledge and skills of medical assistants for the benefit of patients and professional colleagues;
E. participate in additional service activities aimed toward improving the health and well-being of the community.

Medical Assistant Credentials

Employers today prefer or even insist that their medical assistants have credentialing within their discipline. Understanding why employers are aggressively recruiting credentialed medical assistants is of utmost importance for medical assisting educators as well as all medical assistants. Listed here are some explanations as to why obtaining and maintaining a professional credential is becoming so important for a medical assistant's entry into and advancement within the allied health force.

Malpractice

The United States continues to be one of the most litigious nations in the civilized world. Disputes that used to be settled by discussion and mediation are now being referred to attorneys and ending up in courts of law. Lawsuits are particularly acute in the world of health care. Employers of allied health professionals have correctly concluded that having credentialed personnel or staff will lessen the likelihood of a successful legal challenge to the quality of work of employees.

An accredited medical assisting program is competency based; this means that standards are set by the accrediting body, such as the Accrediting Bureau of Health Education Schools (ABHES) or the Commission on Accreditation of Allied Health Education Programs (CAAHEP), for administrative and clinical competencies. It is the duty of the educational institution to ensure that all medical assisting competencies are learned by medical assisting students and that evidence is clearly documented for each student. Periodic evaluations are performed by the accrediting agencies to ensure the effectiveness of the program. The theory of

the competencies as well as the proficiency assessments are components of the CMA (AAMA) examination. For example, administering medications is a competency required of accredited medical assisting programs and is a component of the CMA (AAMA) examination. The CMA (AAMA) credential and the affiliation with a professional organization demonstrate competence and provide evidence of training. They will also lessen the likelihood of a legal challenge to the quality of a medical assistant's work.

Managed Care Organizations

Managed care is a growing trend in today's health-care industry. The cost limitations imposed by **managed care organizations (MCOs)** are causing mergers and buyouts throughout the nation. Small physician practices are being consolidated or merged into larger providers of health care, such as by hospitals or for-profit organizations, which result in decreased operating expenses. These larger health-care providers can make the delivery of health care more cost-effective. Human resource directors of MCOs place great importance in professional credentials for their employees and therefore are more likely to establish certification or registry as a mandatory professional designation for medical assistants.

State and Federal Regulations

Certain provisions of the **OSHA (Occupational Safety and Health Act)** and the **CLIA '88 (Clinical Laboratory Improvement Amendments of 1988)** are making mandatory credentialing for medical assistants a logical step in the hiring process. Presently, OSHA and CLIA '88 do not require that medical assistants be credentialed, but there are various components of these statutes and their regulations that can be met by demonstrating that medical assistants in a clinical setting are certified. For example, some physician offices perform moderately complex laboratory testing on site. The medical assistant can perform moderately complex tests if she or he has the appropriate training and skills. The Certified Office Laboratory Technician (COLT) certification offered by the American Medical Technologists is designed to test health-care professionals for the appropriate skills necessary to perform moderately complex laboratory tests under CLIA regulations.

CMA Certification

The **Certified Medical Assistant (CMA)** credential is awarded by the Certifying Board of the AAMA. The AAMA's certification examination evaluates mastery of medical assisting competencies based on the Occupational Analysis of the CMA (AAMA) and are available at www.aama-ntl.org/medassisting/OA.pdf. The National Board of Medical Examiners (NBME) also provides technical assistance in developing the tests.

CMAs (AAMA) must recertify the CMA (AAMA) credential every 5 years. To be recertified as a CMA (AAMA),

60 contact hours must be accumulated during the five-year period: 10 in the administrative area, 10 in the clinical area, and 10 in the general area, with 30 additional hours in any of the three categories. In addition, 30 of these contact hours must be from an approved AAMA program. This mandate requires you to learn about new medical developments through education courses or participation in an examination. Hundreds of continuing education courses are sponsored by local, state, and national AAMA groups. The AAMA also offers self-study courses through its Continuing Education Department. As described in the AAMA's publication *CMA Today,* the advantages of CMA (AAMA) certification include respect and recognition from peers in the medical assisting profession.

As of June 1998, only applicants of medical assisting programs accredited by the CAAHEP and the ABHES are eligible to take the certification examination. The examination is administered nationwide every January, June, and October at more than 100 test sites. The AAMA offers the *Candidate's Guide to the Certification Examination* to help applicants prepare for the examination. This guide explains the test format and test-taking strategies. It also includes a sample examination with answers and information about study references. As of January 2009, the CMA (AAMA) examination is computerized. You may search the Internet for application and test review materials. Once you have successfully passed the CMA (AAMA) examination you have earned the right to add that credential to your name: Tiffany Heath, CMA (AAMA).

American Medical Technologists (AMT) Organization

The **American Medical Technologists (AMT)** organization, founded in 1939, credentials medical assistants as **Registered Medical Assistants (RMA)**. RMA (AMT) credentialing by the AMT ensures that you have taken and passed the RMA (AMT) certification examination for the RMA (AMT).

The AMT sets forth certain educational and experiential requirements to earn the RMA (AMT) credential. These include:

- Graduation from an accredited high school or acceptable equivalent.
- Graduation from a medical assistant program or institution accredited by the ABHES, from a medical assistant program accredited by a regional accrediting commission, or from a formal medical services training program of the U.S. Armed Forces. Alternatively, the applicant can have been employed in the profession of medical assisting for a minimum of 5 years, not more than 2 of which may have been as an instructor in a postsecondary medical assistant program.
- Passing the AMT examination for RMA (AMT) certification. RMAs (AMT) must accumulate 30 contact hours for continuing education units (CEU) every three years if they were certified after 2006. RMAs (AMT) who were

certified before this date are expected to keep abreast of all the changes and practices in their field through educational programs, workshops, or seminars. However, there are no specific continuing education requirements. Once a medical assistant has passed the AMT exam, he has earned the right to add RMA (AMT) to his name: James Wood, RMA (AMT).

Major Areas of the RMA (AMT)/ CMA (AAMA) Examinations

The RMA (AMT) and CMA (AAMA) qualifying examinations are rigorous. Participation in an accredited program, however, will help you learn what you need to know. The examinations cover several distinct areas of knowledge. These include:

- General medical knowledge, including terminology, anatomy, physiology, behavioral science, medical law, and ethics
- Administrative knowledge, including medical records management, collections, insurance processing, and the **Health Insurance Portability and Accountability Act (HIPAA)**
- Clinical knowledge, including examination room techniques, medication preparation and administration, pharmacology, and specimen collection

Membership in a Medical Assisting Association

Professional associations set high standards for quality and performance in a profession. They define the tasks and functions of an occupation. In addition, they provide members with the opportunity to communicate and network with one another. They also present their goals to the profession and to the general public. Becoming a member of a professional association helps you achieve career goals and further the profession of medical assisting.

Professional Support for CMAs (AAMA)

When you become a member of the AAMA, you will have a large support group of active medical assistants. Membership benefits include:

- Professional publications, such as *CMA Today*
- A large variety of educational opportunities, such as chapter-sponsored seminars and workshops about the latest administrative, clinical, and management topics (Figure 1-2)
- Group insurance
- Legal information

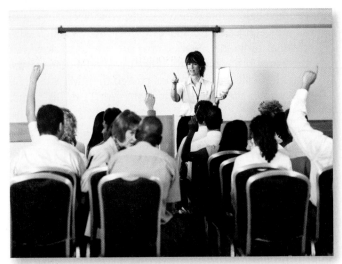

Figure 1-2. In this picture, a representative is giving information concerning certification to students and instructors at a local chapter meeting of AAMA.

- Local, state, and national activities that include professional networking and multiple continuing education opportunities
- Legislative monitoring. The AAMA continually works to protect your right to practice as a medical assistant.
- Access the website at www.aama-ntl.org

Networking

Networking is building alliances, socially and professionally. It starts long before your job search. By attending professional association meetings, conferences, or other functions, medical assistants generate opportunities for employment and personal and professional growth.

Professional Support for RMAs (AMT)

The AMT offers many benefits for RMAs (AMT). These include:

- Professional publications
- Membership in the AMT Institute for Education
- Group insurance programs—liability, health, and life
- State chapter activities
- Legal representation in health legislative matters
- Annual meetings and educational seminars
- Student membership
- Access the website at www.amt1.com

Training Programs and Other Learning Opportunities

Formal programs in medical assisting are offered in a variety of educational settings. They include vocational-technical high schools, postsecondary vocational schools, community and junior colleges, and 4-year colleges and universities. Vocational school programs usually last 9 months to 1 year and award a certificate or diploma. Community and junior college programs are usually 2-year associate degree programs.

Accreditation

Accreditation is the process by which programs are officially authorized. There are two national entities recognized by the U.S. Department of Education that accredit medical assisting educational programs:

1. The Commission on Accreditation of Allied Health Education Programs (CAAHEP). CAAHEP works directly with the Medical Assisting Educational Review Board (MAERB) of Medical Assistants Endowments to ensure that all accredited schools provide a competency-based education. CAAHEP accredits medical assisting programs in both public and private postsecondary institutions throughout the United States that prepare individuals for entry into the medical assisting profession.
2. Accrediting Bureau of Health Education Schools (ABHES). ABHES accredits private postsecondary institutions and programs that prepare individuals for entry into the medical assisting profession.

Accredited programs must cover the following topics: anatomy and physiology; medical terminology; medical law and ethics; psychology; oral and written communications; laboratory procedures; and clinical and administrative procedures. High school students may prepare for these courses by studying mathematics, health, biology, keyboarding, office skills, bookkeeping, and information technology. You may obtain current information about accreditation standards for medical assisting programs from the AAMA.

Medical assisting programs must also include an externship. An **externship** (or practicum) is practical work experience for a specified timeframe in an ambulatory care setting, such as physicians' offices, hospitals, or other health-care facilities.

Additionally, the AAMA lists its minimum standards for accredited programs. This list of standards ensures that all personnel—administrators and faculty—are qualified to perform their jobs.

The AAMA requires that administrative personnel exhibit leadership and management skills. They must also be able to fully perform the functions identified in documented job descriptions. Faculty members must develop and evaluate lesson plans, assess student progress toward the program's objectives, and be knowledgeable regarding course content. They must be qualified through work experience and be able to effectively direct and evaluate student learning and laboratory experiences.

The AAMA also has accreditation requirements for financial and physical resources. Each program's financial resources must meet its obligations to students. Schools must also have adequate physical resources—classrooms, laboratories, clinical and administrative facilities, and equipment and supplies.

The Benefits of Certification/Registration

Certification or registration is not required to practice as a medical assistant. You may practice with a high school diploma or equivalent although opportunities for this type of on-the-job training are becoming less common. Your career options will be greater, however, if you graduate from an accredited school and you become certified or registered.

Graduation from an accredited program helps your career in three ways. First, it shows that you have completed a program that meets nationally accepted standards. Second, it provides recognition of your education by professional peers. Third, it makes you eligible for registration or certification. Students who graduate from an accredited medical assisting program, such as ABHES or CAAHEP, are eligible to take the CMA (AAMA) or RMA (AMT) immediately.

Externships

In an externship you will obtain work experience while completing a medical assisting program. You will practice skills learned in the classroom in an actual medical office environment. Because of this professional experience, you also earn the right to include your externship on your resume under job experience, as long as you title it as "Medical Assistant Externship."

Externship Requirements. Externships are mandatory in accredited schools. The length of your externship will vary, depending on your particular program. Familiarize yourself with the program requirements as soon as possible because as a mandatory part of the program, no matter how good your grades are in class, if the externship is not completed you will not graduate from the program. You may be able to obtain an externship site of your choice either at a practice already affiliated with the school or at a practice you find on your own.

The externship is offered in cooperative medical offices or hospitals for a predetermined period (several weeks to several months). Another experienced medical assistant, nurse manager, or licensed nurse practitioner in the externship office often becomes your mentor. This mentor advises and supervises you during the externship.

Externship Duties. Your duties will be planned to meet your program's requirements for real-world work experience. Approach the externship with a positive attitude. Accept any guidance, constructive criticism, or praise as a learning experience. Figure 1-3 is an example of an externship agreement between a medical assisting school and an externship site. Note that agreements may vary.

Other Professional Memberships and Certification

The National Healthcare Association (NHA) was established in 1989 as an information resource and network for today's active health-care professionals. They offer a variety of certification exams and continuing education. Some of the programs and services of the NHA include:

- Certification development and implementation
- Continuing education curriculum development and implementation
- Program development for unions, hospitals, and schools
- Educational, career advancement, and networking services for members
- Registry of certified professionals

Some of the certification examinations offered by the National Healthcare Association include:

- Phlebotomy Technician (CPT)
- EKG/ECG Technician (CET)
- Billing & Coding Specialist
- Medical Transcriptionist (CMT)
- Medical Administrative Assistant (CCMA)
- Medical Laboratory Assistant

The National Healthcare Association certification exams are developed by health-care educators working in their various fields of study. The NHA is a member of The National Organization of Competency Assurance (NOCA).

The National Center for Competency Testing (NCCT) is another independent agency that certifies the validity of competency and knowledge of the medical profession through examination.

Medical assistants and medical office assistants receive the designation of National Certified Medical Assistant (NCMA) and National Certified Medical Office Assistant (NCMOA) after passing the certification examination.

Volunteer Programs

Volunteering is a rewarding experience. Before you even begin a medical assisting program, you can gain experience in a health-care profession through volunteer work. As a volunteer, you will get hands-on training and learn what it is like to assist patients who are ill, disabled, or frightened.

You may volunteer as an aide in a hospital, clinic, nursing home, or doctor's office, or as a typist or filing clerk in a medical office or medical record room. Some visiting nurse associations and hospices (homelike medical settings that provide medical care and emotional support to terminally ill patients and their families) also offer volunteer opportunities. These experiences may help you decide if you want to pursue a career as a medical assistant.

The American Red Cross also offers volunteer opportunities for the student medical assistant. The Red Cross needs volunteers for its disaster relief programs locally, statewide, nationally, and abroad.

Externship Affiliation Agreement

Name of School: _____

Address of School: _____

AGREEMENT OF AFFILIATION WITH

Name of Facility: _____

Address of Facility: _____

The (*name of school*) has been approved to conduct a (name of program) training program which requires clinical experience in a medical facility. The (*name of facility*) has agreed to provide this supervised clinical experience. Therefore the externship facility, now referred to as the affiliating institution, and the school, enter into the following agreement:

The school will arrange for students to affiliate at (name of affiliating institution) for a period of *160* hours. The specific hours/days will be agreed upon by a designee of each party and each will keep a copy of the schedule. Taking attendance sheets will be given to students and must be faxed every Monday during externship rotations.

(For medical assisting externships only): Before the student begins the supervised clinical experience, he or she will show evidence of physical requirements deemed necessary by agreement of both parties. The school is responsible for insuring that the student has had a physical exam within six months, and all recommended inoculations, before the start of the internship.

(*School/Affiliating Institution*) is responsible for student injury acquired at the affiliation site. Students and instructors will also carry liability insurance and a signed statement indicating that they have a policy covering liability against third parties resulting from this internship.

Students will be under the supervision of the clinical instructor(s) employed by the school, but may also be supervised by the professional staff of the affiliating institution. The school is responsible for providing all theory/practice instruction. Students will have received the necessary classroom and clinical instruction from the school before being authorized to perform patient care. The clinical instructor(s) will make assignments and, with the help of the professional staff of the institution, will evaluate each student's performance using the evaluation instruments provided by the school.

The clinical instructor will be present at all times students are present. The school's program coordinator will make (*frequency*) visits at the externship site.

The school is responsible for the conduct/dress requirements of the students at the affiliation site. A student who does not satisfactorily meet the requirements of this externship may be terminated. Prior to termination, the student will be notified of these deficiencies and will be given (*x*) days to correct these deficiencies.

The agreement will begin on (___/___/___) and will be reviewed annually by both parties before the agreement is renewed. A (Length of time) notice will be given by either party if the agreement will not be renewed. Both parties agree to contact the (name of accrediting agency) immediately upon requesting termination of the contract.

The affiliating institution and the school will not discriminate in regard to student externs, according to state and federal laws.

Affiliating Institute Representative, Name/Title _____

Date: ____/____/_____

School Representative, Name/Title _____

Date: ____/____/_____

Figure 1-3. Externship Affiliation Agreement

As part of a disaster relief team at the site of a hurricane, tornado, storm, flood, earthquake, or fire, volunteers learn first-aid and emergency triage skills. Red Cross volunteers gain valuable work experience that may help them obtain a job.

Because volunteers are not paid, it is usually easy to find work opportunities. Just because you are not paid for volunteer work, however, does not mean the experience is not useful for meeting your career goals.

Include information about any volunteer work on your **résumé**—a computer-generated document that summarizes your employment and educational history. Be sure to note specific duties, responsibilities, and skills developed during the volunteer experience. Refer to the "Externship" chapter (Chapter 54) for examples of résumés.

Multiskill Training

Today many hospitals and health-care practices are embracing the idea of a multiskilled health-care professional (MSHP). An MSHP is a cross-trained team member who is able to handle many different duties.

The AAMA includes the word *multiskilled* in its definition of the profession of medical assisting:

Medical assisting is a multiskilled allied health profession whose practitioners work primarily in ambulatory settings, such as medical offices and clinics. Medical assistants function as members of the healthcare delivery team and perform administrative and clinical procedures.

An MSHP may be trained to perform certain clinical procedures. She or he is not, however, trained to make judgments or interpretations concerning a patient's diagnosis or treatment, as a physician would.

Reducing Health-Care Costs. As a result of health-care reform and downsizing (a reduction in the number of staff members) to control the rising cost of health care, medical practices are eager to reduce personnel costs by hiring multiskilled health professionals. These individuals, who perform the functions of two or more people, are the most cost-efficient employees.

Expanding Your Career Opportunities. Career opportunities are vast if you are self-motivated and willing to learn new skills. If you continue to learn about new administrative and clinical techniques and procedures, you will be an important part of the health-care team.

As you read this book, look for a boxed feature titled Career Opportunities. This feature highlights additional skills medical assistants can learn and integrate into their jobs to make themselves more marketable as multiskilled health professionals. Following are several examples of positions for medical assistants with various experience and certifications:

- Office manager
- Certified Office Laboratory Technician (COLT certification)
- ECG technician
- Medical transcriptionist
- Medical biller
- Hospital admissions coordinator
- A professional who performs physical exams for applicants to insurance companies
- An administrative assistant at insurance companies
- Medical Assisting Instructor (with a specified amount of experience and education)

If you are multiskilled, you will have an advantage when job hunting. Employers are eager to hire multiskilled medical assistants and may create positions for them.

You can gain multiskill training by showing initiative and a willingness to learn every aspect of the medical facility in which you are working. When you begin working within a medical facility, establish goals regarding your career path and discuss them with your immediate supervisor. Indicate to your supervisor that you would like to become **cross-trained** in every aspect of the medical facility. Begin your mastery of the department that you are currently working in and branch out to other departments once you master the skills needed for your current position. This will demonstrate a commitment to your profession as well as a strong work ethic. Cross-training is a valuable marketing tool to include on your résumé.

Daily Duties of Medical Assistants

As a medical assistant, you will be the physician's "right arm." Duties include maintaining an efficient office, preparing and maintaining medical records, assisting the physician during examinations, and keeping examining rooms in order. You may also handle the payroll for the office staff (or supervise a payroll service), obtain equipment and supplies, and serve as the link between the physician and representatives of pharmaceutical and medical supply companies. In small practices you will usually handle all duties. In larger practices you may specialize in a particular duty. As a medical assistant grows in his or her profession, advanced duties may be required, such as Office Practice Management, which may include marketing, and financial and strategic planning.

Entry-Level General Duties

Your general duties may vary according to state law. In an entry-level position, they may include:

- Recognize and respond effectively to verbal, nonverbal, and written communications
- Explaining treatment procedures to patients
- Patient education within scope of practice
- Facilitating treatment for patients from diverse cultural backgrounds and for patients with hearing or vision impairments, or physical or mental disabilities
- Acting as a patient advocate
- Maintain medical records

Certified Office Laboratory Technician

To gain medical assistant credentials, you must fulfill the requirements of either the American Association of Medical Assistants (obtaining CMA certification) or the American Medical Technologists (obtaining RMA certification). After acquiring your CMA or RMA certification, you may wish to acquire additional skills in specialty areas through course work or on-the-job training. The Certified Office Laboratory Technician certification is awarded by the American Medical Technologists to qualified applicants.

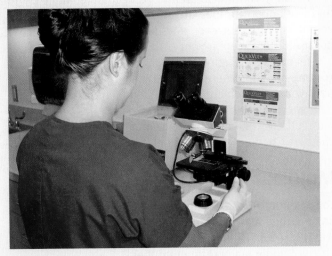

Nature of the Job

The Certified Office Laboratory Technician is a multi-skilled practitioner qualified by education and experience to perform medical laboratory testing, including CLIA-waived and moderately complex testing. This health-care professional is also trained to perform front and back office tasks, as well as a variety of tasks involving direct patient contact. The position's scope of practice covers many areas and it is necessary to have knowledge of all federal and state regulations applicable to the job.

Duties and Skills

- Assists others in performing routine administrative and clinical tasks
- Answers telephones
- Processes laboratory specimens
- Assists in the collection and testing of medical specimens
- Depending on state law, performs chemical, biological, hematological, immunologic, microscopic, and bacteriological tests
- Assists with the processing, reading, and reporting of specimens to determine the presence of bacteria, fungi, parasites, or other microorganisms

Educational Requirements

Applicant must have a high school diploma or the equivalent with acceptable training. Often, Certified Office Laboratory Technicians are medical assistants who have passed the certification examination and have advanced training.

Workplace Settings

Most Certified Office Laboratory Technicians work in a physician's office or clinic. She or he may work a flexible schedule that includes evenings and weekends.

For more information, visit the websites of the following organizations, which are available on the Online Learning Center at www.mhhe.com/medicalassisting4e.

American Medical Technologists

National Healthcare Association

Entry-Level Administrative Duties

In an entry-level position, your administrative duties may include the following:

- Greeting patients
- Handling correspondence
- Scheduling appointments
- Answering telephones
- Creating and maintaining patient medical records
- Handling billing, bookkeeping, and insurance processing
- Performing medical transcription
- Arranging for hospital admissions

Advanced Administrative Duties

Your advanced administrative duties may vary according to the practice and may include:

- Developing and conducting public outreach programs to market the physician's professional services
- Negotiating leases of equipment and supply contracts
- Negotiating nonrisk and risk managed care contracts
- Managing business and professional insurance
- Developing and maintaining fee schedules
- Participating in practice analysis
- Coordinating plans for practice enhancement, expansion, consolidation, and closure

- Performing as a HIPAA compliance officer
- Providing personnel supervision and employment practices
- Providing information systems management

Entry-Level Clinical Duties

Your clinical duties may vary according to state law. In an entry-level position, they may include:

- Assisting the doctor during examinations
- Asepsis and infection control
- Performing diagnostic tests, such as spirometry and ECGs
- Giving injections, where allowed
- Phlebotomy including venipuncture and capillary puncture
- Disposing of **contaminated** (soiled, or stained) supplies
- Performing first aid and cardiopulmonary resuscitation (CPR)
- Preparing patients for examinations
- Preparing and administering medications as directed by the physician, and following state laws for invasive procedures
- Recording vital signs and medical histories
- Removing sutures or changing dressings on wounds
- Sterilizing medical instruments

Other clinical duties may include instructing patients about medication and special diets, authorizing drug refills as directed by the physician, and calling pharmacies to order prescriptions. You may also assist with minor surgery or teach patients about special procedures before laboratory tests, surgery, x-rays, or ECGs.

Advanced Clinical Duties

As with entry-level clinical duties, your advanced clinical duties may vary according to state law. They may include:

- Initiating an IV and administering IV medications with appropriate training and as permitted by state law
- Reporting diagnostic study results
- Assisting patients in the completion of advanced directives and living wills
- Assisting with clinical trials

Entry-Level Laboratory Duties

As an entry-level medical assistant, your laboratory duties may include:

- Performing Clinical Laboratory Improvement Amendments (CLIA)–waived tests, such as a urine pregnancy test, on the premises

- Collecting, preparing, and transmitting laboratory specimens
- Teaching patients to collect specific specimens properly
- Arranging laboratory services
- Meeting safety standards (OSHA guidelines) and fire protection mandates

Advanced Laboratory Duties

As with entry-level laboratory duties, your advanced laboratory duties may vary according to state law. They may include:

- Performing as an OSHA compliance officer
- Performing moderately complex laboratory testing with appropriate training and certification

Specialization

You may also choose to specialize in a specific area of health care. For example, podiatric medical assistants make castings of feet, expose and develop x-rays, and assist podiatrists in surgery. Ophthalmic medical assistants help ophthalmologists (doctors who provide eye care) by administering diagnostic tests, measuring and recording vision, testing the functioning of eyes and eye muscles, and performing other duties. (Chapter 2 fully discusses medical specialties and medical assistant specialties.)

Personal Qualifications of Medical Assistants

There are several personal qualifications that you must have to be an effective and productive medical assistant. You must enjoy working with all types of people, possess good critical thinking skills, and be able to pay attention to detail. Empathy, willingness to learn, flexibility, self-motivation, professionalism, integrity, and sound judgment are other important traits. Additionally, you must have a neat, professional appearance; possess good communication skills; be able to work in a team environment; and know how to remain calm in a crisis.

Critical Thinking Skills

You will develop critical thinking skills over time, as you apply knowledge about and experience with human nature, medicine, and office administration to new situations. Critical thinking skills include quickly evaluating circumstances, solving problems, and taking action.

Critical thinking skills are used every day. One example is prioritizing your work—deciding which are the most important tasks of the day and which are less important. On a day where everything seems to be "top priority," you must use your professional judgment, knowledge of office policies, and experience with physicians and

Recycling in the Medical Office, Hospital, Laboratory, or Clinic

You may easily incorporate recycling procedures into the daily routine of a medical office, hospital, laboratory, or clinic. Medical facilities generate a tremendous amount of recyclable paper material. Recycling may be required by state law. Purchase paper products that can be recycled, or those made of postconsumer recycled materials, and take care in disposing of them. Care should be taken to ensure HIPAA compliance when recycling paper. Shredding is the most effective way to comply with HIPAA regulations.

Some states levy large fines for noncompliance with recycling regulations. It is thus important to have a well-organized office recycling program. There are two essential aspects of recycling: disposal and purchasing. To create a complete recycling program, ensure that materials are disposed of properly and that purchased products have been made from recycled materials.

You may easily call the town's recycling center for guidelines for packaging recycled materials and for a pickup schedule. The recycling center may also provide containers for recyclable materials. You must fulfill all town and state legal recycling requirements.

Most paper products that do not have a glossy coating (like some fax paper) are recyclable. Each recycling center will provide a list of paper materials that can and cannot be recycled.

You must also research disposal techniques for biohazardous materials and follow regulations listed in the office policy manual and OSHA guidelines. These materials cannot be recycled and must be disposed of properly. They must not be mixed with recyclable waste. You will follow the office policy manual and OSHA guidelines for hazardous medical wastes—including blood products, gloves, cotton swabs, body fluids, and sharps (needles or instruments that puncture the skin). These materials must be disposed of following standard guidelines and in a specially designed protective container.

You must keep recycling issues in mind at all times. Always choose products made from recycled materials—including paper (computer paper and letterhead), printer cartridges, pencils, and many other products.

---

coworkers to determine what should get done first, second, third, and so on.

You must use critical thinking skills to assess how to react to emergency situations. If you see a patient suddenly pass out in the physician's waiting room, you must quickly see that the patient receives first aid, notify a physician, and alert the patient's family.

Time Management

Personal and professional time management skills are essential skills for medical assistants. Time management is controlling how you spend your time. People who use time management techniques routinely are the highest achievers in all walks of life, professionally and personally. Using these skills will assist you in functioning exceptionally well in the medical office, even under intense pressure. What's even more important is that you can say goodbye to the often-intense stress of work overload. Concentrating on results, instead of being busy, is the main focus of time management.

Attention to Detail

The profession of medical assisting requires attention to detail. You must check every detail when administering drugs, processing bills and insurance forms, and completing patient charts.

The need for attention to detail is illustrated in the common request to call a patient's pharmacy to order a

prescription. You must accurately relay information from the doctor's prescription to the pharmacist. You must ask the pharmacist to read back the information to ensure that he has heard it correctly. Then you must document, in the chart, what has been ordered and when.

Empathy

Empathy is the ability to "put yourself in someone else's shoes" and to identify with and understand another person's feelings. Patients who are ill, frustrated, or frightened appreciate empathic medical personnel.

Patients require empathy during all medical situations. For example, a patient with the flu may describe how coughing has prevented him from getting a full night's sleep. You may display empathy by saying, "I know how the flu can disrupt sleep but it's important to rest in bed, though, even if you can't always sleep."

Willingness to Learn

You must always display a willingness to learn. You will gain new skills more easily and become better acquainted with the administrative and clinical topics and issues related to the practice in which you work if you are willing to learn. Keep an open mind, listen carefully to the professionals with whom you work, observe procedures carefully, listen actively to others, and do your own homework to learn more about medical topics so you can apply new

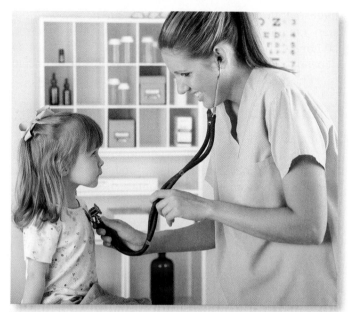

Figure 1-4. A medical assistant who works part-time in a pediatric practice might volunteer one day a week at a preschool to learn more about working with children.

information to your daily activities. For example, if you work in a pediatric practice, you might take a continuing education class on child development at a local community college, at a YWCA, or in a workshop offered by a professional association such as the AAMA or AMT (Figure 1-4).

Flexibility

You will encounter new people and situations every day. An attitude of flexibility will allow you to adapt and to handle them with professionalism.

An example of the need for flexibility occurs when a physician's schedule changes to include evening and weekend hours. The staff may also be asked to change schedules. You must make it a priority to be flexible and to meet the employer's needs.

Self-Motivation

You must be self-motivated and willing to offer assistance with work that needs to be done, even if it is not your assigned job. For example, if you think of a more efficient way to organize patient check-in, discuss it with your supervisor. She/he may agree and be willing to give your idea a try. If a coworker is on vacation, offer to pitch in and work extra time so that patients all receive quality care and to keep the office running smoothly.

Professionalism

You should exhibit courtesy, conscientiousness, and a generally businesslike manner at all times on the job. It is important to act professionally with coworkers, patients, doctors, and others in the work setting. You are an agent of your employer—you represent the doctor or doctors in the practice.

One example of professional behavior includes treating all patients with dignity and kindness. Another is making sure that you have completed and documented all your daily duties before leaving work at the end of each day.

You can start acting like a professional even while you are in the classroom studying to become a medical assistant. Presenting a neat appearance, showing courtesy and respect for peers and instructors, having a good attendance record, and arriving on time to class are all important elements that contribute to professionalism in school and in the workplace.

Neat Appearance

A medical professional always strives to maintain a neat appearance in the workplace. Personal cleanliness is an important part of maintaining a neat appearance. Your appearance is your first impression to your patients, coworkers, and the physicians you work with. Medical facilities and staff are considered "conservative" work environments. Your appearance should reflect a conservative style. Listed here are a few professional guidelines to follow in the medical environment:

- Your uniforms should be clean, pressed crisply, and in good repair. Your uniform should fit your body type and should not be too large or too small.

- Your shoes should be comfortable, white, clean, and in good condition. Laces should be white and clean. Avoid athletic-looking shoes. Polish your shoes on a daily basis. Only leather shoes that are not open are permitted in a patient treatment area.

- Choose a hairstyle that is flattering and conservative.

- Hair should be clean and pulled back from your face and off your collar if long. Natural colors for hair are the only acceptable color in a medical environment.

- Your nails should be a short working length, no more than one-fourth inch. Nail polish should be pale or clear. A French manicure is acceptable. Acrylic nails should be avoided. Many medical facilities are banning acrylic nails because they pose a risk for infection.

- Avoid heavy perfumes, lotions, shampoos, hairsprays, and colognes. Frequently patients and coworkers are allergic to perfumes and cologne.

- Jewelry should be kept to a minimum and in good taste. No more than one ring should be worn. Rings may tear through latex gloves. Ears can be pierced with one hole, and small earrings are appropriate. Any earrings that dangle can be torn off by a patient, such as pediatric patients. Males should not wear earrings in the medical environment.

- Tattoos should never be in a location where they can be seen by a patient.

- Body piercing and tongue piercing are not acceptable in a medical environment. Patients may view this as a visual threat and question your level of competence. Many physicians will rule you out on the first interview if a body piercing (other than ears) is present.

- Bathe or shower daily and use an antiperspirant.
- Brush your teeth at least twice daily and schedule regular dental visits to maintain oral health and hygiene.
- Schedule regular checkups with your personal physician.
- Get plenty of rest and eat a well-balanced diet.
- If you are not required to wear a uniform, choose clothing that is conservative and business-appropriate. Avoid fad fashions. Wear low-heeled or flat, polished shoes and a lab coat if working in a clinical area with patients.

Some activities may make it difficult to maintain a neat appearance—replacing the toner in the copy machine, for example, or filling the developing solution in the x-ray machine. Always store a spare uniform or business outfit at your workplace.

Attitude

Your attitude will leave an impression of the type of person you are. In the medical environment, many people depend on you, including coworkers and patients. Your attitude can make or break your career. Professionals always project a positive, caring attitude. They respond to criticism as a learning experience. They take direction from authority without question. They function as a vital member of a medical team. A negative attitude will not be acceptable in a team-oriented medical environment. Many people do not know they have a negative attitude. Ask yourself these questions, and determine if you need to make improvements in your attitude before you begin your new career.

- Do I have repeated conflict with friends or family?
- Have I had a conflict at work that has resulted in voluntary or involuntary termination?
- Do I have conflict with authority figures, such as my instructors?
- Do people make comments about my attitude?

In the workplace environment, professional medical assistants are pleasant, smiling, and conducting themselves in a businesslike and professional manner.

Integrity and Honesty

People with integrity hold themselves to high standards. Everything they do, every task they complete, is performed with a goal of excellence. Individuals with integrity take extreme pride in everything they do. The characteristics of integrity are honesty, dependability, and reliability. Integrity and honesty are key in providing superior customer service to your patients. You must follow through on everything you say you are going to do. For example, if you tell a patient that you are going to return their call regarding a medication, you must call the patient at the time you

indicated. Professionals with integrity are honest with the staff and physicians they work with. If you make an error, be honest about it. In order to have integrity, you must be dependable and reliable. Your office staff and physician must be able to trust you and the decisions you make.

Diplomacy

Diplomacy is the ability to communicate with patients, coworkers, managers, and physicians in a manner that is not offensive and that both expresses and inspires cooperation. Communicating with diplomacy is communicating with tact. Medical assistants are often exposed to situations that they may not agree with. A professional has the ability to look at both sides of a situation and to handle it with courtesy and professionalism.

Proper Judgment

You should demonstrate proper judgment in every task. Before making an important decision, you must carefully evaluate each possible outcome.

An example of a situation that requires proper judgment is assessing when an exception should be made in a doctor's schedule of patients. Suppose the next patient on the schedule is in the waiting room. She is having a routine checkup. An unscheduled patient comes in with chest pains. You use proper judgment and allow the patient with chest pains to see the doctor first.

Communication Skills

Effective communication involves careful listening, observing, speaking, and writing. Communication even involves good manners—being polite, tactful, and respectful. You must use good communication skills during every patient discussion and in every interaction you have with physicians, other staff members, and other professionals with whom your practice does business. The chapter "Communication with Patients, Families, and Coworkers" (Chapter 4) discusses communication skills in more detail.

Remaining Calm in a Crisis

There is always the potential for a crisis or emergency in the health-care field. During a crisis you must remain calm and be prepared to handle any situation.

An example of the need for calm and effective action occurs when a patient appears to suffer a stroke while sitting in the waiting room of a busy medical office. You must quickly direct your peers to alert the doctor and remove the other patients from the room while you begin emergency first-aid measures.

Willingness to Work as a Team Member

Working with and as a member of the health-care team is critical for the overall efficiency of the medical facility.

Everyone in the facility has an important job that depends on someone else. It is important to remember that the patient comes first and everyone is responsible for the care of that patient. Team dynamics consist of:

- Assisting each other on a daily basis with the duties required
- Avoiding interpersonal conflict with members of the team
- Performing extra responsibilities without questioning or complaining
- Being considerate of all other team members' duties and responsibilities

Ethical Behavior

Ethics is a system of values that determines right or wrong behavior. Our standard of values is learned by our life experiences. Ethical behavior can have a strong, positive impact on the profession of medical assisting and on the overall reputation of medical assistants in the health-care community. Your professional ethics will involve your relationship with patients and families, your relationship with other allied health professionals, and facilities and your community as a whole. The AAMA Code of Ethics is designed to elevate the profession of medical assisting to a profession of dignity and respect.

The AAMA Occupational Analysis

In 1996 the AAMA formed a committee whose goal was to revise and update its standards for the accreditation of programs that teach medical assisting. The committee's findings were published in 1997 as the "AAMA Role Delineation Study: Occupational Analysis of the Medical Assistant Profession." The study included a new Role Delineation Chart that outlined the areas of competence to be mastered as an entry-level medical assistant. The Role Delineation Chart of the CMA (AAMA) was further updated in 2003 to include additional competencies and in 2009 was updated again and was renamed the Occupational Analysis of the CMA (AAMA).

Areas of Competence

The Medical Assistant Occupational Analysis provides the basis for medical assisting education and evaluation. Mastery of the areas of competence listed in this Occupational Analysis is required for all students in accredited medical assisting programs. The Occupational Analysis shows three areas of competence: administrative, clinical, and general. Each of these three areas is divided into two or more narrower areas, for a total of ten specific areas of competence. Within each area, a bulleted list of statements describes the medical assistant's role.

Uses of the Occupational Analysis

According to the AAMA, Occupational Analysis may be used to:

- Describe the field of medical assisting to other health-care professionals
- Identify entry-level areas of competence for medical assistants
- Help practitioners assess their own current competence in the field
- Aid in the development of continuing education programs
- Prepare appropriate types of materials for home study

Scope of Practice

Medical assistants are not "licensed" health-care professionals and most often work under another licensed health-care provider, such as a nurse or physician. Licensed health-care professionals may delegate certain duties to a medical assistant, providing she or he has had the appropriate training through an accredited medical assisting program or through on-the-job training provided by the medical facility or physician. Questions often arise regarding the kinds of duties a medical assistant can perform, such as:

- What kinds of clinical duties can a medical assistant lawfully perform?
- Is a medical assistant permitted to start an IV?
- Can a medical assistant run lab tests? If so, which tests are allowed?

There is no universal answer to any of the above questions. There is no single national definition of a medical assistant's scope of practice. Therefore, the medical assistant must research the state in which he or she works to learn about the scope of practice in his or her state. In general, a medical assistant may not perform procedures for which he or she was not educated or trained. The AAMA and AMT are good resources to assist you in your research. The AAMA Occupational Analysis is also a good reference source that identifies the procedures that medical assistants are educated to perform.

Summary

1.1 The responsibility of a medical assistant varies from entry-level administrative duties to entry-level laboratory duties.

1.2 Professional training for medical assistants includes formal training in a variety of educational settings (i.e., postsecondary vocational schools, four-year colleges).

1.3 Some of the personal characteristics of medical assistants are flexibility, attentiveness to detail, and excellent communication skills.

1.4 Cross-training becomes more crucial as organizations downsize. Medical assistants are much more marketable if they are multiskilled.

1.5 Continuing education keeps you abreast of changing technology, procedures, and state, local, and federal regulations.

1.6 Certification and registration provide recognition of your education by peers and for advancement in your career.

1.7 Professional membership affiliation provides networking opportunities and access to potential employers.

REVIEW

CHAPTER 1

CASE STUDY QUESTIONS

Now that you have completed this chapter, review the case study at the beginning of the chapter and answer the following questions:

1. How are the three jobs different?
2. How are the three jobs the same?
3. How do these three medical assistants function as multiskilled health-care professionals?

Multiple-Choice Questions

1. Two accrediting bodies for medical assisting programs are
   a. ABHES and OSHA.
   b. OSHA and AAMA.
   c. ABHES and CAAHEP.
   d. CAAHEP and CLIA.
2. Entry-level clinical duties for a medical assistant include
   a. patient education, drawing blood, and negotiating leases.
   b. taking vital signs and prescribing medicine.
   c. assisting the doctor during exams, performing diagnostic tests, and sterilizing medical instruments.
   d. performing ECGs, infection control, and billing and coding.
3. The personal qualifications of a medical assistant are
   a. great clinical and administrative skills.
   b. attentiveness to detail, professionalism, diplomacy, and empathy.
   c. the ability to expand your career opportunities.
   d. graduating from an accredited school.
4. The main purpose of the American Association of Medical Assistants (AAMA) is to
   a. raise the standards of professionalism.
   b. assist with malpractice lawsuits.

c. provide externships.
d. use their resources to support CMAs' (AAMA) and RMAs' (AMT) continuing education.

5. The increase in job opportunities for medical assistants is due to
   a. population increase, wage increases, and increases in births.
   b. the growth of outpatient clinics and HMOs.
   c. patient education and professional membership.
   d. the ability to handle patients' privacy.

Discussion Questions

1. Why are more employers recruiting credentialed medical assistants?
2. Explain the importance of continuing education for medical assistants.
3. What is the purpose of the AAMA Occupational Analysis?
4. Discuss why volunteer work will enhance a medical assistant's career.

Critical Thinking Questions

1. Describe an effective medical assistant, and explain two ways a new medical assistant may learn to be an efficient and effective employee.
2. How will the "aging boom" affect health care and the profession of medical assisting in the future?
3. What is a self-directed, lifelong learner? How can a medical assistant achieve this goal?
4. Why is it important to stay current on changes in technology and health care?

1. With a partner, pick one of the following two situations. Without showing your partner, write a description of how you would display the personal attribute stated at the end of the scenario. After you and your partner have written your descriptions, compare them with each other.

   Patient Situation

   Patient says: "I have such a horrible headache. I've been feeling tired lately too."

   Attribute You Wish to Display

   Empathy

   Patient Situation

   Doctor: "I'm really backed up on paperwork. Could you come in an hour early tomorrow morning to help me organize it? You will be paid for the overtime."

   Attribute You Wish to Display

   Flexibility

2. Chose a mentor who displays the personal attributes listed in this chapter and write a few sentences to explain why these attributes apply to her or him.

3. A. Think of all the personal qualifications you possess. List those that will help you as a medical assistant.

   B. List all of the personal qualifications you need to develop or improve in order to work successfully in the career of medical assisting.

   C. Describe the actions you will take to acquire the personal qualifications to become a multiskilled medical assistant.

Virtual Fieldtrip

Visit the McGraw-Hill Higher Education Medical Assisting website at www.mhhe.com/medicalassisting4e to complete the following activity:

Prepare an oral presentation regarding topics such as certification examinations, scope of practice, or accreditation agencies such as ABHES or CAAHEP. Prepare a report using a specified number of references and citations and present your report to the class. Schedule the presentations throughout the course and use available multimedia such as PowerPoint slides or an overhead projector for the student presentations. Visit the websites of The American Association of Medical Assistants or American Medical Technologists for possible report topics.

Open the CD and complete this chapter's practice activities, play the games, listen to the key terms, and test yourself with the interactive review. E-mail, print, and/or save your results to document your proficiency.

CHAPTER 2

Types of Medical Practice

LEARNING OUTCOMES

After completing Chapter 2, you will be able to:

2.1 Describe medical specialties and specialists.

2.2 Explain the purpose of the American Board of Medical Specialties.

2.3 Explain the duties of several types of allied health professionals with whom medical assistants may work.

2.4 Differentiate the professional associations that may help advance a medical assistant's career.

MEDICAL ASSISTING COMPETENCIES

CAAHEP	ABHES

IX. C (7) Compare and contrast physician and medical assistant roles in terms of standard of care
IX. P (2) Perform within scope of practice
	1. General Orientation
	  b. Compare and contrast the allied health professions and understand their relation to medical assisting
	  d. Have knowledge of the general responsibilities of the medical assistant
	  e. Define scope of practice for the medical assistant, and comprehend the conditions for practice within the state that the medical assistant is employed
	
	11. Career Development
	Demonstrate professionalism by:
	  4) Being cognizant of ethical boundaries
	  9) Conducting work within scope of education, training, and ability

MEDICAL ASSISTING MEDIA

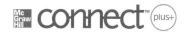 **Connect Plus+™**
connect.mcgraw-hill.com

- Electronic Health Records (E.H.R.) SpringCharts®
- eBook

SpringCharts®
Electronic Health Records

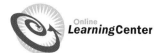 **LearnSmart™**
www.mhhe.com/learnsmart

Complete Learning Module: Types of Medical Practice

 Student CD-ROM

Online Learning Center™
www.mhhe.com/medicalassisting4e

KEY TERMS

acupuncturist	endocrinologist	oncologist	plastic surgeon
allergist	family practitioner	orthopedist	podiatrist
anesthetist	gastroenterologist	osteopathic manipulative	primary care physician
autopsy	gerontologist	medicine (OMM)	proctologist
biopsy	gynecologist	otorhinolaryngologist	radiologist
cardiologist	internist	pathologist	surgeon
chiropractor	massage therapist	pediatrician	triage
dermatologist	nephrologist	physiatrist	urologist
doctor of osteopathy	neurologist	physician assistant (PA)	

CHAPTER OUTLINE

- Medical Specialties
- Working with Other Allied Health Professionals
- Specialty Career Options
- Professional Associations

PREPARATION FOR CERTIFICATION

RMA (AMT) Exam
- Ethical conduct
- Licensure, certification, registration

CMAs Exam
- Participate in appropriate continuing education

CMA (AAMA) Exam
- Professionalism

Introduction

Medical assistants are an integral part of a health-care delivery team. It is important to recognize the many different physician specialists and allied health professions. Medical assistants are often asked to call and process insurance referrals to different specialties and diagnostic departments. Therefore, a working knowledge of the different specialties and allied health professionals demonstrates professionalism and competence.

Susan has worked as a medical assistant for 12 years. She is considering furthering her educational background in a different allied health profession. She has a strong interest in nursing and in the laboratory.

As you read this chapter, consider the following questions:
1. What are Susan's career options in nursing? How much further education would she need in order to become a nurse?
2. What are Susan's career options in a laboratory setting? How much further education would she need in order to work in a laboratory?

 # Medical Specialties

Since the beginning of the 20th century, some physicians have specialized in particular areas of study. There are now approximately 24 major medical specialties approved in the United States. Within each specialty are several subspecialties. For example, cardiology is a major specialty; pediatric cardiology is a subspecialty. As advances in the diagnosis and treatment of diseases and disorders unfold, the demand for specialized care increases and more medical specialties emerge.

If you graduate from an accredited medical assisting program, you will be well equipped to work with a physician specialist. If you work in the office of a physician specialist, you must continue to learn all the new skills that apply to that specialty. First, however, it is helpful to understand the education and licensing process any medical doctor must undergo to become a board-certified physician.

Physician Education and Licensure

The educational requirements for physicians are rigorous and take several years to complete. To earn the title MD (doctor of medicine), thereby qualifying as a licensed physician, a student must complete a bachelor's degree with a concentration typically in the sciences. Then she must attend a medical school accredited by the Liaison Committee on Medical Education (LCME). Upon completing medical school, she is awarded the degree of MD, but this is not the end of her required medical training. She must also pass the U.S. Medical Licensing Examination (USMLE). This examination, commonly known as medical boards, has three parts. Part 1 is usually taken after the second year of medical school, part 2 during the fourth year of medical school, and part 3 during the first or second year of postgraduate medical training.

After medical school an MD begins a residency—a period of practical training in a hospital. The first year of residency is known as an internship. Once it is completed an MD can become certified by the National Board of Medical Examiners (NBME). After completing an internship and passing her medical boards, the MD becomes certified as an NBME Diplomate. If she wishes to specialize in a particular branch of medicine, she must complete an additional 2 to 6 years of residency. She also will apply to the American Board of Medical Specialties (ABMS) to take an examination in her specialty area. After passing the examination, she will be board-certified in her area of specialization. For example, a physician who specializes in pediatrics would receive certification from the American Board of Pediatrics.

The ABMS is an organization of many different medical specialty boards. Its primary purpose is to maintain and improve the quality of medical care and to certify doctors in various specialties. This organization helps the member boards develop professional and educational standards for physician specialists.

Family Practice

Family practitioners (sometimes called general practitioners) are MDs or DOs who are generalists and treat all types of illnesses and ages of patients. They do not specialize in a particular branch of medicine. Many patients seek medical care from a family practitioner and may never have visited a medical specialist. Family practitioners are called **primary care physicians** (PCPs) by insurance companies. The term refers to individual doctors who oversee patients' long-term health care. Some people, however, have internists or OB/GYNs as their primary care physician.

A family practitioner sends a patient to a specialist when the patient has a specific condition or disease that requires advanced care. For example, a family practitioner refers a patient with a lump in her breast to an **oncologist,** a specialist who treats tumors, or to a general surgeon. Either of these doctors may order a mammogram or perform a needle biopsy of the lump to determine if it is malignant.

If you work in a general practice, you will encounter patients with many different conditions and illnesses. As in any medical setting, you must become knowledgeable about preventing the transmission of viruses. This important topic is discussed in several parts of this book.

If you work for a general practitioner, you will often be responsible for arranging patient appointments with specialists. It is important, therefore, for you to know about the duties of each medical specialist. One or more of these specialties may interest you, and you may decide to seek a position as a medical assistant for a physician in that specialty.

Allergy

Allergists diagnose and treat physical reactions to substances, including mold, dust, fur, and pollen from plants or flowers. An individual with allergies is hypersensitive to substances such as drugs, chemicals, or elements in nature. An allergic reaction may be minor, such as a rash; serious, such as asthma; or life-threatening (capable of producing anaphylactic shock), such as swelling of the airways or nasal passages.

Anesthesiology

Anesthesiologists and **anesthetists** use medications that cause patients to lose sensation or feeling during surgery. These health-care practitioners administer anesthetics before, during, and sometimes even after surgery. They also educate patients regarding the anesthetic that will be used and its possible postoperative effects. An anesthesiologist is an MD. A certified registered nurse anesthetist (CRNA) is a registered nurse who has completed an additional program of study recognized by the American Association of Nurse Anesthetists.

Bariatrics

Bariatrics is the specialty of medicine that deals with the medical and surgical treatment of obesity. Specialists in surgical bariatrics are called bariatric surgeons. Bariatric surgery may be recommended for extremely obese patients who may suffer impaired health as a result of their weight. Prior to undergoing any type of bariatric surgery, candidates must first undergo counseling and other treatment options for weight management. Therapy before and after bariatric surgery is necessary due to the extreme life changes that the patients must maintain to be successful in their weight loss and health goals. There are several options available in bariatric surgery, such as gastric banding and gastric bypass.

Cardiology

Cardiologists diagnose and treat cardiovascular diseases (diseases of the heart and blood vessels). Cardiologists also read electrocardiograms (ECGs, which are sometimes referred to as EKGs) for hospital cardiology departments. They educate patients about the positive role healthy diet and regular exercise play in preventing and controlling heart disease.

Dermatology

Dermatologists diagnose and treat diseases of the skin, hair, and nails. Their patients have conditions ranging from warts and acne to skin cancer. Dermatologists treat boils, skin injuries, and infections. They remove growths—such as moles, cysts, and birthmarks—and they treat scars and perform hair transplants.

Doctor of Osteopathy

Doctors of osteopathy, who hold the title of DO, practice a "whole-person" approach to health care. DOs believe that patients are more than just a sum of their body parts, and they treat the patient as a whole person instead of concentrating on specific symptoms. Osteopathic physicians understand how all the body's systems are interconnected and how each one affects the other. They focus special attention on the musculoskeletal system, which reflects and influences the condition of all other body systems.

One key concept that DOs believe is that structure influences function. If a problem exists in one part of the body, it may affect the function in both that area and other areas. DOs focus on the body's ability to heal itself and they actively engage patients in the healing process. By using **osteopathic manipulative medicine (OMM)** techniques, DOs can help restore motion to these areas of the body, thus improving function and often restoring health.

Emergency Medicine

Physicians who specialize in emergency medicine work in hospital emergency rooms and outpatient emergency care centers. They diagnose and treat patients with conditions resulting from an unexpected medical crisis or accident. Common emergencies include trauma, such as gunshot wounds or serious injuries from car accidents; other injuries, such as severe cuts; and sudden illness, such as alcohol or food poisoning. Emergency medicine practitioners stabilize the patient so they can then be managed by their PCP or other specialist.

Endocrinology

Endocrinologists diagnose and treat disorders of the endocrine system. This system regulates many body functions by circulating hormones that are secreted by organs and glands throughout the body. An example of a disorder treated by an endocrinologist is hyperthyroidism, an abnormality of the thyroid gland causing excess production of thyroid hormone. Symptoms include weight loss, shakiness, and weakness.

Gastroenterology

Gastroenterologists diagnose and treat disorders of the gastrointestinal tract. These disorders include problems related to the functioning of the stomach, intestines, and associated organs.

Gerontology

Gerontologists study the aging process. Geriatrics is the branch of medicine that deals with the diagnosis and treatment of problems and diseases of the older adult. A specialist in geriatrics may also be called a geriatrician. As the population of older adults continues to increase, there will be greater need for physicians who specialize in diagnosing and treating diseases of the elderly.

Gynecology

Gynecology is the branch of medicine that is concerned with diseases of the female genital tract. **Gynecologists** perform routine physical care and examination of the female reproductive system. Many gynecologists are also obstetricians.

Internal Medicine

Internists specialize in diagnosing and treating problems related to the internal organs. The internal medicine subspecialties include cardiology, critical care medicine, diagnostic laboratory immunology, endocrinology and metabolism, gastroenterology, geriatrics, hematology, infectious diseases, medical oncology, nephrology, pulmonary disease, and rheumatology. Internists must be certified as specialists in these areas.

Nephrology

Nephrologists study, diagnose, and manage diseases of the kidney. They may work in either a clinic or hospital setting. A medical assistant working with a nephrologist may assist in the operation of a dialysis unit for the treatment of patients with kidney failure (ESRD). In a rural setting a medical assistant might help a doctor operate a mobile dialysis unit that can be taken to the patient's home or to a medical practice that does not have this technology.

Neurology

Neurology is the branch of medical science that deals with the nervous system. **Neurologists** diagnose and treat disorders and diseases of the nervous system, such as strokes. The nervous system is made up of the brain, spinal cord, and nerves that receive, interpret, and transmit messages throughout the body.

Nuclear Medicine

Nuclear medicine is a fast-growing specialty related to radiology. Both fields use radiation to diagnose and treat disease, but radiology beams radiation through the body from an outside source, whereas nuclear medicine introduces a small amount of a radioactive substance into the body and forms an image by detecting radiation as it leaves the body. The radiation that patients are exposed to is comparable to that of a diagnostic x-ray. Radiology reveals interior anatomy whereas nuclear medicine reveals organ function and structure. Noninvasive, painless nuclear medicine procedures are used to identify heart disease, assess organ function, and diagnose and treat cancer.

Obstetrics

Obstetrics involves the study of pregnancy, labor, delivery, and the period following labor called postpartum (Figure 2-1). This field is often combined with gynecology.

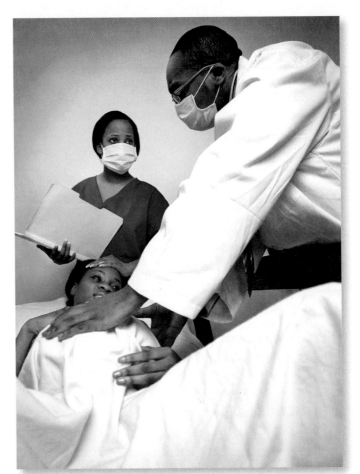

Figure 2-1. Obstetricians who are part of a private practice are usually connected with a specific hospital where they help their patients through labor and delivery.

A physician who practices both specialties is referred to as an obstetrician/gynecologist, or OB/GYN.

Oncology

Oncologists, as stated earlier in the chapter, identify tumors, determine if they are benign or malignant, and treat patients with cancer. Treatment may involve chemotherapy, which is the administration of drugs to destroy cancer cells. Treatment may also involve radiation therapy, which kills cancer cells through the use of x-rays. Newer therapies include immune therapy and transplant techniques to urge the body to create healthy tissues to replace those affected by cancer. Oncologists treat both adults and children.

Ophthalmology

An ophthalmologist is an MD who diagnoses and treats diseases and disorders of the eye. This physician specialist examines patients' eyes for poor vision or disease. Other responsibilities include prescribing corrective lenses or medication, performing surgery, and providing follow-up care after surgery. The specialty of ophthalmology includes two other practitioners who are not MDs. An optometrist obtains the credential of OD (optometric doctor). An optometrist specializes in diagnosing and treating visual defects with glasses and contacts. An optician is the specialist who works with ophthalmologists and optometrists by filling the prescriptions written by them for glasses and contact lenses.

Orthopedics

Orthopedics is a branch of medicine specializing in maintaining the function of the musculoskeletal system and its associated structures. An **orthopedist** diagnoses and treats diseases and disorders of the muscles and bones. Some orthopedists concentrate on treating sports-related injuries, either exclusively for professional athletes or for nonprofessionals of all ages. They are called sports medicine specialists.

Otorhinolaryngology

Otorhinolaryngology involves the study of the ear, nose, and throat. An **otorhinolaryngologist** diagnoses and treats diseases of these body structures. This physician specialist is also referred to as an ear, nose, and throat (ENT) specialist. Otorhinolaryngology is also called otolaryngology according to the American Academy of Otolaryngology.

Pathology

Pathology is the study of disease. It provides the scientific foundation for all medical practice. The **pathologist** studies the changes a disease produces in the cells, fluids, tissues, and processes of the entire body. These samples often come from biopsies, cultures, and tissue samples, but some pathologists also perform **autopsies,** examinations of the bodies of the deceased, to determine the cause of a patient's death and to advance the clinical practice of medicine.

There are two basic types of pathologists. Governments and police departments use forensic pathologists to determine facts about unexplained or violent deaths. Anatomic pathologists often work at hospitals in a research capacity, and they may read **biopsies** (samplings of cells that could be malignant).

Pediatrics and Adolescent Medicine

Pediatrics is concerned with the development and care of children from birth until 18 (in some practices, up to 21) years and the diseases and conditions that affect children and adolescents. A **pediatrician** diagnoses and treats childhood diseases and teaches parents skills to keep their children healthy.

Physical Medicine

Physical medicine specialists (**physiatrists**) are physicians who specialize in physical medicine and rehabilitation. They are certified by the American Board of Physical Medicine and Rehabilitation to diagnose and treat diseases and disorders such as sore shoulders and spinal cord injuries.

Physiatrists offer an aggressive, nonsurgical approach to pain and injury. Physical medicine specialists' patients include both adults and children.

Podiatry

Podiatry is practiced by a licensed doctor of podiatric medicine (D.P.M.). A **podiatrist** is a podiatry professional devoted to the study and treatment of the foot and ankle. A podiatrist's education consists of an undergraduate degree plus a doctoral level 4-year program followed by a 2- or 3-year residency. Podiatrists may independently diagnose, treat, prescribe medication, and perform surgery for disorders of the foot and, in some states, the ankle and leg. There are three board certification possibilities for podiatrists. The Board of Primary Care and Orthopedics is a nonsurgical Board Certification. The Surgical Board of Certification is divided into foot surgery and rear foot and ankle reconstruction surgery. The rear foot and ankle Board Certification requires at least a 3-year residency to qualify.

Plastic Surgery

A **plastic surgeon** performs the reconstruction, correction, or improvement of body structures. Patients may be accident victims or disfigured due to disease or abnormal development. Plastic surgery includes facial reconstruction, face-lifts, and skin grafting. Plastic surgery is also used to repair problems like cleft lip and cleft palate, as well as disfigurement and restrictive scarring due to trauma.

Proctology

Proctology is the branch of medicine that diagnoses and treats disorders of the anus, rectum, and intestines. **Proctologists** treat conditions such as colitis, hemorrhoids, fistulas, tumors, and ulcers. Proctologists often work closely with urologists.

Radiology

Radiology is the branch of medical science that uses x-rays and radioactive substances to diagnose and treat disease. **Radiologists** specialize in taking and reading x-rays.

Sports Medicine

Sports medicine is an interdisciplinary subspecialty of medicine that deals with the treatment and preventative care of amateur and professional athletes. Sports medicine teams consist of specialty physicians and surgeons, athletic trainers, and physical therapists. Sports medicine is more than treating injuries to the musculoskeletal system. Sports medicine can include an array of treatments, such as prevention and nutritional health. Sports medicine was recognized by the American Board of Medical Specialties in 1989 and continues to grow today.

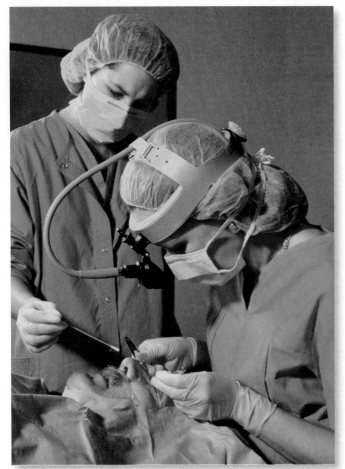

Figure 2-2. Most surgeons specialize in a particular type of surgery, such as heart surgery or eye surgery.

Surgery

Surgeons use their hands and medical instruments to diagnose and correct deformities and treat external and internal injuries or disease (Figure 2-2). They work with many different specialists to surgically treat a broad range of disorders. General surgeons may, for example, perform operations as diverse as breast lumpectomy and repair of a pacemaker. There are also subspecialties of surgery, such as neurosurgery, vascular surgery, and orthopedic surgery.

Urology

A **urologist** diagnoses and treats diseases of the kidney, bladder, and urinary system. A urologist's patients include infants, children, and adults of all ages. Urologists also treat male reproductive diseases.

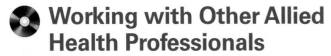 Working with Other Allied Health Professionals

You will always work as a member of a health-care team. That health-care team will include doctors, nurses, specialists, and the patients themselves. You must know the duties of the other allied health professionals in your workplace. Even if you do not work with other allied health professionals in the office, you may contact them through correspondence or by telephone. Understanding the duties of other health-care team members will help make you a more effective medical assistant.

Acupuncturist

Acupuncturists treat people with pain or discomfort by inserting thin, hollow needles under the skin. The points used for insertion are selected to balance the flow of *qi* (pronounced *chee*), or life energy, in the body. The theory of acupuncture relates to Chinese beliefs about how the body works. Qi is composed of two opposite forces called yin and yang. If the flow of qi is unbalanced, insufficient, or interrupted, then emotional, spiritual, mental, and physical problems will result. The acupuncturist works to balance these two forces in perfect harmony. Although there are variations in types of acupuncture—Chinese, Korean, and Japanese—all practitioners will focus on many pulse points along different meridians, the channels through which qi flows.

Chiropractor

Chiropractors treat people who are ill or in pain without using drugs or surgery. They primarily use manual treatments, although they may also employ physical therapy treatments, exercise programs, nutritional advice, and lifestyle modification to help correct the problem causing the pain. The manual treatments, called adjustments, realign the vertebrae in the spine and restore the function of spinal nerves. Chiropractors use diagnostic testing such as x-rays, muscle testing, and posture analysis to determine the location of spinal misalignments, also called *subluxations*. They then develop a treatment plan based on these findings. The treatment plan generally requires several adjustments per week for several weeks or months. Because the treatment does not involve drugs or surgery, the body needs time for healing and correction to occur.

Electroencephalographic Technologist

Electroencephalography (EEG) is the study and recording of the electrical activity of the brain. It is used to diagnose diseases and irregularities of the brain. The EEG technologist (sometimes called a technician) attaches electrodes to the patient's scalp and connects them to a recording instrument. The machine then provides a written record of the electrical activity of the patient's brain. EEG technologists work in hospital EEG laboratories, clinics, and physicians' offices.

Electrocardiograph Technician

The electrocardiograph (ECG/EKG) technician is a trained professional who operates an electrocardiograph machine, as pictured in Figure 2-3. An ECG records the electrical impulses reaching the heart muscles. Physicians and

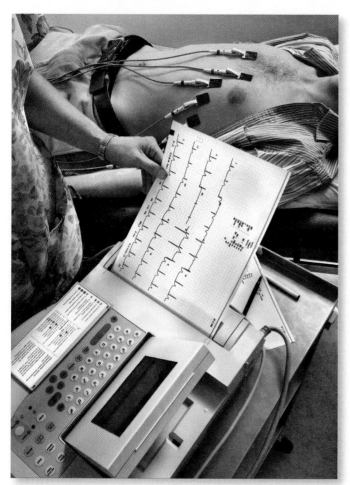

Figure 2-3. The electrocardiograph (ECG) technician is responsible for operating an electrocardiograph machine, which detects heart abnormalities and monitors patients with cardiac problems.

cardiologists use the readings from this machine to detect heart abnormalities and to monitor patients with known cardiac problems. Electrocardiograph technicians generally work in hospitals and large clinics.

Massage Therapist

Massage therapists use pressure, kneading, stroking, vibration, and tapping to promote muscle and full-body relaxation as well as to increase circulation and lymph flow. Increasing circulation helps remove blood and waste products from injured tissues and brings fresh blood and nutrients to the areas to speed healing. Massage is one of the oldest methods of promoting healing and is used to treat strains, bruises, muscle soreness or tightness, lower back pain, and dislocations. It can also relieve muscle spasm, restore motion and function to a body part, and decrease edema.

Medical Administrative Assistant

A medical administrative assistant assists medical, professional, and technical personnel by providing administrative support. These functions include transcribing dictation and composing correspondence. A medical administrative assistant should also be familiar with application software, such as Microsoft Office. Other functions include maintaining medical and administrative files. A medical administrative specialist may work in a hospital, nursing home, physician's office, or clinic.

Medical Billing and Coding

Professional medical billers and coders are in very high demand. They perform duties that encompass a wide variety of skills. Medical billers are very knowledgeable in health insurance products offered to patients. They perform a variety of functions, including:

- Reviewing patient insurance coverage
- Educating patients regarding their insurance coverage
- Estimating insurance reimbursement for procedures
- Preparing accurate health-care claims
- Preparing bills and statements
- Working with collection agencies

Medical coders are responsible for abstracting medical information from patient records. They assign internationally recognized and alphanumeric codes that correlate to procedures and diagnoses to reimbursement documents such as a CMS-1500 claim form. A physician will depend on medical coders to accurately code the patient's medical record so that the biller may accurately prepare the claim form for submission to the insurance carrier. Accurate coding and clean claim forms maximize reimbursement and help to ensure ethical standards in medical billing and coding.

Medical Records Technologist

There are two types of medical records technologists: the Registered Health Information Administrator (RHIA) and the Registered Health Information Technician (RHIT). These technologists are responsible for organizing, analyzing, and evaluating medical records. Other responsibilities include compiling administrative and health statistics, coding symptoms, and inputting and retrieving computerized health data. These positions involve typing medical reports, preparing statistical reports on patient treatments, and supervising clerical personnel in the medical records department. Registered Health Information Technicians and Registered Health Information administrators work in hospitals, nursing homes, health maintenance organizations, physicians' offices, and government agencies.

Medical Technology

Medical technology is an umbrella term that refers to the development and design of clinical laboratory tests (such as diagnostic tests), procedures, and equipment. Two types of allied health professionals who work in medical technology are the clinical laboratory technician and the medical technologist.

Clinical Laboratory Technician. Clinical laboratory technicians (CLTs) have 1- to 2-year degrees and are

Medical Office Administrator or Manager

To gain medical assistant credentials, you must fulfill the requirements of either the American Association of Medical Assistants (for a Certified Medical Assistant) or the American Medical Technologists (for a Registered Medical Assistant). After obtaining your medical assistant certification, you may wish to acquire additional skills in specialty areas through course work or on-the-job training. Although this course work or training may not lead to an additional certification or degree, it will enable you to expand your role in the medical office and advance your career as the demand for skilled health professionals increases.

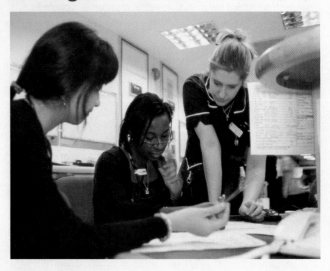

Skills and Duties

A medical office administrator or manager manages the practice of a single physician (solo practice) or of a group practice. His duties are determined, in part, by the size of the practice. If the practice is large, he may have more managerial duties. If it is small, he may act as the receptionist, secretary, and records clerk. (Occasionally, in a solo practice, the practice nurse performs many or all of these functions.) Large group practices with 10 to 15 physicians may have one medical office administrator or manager, while larger group practices with 40 to 50 physicians (such as managed care organizations) may have a highly trained practice administrator or manager who oversees and coordinates the work of several administrators at multiple practice locations.

The medical office administrator's or manager's reception duties begin with greeting and welcoming new patients. He may provide a medical history form for patients and answer any questions they may have. The administrator must have knowledge of medical terminology in order to answer patients' questions.

This office manager coordinates the practice's records and filing. For example, he ensures that x-rays and test results are attached to the appropriate records and that insurance information is up to date. The medical office administrator or manager may also schedule appointments for patients as well as referrals with other specialists. He may also keep track of the medical and nursing staff schedule. Sometimes the administrator or manager is the person who calls patients ahead of time to confirm their appointments.

In a solo or small practice, the medical office administrator or manager may perform general secretarial tasks, such as handling the mail and answering the telephone. He must have strong computer and application software skills, such as spreadsheet applications and advanced document processing skills, as well as solid accounting skills. In a large practice, the administrator or manager may train and supervise the office staff. It is important that this administrator be knowledgeable in all employment practice laws when in a managerial role. The office administrator may also be responsible for recruiting and hiring medical staff.

Workplace Settings

Medical office administrators or managers may work in solo practices, group practices, or medical clinics. Specialized health-care facilities, such as nursing homes, may also employ medical office administrators.

Education

Although medical office administrators or managers may learn the medical terminology they need on the job, they usually acquire their secretarial and clerical background through course work, either in a business/ vocational school or in a junior or community college. The educational requirements for a medical office administrator vary with the size of the practice and the extent of the administrator's responsibilities. Upper-level positions require a graduate degree.

For more information, visit the websites of the following organizations, which are available on the Online Learning Center at www.mhhe.com/medicalassisting4e.

American Academy of Medical Administrators
Medical Group Management Association
National Association of Medical Staff Services

responsible for clinical tests performed under the supervision of a physician or medical technologist. They perform tests in the areas of hematology, serology, blood banking, urinalysis, microbiology, and clinical chemistry. Clinical laboratory technicians work in hospital laboratories, commercial laboratories, medical clinics, and physicians' offices.

Medical Technologist. Medical technologists perform laboratory tests and procedures with clinical laboratory equipment. They examine specimens of human body tissues and fluids, analyze blood factors, and culture bacteria to identify disease-causing organisms. They also supervise and train technicians and laboratory aides. Medical technologists have 4-year degrees and may specialize in areas such as blood banking, microbiology, and chemistry. These technologists are employed in clinics, hospitals, private practices, colleges, pharmaceutical companies, government, research, and industry.

Medical Transcriptionist

Medical transcriptionists translate a physician's dictation about patient treatments into comprehensive, typed records. Attorneys, insurance companies, and medical specialists need accurate medical records. Medical transcriptionists work in doctors' offices, hospitals, clinics, laboratories, and radiology departments and for medical transcription services and insurance companies. Medical assistants often have medical transcription duties.

Mental Health Technician

A mental health technician, sometimes called a psychiatric aide or counselor, works in a variety of health-care settings with emotionally disturbed and mentally challenged patients. This health professional assists the psychiatric team by observing behavior and providing information to help in the planning of therapy. The mental health technician also participates in supervising group therapy and counseling sessions. This technician may work in a psychiatric clinic, specialized nursing home, psychiatric unit of a hospital, or community health center. Other places of employment include crisis centers and shelters. Training varies widely, from on-the-job training to advanced degrees, depending medical setting insurance carrier credentialing mandates, as well as state and federal laws.

Nuclear Medicine Technologist

A nuclear medicine technologist performs tests to oversee quality control, to prepare and administer radioactive drugs, and to operate radiation detection instruments. This allied health professional is also responsible for correctly positioning the patient, performing imaging procedures, and preparing the information for use by a physician. A nuclear medicine technologist may work in a hospital, public health institution, or physician's office or—with appropriate clinical experience—in a teaching position at a college or university. There are 2- and 4-year training programs. The registration examination is administered by the American Registry of Radiologic Technologists.

Occupational Therapist

An occupational therapist works with patients who have physical injuries or illnesses, psychologic or developmental problems, or problems associated with the aging process. This health professional helps patients attain maximum physical and mental health by using educational, vocational, and rehabilitation therapies and activities. The occupational therapist may work in a hospital, clinic, extended care facility, rehabilitation hospital, or government or community agency. To become an occupational therapist, you need a 4-year degree, followed by a 9- to 12-month internship at an accredited hospital. Then you must pass the national board examination in order to earn the title of OTR—registered occupational therapist.

Pharmacist

Pharmacists are professionals who have studied the science of drugs and who dispense medication and health supplies to the public. Pharmacists know the chemical and physical qualities of drugs and are knowledgeable about the companies that manufacture drugs.

Pharmacists inform the public about the effects of prescription and nonprescription (over-the-counter) medications. Pharmacists are employed in hospitals, clinics, and nursing homes. They may also work for government agencies, pharmaceutical companies, privately owned pharmacies, or chain store pharmacies. Some pharmacists own their own stores. There are three levels of pharmacists, each with different training requirements. A pharmacy technician (CPhT) can typically receive on-the-job training. Formal training, although not yet required by most states, includes certificate programs and 2-year college programs offering associate degrees in science. Voluntary certification is by examination. A registered pharmacist (RPh) requires 5 years of college training with a bachelor's degree in science. Pharmacists must be registered by the state and must pass a state board examination. A doctor of pharmacy (PharmD) requires 6 to 7 years of college training, which may be followed by a residency in a hospital setting.

Phlebotomist

Phlebotomists are allied health professionals trained to draw blood for diagnostic laboratory testing. They work in medical clinics, laboratories, and hospitals. Although medical assistants are also trained to draw blood for standard types of tests, phlebotomists are trained at a more advanced level to be able to draw blood under difficult circumstances or in special situations. For example, if a blood sample is needed for an ammonia-level test, it must be drawn and stored in a particular manner that only phlebotomists are trained to do. In most states phlebotomists must be certified by the National Phlebotomy Association or registered by the American Society of Clinical Pathologists.

Physical Therapist

A physical therapist (PT) plans and uses physical therapy programs for medically referred patients. The PT helps these patients to restore function, relieve pain, and prevent disability following disease, injury, or loss of body parts. A physical therapist uses various treatment methods, which include therapy with electricity, heat, cold, ultrasound, massage, and exercise. The physical therapist also helps patients accept their disabilities. A physical therapist may work in a hospital, outpatient clinic, rehabilitation center, home-care agency, nursing home, voluntary health agency, private practice, or sports medicine center. A physical therapist must have a master's degree in physical therapy and must pass a state board examination.

Physician Assistant

A **physician assistant (PA)** is a health-care provider who practices medicine under the supervision of a physician. Physician assistants are licensed by the state in which they practice. PAs are trained in medicine with a curriculum similar in content but shorter in duration than medical school. Most physician assistants are nationally certified and hold the title PA-C. National certification is maintained through cycles of examinations and continuing medical education.

The scope of the physician assistant's practice corresponds to the supervising physician's practice. Duties may include taking patient histories, performing physical examinations, ordering and interpreting laboratory tests, performing procedures, assisting in surgery, diagnosing medical conditions, and developing and carrying out treatment plans. Physician assistants can prescribe medication in most states. PAs work in a wide variety of healthcare settings, including hospitals, clinics, private physician offices, schools, prisons, and governmental agencies. They also serve as faculty in physician assistant programs. Medical assistants may work with physician assistants, particularly in outpatient settings.

Radiographer

A radiographer (x-ray technician) is one of the most common positions for individuals whose education is in radiologic technology. The radiographer assists a radiologist in taking x-ray films. These films are used to diagnose broken bones, tumors, ulcers, and disease. A radiographer usually works in the radiology department of a hospital. The x-ray technician may, however, use mobile x-ray equipment in a patient's room or in the operating room. A radiographer may be employed in a hospital, laboratory, clinic, physician's office, government agency, or industry.

Registered Dietitian

Registered dietitians help patients and their families make healthful food choices that provide balanced, adequate

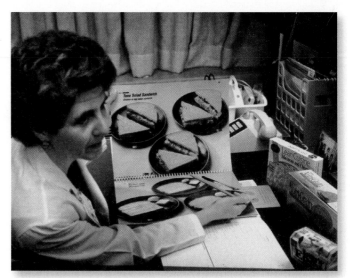

Figure 2-4. Registered dietitians work closely with patients who need to modify their food choices for better health.

nutrition particularly when disease or illness makes known what to eat to help fight the disease difficult (Figure 2-4). Dietitians are sometimes confused with nutritionists. Where a dietician has specialized training to assist ill patients with their nutritional needs, a nutritionist's goal is for those of us who are healthy to maintain a lifestyle of healthful eating. Dietitians may assist food-service directors at health-care facilities and prepare and serve food to groups. They may also participate in food research and teach nutrition classes. Dietitians work in community health agencies, hospitals, clinics, private practices, and managed care settings. They may also teach at colleges and universities, and they serve as consultants to organizations and individuals.

Radiologic Technologist

A radiologic technologist is a health-care professional who has studied the theory and practice of the technical aspects of the use of x-rays and radioactive materials in the diagnosis and treatment of disease. A radiologic technologist may specialize in radiography, radiation therapy, or nuclear medicine. Radiologic technologists generally work in hospitals; some work in medical laboratories, medical practices, and clinics.

Respiratory Therapist

A respiratory therapist evaluates, treats, and cares for persons with respiratory problems. The respiratory therapist works under the supervision of a physician and performs therapeutic procedures based on observation of the patient. Using respiratory equipment, the therapist treats patients with asthma, emphysema, pneumonia, and bronchitis. The respiratory therapist plays an active role in newborn, pediatric, and adult intensive care units. The therapist may work in a hospital, nursing home, physician's office, or commercial company that provides emergency oxygen equipment and services to home-care patients.

Nursing Aide/Assistant

Nursing aides assist in the direct care of patients under the supervision of the nursing staff. Typical functions include making beds, bathing patients, taking vital signs, serving meals, and transporting patients to and from treatment areas. Nursing assistants are often employed in psychiatric and acute care hospitals, nursing homes, and home health agencies. On-the-job training can range from 1 week to 3 months. Certification as a certified nursing assistant (CNA) is available and is required by many health care facilities, especially long-term care facilities.

Practical/Vocational Nurse

Licensed practical nurses (LPNs) and licensed vocational nurses (LVNs) provide nursing care to the sick. Both terms refer to the same type of nurse. Duties involve taking and recording patient temperatures, blood pressure, pulse, and respiration rates. They also include administering some medications under supervision, dressing wounds, and applying compresses. LPNs and LVNs are not allowed, however, to perform certain other duties, such as some intravenous (IV) procedures or the administration of certain medications. LPNs/LVNs can obtain additional training to become certified in IV therapy.

Practical/vocational nurses assist registered nurses and physicians by observing patients and reporting changes in their conditions. LPNs/LVNs work in hospitals, nursing homes, clinics, and physicians' offices and in industrial medicine. To meet the needs of the growing aging population in this country, employment opportunities for LPNs and LVNs in long-term care settings have increased.

LPNs/LVNs must graduate from an accredited school of practical (vocational) nursing (usually a 1-year program). They are also required to take a state board examination for licensure as LPNs/LVNs.

Associate Degree Nurse

Associate degrees in nursing (ADNs) are offered at many junior colleges and community colleges and at some universities. These programs combine liberal arts education and nursing education. The length of the ADN program is typically 2 years. ADNs are also considered RNs if they pass the state boards.

Diploma Graduate Nurse

Diploma programs are usually 3-year programs designed as cooperative programs between a community college and a participating hospital. The programs combine course work and clinical experience in the hospital.

Baccalaureate Nurse

A baccalaureate degree refers to a 4-year college or university program. Graduates of a 4-year nursing program are awarded a bachelor of science in nursing (BSN) degree. The curriculum includes courses in liberal arts, general education, and nursing courses. Graduates are prepared to function as nurse generalists and in positions that go beyond the role of hospital staff nurses. BSNs are also considered RNs if they pass the state boards.

Registered Nurse

A nurse who graduates from a nursing program and passes the state board examination for licensure is considered an RN, indicating formal, legal recognition by the state. The RN is a professional who is responsible for planning, giving, and supervising the bedside nursing care of patients. An RN may work in an administrative capacity, assist in daily operations, oversee programs in hospital or institutional settings, or plan community health services.

Registered nurses work in a variety of settings. These settings include hospitals, nursing homes, public health agencies, industry, physicians' offices, government agencies, and educational settings. Some RNs continue their education to earn master's or doctoral degrees.

Nurse Practitioner

A nurse practitioner (NP) is an RN who functions in an expanded nursing role. The NP usually works in an ambulatory patient care setting alongside physicians. An NP may work in an independent nurse practitioner practice without physicians. An independent nurse practitioner takes health histories, performs physical exams, conducts screening tests, and educates patients and families about disease prevention.

An NP who works in a physician's practice may perform some duties that a physician would, such as administering physical exams and treating common illnesses and injuries (Figure 2-5). For example, in an OB/GYN practice the NP can perform a standard annual gynecologic exam, including taking a Pap smear or a culture to test for yeast

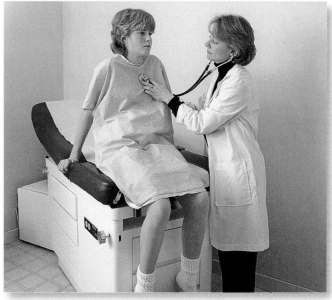

Figure 2-5. Many nurse practitioners work in physicians' offices and are trained to perform routine examinations.

infection or a bacterial infection. The nurse practitioner usually emphasizes preventive health care.

The NP must be an RN with at least a master's degree in nursing and must complete 4 to 12 months of an apprenticeship or formal training. With specific formal training the student may become a pediatric nurse practitioner, an obstetric nurse practitioner (midwife), or a psychiatric nurse practitioner.

Specialty Career Options

The various medical specialties can open up many career possibilities for medical assistants. Deciding to specialize may become one of your career goals 5 or more years from now. Remember that you may need additional training or education for some of these positions. Your hard work will be rewarded, however, as you gain additional job responsibilities.

Choosing an area in which to specialize involves research and careful thought. Local and medical college libraries can supply a great deal of information about the areas in which you may specialize. State employment agencies or schools can help you make career choices.

It is also helpful to check the help-wanted section in local newspapers for information about jobs in specialized areas. Many newspapers separate health-care career opportunities into easy-to-find boxed sections. You may also directly contact companies you would like to work for. Ask about job opportunities, and find out what skills and training the employer requires.

Anesthetist's Assistant

Anesthetist's assistants provide anesthetic care under an anesthetist's direction. Hospitals and high-technology surgical centers frequently employ anesthetist's assistants. These assistants gather patient data and assist in evaluation of patients' physical and mental status. They also record planned surgical procedures, assist with patient monitoring, draw blood samples, perform blood gas analyses, and conduct pulmonary function tests.

Certified Laboratory Assistant

Certified laboratory assistants perform routine procedures in bacteriology, chemistry, hematology, parasitology, serology, and urinalysis. Laboratory assistants work under the supervision of a medical technologist or hospital anatomic pathologist. They work in laboratories at hospitals, clinics, and physicians' offices and in independent laboratories. One-year training programs are offered by hospitals, vocational schools, and community colleges. Some certified laboratory assistants are medical assistants with advanced training in laboratory testing.

Dental Assistant

A dental assistant can practice without formal education or training. In this case, on-the-job training is provided. A dental assistant performs many administrative and laboratory functions that are similar to the duties of a medical assistant. For example, a dental assistant may serve as chair-side assistant, provide instruction in oral hygiene, and prepare and sterilize instruments. To perform expanded clinical and chair-side functions such as those of a hygienist, a dental assistant must have at least 1 year of training in theory and clinical application. This formal education also requires work experience in a dental office.

Dental assistants often work in a private practice. They also work in clinics, dental schools, and local health agencies. Insurance companies hire dental assistants to process dental claims.

Emergency Medical Technician/Paramedic

An emergency medical technician (EMT), sometimes called a paramedic, works under the direction of a physician through a radio communication network. This health professional assesses and manages medical emergencies that occur away from hospitals or other medical settings, such as in private homes, schools, offices, or public areas. An EMT is trained to **triage** patients (to assess the urgency and type of condition presented as well as the immediate medical needs) and to initiate the appropriate treatment for a variety of medical emergencies. While transporting patients to the medical facility, an EMT records, documents, and radios the patient's condition to the physician, describing how the injury occurred. An EMT may work for an ambulance service, fire department, police department, hospital emergency department, private industry, or voluntary care service. Training requirements vary by state but typically require a high school diploma and driver's license, 100 hours of classroom training, and an average of 6 months of practical training on an ambulance squad or in a hospital emergency room.

Occupational Therapist Assistant

Occupational therapist assistants work under the supervision of an occupational therapist. They help individuals with mental or physical disabilities reach their highest level of functioning through the teaching of fine motor skills, trades (occupations), and the arts. Duties include preparing materials for activities, maintaining tools and equipment, and documenting the patient's progress. Occupational therapist assistants must earn a 2-year degree (OTA).

Ophthalmic Assistant

An ophthalmic assistant aids ophthalmologists and optometrists with the routine functions of the practice. This health professional performs simple vision testing, takes medical histories, administers eyedrops, and changes dressings. There are three levels in this category of allied health professional (from most senior to least senior): ophthalmic technologist, ophthalmic technician, and ophthalmic assistant. Duties are determined by the supervising ophthalmologist.

Medical assistants can obtain on-the-job training to become an ophthalmic assistant. Although no states currently require certification for these positions, certification examinations are available for each type of category.

Pathologist's Assistant

Pathologist's assistants work under the supervision of a pathologist. Pathologist's assistants sometimes work with forensic pathologists—professionals who study the human body and diseases for legal purposes, in cooperation with government or police investigations. They may prepare frozen sections of dissected body tissue. Assistants working for anatomic pathologists (professionals who study the human body and diseases in a research capacity) may maintain supplies, instruments, and chemicals for the anatomic pathology laboratory. Pathologist's assistants perform laboratory work about 75% of the workday. Assistants also perform a variety of administrative duties. They work in community hospitals, university medical centers, and private laboratories.

Pediatric Medical Assistant

A pediatric medical assistant assists the pediatrician in administrative and clinical duties (Figure 2-6). These duties include obtaining medical histories and preparing patients for examination. Other duties include performing routine tests, sterilizing supplies and equipment, typing, filing, and clerical work. This health professional also educates patients and their parents or guardians about follow-up care and maintains patients' records. A pediatric medical assistant should be able to communicate well with children. Other helpful skills include patience and organizational skills. Pediatric medical assistants work with pediatricians in private practice, hospitals, and clinics.

Pharmacy Technician

Pharmacy technicians perform specific routine tasks related to record keeping and preparing and dispensing drugs. Duties include preparing medications for administration and making sure patients receive the correct medication. Pharmacy technicians usually work in hospitals or similar facilities under the supervision of a nurse, pharmacist, or other health-care professional. In a commercial pharmacy they work under the pharmacist's supervision. Opportunities are also available with pharmaceutical firms and wholesale pharmaceutical distributors.

Training can be on the job or through certificate programs and 2-year college programs (associate degree). National certification is voluntary by examination and earns the title CPhT (certified pharmacy technician).

Physical Therapy Assistant

A physical therapy assistant (PTA) works under the direction of a physical therapist to assist with patient treatment. The assistant follows the patient care program created by the physical therapist and physician. This health professional performs tests and treatment procedures, assembles or sets up equipment for therapy sessions, and observes and documents patient behavior and progress (Figure 2-7). A physical therapy assistant may practice in a hospital, nursing home, rehabilitation center, or community or government agency.

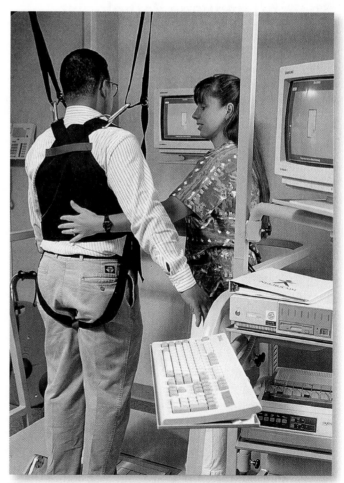

Figure 2-7. Physical therapy assistants provide guidance and support to patients who are recovering from a physical injury or from surgery on a limb or joint.

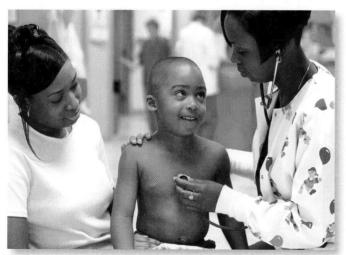

Figure 2-6. If you enjoy working with children, you might consider working as a pediatric medical assistant.

Radiation Therapy Technologist

A radiation therapy technologist assists the radiologist. He may, for example, assist with administering radiation treatment to patients who have cancer. He may also be responsible for maintaining radiation treatment equipment. The technologist shares responsibility with the radiologist for the accuracy of treatment records. A radiation therapy technologist may work in a hospital, laboratory, clinic, physician's office, or government agency. Training requires a high school diploma and graduation from a 2- or 4-year program in radiography.

Respiratory Therapy Technician

Respiratory therapy technicians work under the supervision of a physician and a respiratory therapist. Respiratory therapists perform procedures such as artificial ventilation. They also clean, sterilize, and maintain the respiratory equipment and document the patient's therapy in the medical record. Respiratory therapy technicians work in hospitals, nursing homes, physicians' offices, and commercial companies that provide emergency oxygen equipment and therapeutic home care.

Speech/Language Pathologist

A speech/language pathologist treats communication disorders, such as stuttering, and associated disorders, such as hearing impairment. This health professional evaluates, diagnoses, and counsels patients who have these problems. A speech/language pathologist may work in a school, hospital, research setting, or private practice or may teach at a college or university.

Speech/language pathologists usually have a master's degree in speech/language pathology or audiology. Certification and licensing requirements vary by state, usually depending on the work setting (public school, private practice, clinic, and so on).

Surgical Technician

A surgical technician provides patient services under the direction, supervision, and responsibility of a licensed surgeon. This health professional's tasks include obtaining a patient's history and physical data. She then discusses the data with a physician or surgeon to determine what procedures to use to treat the problem. A surgical technician may also assist in performing diagnostic and therapeutic procedures. She must be calm and have good judgment in the high-pressure environment of the operating room. Surgical technicians work primarily in hospitals and outpatient surgery centers.

Training programs for this position are usually affiliated with 2- and 4-year colleges and with university schools of medicine and allied health. These programs include practical work in the surgery unit of an affiliated hospital.

Professional Associations

Membership in a professional association enables you to become involved in the issues and activities relevant to your field and presents opportunities for continuing education. It is a good idea to become informed about such associations, even those, such as the American Medical Association, that are open to physicians only. The physician you work for may ask you to obtain information about the group's activities and meetings. Table 2-1 summarizes professional associations related to the field of medicine and medical assisting.

American Association of Medical Assistants

The American Association of Medical Assistants (AAMA), as described in Chapter 1, was created to serve the interests of medical assistants and to further the medical assisting profession. The AAMA offers self-paced continuing education classes; workshops and seminars at the local, state, and national levels; and job networking opportunities. Other benefits include legal counsel, group health insurance, professional recognition, and member discounts.

The Association for Healthcare Documentation Integrity

The Association for Healthcare Documentation Integrity (AHDI) is the professional organization for the advancement of medical transcription. The AHDI also educates medical transcriptionists as medical language specialists. The AHDI offers advice and support to the many medical transcriptionists who are self-employed.

American College of Physicians

Founded in 1915, the American College of Physicians (ACP) is the largest medical specialty organization in the world. It is the only society of internists dedicated to providing education and information resources to the entire field of internal medicine and its subspecialties.

American Hospital Association

The American Hospital Association (AHA) is the nation's largest network of institutional health-care providers. These providers represent every type of hospital: rural and city hospitals, specialty and acute care facilities, freestanding hospitals, academic medical centers, and health systems and networks. The AHA works to support and promote the interests of hospitals and health-care organizations across the country. Organizations as well as individual professionals may join the AHA. Membership benefits include use of the AHA consultant referral service, accessed, for example, by hospitals that need experts in areas not addressed by in-house personnel. Members also have access to AHA's health-care information resources, including teleconferencing and AHA database services.

TABLE 2-1 Professional Medical Organizations

Professional Organization	Membership Requirements	Advantages of Membership
American Association of Medical Assistants (AAMA) www.aama-ntl.org (312) 899-1500	Interested individuals, including medical assisting students and those who practice medical assisting, may join the AAMA.	Offers flexible continuing education programs; publishes *CMA Today;* offers legal counsel, professional recognition, and various member discounts
Association of Healthcare Documentation Integrity (AHDI) www.ahdionline.org (800) 982-2182	Interested individuals and those who practice medical transcription may join the AHDI.	Educates and develops medical transcriptionists as medical language specialists; offers advice and support for self-employed medical transcriptionists
American College of Physicians (ACP) www.acponline.org (800) 523-1546	Physicians and medical students may join.	Provides education and information resources to the field of internal medicine and its subspecialties
American Hospital Association (AHA) www.aha.org (312) 442-3000	Institutional health-care providers and other individuals may join.	Provides consultant referral service and access to health-care information resources
American Medical Association (AMA) www.ama-assn.org (800) 621-8353	Physicians and medical students may join.	Provides large information source; publishes *Journal of the American Medical Association (JAMA);* offers AMA/Net
American Medical Technologists (AMT) www.amt1.com (800) 275-1268	Medical assistants, medical technologists, medical laboratory technicians, dental assistants, and phlebotomy technicians may join.	Offers national certification as Registered Medical Assistant (RMA); offers certification to other health-care professionals, publications, state chapter activities, continuing education programs
American Pharmacists Association (APhA) www.pharmacists.com (202) 628-4410	Pharmaceutical professionals and physicians may join.	Helps members improve skills; active in pharmacy policy development, networking, publishing, research, public education
American Society of Clinical Pathology (ASCP) www.ascp.org (800) 267-2727	Any professional involved in laboratory medicine or pathology may join.	Resource for improving the quality of pathology and laboratory medicine; offers educational programs and materials; certifies technologists and technicians
American Society of Phlebotomy Technicians (ASPT) www.aspt.org (828) 294-0078	Interested individuals and those who practice phlebotomy may join.	Offers national certification as a phlebotomy technician and continuous education programs
National Healthcare Association (NHA) 7 Ridgedale Ave., Suite 203 Cedar Knolls, NJ 07927 Phone: 973-605-1881 Toll Free: 800-499-9092 www.nhanow.com	Member or Student of Allied Health Field Career	Healthcare Job Search Assistance Free Seminars and Workshops for continuing education Certification for certified clinical medical assistant (CCMA) Certification for certified medical administrative assistant (CMAA)

The Joint Commission (TJC)

The Joint Commission, previously known as The Joint Commission on Accreditation of Healthcare Organizations (JCAHO), is a U.S.-based nonprofit organization. It was formed in 1951 with a goal of maintaining and elevating the standards of health-care delivery through the evaluation and accreditation of health-care organizations. TJC employs surveyors who are sent to health-care organizations to evaluate their operational practices and facilities. Organizations are given a score from 1 to 100, with 100 being a perfect score. Healthcare organizations are highly motivated to do well during a survey because accreditation by TJC is a significant factor in gaining reimbursement from Medicare and managed care organizations. In January 2004, TJC expanded their focus to include patient safety requirements, to:

- Improve the accuracy of patient identification
- Improve the safety of high-alert medications, such as electrolyte concentrations
- Eliminate the wrong site, wrong patient, wrong procedure, or wrong surgery
- Improve the safety of using infusion pumps
- Improve the effectiveness of clinical alarm systems
- Reduce the risk of health-care-acquired infections

TJC established these requirements to help accredited health-care organizations address issues of patient safety that can lead to adverse events that can result in lawsuits.

Council of Ethical and Judicial Affairs (CEJA)

The Council of Ethical and Judicial Affairs (CEJA) develops ethics policy for the AMA. It is composed of seven practicing physicians, a resident or fellow, and a medical student. The Council prepares reports that analyze and address timely ethical issues that confront physicians and the medical profession. CEJA maintains and updates the AMA Code of Medical Ethics. This code is widely recognized as the most comprehensive ethics guide for physicians who strive to practice ethically.

American Medical Association

The American Medical Association (AMA) was founded in 1847. Its members include 300,000 physicians from every medical specialty. The AMA promotes science and the art of medicine and works to improve public health. The AMA is the world's largest publisher of scientific and medical information and publishes 10 monthly medical specialty journals. The AMA also accredits medical programs in the United States and Canada.

The AMA provides an online service called AMA/Net for physicians and medical assistants, offering up-to-date information about current medical topics. To use the AMA/Net, the medical office must have a computer, telephone, and modem.

American Medical Technologists

American Medical Technologists (AMT) was established in 1939 as a not-for-profit organization. The AMT offers national certification as a Registered Medical Assistant (RMA) to medical assisting practitioners. It also offers certification to medical technologists, clinical laboratory technicians, dental assistants, medical administrative specialists, and phlebotomy technicians. Membership benefits include continuing education classes, workshops and seminars, and job networking opportunities.

American Pharmacists Association

The American Pharmacists Association (APhA), the national professional society of pharmacists, was founded in 1852. The APhA represents the interests of pharmaceutical professionals, and it strives to help individual members improve their skills. The APhA works to advance the field of pharmacy and the safety of patients. The APhA is active in pharmacy policy development, networking, publishing, research, and public education.

Summary

2.1 Today there are approximately 22 major medical specialties. Within these specialties are several subspecialties. Medical specialties range from cardiology to oncology. A subspecialty in the area of cardiology is pediatric cardiology. As new medical advances occur, the demand for more specialty areas will emerge.

2.2 The American Board of Medical Specialties is an organization of many different medical specialty boards. Its primary purpose is to maintain and improve the quality of medical care and to certify doctors in various specialties.

2.3 Medical assistants are members of a health-care team. The health-care team includes doctors, nurses, physical therapists, other allied health professionals, and patients. Understanding other health-care professionals' duties will assist the medical assistant as a professional. Even if you do not work with some of the team members directly, you may have to contact them on the telephone or through written correspondence.

2.4 Membership in professional associations enables medical assistants to become involved in activities relevant to their field. These organizations were created to further the careers and education of those in the medical assisting field. The American Association of Medical Assistants is a key professional organization for medical assistants.

CASE STUDY QUESTIONS

Now that you have completed this chapter, review the case study at the beginning of the chapter and answer the following questions:

1. What are Susan's career options in nursing? How much further education would she need in order to become a nurse?
2. What are Susan's career options in a laboratory setting? How much further education would she need in order to work in a laboratory?

Multiple-Choice Questions

1. _____ are medical specialists that deal with the medical and surgical treatment of obesity.
   a. Gastroenterologists   c. Gynecologists
   b. Allergists   d. Bariatric surgeons

2. The abbreviation for a licensed doctor of podiatric medicine is
   a. D. P. M.   c. M. D.
   b. D. V. M.   d. O. D.

3. The Joint Commission (TJC) is a U.S.-based organization that
   a. offers continuing education for medical assistants.
   b. provides credentialing for physicians.
   c. maintains and elevates the standards of health-care delivery through credentialing and accreditation.
   d. obtains information for medical groups.

4. The first year of residency for a new physician is known as
   a. student practice.
   b. credentialing of medical training.
   c. diplomatic certification.
   d. an internship.

5. An _____ is an M.D. who diagnoses and treats diseases and disorders of the eye.
   a. optometrist   c. ophthalmologist
   b. orthopedist   d. optician

Discussion Questions

1. Discuss the different types of physicians, such as podiatrist, chiropractor, MD, and DO. What are the differences in training, education, and board certification?
2. Medical assistants can perform many roles. Discuss the different allied health careers that medical assistants can receive training in, such as phlebotomy assistant, ophthalmic medical assistant, administrative roles, and other positions.
3. How do professional organizations help medical assistants perform their job duties?

Critical Thinking Questions

1. How might a medical assistant's experience working with a medical specialist differ from her experience working with a general practitioner, in terms of learning about medicine?
2. Why is it important for a medical assistant to be knowledgeable about other allied health-care professionals and their primary duties?
3. How can medical assistants enhance their careers by joining professional organizations such as the AMT or AAMA?

Application Activities

1. Interview a medical assistant, such as an ophthalmic medical assistant, who has chosen a specialty career option. What additional education or training did she need to obtain the position? What are her administrative and clinical duties? What does she like about her job? What does she find most challenging? How did she come to choose the specialty? Report your findings to the class.
2. Invite a guest speaker to your class who is currently working in an allied health career, such as a pharmacy technician or phlebotomist, to talk about his or her job duties, certifications, and overall involvement in the medical community.
3. Pick three medical specialties and identify the skills required for a medical assistant in each specialty.

Virtual Fieldtrip

Visit the McGraw-Hill Higher Education Medical Assisting website at www.mhhe.com/medicalassisting4e to complete the following activity:

Research a professional organization that interests you the most and research the opportunities that interest you. One opportunity is the professional credentialing offered by the various organizations. Share your research with your classmates.

Open the CD and complete this chapter's practice activities, play the games, listen to the key terms, and test yourself with the interactive review. E-mail, print, and/or save your results to document your proficiency.

CHAPTER 3

Legal and Ethical Issues in Medical Practice, Including HIPAA

LEARNING OUTCOMES

After completing Chapter 3, you will be able to:

3.1 Clarify ethics, bioethics, and medical law.

3.2 Describe the measures a medical practice must take to avoid malpractice claims.

3.3 Explain medical documentation and how it applies to medical law.

3.4 Explain the various types of health-care legislation.

3.5 Explain Occupational Safety and Health Administration (OSHA) requirements for a medical office.

3.6 Explain the impact that Health Insurance Portability and Accountability Act (HIPAA) regulations have in the medical office.

(continued)

MEDICAL ASSISTING COMPETENCIES

CAAHEP

IX. C (1) Discuss legal scope of practice for medical assistants

IX. C (2) Explore issue of confidentiality as it applies to the medical assistant

IX. C (3) Describe the implications of HIPAA for the medical assistant in various medical settings

IX. C (4) Summarize the Patient Bill of Rights

IX. C (13) Discuss all levels of governmental legislation and regulation as they apply to medical assisting practice, including FDA and DEA regulations

IX. C (14) Describe the process to follow if an error is made in patient care

IX. P (1) Respond to issues of confidentiality

IX. P (2) Perform within scope of practice

IX. P (3) Apply HIPAA rules in regard to privacy/release of information

IX. A (2) Demonstrate awareness of the consequences of not working within the legal scope of practice

IX. A (3) Recognize the importance of local, state, and federal legislation and regulations in the practice setting

X. C (1) Differentiate between legal, ethical, and moral issues affecting health care

X. C (2) Compare personal, professional, and organizational ethics

X. C (3) Discuss the role of cultural, social, and ethnic diversity in ethical performance of medical assisting practice

IX. P (1) Report illegal and/or unsafe activities and behaviors that affect health, safety, and welfare of others to proper authorities

(continued)

ABHES

4. Medical Law and Ethics
  a. Document accurately
  b. Institute federal and state guidelines when releasing medical records or information
  c. Follow established policies when initiating or terminating medical treatment
  d. Understand the importance of maintaining liability coverage once employed in the industry
  e. Perform risk management procedures
  f. Comply with federal, state, and local health laws and regulations

6. Pharmacology
  d. Understand legal aspects of writing prescriptions, including federal and state laws

11. Career Development
  Demonstrate professionalism by:
  1) Exhibiting dependability, punctuality, and a positive work ethic
  2) Exhibiting a positive attitude and a sense of responsibility
  3) Maintaining confidentiality at all times
  4) Being cognizant of ethical boundaries
  9) Conducting work within scope of education, training, and ability

CAAHEP	ABHES
X. A (1) Apply ethical behaviors, including honesty/integrity in performance of medical assisting practice **X. A (2)** Examine the impact personal ethics and morals may have on the individual's practice **X. A (3)** Demonstrate awareness of diversity in providing patient care **XI. C (1)** Describe personal protective equipment **XI. C (2)** Identify safety techniques that can be used to prevent accidents and maintain a safe work environment **XI. C (9)** Discuss requirements for responding to hazardous material disposal	

MEDICAL ASSISTING MEDIA

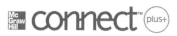 **Connect Plus+™**
connect.mcgraw-hill.com

- Elecronic Health Records (E.H.R.) SpringCharts®
- eBook

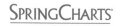

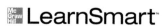 **LearnSmart™**

www.mhhe.com/learnsmart

Complete Learning Module(s): Legal and Ethical Issues in Medical Practice, Including HIPAA

 Student CD-ROM

 Online Learning Center™

www.mhhe.com/medicalassisting4e

KEY TERMS

abandonment	crime	ethics	living will
agent	criminal law	expressed contract	malpractice claim
arbitration	defamation	felony	minors
assault	disclosure	fraud	misdemeanor
authorization	discrimination	group practice	moral values
battery	doctrine of informed consent	implied consent	negligence
bioethics		implied contract	Notice of Privacy Practices (NPP)
breach of contract	doctrine of professional discretion	informed consent	
civil law		law	partnership
consent	durable power of attorney	law of agency	Privacy Rule
contract	electronic transaction record	liable	protected health information (PHI)
corporation		libel	

qui tam	slander	subpoena testificandum	uniform donor card
res ipsa loquitur	sole proprietorship	tort	use
respondeat superior	subpoena	treatment, payment, and	void
Security Rule	subpoena duces tecum	operations (TPO)	

CHAPTER OUTLINE

- Medical Law and Ethics
- The Patient-Physician Contract
- Special Circumstances for Physician Practices
- Preventing Lawsuits
- Federal Legislation Affecting Health Care
- OSHA Regulations
- Laws That Protect the Employee

- HIPAA
- Risk Management
- Confidentiality Issues and Mandatory Disclosure
- Code of Ethics
- Managing Contracts
- Labor and Employment Laws
- Legal Medical Practice Models

PREPARATION FOR CERTIFICATION

RMA (AMT) Exam
- Medical ethics
- Compliance with OSHA guidelines and regulation of office safety
- Principles of medical ethics

CMA (AAMA) Exam
- Displaying professional attitude
- Legislation
- Maintaining confidentiality
- Working as a team member to achieve goals

CMAS Exam
- Professionalism
- Legal and ethical considerations
- Confidentiality

Introduction

Medical law plays an important role in medical facility procedures and the way we care for patients. We live in a litigious society, where patients, relatives, and others are inclined to sue health-care practitioners, health-care facilities, manufacturers of medical equipment and products, and others when medical outcomes are not acceptable. It is important for a medical professional to understand medical law, ethics, and protected health information as it pertains to the Health Insurance Portability and Accountability Act (HIPAA) of 1996. There are two main reasons for medical professionals to study law and ethics: The first is to help you function at the highest professional level by providing competent, compassionate health care to patients and the second is to help you avoid legal problems that can threaten your ability to earn a living.

A knowledge of medical law and ethics can help you gain perspective in the following three areas:

1. *The rights, responsibilities, and concerns of health-care consumers.* Not only do health-care professionals need to be concerned about how law and ethics impact their respective professions, they must also understand how legal and ethical issues affect patients. As medical technology advances and the use of computers increases, patients want to know more about their options and rights as well as more about the responsibilities of health-care practitioners. Patients want to know who uses their information, how it is used, and what the options they have regarding health-care treatments. Patients have come to expect favorable outcomes from medical treatment, and when these expectations are not met, lawsuits may result.

2. *The legal and ethical issues facing society, patients, and health-care professionals as the world changes.* Every day new technologies emerge with solutions to biological and medical issues. These solutions often involve social issues, and we are faced with decisions, for example, regarding reproductive rights, fetal stem cell research, and confidentiality with sensitive medical records.

3. *The impact of rising costs on the laws and ethics of health-care delivery.* Rising costs, both of health-care insurance and of medical treatment in general, can lead to questions concerning access to health-care services and the allocation of medical treatment. For example, should everyone, regardless of age or lifestyle, have the same access to scarce medical commodities such as transplant organs or very expensive drugs.

In today's society, medical treatment and decisions surrounding health care have become complex. It is therefore important to be knowledgeable about and aware of the ethical issues and the laws that govern patient care.

A medical assistant is very busy on a Monday morning. She has drawn blood on a patient that she has known for years and has been very comfortable chatting with this patient. The patient is checking out at the front desk in the reception area, and she notices that he forgot his prescription for Dilantin, a medication for seizure control. She rushes up to the front area and, as he is opening the door, says to him, "Mr. Doe, you forgot your prescription for Dilantin."

As you read this chapter, consider the following questions:
1. Does the medical assistant's comment represent a breach of confidentiality?
2. Has any HIPAA rule been violated? If so, which one?

Medical Law and Ethics

In order to understand medical law and ethics, it is helpful to understand the differences between laws and ethics. A **law** is defined as a rule of conduct or action prescribed or formally recognized as binding or enforced by a controlling authority, such as local, state, and federal governments. **Ethics** is considered a standard of behavior and a concept of right and wrong beyond what the legal consideration is in any given situation. **Moral values** serve as a basis for ethical conduct. Moral values are formed through the influence of the family, culture, and society.

Classifications of Law

There are two types of law that pertain to health-care practitioners: criminal law and civil law.

Criminal Law. A **crime** is any offense committed or omitted in violation of a public law. **Criminal law** involves crimes against the state. When a state or federal criminal law is violated, the government brings criminal charges against the alleged offender, for example, *Ohio v. John Doe*. Criminal laws prohibit such crimes as murder, arson, rape, and burglary. A criminal act may be classified as a felony or misdemeanor. A **felony** is a crime punishable by death or by imprisonment in a state or federal prison for more than 1 year. Some examples of a felony include abuse (child, elder, or domestic violence), manslaughter, fraud, attempted murder, and practicing medicine without a license.

Misdemeanors are less serious crimes than felonies. They are punishable by fines or by imprisonment in a facility other than a prison for 1 year or less. Some examples of misdemeanors are thefts under a certain dollar amount, attempted burglary, and disturbing the peace.

Civil Law. **Civil law** involves crimes against the person. Under civil law, a person can sue another person, a business, or the government. Court judgments in civil cases often require the payment of a sum of money to the injured party. Civil law includes a general category of law known as torts. A **tort** is broadly defined as a civil wrong committed against a person or property that causes physical injury or damage to someone's property or that deprives someone of his or her personal liberty and freedom. Torts may be intentional (willful) or unintentional (accidental).

Intentional Torts. When one person intentionally harms another, the law allows the injured party to seek a remedy in a civil suit. The injured party can be financially compensated for any harm done by the person guilty of committing the tort. If the conduct is judged to be malicious, punitive damages may also be awarded. Examples of intentional torts include the following:

- Assault. Assault is the open threat of bodily harm to another, or acting in such a way as to put another in the "reasonable apprehension of bodily harm."

- Battery. **Battery** is an action that causes bodily harm to another. It is broadly defined as any bodily contact made without permission. In health-care delivery, battery may be charged for any unauthorized touching of a patient, including such actions as suturing a wound, administering an injection, or performing a physical examination.

- Defamation of character. Damaging a person's reputation by making public statements that are both false and malicious is considered **defamation** of character. Defamation of character can take the form of slander and libel. **Slander** is speaking damaging words intended to negatively influence others against an individual in a manner that jeopardizes his or her reputation or means of livelihood. **Libel** is publishing in print damaging words, pictures, or signed statements that will injure the reputation of another.

- False imprisonment. False imprisonment is the intentional, unlawful restraint or confinement of one person by another. Preventing a patient from leaving the facility might be seen as false imprisonment.

- Fraud. **Fraud** consists of deceitful practices in depriving or attempting to deprive another of his or her rights. Health-care practitioners might be accused of fraud for promising patients "miracle cures" or for accepting fees from patients while using mystical or spiritual powers to heal.

- Invasion of privacy. Invasion of privacy is the interference with a person's right to be left alone. Entering an exam room without knocking can be considered an invasion of privacy. The improper use of or a breach of confidentiality of medical records may be seen as an invasion of privacy.

Unintentional Torts. The most common torts within the health-care delivery system are those committed unintentionally. Unintentional torts are acts that are not intended to cause harm but are committed unreasonably or with a disregard for the consequences. In legal terms, such acts constitute negligence. **Negligence** is charged when a health-care practitioner fails to exercise ordinary care and the patient is injured. The accused may have performed an act or failed to perform an act that a reasonable person would or would not have performed. Under the principles of negligence, civil liability exists only in cases in which the act is judicially determined to be wrongful. Health-care practitioners, for example, are not necessarily liable for a poor-quality outcome in delivering health care. Practitioners become liable only when their conduct is determined to be malpractice, the negligent delivery of professional services.

Contracts

A **contract** is a voluntary agreement between two parties in which specific promises are made for a consideration. The elements of a contract are important to health-care practitioners because health-care delivery takes place under various types of contracts. To be legally binding, four elements must be present in a contract:

1. Agreement—One party makes an offer and another party accepts it. Certain conditions pertain to the offer:

   - It can relate to the present or the future.
   - It must be communicated.
   - It must be made in good faith and not under duress or as a joke.
   - It must be clear enough to be understood by both parties.
   - It must define what both parties will do if the offer is accepted.

   For example, a physician offers a service to the public by obtaining a license to practice medicine and opening or business. Patients accept the physician's offer by scheduling appointments, submitting to physical examinations, and allowing the physician to prescribe or perform medical treatment. The contract is complete when the physician's fee is paid.

2. Consideration—Something of value is bargained for as part of the agreement. The physician's consideration is providing service; the patient's consideration is payment of the physician's fee.

3. Legal subject matter—Contracts are not valid and enforceable in court unless they are for legal services or purposes. For example, a contract entered into by a patient to pay for services of a physician in private practice would be **void** (not legally enforceable) if the physician was not licensed to practice medicine.

Breach of contract may be charged if either party fails to comply with the terms of a legally valid contract.

4. Contractual capacity—Parties who enter into the agreement must be capable of fully understanding all its terms and conditions. For example, a mentally incompetent individual or a person under the influence of drugs or alcohol cannot enter into a contract.

Types of Contracts. The two main types of contracts are expressed contracts and implied contracts. An **expressed contract** is clearly stated in written or spoken words. A payment contract is an example of an expressed contract. **Implied contracts** are those in which the acceptance or conduct of the parties, rather than expressed words, creates the contract. A patient who rolls up a sleeve and offers an arm for an injection is creating an implied contract.

Legal Elements of a Contract. An employment contract is a legal agreement between two or more people to perform an act in exchange for payment. To be binding, the contract must include these main elements:

- An agreement between two or more competent people to do something legal
- Names and addresses of the people involved
- Consideration (whatever is given in exchange, such as money, work, or property)
- Starting and ending dates, as well as date(s) the contract was signed
- Signature of the employer and employee

A Medical Assistant Contract. Some medical practices use employment contracts for medical assistants. This type of contract would include these elements:

- A description of your duties and your employer's duties
- Plans for handling major changes in job responsibilities
- Salary, bonuses, and other forms of compensation
- Benefits, such as vacation time, sick days, life insurance, and participation in pension plans
- Grievance procedures
- Exceptional situations under which the contract may be terminated by either you or your employer
- Termination procedures and compensation
- Special provisions, such as job sharing, medical examinations, or liability coverage

If you are offered an employment contract, study it closely. Consider any local laws that may apply, and have a lawyer or business adviser review the contract.

The Patient-Physician Contract

A physician has the right, after forming a contract or agreeing to accept a patient under his or her care, to make reasonable limitations on the contractual relationship. The physician is under no legal obligations to treat patients who may wish to exceed those limitations. Under the patient-physician contract, both parties have certain rights and responsibilities.

Physician Rights and Responsibilities

Physicians have the right to:

- Set up a practice within the boundaries of his or her license to practice medicine
- Set up an office where he or she chooses and to establish office hours
- Specialize
- Decide which services he or she will provide and how those services will be provided

While practicing within the context of an implied contract with the patient, the physician is not bound to:

- Treat every patient with medical care. A physician is free to use his or her discretion to form contracts within his or her practice, with one exception: If a physician is providing care to patients in a hospital emergency room or free clinic, then the physician must treat every patient who comes for treatment.
- Restore the patient to his or her original state of health
- Make a correct diagnosis in every case
- Guarantee the successful result of any treatment or operation. In fact, guarantees of "cures" may constitute fraud on the part of the physician.

Under an implied contract with the patient, the physician has the obligation or responsibility to:

- Use due care, skill, judgment, and diligence in treating patients that peers in the same specialty use
- Stay informed of the best methods of diagnosis and treatment
- Perform to the best of his or her ability, whether or not he or she is to receive a fee
- Furnish complete information and instructions to the patient about diagnoses, options, methods of treatment, and fees for services

Liability. All competent adults are liable or legally responsible for their actions, in both their personal lives and their professional careers. It is important as a medical assistant to know and understand your scope of practice within the state you are working. As health-care providers, medical assistants have general liability in the duties they perform, as well as the facility in which they work. By understanding the standard of care and the duty of care, medical assistants can function ethically and legally within their job scope. Medical assistants are held to the "reasonable person standard," which means to carry out your professional and interpersonal relationships without causing harm.

Patient Rights and Responsibilities

Patients have the right to choose a physician, although some managed care plans may limit choices. Patients also have the right to terminate a physician's services if they wish. Most states have adopted a version of the American Hospital Association's *Patient Care Partnership* (formerly called the Patient's Bill of Rights). The Patient Care Partnership is a list of standards that patients can expect in health care. TJC requires hospitals to post a copy of these standards and most managed care organizations also require contracted physicians to post a copy of them as well.

Patient Responsibilities. Patients are also part of the medical team involved in their treatment. Patients have the responsibility under an implied contract to:

- Follow any instructions given by the physician and cooperate as much as possible
- Give all relevant information to the physician in order to reach a correct diagnosis. If a patient fails to inform a physician of any medical conditions he or she may have and an incorrect diagnosis is made, the physician is not liable.
- Follow the physician's orders for treatment
- Pay the fees charged for services provided

Consent. **Consent** means that the patient has given permission, either expressed or implied, for the physician to examine him or her, to perform tests that aid in diagnoses, or to treat for a medical condition. When the patient makes an appointment to be examined by a physician, the patient has given **implied consent** to the examination and any diagnostic testing procedures needed for treatment.

Informed Consent. **Informed consent** involves the patient's right to receive all information relative to his or her condition and to make a decision regarding treatment based upon that knowledge. The **doctrine of informed consent** is the legal basis for informed consent and is usually outlined in a state's medical practice acts. Informed consent implies that the patient understands:

- Proposed treatment modes
- Why the treatment was necessary
- The risks involved in the proposed treatment
- Available alternative modes of treatment
- The risks of alternative treatments
- The risks involved if treatment is refused

Adult patients who are of sound mind are usually able to give informed consent. In the case of emancipated minors, courts have ruled that they understand as a competent adult would, and therefore are able to make decisions on their own. Mature minors are able to understand the courts' decisions and what is happening to and for them.

Those patients who cannot give informed consent include the following:

- **Minors** and persons under the age of majority, which excludes married minors
- The mentally incompetent
- Those who speak a foreign language—interpreters may be necessary

Informed consent is a vital part of the practice of medicine today. Physicians are often sued for negligence because of the failure to adequately inform patients of adverse surgical complications, drug reactions, and alternative treatment modes.

Special Circumstances for Physician Practices

Distressful economic circumstances may happen when a medical practice has to terminate and close its services to its patients. If this becomes necessary, make sure the medical staff and all physicians

- Comply with all HIPAA laws for maintaining confidentiality.
- Write letters to all patients, giving them knowledge that your practice will be closing (Figure 3-1).
- Give patients an option of choosing another physician, or make referrals. If the patient chooses another physician to take over his care, get written consent that their charts will be transferred to that physician properly.

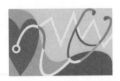

TOTAL CARE MEDICAL GROUP, INC.

10 Cedarfield Drive, Springfield, MA 01107 30031
(413) 788-0123 Phone   (413) 788-3210 Fax

Brendan M. Whalen, MD
Matthew D. Whalen, MD

Alexis N. Wyman, MD

LETTER OF TERMINATION OF SERVICES DUE TO CLOSING OF PRACTICE

May 23, 200X

Ms. Gisele Monagon
234 Cutter Lane
Monson, MA 01057

Dear Ms. Monagon:

I find it necessary to inform you that our medical practice will be closing on July 15, 200X. My medical practice will be purchased by The Vaughn Group, 2345 Williamsburg Ct., Springfield, MA 01118

If you wish to use this group of medical practitioners, please sign the enclosed authorization release form so that your files can be sent to them promptly.

If you choose not to use this group of physicians, you may send me a letter with your signature, authorizing the release of your files to the physician of your choice.

It has been a pleasure serving you.

Sincerely,

Alexis N. Wyman, MD

Alexis N. Wyman, MD
mng
Enclosure: Authorization Form

Figure 3-1. Sample of a letter of termination.

- Keep all files in a secured location for the maximum amount of time files should be saved if contacts cannot be made to patients. You will have to choose a vendor that stores files. Make sure you choose a reputable vendor
- Shred files if necessary; make sure you choose reputable vendors.
- Are up-to-date on any HIPAA laws that will affect the practice.

Preventing Lawsuits

Malpractice litigation not only adds to the cost of health care, it takes a psychological toll on both patients and health-care practitioners. Both sides would probably agree that prevention is preferable to litigation. Health-care practitioners who use reasonable care in preventing professional liability claims are least likely to be faced with defending themselves against malpractice claims.

Malpractice

Malpractice claims are lawsuits by a patient against a physician for errors in diagnosis or treatment. Negligence cases are those in which a person believes that a medical professional did not perform an essential action or performed an improper one, thus harming the patient.

Following are some examples of malpractice:

- Postoperative complications. For example, a patient starts to show signs of internal bleeding in the recovery room. The incision is reopened, and it is discovered that the surgeon did not complete closure (cauterization) of all the severed capillaries at the operation site.
- *Res ipsa loquitur.* This Latin term, which means "the thing speaks for itself," refers to a case in which the doctor's fault is completely obvious. For example, a case in which a surgeon accidentally leaves a surgical-instrument inside the patient.

Following are examples of negligence:

- Abandonment. A health-care professional who stops care without providing an equally qualified substitute can be charged with **abandonment.** For example, a labor and delivery nurse is helping a woman in labor. The nurse's shift ends, but all the other nurses are busy and her replacement is late for work. Leaving the woman would constitute abandonment.
- Delayed treatment. A patient shows symptoms of some illness or disorder, but the doctor decides, for whatever reason, to delay treatment. If the patient later learns of the doctor's decision to wait, the patient may believe he has a negligence case.

Negligence cases are sometimes classified using the following three legal terms.

1. *Malfeasance* refers to an unlawful act or misconduct.
2. *Misfeasance* refers to a lawful act that is done incorrectly.
3. *Nonfeasance* refers to failure to perform an act that is one's required duty or that is required by law.

The Four Ds of Negligence. The American Medical Association (AMA) lists the following four Ds of negligence:

1. Duty. Patients must show that a physician-patient relationship existed in which the physician owed the patient a duty.
2. Derelict. Patients must show that the physician failed to comply with the standards of the profession. For example, a gynecologist has routinely taken Pap smears of a patient and then, for whatever reason, does not do so. If the patient then shows evidence of cervical cancer, the physician could be said to have been derelict.
3. Direct cause. Patients must show that any damages were a direct cause of a physician's breach of duty. For example, if a patient fell on the sidewalk and damaged her cast, she could not prove that the cast was damaged because it was incorrectly or poorly applied by her physician. It would be clear that the damage to the cast resulted from the fall. If, however, the patient's leg healed incorrectly because of the way the cast had been applied, she might have a case.
4. Damages. Patients must prove that they suffered injury.

To go forward with a malpractice suit, a patient must be prepared to prove all four Ds of negligence.

Malpractice and Civil Law. Malpractice (negligence) lawsuits are part of civil law coming under the heading of torts. A tort is defined as the breach of an obligation that causes harm or injury and may intentional or unintentional. A breach of contract is the failure of one of the parties to adhere to the terms of the contract.

In the case of medical care contracts, which are often implied contracts, either the provider or the patient may breach the contract. The provider may breach the contract by not maintaining patient confidentiality or by not providing adequate medical care (negligence). The patient may breach the contract by not showing for appointments or by not following the physician's plan of care.

Settling Malpractice Suits. Malpractice suits often require a trial in a court of law. Sometimes, however, they are settled through arbitration. **Arbitration** is a process in which the opposing sides choose a person or persons outside the court system, often with special knowledge in the field, to hear and decide the dispute. (Your local or state medical society has information about your state's policy on arbitration.) If injury, failure to provide reasonable care, or abandonment of the patient is proved to have occurred, the doctor must pay damages (a financial award) to the injured party.

If the doctor you work with becomes involved in a lawsuit, you should be familiar with subpoenas. A **subpoena** is a written court order addressed to a specific person, requiring that person's presence in court on a specific date at a specific time. If you were directly involved in the patient case or have knowledge of the events that precipitated the lawsuit, you might be subpoenaed to provide testimony under penalty, known as *subpoena testificandum.* Another important term to know is *subpoena duces tecum,* which is a court order to produce specific, requested documents required at a certain place and time to enter into court records. If you are in charge of patient records at the practice, you will be required to locate, assemble, photocopy, and arrange for delivery of the requested records or be charged with contempt of court if you do not comply.

Law of Agency. According to the **law of agency,** an employee is considered to be acting as a doctor's **agent** (on the doctor's behalf) while performing professional tasks. The Latin term *respondeat superior,* or "let the master answer," is sometimes used to refer to this relationship. For example, the employee's word is as binding as if it were the doctor's (so you should never, for example, promise a patient a cure). Therefore, the doctor is responsible, or **liable,** for the negligence of employees. A negligent employee, however, may also be sued directly because individuals are legally responsible for their own actions. Therefore, a patient can sue both the doctor and the involved employee for negligence. The employer, or the employer's insurance company, can also sue the employee. Most likely, in a case of negligence, the doctor would be sued (because you as an employee are acting on the doctor's behalf), and you are usually covered by the doctor's malpractice insurance. Some medical assistants choose to obtain malpractice insurance. Obtaining personal malpractice insurance is a professional decision that depends on the type of work or facility in which you are employed. The American Association of Medical Assistants offers medical assisting malpractice insurance through various insurance companies at reduced rates.

Courtroom Conduct. Most health-care practitioners will never have to appear in court. If you should be asked to appear, the following suggestions may prove helpful:

- Attend court proceedings as required. Failure to appear in court could result in either charges of contempt of court or the case being forfeited.
- Do not be late for scheduled hearings.
- Bring required documents to court and present them only when requested to do so.
- Before testifying, refresh your memory concerning all the facts observed about the matter in question, such as dates, times, words spoken, and circumstances.
- Speak slowly, clearly, and professionally. Do not use medical terms. Do not lose your temper or attempt to be humorous.

- Answer all questions in a straightforward manner, even if the answers appear to help the opposing side.
- Answer only the question asked, no more and no less.
- Appear well groomed, and dress in clean, conservative clothing.

Professional Liability Coverage. Professional liability coverage is specialty coverage. It protects the physician and staff against financial losses from lawsuits filed against them by their clients or others. It protects the physician if she is determined negligent in her actions, and it protects the physician and her staff if it is determined that the staff are negligent in their actions as well.

Reasons Patients Sue

The following reasons were researched by interviewing families and patients who have sued health-care practitioners:

1. Unrealistic expectations. With the advancements in medical technology today, patients often expect perfection in medical outcomes. They may feel betrayed by the health-care system when a medical outcome is not what was expected.

2. Poor rapport and poor communication. Patients usually do not sue health-care practitioners that they like and trust. Health-care providers who do not return telephone calls or are otherwise unavailable to a patient's family members may be perceived as arrogant, cold, or uncaring. When such perceptions exist, patients and family members are more likely to sue if something goes wrong.

3. Greed and our litigious society. Financial gain is seldom the reason for medical malpractice, but in some cases it may be an influencing factor. Malpractice attorneys sometimes make it very easy for patients to retain their services, such as contingency arrangements.

4. Poor quality of care. Poor quality means that a patient is truly not receiving quality care. Poor quality in "perception" means that the patient believes he or she is not receiving quality care, even if it is not true. Either situation can lead to a malpractice lawsuit.

Statute of Limitations. Statutes of limitations are laws that set the deadline or maximum period of time within which a lawsuit or claim may be filed. The most common length of time is two years. The deadlines may vary depending on the circumstances and the type of case or claim. The periods of time also vary from state to state and depending on whether they are filed in federal or state court. The lawsuit or claim is barred if not filed before the statutory deadline. Under certain circumstances, a statute of limitations will be extended beyond its deadline. The following are examples for a civil claim for professional malpractice:

- *Medical:* 1 to 4 years from the act or occurrence of injury, or 6 months to 3 years from discovery; certain circumstances will extend the statute, including if the party is a minor, when a foreign object is involved, or in cases of fraud

- *Legal:* 1 to 3 years from date of discovery, or a maximum of 2 to 5 years from the date of the wrongful act

Four Cs of Medical Malpractice Prevention

1. *Caring.* As a health-care professional, caring about your patients and colleagues is your most important asset. Showing patients that you care about them may result in an improvement in their medical condition and, if you are sincere, decreases the likelihood that patients will feel the need to sue if treatment has unsatisfactory results or adverse events occur.
2. *Communication.* If you communicate in a professional manner and clearly ask for confirmation that you have been understood, you will earn respect and trust with your patients and other members of the allied health team.
3. *Competence.* Be competent in your skills and job knowledge and maintain and update your knowledge and skills frequently through continuing education.
4. *Charting.* Documentation is proof of competence. Make sure that all current reports and consultations have been reviewed by the physician and are evident in the chart. Chart every conversation or interaction you have with a patient.

How Effective Communication Can Help Prevent Lawsuits. Patients who see the medical office as a friendly place are generally less likely to sue. Physicians, medical assistants, and other medical office staff who have pleasant personalities and are competent in their jobs will have less risk of being sued. Medical assistants can help by:

- Developing good listening skills and nonverbal communication techniques so that patients feel the time spent with them is not rushed
- Setting aside a certain time during the day for returning patients' phone calls
- Checking to be sure that all patients or their authorized representatives sign informed consent forms before they undergo medical or surgical procedures
- Avoiding statements that could be construed as an admission of fault on the part of the physician or other medical staff
- Using tact, good judgment, and professional ability in handling patients
- Making every effort to reach an understanding about fees with the patient before treatment so that billing does not become a point of contention

Terminating Care of a Patient

A physician may wish to terminate care of a patient. Terminating care is sometimes called withdrawing from a case. The following are some typical reasons a physician may choose to withdraw from a case:

- The patient refuses to follow the physician's instructions.
- The patient's family members complain incessantly to or about the physician.
- A personality conflict develops between the physician and patient that cannot be reasonably resolved.
- The patient habitually does not pay for or fails to make satisfactory arrangements to pay for medical services. A physician may stop treatment of such a patient and end the physician-patient relationship only if adequate notice is given to the patient.
- The patient fails to keep scheduled appointments. To protect the physician from charges of abandonment, all missed and cancelled appointments should be noted in the patient's chart.

A physician who terminates care of a patient must do so in a formal, legal manner, following these four steps.

1. Write a letter to the patient, expressing the reason for withdrawing from the case and recommending that the patient seek medical care from another physician as soon as possible. Thirty days is the usual norm for finding another physician. Figure 3-2 shows an example of a letter of termination.
2. Send the letter by certified mail with a return receipt requested. This will provide evidence that the patient received the notification by providing a signature on the return receipt.
3. Place a copy of the letter (and the return receipt, when received) in the patient's medical record.
4. Summarize in the patient record the physician's reason for terminating care and the actions taken to inform the patient.

Standard of Care

You are expected to fulfill the standards of the medical assisting profession for applying legal concepts to practice. According to the AAMA, medical assistants should uphold legal concepts in the following ways:

- Maintain confidentiality
- Practice within the scope of training and capabilities
- Prepare and maintain medical records
- Document accurately
- Use appropriate guidelines when releasing information
- Follow legal guidelines and maintain awareness of health-care legislation and regulations
- Maintain and dispose of regulated substances in compliance with government guidelines

LETTER OF WITHDRAWAL FROM CASE

December 12, 2012

Jack Smallwood
Box 3457C
Rogersville, TN 37878

Dear Mr. Smallwood:

This is to inform you of our intent to discontinue medical care to you due to the habitual and continued noncompliance in your medical care. Our records indicate that you have missed several appointments and have not complied with ordered testing. This discontinuance will go into effect 30 days from the date of this letter in order to allow you sufficient time to locate another physician. We will be happy to forward your medical records to the physician of your choice. There is 24-hour medical care available to you at the hospital.

If you need assistance in locating a new physician, please contact your insurance carrier or the Tennessee Medical Society at 1-800-666-9898.

Sincerely,

John Doe, MD

Figure 3-2. Physicians are required to inform patients in writing if they wish to withdraw from a case.

- Follow established risk-management and safety procedures
- Meet the requirements for professional credentialing

Often, state laws dictate what medical assistants may or may not do. For instance, in some states it is illegal for medical assistants to draw blood. No states consider it legal for medical assistants to diagnose a condition, prescribe a treatment, or let a patient believe that a medical assistant is a nurse. In addition to what is stated by law, you and the physician must establish the procedures that are appropriate for you to perform (known as scope of practice).

Administrative Duties and the Law

Many of a medical assistant's administrative duties are related to legal requirements. Paperwork for insurance billing, patient consent forms for surgical procedures, and correspondence (such as a physician's letter of withdrawal from a case) must be handled correctly to meet legal standards. Documentation, such as making appropriate and accurate entries in a patient's medical record, is legally important. You may also maintain the physician's appointment book. The appointment book is considered a legal document, especially for tracking missed or canceled appointments.

You may also be responsible for handling certain state reporting requirements. Items that must be reported include births; certain communicable diseases such as acquired immunodeficiency syndrome (AIDS) and STDs; drug abuse; suspected child abuse or abuse of the elderly; injuries caused by violence, such as knife and gunshot wounds; and deaths. Reports are sent to various state departments, depending on the content of the report. For example, suspected child and elder abuse cases are reported to the state department of social services. Addressing these state requirements is called the physician's public duty.

Phone calls must be handled with an awareness of legal issues. For example, if the physician asks you to contact a patient by phone and you call the patient at work, you should not identify yourself or the physician by name to someone else without the patient's permission. You can say, for example, "Please tell Mrs. Arnot that her doctor's office is calling." If you do not take this precaution, the physician can be sued for invasion of privacy. You must abide by similar guidelines if you are responsible for making follow-up calls to a patient after a procedure or office visit and when leaving messages on answering machines where the message may be picked up by someone other than the person you are attempting to reach.

Documentation

Patient records are often used as evidence in professional medical liability cases, and improper documentation can contribute to or cause a case to be lost. Physicians should keep records that clearly show what treatment was performed and when it was done. It is important that physicians be able to demonstrate that nothing was neglected and that the care given fully met the standards demanded by law. One cliché to remember is "If it is not written down, then it was not done." Pay attention to spelling in charts and keep a medical dictionary handy if you are not sure of a spelling. Today's health-care environment requires complete documentation of actions taken and actions not taken. Medical staff members should pay particular attention to the following situations.

Referrals. Make sure the patient understands whether the referring physician's staff will make the appointment and notify the patient, or whether the patient must call to set up the appointment. Document in the chart that the patient was referred and the time and date of the appointment, and follow up with the specialist to verify that the appointment was scheduled and kept. If a paper referral is necessary, make sure a hard copy is placed in the patient's chart. Note whether reports of the consultation were received in your office, and document any further care of the patient from the referring physician.

Missed Appointments. At the end of the day, a designated person in the medical office should gather all patient charts of those who missed or canceled appointments without rescheduling. Charts should be dated, stamped, and documented "No Call/No Show" or "Canceled/No Reschedule." The appointment book is also considered a legal document; make sure that all missed appointments are documented on the appointment book or in the computer. The treating physician should review these records and note whether follow-up is indicated.

Dismissals. To avoid charges of abandonment, the physician must formally withdraw from a case. Be sure that a letter of withdrawal or dismissal has been filed in the patient's records. All mailing confirmations should be filed in the record, such as the return receipt from certified mail.

All Other Patient Contact. Patient records should include reports of all tests, procedures, and medications prescribed, including prescription refills. Make sure all necessary informed consent papers have been signed and filed in the chart. Make entries into the chart of all telephone conversations with the patient. Correct documentation requires the initials or signature of the person making the notation on the patient's chart as well as the date and time.

Medical Record Correction. Errors made when making an entry in a medical record or errors discovered later can be corrected, but corrections must be made in a certain manner so that if the medical records are ever used in a medical malpractice lawsuit, it will not appear that they were falsified. When deleting information, never black it out, never use correction fluid to cover it up, and never in any other way erase or obliterate the original wording. Draw a line through the original information so that it is still legible. Write or type in the correct information above or below the original line or in the margin. The "Maintaining Patient Records" chapter (Chapter 9) describes the proper procedure for correcting chart errors.

Ownership of the Patient Record. Patients' medical records are considered the property of the owners of the facility where they were created. A physician in a private practice owns his or her charts or records, while records in a hospital or clinic belong to the facility. The facility in which the records were created owns the records, but the patient owns the information they contain. Upon signing a release, patients may usually obtain access to or copies of their medical records depending upon state law. Under HIPAA, patients who ask to see or copy their medical records must be accommodated with few exceptions, such as in mental health records where the physician decides if it may be harmful to the patient to see the record. The physician is protected under the **doctrine of professional discretion.**

Retention and Storage of the Patient Record. As a protection against legal litigation, records should be kept until the applicable statute of limitations period has elapsed, which is generally 2 to 7 years. In some cases, this involves keeping the medical records for minor patients for a specified length of time after they reach legal age. Some states have enacted statutes for the retention of medical records. Most physicians retain records indefinitely to provide evidence in medical professional liability suits or for tax purposes. The medical record may provide the patient's medical history for future medical treatment.

Controlled Substances and the Law

It is important to know the right dosages and potential complications of these drugs, as well as prescription refill rules, in order to understand and interpret the directions of the physician in a legally responsible manner.

The Controlled Substances Act (CSA) of 1970 maintains that facilities have close control of drugs. Since there is great potential for abuse, medical staff must follow correct procedure for disposal. Medical assistants oftentimes have to discard outdated medicines that are in this category. Your medical facility should have enacted policies and procedures for removal of controlled substances.

If the medical assistant has any questions in regards to disposal, he or she should call the U.S. Department of Drug Enforcement or go to the website. The website offers an array of information, and you can download the Form 41 (Registrants Inventory of Drugs Surrendered). There are directions that you must follow explicitly for completion of this form (see Figure 3-3).

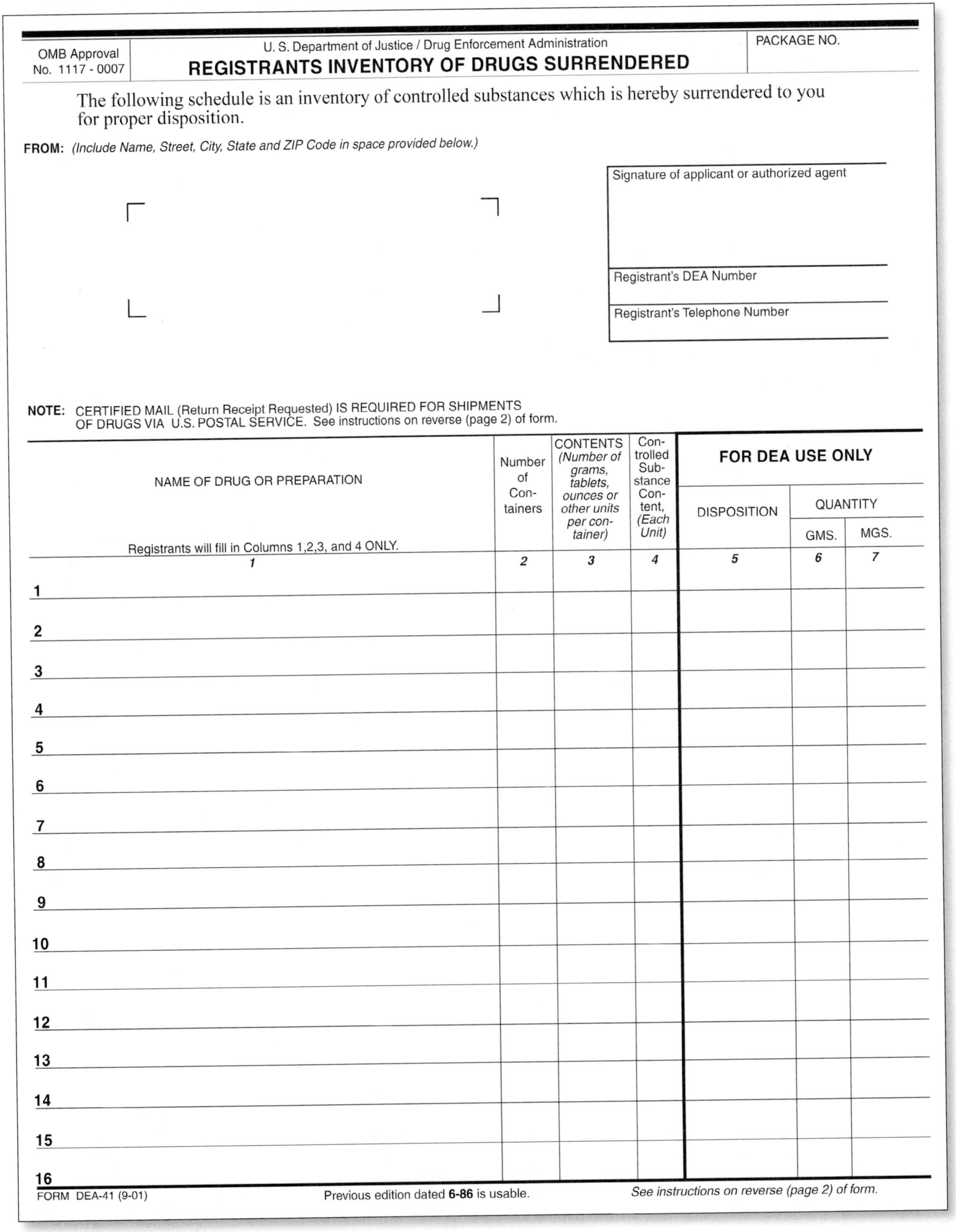
OMB Approval No. 1117 - 0007

U. S. Department of Justice / Drug Enforcement Administration

REGISTRANTS INVENTORY OF DRUGS SURRENDERED

PACKAGE NO.

The following schedule is an inventory of controlled substances which is hereby surrendered to you for proper disposition.

FROM: *(Include Name, Street, City, State and ZIP Code in space provided below.)*

Signature of applicant or authorized agent

Registrant's DEA Number

Registrant's Telephone Number

NOTE: CERTIFIED MAIL (Return Receipt Requested) IS REQUIRED FOR SHIPMENTS OF DRUGS VIA U.S. POSTAL SERVICE. See instructions on reverse (page 2) of form.

NAME OF DRUG OR PREPARATION Registrants will fill in Columns 1,2,3, and 4 ONLY.	Number of Containers	CONTENTS *(Number of grams, tablets, ounces or other units per container)*	Controlled Substance Content, *(Each Unit)*	FOR DEA USE ONLY DISPOSITION	QUANTITY GMS.	MGS.
1	*2*	*3*	*4*	*5*	*6*	*7*
1						
2						
3						
4						
5						
6						
7						
8						
9						
10						
11						
12						
13						
14						
15						
16						

FORM DEA-41 (9-01) Previous edition dated **6-86** is usable. *See instructions on reverse (page 2) of form.*

Figure 3-3. DEA form.

NAME OF DRUG OR PREPARATION	Number of Containers	CONTENTS (Number of grams, tablets, ounces or other units per container)	Controlled Substance Content, (Each Unit)	FOR DEA USE ONLY		
				DISPOSITION	QUANTITY	
Registrants will fill in Columns 1,2,3, and 4 ONLY.					GMS.	MGS.
1	2	3	4	5	6	7
17						
18						
19						
20						
21						
22						
23						
24						

The controlled substances surrendered in accordance with Title 21 of the Code of Federal Regulations, Section 1307.21, have been received in _____ packages purporting to contain the drugs listed on this inventory and have been: ** (1) Forwarded tape-sealed without opening; (2) Destroyed as indicated and the remainder forwarded tape-sealed after verifying contents; (3) Forwarded tape-sealed after verifying contents.

DATE _____   DESTROYED BY: _____

** *Strike out lines not applicable.*   WITNESSED BY: _____

INSTRUCTIONS

1. List the name of the drug in column 1, the number of containers in column 2, the size of each container in column 3, and in column 4 the controlled substance content of each unit described in column 3; e.g., morphine sulfate tabs., 3 pkgs., 100 tabs., 1/4 gr. (16 mg.) or morphine sulfate tabs., 1 pkg., 83 tabs., 1/2 gr. (32mg.), etc.

2. All packages included on a single line should be identical in name, content and controlled substance strength.

3. Prepare this form in quadruplicate. Mail two (2) copies of this form to the Special Agent in Charge, under separate cover. Enclose one additional copy in the shipment with the drugs. Retain one copy for your records. One copy will be returned to you as a receipt. No further receipt will be furnished to you unless specifically requested. Any further inquiries concerning these drugs should be addressed to the DEA District Office which serves your area.

4. There is no provision for payment for drugs surrendered. This is merely a service rendered to registrants enabling them to clear their stocks and records of unwanted items.

5. Drugs should be shipped tape-sealed via prepaid express or certified mail (**return receipt requested**) to Special Agent in Charge, Drug Enforcement Administration, of the DEA District Office which serves your area.

PRIVACY ACT INFORMATION

AUTHORITY: Section 307 of the Controlled Substances Act of 1970 (PL 91-513).
PURPOSE: To document the surrender of controlled substances which have been forwarded by registrants to DEA for disposal.
ROUTINE USES: This form is required by Federal Regulations for the surrender of unwanted Controlled Substances. Disclosures of information from this system are made to the following categories of users for the purposes stated.
    A. Other Federal law enforcement and regulatory agencies for law enforcement and regulatory purposes.
    B. State and local law enforcement and regulatory agencies for law enforcement and regulatory purposes.
EFFECT: Failure to document the surrender of unwanted Controlled Substances may result in prosecution for violation of the Controlled Substances Act.

Under the Paperwork Reduction Act, a person is not required to respond to a collection of information unless it displays a currently valid OMB control number. Public reporting burden for this collection of information is estimated to average 30 minutes per response, including the time for reviewing instructions, searching existing data sources, gathering and maintaining the data needed, and completing and reviewing the collection of information. Send comments regarding this burden estimate or any other aspect of this collection of information, including suggestions for reducing this burden, to the Drug Enforcement Administration, FOI and Records Management Section, Washington, D.C. 20537; and to the Office of Management and Budget, Paperwork Reduction Project no. 1117-0007, Washington, D.C. 20503.

Figure 3-3. (*Continued*)

Legal Documents and the Patient

You need to be aware of two legal documents that are typically completed by a patient prior to major surgery or hospitalization: the living will and the uniform donor card. Traditionally, these documents were completed outside the medical office or in the hospital. The current trend, however, is for medical practice personnel, including medical assistants, to assist patients in developing these important documents. Contact your state's Public Health Department website for additional information.

Living Wills. A **living will,** consists of two documents. An advance medical directive, is a legal document addressed to the patient's family and health-care providers stating what type of treatment the patient wishes or does not wish to receive if she becomes terminally ill, unconscious, or permanently comatose (sometimes referred to as being in a persistent vegetative state). For example, an advance directive typically states whether a patient wishes to be put on life-sustaining equipment should she become permanently comatose. Some directives contain DNR (do not resuscitate) orders. These orders mean the patient does not wish medical personnel to try to resuscitate her should the heart stop beating. Advance medical directives are a means of helping families of terminally ill patients deal with the inevitable outcome of the illness and may help limit unnecessary medical costs.

The directive is signed when the patient is mentally and physically competent to do so. It must also be signed by two witnesses. Medical practices can help patients develop an advance medical directive, sometimes in conjunction with organizations that make available preprinted living will forms. The Partnership for Caring (based in Washington, D.C.) is one such organization.

Patients who have living wills are asked to name, in the second document called a **durable power of attorney** (also known as a healthcare proxy), someone who will make decisions regarding medical care on their behalf if they are unable to do so.

The Uniform Donor Card. In 1968 the Uniform Anatomical Gift Act was passed, setting forth guidelines for all states to follow in complying with a person's wish to make a gift of one or more organs (or the whole body) upon death. An anatomical gift is typically designated for medical research, organ transplants, or placement in a tissue bank. The **uniform donor card** is a legal document that states one's wish to make such a gift. People often carry the uniform donor card in their wallets. Many medical practices offer the service of helping their patients obtain and complete a uniform donor card. In some states the Department of Motor Vehicles makes the process simple by asking you if you would like to be an organ donor at the time you renew your driver's license with a card being issued to you at that time. The patient's family should be aware of his wish to be an organ donor so that the wishes are carried out upon his death.

Federal Legislation Affecting Health Care

Congress has passed legislation intended to improve the quality of health care in the United States, to reduce fraud, and to ensure that patients will not be discriminated against by insurance providers. The most significant health-care laws passed in recent years are the Health Care Quality Improvement Act of 1986, the Federal False Claims Act, and the Health Insurance Portability and Accountability Act (HIPAA) of 1996. HIPAA is discussed in detail in the chapter. The Occupational Safety and Health Administration (OSHA) regulations, which are vitally important to the practice of health care, are also discussed in detail in this chapter.

Health Care Quality Improvement Act of 1986

The Health Care Quality Improvement Act of 1986 (HCQIA) is a federal statute passed to improve the quality of medical care nationwide. Congress created HCQIA because they found that there was an increasing occurrence of medical malpractice and a need to improve the quality of medical care. The act requires professional peer review in certain cases, limits damages to professional reviewers, and protects from liability those who provide information to professional review bodies. One of the most important provisions of the HCQIA was the establishment of the National Practitioner Data Bank. The use of the National Practitioner Data Bank was intended to improve the quality of medical care nationwide by encouraging effective professional peer review of physicians. Information that must be reported to the National Practitioner Data Bank includes medical malpractice payments, adverse licensure actions, adverse clinical privilege actions, and adverse professional membership actions. This data bank is a resource to assist state licensing boards, hospitals, and other health-care entities in investigating qualifications of physicians and other health-care practitioners.

Federal False Claims Act

The Federal False Claims Act is a law that allows individuals to bring civil actions on the behalf of the U.S. government for false claims made to the federal government, under a provision of the law call *qui tam* (from Latin meaning to bring an action for the king and for one's self). The law was enacted because of the rising cost of health care, fraud, and abuse within the health-care industry. As a result, laws have been passed to control three types of illegal conduct:

1. False billing claims. Fraudulently billing for services not performed is prohibited.
2. Kickbacks. Giving financial incentives to a health-care provider for referring patients or for recommending

services or products is prohibited under the federal Anti-Kickback Law and by state laws.

3. **Self-referrals.** Referring patients to any service or facility where the health-care provider has financial interests is prohibited by the Federal Ethics in Patient Referral Act and other federal and state laws.

Violations of laws against health-care fraud and abuse can result in imprisonment and fines, a loss of professional license, a loss of health-care facility staff privileges, and exclusion from participating in federal health-care programs.

OSHA Regulations

The Occupational Safety and Health Administration (OSHA), a division of the U.S. Department of Labor, has created federal laws to protect health-care workers from health hazards on the job. Medical personnel may accidentally contract a dangerous or even fatal disease by coming into contact with a virus a patient is carrying. Medical assistants may also be exposed to toxic substances in the office. OSHA regulations describe the precautions a medical office must take with clothing, housekeeping, record keeping, and training to minimize the risk of disease or injury.

Some of the most important OSHA regulations are those for controlling workers' exposure to infectious disease. These regulations are set forth in the OSHA Bloodborne Pathogens Protection Standard of 1991. A pathogen is any microorganism that causes disease. Microorganisms are microscopic living bodies such as viruses or bacteria that may be present in a patient's blood or other body fluids (saliva or semen).

Of particular concern to medical workers are the human immunodeficiency virus (HIV), which causes AIDS, and the hepatitis B virus (HBV). AIDS damages the body's immune system and thus its ability to fight disease. AIDS is almost always fatal. HBV is a highly contagious disease that is potentially fatal. It causes inflammation of the liver and may cause liver failure. Every year, about 8700 healthcare workers become HBV-infected at work, and about 200 die from the disease.

OSHA requires that medical professionals in medical practices follow what are called Standard Precautions. They were developed by the Centers for Disease Control and Prevention (CDC) to prevent medical professionals from exposing themselves and others to blood-borne pathogens. Exposure can occur, for example, through skin that has been broken from a needle puncture or other wound and through mucous membranes, such as those in the nose and throat. If these areas come into contact with a patient's (or coworker's) blood or body fluids, a virus could be transferred from one person to another.

Laws That Protect the Employee

Medical facilities are required to have an exposure plan to safeguard their employees. This plan must include the following safeguards:

- Personal protective equipment or gear
- Immunizations against hepatitis B virus (HBV)
- Information on what to do in case of exposure
- Information on decontamination of waste products
- Information on how to dispose of sharp equipment (needles, etc.)
- Information on post-exposure evaluation and follow-up
- Information on how to keep an inventory of hazardous materials
- Labeling for biohazardous wastes
- Training and annual updates regarding hazardous materials and infectious substances
- Recordkeeping and documentation to protect the legal rights and safety of employees

All employees are entitled to be informed about hazardous substances in the workplace and to be trained in how to use them safely.

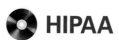 # HIPAA

Today, health care is considered a trillion-dollar industry, growing rapidly with technology and employing millions of health-care workers in numerous fields. The U.S. Department of Labor recognizes 400 different job titles in the health-care industry.

On August 21, 1996, the U.S. Congress passed the Health Insurance Portability and Accountability Act (HIPAA). The primary goals of the act are to improve the portability and continuity of health-care coverage in group and individual markets; to combat waste, fraud, and abuse in health-care insurance and health-care delivery; to promote the use of medical savings accounts; to improve access to long-term care services and coverage; and to simplify the administration of health insurance.

The purposes of the act are to:

- Improve the efficiency and effectiveness of health-care delivery by creating a national framework for health privacy protection that builds on efforts by states, health systems, and individual organizations and individuals
- Protect and enhance the rights of patients by providing them access to their health information and controlling the inappropriate use or disclosure of that information
- Improve the quality of health care by restoring trust in the health-care system among consumers, health-care professionals, and the multitude of organizations and individuals committed to the delivery of care

HIPAA is divided into two main sections of law: Title I, which addresses health-care portability, and Title II, which covers the prevention of health-care fraud and abuse, administrative simplification, and medical liability reform. Although in this text we will discuss Titles I and II in detail, you should also be aware of three other titles included in HIPAA regulations: Title III—Tax-related health provisions governing medical savings accounts, Title IV—Application and enforcement of group health insurance requirements, and Title V—Revenue offset governing tax deductions for employers providing company-owned life insurance premiums.

Title I: Health-Care Portability

The issue of portability deals with protecting health-care coverage for employees who change jobs, allowing them to carry their existing plans with them to new jobs. HIPAA provides the following protections for employees and their families:

- Increases workers' ability to get health-care coverage when starting a new job.
- Reduces workers' probability of losing existing health-care coverage.
- Helps workers maintain continuous health-care coverage when changing jobs.
- Helps workers purchase health insurance on their own if they lose coverage under an employer's group plan and have no other health-care coverage available.

The specific protections of this title include the following:

- Limits the use of exclusions for preexisting conditions.
- Prohibits group plans from discriminating by denying coverage or charging extra for coverage based on an individual's or a family member's past or present poor health.
- Guarantees certain small employers, as well as certain individuals who lose job-related coverage, the right to purchase health insurance.
- Guarantees, in most cases, that employers or individuals who purchase health insurance can renew the coverage regardless of any health conditions of individuals covered under the insurance policy.

Title II: Prevention of Health-Care Fraud and Abuse, Administrative Simplification, and Medical Liability Reform

HIPAA Privacy Rule. The HIPAA Standards for Privacy of Individually Identifiable Health Information provide the first comprehensive federal protection for the privacy of health information. The **Privacy Rule** is designed to provide strong privacy protections that do not interfere with patient access to health care or the quality of health-care delivery. This act creates, for the first time, national standards to protect individuals' medical records and other personal health information. The privacy rule is intended to:

- Give patients more control over their health information
- Set boundaries on the use and release of health-care records
- Establish appropriate safeguards that health-care providers and others must achieve to protect the privacy of health information
- Hold violators accountable, with civil and criminal penalties that can be imposed if they violate patients' privacy rights
- Strike a balance when public responsibility supports disclosure of some forms of data—for example, to protect public health

Before the HIPAA Privacy Rule, the personal information that moves across hospitals and doctors' offices, insurers or third-party payers, and state lines fell under a patchwork of federal and state laws. This information could be distributed—without either notice or authorization—for reasons that had nothing to do with a patient's medical treatment or health-care reimbursement. For example, unless otherwise forbidden by state or local law, without the Privacy Rule, patient information held by a health plan could, without the patient's permission, be passed on to a lender who could then deny the patient's application for a home mortgage or a credit card or could be given to an employer who could use it in personnel decisions.

Individually identifiable health information includes:

- Name
- Address
- Phone numbers
- Fax number
- Dates (birth, death, admission, discharge, etc.)
- Social Security number
- E-mail address
- Medical record numbers
- Health plan beneficiary numbers
- Account numbers
- Certificate or license numbers
- Vehicle identifiers and serial numbers, including license plate numbers
- Device identifiers and serial numbers
- Web Universal Resource Locators (URLs)
- Internet Protocol (IP) address numbers

The core of the HIPAA Privacy Rule is the protection, use, and disclosure of **protected health information (PHI).** Protected health information means individually identifiable health information that is transmitted or maintained by electronic or other media, such as computer storage devices. The Privacy Rule protects all PHI held or transmitted by a covered entity, which includes health-care providers, health plans, and health-care clearinghouses. Other covered entities include employers, life insurers, schools or universities, and public health authorities. Protected health information can come in any form or media, such as electronic, paper, or oral, including verbal communications among staff members, patients, and other providers. *Use* and *disclosure* are the two fundamental concepts in the HIPAA Privacy Rule. It is important to understand the differences between these terms.

Use. **Use** refers to performing any of the following actions to individually identifiable health information by employees or other members of an organization's workforce:

- Sharing
- Employing
- Applying
- Utilizing
- Examining
- Analyzing

Information is used when it moves within an organization.

Disclosure. **Disclosure** occurs when the entity holding the information performs any of the following actions so that the information is outside the entity:

- Releasing
- Transferring
- Providing access to
- Divulging in any manner

Information is disclosed when it is transmitted between or among organizations.

Under HIPAA, *use* limits the sharing of information within a covered entity, whereas *disclosure* restricts the sharing of information outside the entity holding the information.

The Privacy Rule covers the following PHI:

- The past, present, or future physical or mental health or condition of an individual
- Health care that is provided to an individual
- Billing or payments made for health care provided

Information that is not individually identifiable or unable to be tied to the identity of a particular patient is not subject to the Privacy Rule.

Managing and Storing Patient Information. Medical facilities have undergone many changes to the way they manage and store patient information. The Privacy Rule compliance was enforced in April of 2003. Many facilities contracted consultants that specialized in HIPAA and

became certified in HIPAA compliance. For the health-care provider, the Privacy Rule requires activities such as:

- Notifying patients of their privacy rights and how their information is used
- Adopting and implementing privacy procedures for its practice, hospital, or plan
- Training employees so that they understand the privacy procedures
- Designating an individual to be responsible for seeing that the privacy procedures are adopted and followed
- Securing patient records containing individually identifiable health information so that they are not readily available to those who do not need them

Under HIPAA, patients have an increased awareness of their health information privacy rights, which includes the following:

- The right to access, copy, and inspect their health-care information
- The right to request an amendment to their health-care information
- The right to obtain an accounting of certain disclosures of their health-care information
- The right to alternate means of receiving communications from providers
- The right to complain about alleged violations of the regulations and the provider's own information policies

Sharing Patient Information. When sharing patient information, HIPAA will allow the provider to use health-care information for **treatment, payment, and operations (TPO).**

- Treatment. Providers are allowed to share information in order to provide care to patients
- Payment. Providers are allowed to share information in order to receive payment for the treatment provided
- Operations. Providers are allowed to share information to conduct normal business activities, such as quality improvement

If the use of patient information does not fall under TPO, then written authorization must be obtained before sharing information with anyone.

Patient information may be disclosed without authorization to the following parties or in the following situations:

- Medical researchers
- Emergencies
- Funeral directors/coroners
- Disaster relief services
- Law enforcement
- Correctional institutions
- Abuse and neglect
- Organ and tissue donation centers

- Work-related conditions that may affect employee health
- Judicial/administrative proceedings at the patient's request or as directed by a subpoena or court order

When using or disclosing PHI, a provider must make reasonable efforts to limit the use or disclosure to the minimum amount of PHI necessary to accomplish the intended purpose. Providing only the minimum necessary information means taking reasonable safeguards to protect an individual's health information from incidental disclosure. State laws may impose more stringent requirements regarding the protection of patient information. Healthcare providers and staff should only have access to information they need to fulfill their assigned duties. The minimum necessary standard does not apply to disclosures, including oral disclosures, among health-care providers for treatment purposes. For example, a physician is not required to apply the minimum necessary standard when discussing a patient's medical chart information with a specialist at another hospital.

Patient Notification. Since the effective date of the HIPAA Privacy Rule, medical facilities have made major changes in how they inform patients of their HIPAA compliance. You may have noticed, as a patient yourself, the forms and information packets that are now provided by your health-care providers. The first step in informing patients of HIPAA compliance is the communication of patient rights. These rights are communicated through a document called **Notice of Privacy Practices (NPP).** A notice must:

- Be written in plain, simple language.
- Include a header that reads: "This Notice describes how medical information about you may be used and disclosed and how you can get access to this information. Please review carefully."
- Describe the covered entity's uses and disclosures of PHI
- Describe an individual's rights under the Privacy Rule.
- Describe the covered entity's duties.
- Describe how to register complaints concerning suspected privacy violations.
- Specify a point of contact
- Specify an effective date.
- State that the entity reserves to right to change its privacy practices.

The second step in patient notification is to implement a document that explains the policy of the medical facility on obtaining **authorization** for the use and disclosure of patient information for purposes other than TPO. The authorization form must be written in plain language. Some of the core elements of an authorization form include:

- Specific and meaningful descriptions of the authorized information

- Persons authorized to use or disclose protected health information
- Purpose of the requested information
- Statement of the patient's right to revoke the authorization
- Signature and date of the patient

Security Measures. Health-care facilities can undertake a number of measures in order to help reduce a breach of confidentiality, including for information that is either stored or delivered electronically (that is, stored in computers or computer networks, or delivered via computer networks or the Internet).

HIPAA Security Rule. In February 2003, the final regulations were issued regarding the administrative, physical, and technical safeguards to protect the confidentiality, integrity, and availability of health information covered by HIPAA. The **Security Rule** specifies how patient information is protected on computer networks, the Internet, disks, and other storage media and extranets. The rapidly increasing use of computers in health-care today has created new dangers for breaches of confidentiality. The Security Rule mandates that:

- A security officer must be assigned the responsibility for the medical facility's security
- All staff, including management, receives security awareness training
- Medical facilities must implement audit controls to record and examine staff who have logged into information systems that contain PHI
- Organizations limit physical access to medical facilities that contain electronic PHI
- Organizations must conduct risk analyses to determine information security risks and vulnerabilities
- Organizations must establish policies and procedures that allow access to electronic PHI on a need-to-know basis

Computers are not the only concern regarding security of the workplace. The facility layout can propose a possible violation if not designed correctly. All facilities must take measures to reduce the identity of patient information. Some examples of facility design that can help reduce a breach of confidentiality include the security of patient charts, the reception area, the clinical station, and faxes sent and received.

Chart Security. Patient charts can be kept confidential by following these rules:

- Charts that contain a patient's name or other identifiers cannot be in view at the front reception area or nurse's station. Some offices have placed charts in plain jackets to prevent information from being seen.
- Charts must be stored out of the view of a public area so that they cannot be seen by unauthorized individuals.

- Charts should be placed on the filing shelves without the patient name showing.
- Charts should be locked when not in use. Many facilities have purchased filing equipment that can be locked and unlocked without limiting the availability of patient information.
- Every staff member who uses patient information must be logged and a confidentiality statement signed. Signatures of staff should be on file with the office.

Reception Area Security. The following steps can be taken to secure the reception area:

- Log off or lock your computer or terminal, shutting off the monitor when leaving your terminal or computer.
- The computer must be placed in an area where other patients cannot see the screen.
- Many facilities are purchasing flat screen monitors to prevent visibility of the screen.
- The sign-in sheet must be monitored and not left out in patient view. The names of patients must be blacked out so the next patient cannot read the names. It is best to put another system in place and to eliminate the sign-in sheet.
- Many offices are reviewing the reception area with regard to phone conversations. Some offices are creating call centers away from the reception/waiting area.

Medical Assistant Clinical Station Security. Medical assistants should follow these guidelines to protect PHI at the clinical station:

- Log off or lock your terminal or computer turning your monitor off when leaving your terminal or computer.
- When placing charts in exam room racks or in shelves, the name of the patient or other identifiers must be concealed from other patients.
- HIPAA does not have a regulation about calling patients' names in the reception area, but to increase privacy in your facility, you may suggest a numbering system to identify patients.
- When discussing a patient with another staff member or with the physician, make sure your voice is lowered and that all doors to the exam rooms are closed. Avoid discussing patient conditions in heavy traffic areas.
- When discussing a condition with a patient, make sure that you are in a private room or area where no one can hear you.
- Avoid discussing patients in lunchrooms, hallways, or any place in a medical facility where someone can overhear you.

Fax Security. A lot of information is exchanged over the fax machine in a medical office. The fax machine is a vital link among physicians, hospitals, insurance companies, and other medical staff members. Private health information can be exchanged via faxes sent to covered entities.

Here are some recommendations to help safeguard information exchanged via fax machines:

- Fax cover page. State clearly on the fax cover sheet that confidential and protected health information is included. Further state that the information included is to be protected and must not be shared or disclosed without the appropriate authorizations from the patient.
- Location of the fax machine. Keep the fax machine in an area that is not accessible by individuals who are not authorized to view PHI.
- Faxes with protected health information. Faxes that your office receives with PHI must be stored promptly in a protected, secure area.
- Fax number. Always confirm the accuracy of fax numbers to minimize the possibility of faxes being sent to the wrong person. Call people to tell them the fax is being sent.
- Confirmation. Program the fax machine to print a confirmation for all faxes sent, and staple the confirmation sheet to each document sent.
- Training. Train all staff members to understand the importance of safeguarding PHI sent or received via fax.

Copier Security. Medical assistants should follow these guidelines to protect PHI at the copier:

- Do not leave confidential documents anywhere on the copier where others can read the information.
- Do not discard copies in a shared trash container—shred them.
- If a paper jam occurs, be sure to remove from the copier the copy or partial copy that caused the jam.

Printer Security. To maintain the confidentiality of printed materials, medical assistants should follow these guidelines:

- Do not print confidential material on a printer shared by other departments or in an area where others can read the material.
- Do not leave the printer unattended while printing confidential material.
- Before leaving the printing area, make sure all computer disks containing confidential information and all printed material have been collected.
- Be certain that the print job is sent to the right printer location.
- Do not discard printouts in a shared trash container—shred them.

Violations and Penalties. Every staff member is responsible for adhering to HIPAA privacy and security regulations to ensure that PHI is secure and confidential. Anyone who uses or shares patient information is ethically obligated to comply with HIPAA. If PHI is abused or confidentiality is breached, the medical facility can incur substantial penalties or even the incarceration of staff. Violations of HIPAA law can result in both civil and criminal penalties.

Civil Penalties. Civil penalties for HIPAA privacy violations can be up to $100 for each offense, with an annual cap of $25,000 for repeated violations of the same requirement.

Criminal Penalties. Criminal penalties for the knowing, wrongful misuse of individually identifiable health information can result in the following penalties:

- For the knowing misuse of individually identifiable health information: up to $50,000 and/or one year in prison.
- For misuse under false pretenses: up to $100,000 and/or 5 years in prison.
- For offenses to sell for profit or malicious harm: up to $250,000 and/or 10 years in prison.

Administrative Simplification. The main key to the set of rules established for HIPAA administrative simplification is standardizing patient information throughout the health-care system with a set of transaction standards and code sets. The codes and formats used for the exchange of medical data are referred to as **electronic transaction records**. Regulated transaction information is given a transaction set identifier. For example, a health-care professional claim would be given an identifier of ASC X12N 837. This is a standard transaction code given to any facility that submits a health-care claim to an insurance company.

Standardized code sets are used for encoding data elements. The following books are used for the standardized code sets for all health-care facilities:

- *ICD-9-CM*, Volumes 1 and 2. This book is used to identify diseases and conditions.
- *CPT 4*. This book is used to identify physician services or procedures.
- *HCPCS*. This book is used to identify health-related services and procedures, such as radiology or hearing and vision services that are not included in the CPT manual.

Frequently Asked Questions About HIPAA

1. May one physician's office send a patient's medical records to another physician's office without the patient's consent?

   Yes.

2. Does the HIPAA Privacy Rule prohibit or discourage doctor/patient e-mails?

   Health-care practitioners can continue to correspond with patients via e-mail, but appropriate electronic safeguards must be in place.

3. May a patient be listed in a hospital's directory without the patient's consent, and may the directory be shared with the public?

   The HIPAA Privacy Rule allows hospitals to continue providing directory information to the public unless the patient has specifically chosen not to be included. Hospital directories can include the patient's name, location in the facility, and general condition.

4. May a patient's family member pick up prescriptions for the patient?

   The Privacy Rule allows family members to pick up prescriptions, medical supplies, x-rays, or other similar forms of protected health information.

5. Is a hospital allowed to share patient information with the patient's family without the patient's expressed consent?

   HIPAA provides that a health-care provider may "disclose to a family member, other relative, or a close personal friend of the individual, or any other person identified by the individual" medical information directly relevant to such a person's involvement with the patient's care or payment related to the patient's care.

6. Can patients sue health-care providers who do not comply with the HIPAA Privacy Rule?

   The HIPAA Privacy Rule does not give patients the express right to sue. The patient can file a written complaint with the secretary of Health and Human Services (HHS) through the Office for Civil Rights. The HHS secretary then decides whether or not to investigate the complaint.

7. If a patient refuses to sign an acknowledgment stating that he or she received the health-care provider's notice of privacy practices, must the health-care provider refuse to provide services?

   The Privacy Rule gives the patient a "right of notice" of privacy practices for protecting identifiable health information. It requires that providers make a "good faith effort" to have patients acknowledge receipt of the notice, but the law does not give health-care practitioners the right to refuse treatment to people who do not sign the acknowledgment.

Risk Management

Risk management is the act or practice of controlling risk. This process includes identifying and tracking risk areas, developing risk improvement plans as part of risk handling, monitoring risks, and performing risk assessments to determine how risks have changed.

Proper documentation, patient satisfaction, appropriate behavior, proper medical procedures, and safeguards against exposure assist with decreasing the risk of malpractice lawsuits brought against the medical facility and their staff.

Confidentiality Issues and Mandatory Disclosure

Related to law, ethics, and quality care is the issue of when the medical assistant can disclose information and when it must be kept confidential. The incidents that doctors are legally required to report to the state were outlined earlier in the chapter. A doctor can be charged with criminal action for not following state and federal laws.

Ethics and professional judgment are always important. Consider the question of whether to contact the partners of a patient who has a sexually transmitted disease (STD) and whether to keep the patient's name from those people. The law says that the physician must instruct patients on how to notify possibly affected third parties and give them referrals to get the proper assistance. If the patient refuses to inform involved outside parties, then the doctor's office may offer to notify current and former partners. The Caution: Handle with Care section addresses this issue.

In general, the patient's ethical right to confidentiality and privacy is protected by law. Only the patient can waive the right to confidentiality. A physician cannot publicize a patient case in journal articles or invite other health professionals to observe a case without the patient's written consent. Most states also prohibit a doctor from testifying in court about a patient without the patient's approval. When a patient sues a physician, however, the patient automatically gives up the right to confidentiality.

Following are six principles for preventing improper release of information from the medical office.

1. When in doubt about whether to release information, it is better not to release it.
2. It is the patient's, not the doctor's, right to keep patient information confidential. If the patient wants to

---

CAUTION *Handle with Care*

Notifying Those at Risk for Sexually Transmitted Disease

Few things are more difficult for a patient with an STD than telling current and former partners about the diagnosis. In fact, some patients elect not to do so. When patients refuse to alert their partners, the medical office can offer to make those contacts. Often that responsibility lies with the medical assistant.

You are most likely to encounter such a situation if you are a medical assistant working in a family practice, an obstetrics/gynecology practice, or a clinic. Becoming familiar with all facets of the situation—from ensuring patient confidentiality to handling potentially difficult confrontations—will help you best serve the patient.

The first step is to get the appropriate information from the patient who has contracted the STD. Because the patient may be sensitive about revealing former and current partners, help him feel more comfortable. First, spend some time talking about the STD. How much does the patient know about it? Educate him about implications, including the probable short- and long-term effects of the disease. Explain how the STD is transmitted. Alert the patient as to precautions to take so he will not continue to transmit the disease to others. Help the patient understand why it is important for people who may have contracted the disease from him to be told they may have it.

Then, offer to contact the patient's former and current partners. Fully explain each step in the notification process, assuring the patient that his name will not be revealed under any circumstances. Answer any questions and address any concerns about the notification process. If the patient is still reluctant to provide information, give him some time to think about it away from the office, and follow up periodically with a phone call.

Once the patient agrees to reveal names, write down the names and other information, and preferably phone numbers. To make sure you have correct information, read it back to the patient, spelling each person's name in turn and reciting the phone number or address. Write down the phonetic pronunciations of any difficult names. Tell the patient when you will make the notifications.

You now are ready to contact these individuals. Professionals who work with STD patients recommend guidelines for contacting current and former partners to alert them about potential exposure to an STD. Note that these guidelines are applicable only to STDs other than AIDS.

Determine how you will contact each individual: in writing, in person, or by phone.

1. If you use U.S. mail, mark the outside of the addressed envelope "Personal." On a note inside, simply ask the person to call you at the medical office. Do not put the topic of the call in writing.

continued ⟶

Legal and Ethical Issues in Medical Practice, Including HIPAA

CAUTION *Handle with Care*

Notifying Those at Risk for Sexually Transmitted Disease *(concluded)*

2. If you make the contact in person, ask where you can talk privately. Even if the person appears to be alone, others may still be able to overhear the conversation.

3. If you use the phone, identify yourself and your office, and ask for the specific individual. Do not reveal the nature of your call to anyone but that person. If pressed, tell the person who answers the phone that you are calling regarding a personal matter.

Once on the phone or alone with the person, confirm that you are talking to the correct person. Mention that you wish to talk about a highly personal matter, and ask if it is a good time to continue the discussion. If not, arrange for a more appropriate time.

Inform the individual that she has come in contact with someone who has an STD. Recommend that the person visit a doctor's office or clinic to be tested for the disease.

Be prepared for a variety of reactions, from surprise to anger. Respond calmly and coolly. Expect to respond to questions and statements such as:

- Who gave you my name?
- Do I have the disease?
- Am I really at risk? I haven't had intercourse recently (or) I've only had intercourse with my spouse.

- I feel fine. I just went to my doctor recently.

Let the person know that you cannot reveal the name of the partner because the information is strictly confidential. Assure the person that you will not reveal her name to anyone either.

Explain that exposure to the disease does not mean a person has contracted it. Encourage the person to get tested to know for sure.

Tell the person that she is still at risk, even if she hasn't had intercourse recently or has had it only with a spouse. Let the person know that someone with whom she came in close contact at some point has contracted the disease.

Even if the person says, "I feel fine," she may still have the disease. Again, stress the importance of getting tested.

Provide your name and phone number for contact about further questions. Recommend local offices and clinics for testing, and provide phone numbers. If the person will come to your office, offer to make the appointment.

Finally, document the results of your call. Log in the original patient's file the date that you completed notification. Include any pertinent details about the notification. Alert the patient when all people on the list have been notified.

---

disclose the information, it is unethical for the physician not to do so.

3. All patients should be treated with the same degree of confidentiality, whatever the health-care professional's personal opinion of the patient might be.

4. You should be aware of all applicable laws and of the regulations of agencies such as public health departments.

5. When it is necessary to break confidentiality and when there is a conflict between ethics and confidentiality, discuss it with the patient. If the law does not dictate what to do in the situation, the attending physician should make the judgment based on the urgency of the situation and any danger that might be posed to the patient or others.

6. Get written approval from the patient before releasing information. For common situations, the patient should sign a standard release-of-records form.

The AMA has several standard forms for authorization of disclosure and includes disclosure clauses in many other forms. For example, the consent-to-surgery form includes a clause about consenting to picture taking and observation during the surgery. When using a standard form, cross out anything that does not apply in that particular situation. Medical practices often develop their own customized forms.

Code of Ethics

Medical ethics is a vital part of medical practice and following an ethical code is an important part of your job. Ethics deals with general principles of right and wrong, as opposed to requirements of law. A professional is expected to act in ways that reflect society's ideas of right and wrong, even if such behavior is not enforced by law. Often, however, the law is based on ethical considerations.

Bioethics: Social Issues

Bioethics deals with issues that arise related to medical advances. Here are three examples of bioethical issues.

1. A treatment for Parkinson disease was developed that uses fetal tissue. Some women, upon learning about this treatment, might get pregnant just to have an abortion and sell the fetal tissue. Is this ethical?

2. If a couple cannot have a baby because of a medical condition of the mother, using a surrogate mother is an option some couples choose. The surrogate mother is artificially inseminated with the sperm of the husband and carries the baby to term. The couple then raises the child. Ethically speaking, who is the real mother, the woman who bears the child or the woman who raises the child? If the surrogate mother wants to keep the baby after it is born, does she have a right to do so?

3. When a liver transplant is needed by both a famous patient who has had a history of alcohol abuse and a woman who is a recipient of public assistance, what criteria are considered when determining who receives the organ? Who makes the decision? Ethically, treating physicians should not make the decision of allocating limited medical resources. Decisions regarding the allocation of limited medical resources should consider only the likelihood of benefit, the urgency of need, and the amount of resources required for successful treatment. Nonmedical criteria such as ability to pay, age, social worth, perceived obstacles to treatment, patient's contribution to illness, or the past use of resources should not be considered.

Practicing appropriate professional ethics has a positive impact on your reputation and the success of your employer's business. Many medical organizations, therefore, have created guidelines for the acceptable and preferred manners and behaviors, or etiquette, of medical assistants and physicians.

The principles of medical ethics have developed over time. The Hippocratic oath, in which medical students pledge to practice medicine ethically, was developed in ancient Greece (see http://wikipedia.org/wiki/Hippocratic_Oath). It is still used today and is one of the original bases of modern medical ethics. Hippocrates, the 4th century BC Greek physician commonly called the "father of medicine," is traditionally considered the author of this oath, but its authorship is actually unknown.

Among the promises of the Hippocratic oath are to use the form of treatment believed to be best for the patient, to refrain from harmful actions, and to keep a patient's private information confidential.

The AMA defines ethical behavior for doctors in *Code of Medical Ethics: Current Opinions with Annotations* (Chicago: American Medical Association, 1996). Medical assistants as well as doctors need to be aware of these principles.

A physician shall be dedicated to providing competent medical service with compassion and respect for human dignity.

This concept means that medical professionals will respect all aspects of the patient as a person, including intellect and emotions. The doctor must decide what treatment would result in the best, most dignified quality of life for the patient, and the doctor must respect a patient's choice to forgo treatment.

A physician shall deal honestly with patients and colleagues and strive to expose those physicians deficient in character or competence or who engage in fraud or deception.

Medical professionals, including medical assistants, should respect colleagues, but they must also respect and protect the profession and public welfare enough to report colleagues who are breaking the law, acting unethically, or unable to perform competently. Dilemmas may arise where one suspects, but is not able to prove, for instance, that a coworker has a substance abuse problem or another problem that is affecting performance. Ignoring such a situation in medical practice could cost someone's life as well as lead to lawsuits.

In terms of billing, a doctor should bill only for direct services, not for indirect ones, such as referrals. The doctor also should not bill for services that do not really pertain to the practice of medicine, such as dispensing drugs.

It is also unethical for the doctor to influence the patient about where to fill prescriptions or obtain other medical services when the doctor has a personal financial interest in any of the choices.

A physician shall respect the law and also recognize a responsibility to seek changes in requirements that are contrary to the patient's best interests.

Several legal or employer requirements have come under scrutiny as being contrary to a patient's best interests. Among them are discharging patients from the hospital after a certain time limit for certain procedures, which may be too soon for many patients. Insurance company payment policies have sometimes been criticized as unfair. So have health maintenance organization (HMO) financial policies that may conflict with a doctor's preference in treatment.

A physician shall respect the rights of patients, of colleagues, and of other health professionals and shall safeguard patient confidences within the constraints of law.

A document called the Patient's Bill of Rights (which has now been replaced with the Patient Care Partnership: Understanding Expectations, Rights, and Responsibilities), established by the American Hospital Association in 1973 and revised in 1992, lists ethical principles protecting the patient. Some states have even passed this code of ethics into law. Among a patient's rights are the right to information about alternative treatments, the right to refuse to participate in research projects, and the right to privacy.

Points on Practice

AAMA Code of Ethics

The Code of Ethics of the AAMA shall set forth principles of ethical and moral conduct as they relate to the medical profession and the particular practice of medical assisting.

Members of the AAMA dedicated to the conscientious pursuit of their profession, and thus desiring to merit the high regard of the entire medical profession and the respect of the general public which they serve, do pledge themselves to strive always to:

A. Render service with full respect for the dignity of humanity

B. Respect confidential information obtained through employment unless legally authorized

or required by responsible performance of duty to divulge such information

C. Uphold the honor and high principles of the profession and accept its disciplines

D. Seek to continually improve the knowledge and skills of medical assistants for the benefit of patients and professional colleagues

E. Participate in additional service activities aimed toward improving the health and wellbeing of the community

---

A physician shall continue to study; apply and advance scientific knowledge; make relevant information available to patients, colleagues, and the public; obtain consultation; and use the talents of other health professionals when indicated.

Keeping up with the latest advancements in medicine is crucial for providing high-quality, ethical care. Most states require doctors to accumulate "continuing education units" to maintain a license to practice. These units are earned by means of educational activities such as courses and scientific meetings. The AAMA requires medical assistants to renew their certification every 5 years, by either accumulating continuing education credits through the AAMA or retaking the certification examination.

A physician shall, in the provision of appropriate patient care, except in emergencies, be free to choose whom to serve, with whom to associate, and the environment in which to provide medical services.

Ethically, doctors can set their hours, decide what kind of medicine to practice and where, decide whom to accept as a patient, and take time off as long as a qualified substitute performs their duties. Doctors may decline to accept new patients because of a full workload. In an emergency, however, a doctor may be ethically obligated to care for a patient, even if the patient is not of the doctor's choosing. The doctor should not abandon that patient until another physician is available.

A physician shall recognize a responsibility to participate in activities contributing to an improved community. This ethical obligation holds true for the allied health professions as well.

In addition to knowing the physician's codes of ethics, medical assistants should follow the AAMA's Code of Ethics (see the Points on Practice box).

Labor and Employment Laws

More often than not, medical assistants often find themselves in a supervisory or management role within the medical office. It is not uncommon for a medical assistant to become promoted to an office manager within a medical facility, sometimes in a short period of time after initial employment. It is important to know certain employment and labor laws in order to perform the managerial tasks within legal and ethical guidelines.

Title VII of the Civil Rights Act of 1964

This act applies to businesses with 15 or more employees working at least 20 weeks of the year. The law prevents employers from discriminating in hiring or firing or firing on the basis of race, color, religion, sex, or national origin. Some states have laws that also prohibit **discrimination** based on marital status, parenthood, mental health, mental retardation, sexual orientation, personal appearance, or political affiliation. Title VII also addresses and defines sexual harassment.

Sexual Harassment

Sexual harassment occurs in a variety of circumstances, and anyone may be sexually harassed. A man or a woman may be the victim or harasser, and the victim does not have to be the opposite sex. The victim may be the person being harassed or even a coworker who overhears the harassment. The victim has the responsibility to let the harasser know that the conduct is offensive. The victim should also report any instance of sexual harassment to a supervisor or personnel department. A formal definition of sexual harassment is as follows:

> Unwelcome sexual advances, requests for sexual favors, and other verbal or physical conduct of a sexual nature . . . when submission to such conduct is made either explicitly or implicitly a term or condition of an individual's employment, submission to or rejection of such conduct by an individual is used as the basis for employment decisions affecting such individual, or such conduct has the purpose or effect of unreasonably interfering with an individual's work performance or creating an intimidating, hostile, or offensive working environment. (Lindgren and Taub, 1993)

Age Discrimination in Employment Act (ADEA) of 1967

This act applies to businesses with 20 or more employees working at least 20 weeks of the year. It prohibits discrimination in hiring or firing based on age for persons aged 40 or older.

1976 Pregnancy Discrimination Act

This is an amendment to Title VII of the Civil Rights Act that makes it illegal to fire an employee based on pregnancy, childbirth, or related medical conditions.

The Civil Rights Act of 1991

This act provides monetary damages in cases of intentional employment discrimination.

Titles I and III of the Americans with Disabilities Act of 1990

This act applies to all employers with 15 or more employees working at least 20 weeks during the year. Titles I and III of the act ban discrimination against disabled persons in the workplace, mandate equal access for the disabled to certain public facilities, and require all commercial firms to make existing facilities and grounds more accessible to the disabled.

1938 Fair Labor Standards Act

This act prohibits child labor and the firing of employees for exercising their rights under the act's wage and hour standards. It also provides for overtime pay and a minimum wage. New Fair Pay regulations under the act went into effect on August 23, 2004. The new rules guarantee overtime protection to workers earning less that $23,600 annually and continue exemptions of the overtime rule for certain "learned professional employees." Some nurses may receive overtime pay, depending on how they are paid—hourly or salary—and LPNs and other similar health-care employees are guaranteed overtime pay under the new Fair Pay regulations.

Equal Pay Act of 1963

As an amendment to the Fair Labor Standards Act, this act requires equal pay for men and women doing equal work.

Family Leave Act of 1991

This act applies to employers with 50 or more employees. It mandates allowing employees to take unpaid leave time for maternity, for adoption, or for caring for ill family members. This law has many restrictions. Go to www.fmlaonline.com for further information.

Legal Medical Practice Models

There are five basic types of medical practice:

- Sole proprietorship
- Partnership
- Group practice
- Professional corporation
- Clinics

Laws governing the various types of practice vary, but medical office personnel should be aware of the laws that apply to their employers' practice management models.

Sole Proprietorship

This type of practice is often referred to as a "solo practice." In this type of practice, a physician practicing alone assumes all the benefits for and liabilities of the business. **Sole proprietorship** practice management is not a popular option as a result of the increased expenses and decreased insurance reimbursements. Therefore, more physicians are joining group practices or professional corporations.

Partnership

When two or more physicians decide to practice together, they may form a **partnership,** based on a legal contract that specifies the rights, obligations, and responsibilities of each partner. Advantages of partnerships include sharing the workload, expenses, profits, and assets. A disadvantage is that each partner has equal liability for acts of misconduct, losses, and deficits of the practice, unless specified as a contingency in the contract.

Group Practice

Group practice is a medical practice model in which three or more licensed physicians share the collective income, expenses, facilities, equipment, records, and personnel for the practice. Physicians in group practice may be engaged in the same specialty, calling themselves, for example, Associates in Cardiology, or they can be several physicians offering similar specialties, such as ob/gyn and pediatrics.

Professional Corporations

A **corporation** is a body formed and authorized by state law to act as a single entity. Physicians who form corporations are shareholders and employees of the organization. There are financial and tax advantages to forming a corporation and the fringe benefits for employees may be greater than in a sole proprietorship or partnership.

In forming a corporation, the incorporators and owners have limited liability in case lawsuits are filed. Sometimes medical practices are "managed" by forprofit corporations that are either formed by outside business interests or subsidiary corporations organized by hospitals. Physicians are hired as salaried employees with bonus options. The management corporation provides the facility, office personnel, employee benefits, human resource services, and operating expenses.

Clinics

Patients can be admitted to clinics for special circumstances and research. Clinics are hard to distinguish from large medical facilities.

Clinics are broad in their range of specialties and subspecialties. They often have sophisticated medical equipment and renowned medical practitioners. Clinics may be housed inside of a hospital or may be free-standing. Urgent care centers, also known as walk-in clinics, exist so that patients will have the option of being seen without an appointment.

In-store clinics are becoming more prevalent. They are housed in large major chain stores, and sometimes in chain pharmacies. They offer smaller medical services such as vaccinations, flu shots, and eye exams. These types of clinics are quickly emerging.

Summary

3.1 Ethics deals with general principles of right and wrong. Allied health professionals are expected to do the right thing in all aspects. Bioethics arise from issues that deal with medical advances (e.g., stem cell research) in which medical laws are sometimes questioned and come under scrutiny.

3.2 The Four Cs of medical malpractice are (1) caring about your patients and colleagues, (2) communicating clearly and professionally, (3) being competent in your skills and job knowledge, and (4) charting properly; this is proof of competence.

3.3 Medical documentation is essential. Improper documentation can contribute to or cause a medical liability case to be lost.

3.4 Federal legislation affects health care. Two of the most important laws that have been passed are the Healthcare Quality Improvement Act of 1986 and the Federal False Claims Act.

3.5 OSHA regulations state that the medical assistants must (a) have protective gear, (b) know how to properly decontaminate, (c) know how to dispose properly of sharp equipment, (d) notify officials of exposure incidents, (e) have post-exposure evaluation and follow-up procedures in case they have been exposed to infections, (f) know how to handle potentially infectious laundry, (g) be informed about hazardous substances in the workplace through MSDS, and (h) be given free information and training at least once a year on OSHA regulations.

3.6 HIPAA (Health Insurance Portability and Accountability Act) regulations have a great impact in the medical office today because they address issues such as health-care fraud and abuse, medical liability reform, and standardizing patient information throughout the health-care system.

3.7 Six principles are crucial for protecting patients' confidentiality and avoiding lawsuits. They are (a) treat all patients with the same degree of confidentiality; (b) discuss situations with patients when it is necessary to break confidentiality; (c) get written approval from patients to release their information; (d) be aware of all applicable laws; (e) when in doubt, do not release information; and (f) remember that it is the patient's right to keep information confidential, not the physician's.

3.8 There are five basic types of practice management models: (a) sole proprietorship (one physician); (b) partnership (two or more physicians); (c) group practice (three or more physicians); (d) professional corporation (a body formed and authorized by state law to act as a single entity; physicians are stakeholders and employees of the organization); and (f) clinics.

CASE STUDY QUESTIONS

Now that you have completed this chapter, review the case study at the beginning of the chapter and answer the following questions:

1. Does the medical assistant's comment represent a breach of confidentiality?
2. Has any HIPAA rule been violated? If so, which one?

Multiple-Choice Questions

1. A standard of conduct that is generally accepted as a moral guide for moral values for behavior is
   a. civil law.
   b. professional medical ethics.
   c. medical etiquette.
   d. classification of law.
2. The two types of law that pertain to health-care professionals are
   a. contract law and agency law.
   b. civil law and criminal law.
   c. civil law and medical law.
   d. litigation and malpractice.
3. The main federal legislations that affect health care are
   a. OSHA regulations and HIPAA.
   b. the Healthcare Quality Improvement Act of 1986 and the Federal False Claims Act.
   c. HIPAA and Mandatory Disclosures.
   d. ADEA of 1987 and the Fair Labor Standards Act.
4. The Controlled Substance Act (CSA) of 1970 maintains that medical facilities keep drugs under close control, and they list them in _____ categories
   a. two   c. ten
   b. five   d. seven
5. Informed consent requires that the patient understand
   a. the proposed treatment modes.
   b. the risks of alternative treatment.
   c. the risks involved in the proposed treatment.
   d. all of the above.

Discussion Questions

1. How does the law of agency make it possible for a patient to sue both the medical assistant and the physician for an act of negligence committed by the medical assistant?

2. Under HIPAA, what rights do patients have regarding confidentiality and ownership of their medical records? When does a patient give up the right to confidentiality?
3. How can you prove that the patient gave informed consent?
4. What are two scenarios that would void a contract between physician and patient?
5. Why can't patients schedule appointments at any time of the day?

Critical Thinking Questions

1. What is an example of a bioethical issue? Give two opposing views of the issue.
2. Explain why a medical record entry that is corrected improperly could damage a malpractice suit against the physician.
3. Describe implied consent and two ways that a patient can accept treatment by implied consent.
4. Discuss the "implied" contract between a physician and a patient.

Application Activities

When completing these activities, search the Internet for your choice of topics.

1. Research a controversial topic from the following list:
   - Euthanasia
   - Surrogacy
   - Abortion
   - Fetal stem cell research
   - Cloning
   - Emergency contraceptive (morning-after pill)

   Write a three-page report that presents both the pro side and the con side of the issue. Write a closing paragraph that gives your personal opinion and views and how you have been conditioned in that belief, for example, social, cultural, and religious beliefs.
2. Choose teams of four people, and stage debates on the controversial topics listed in question 1. Research your topics thoroughly and present arguments on both sides. Your purpose is to state facts and persuade your audience to your beliefs.
   Rules for the debate:
   - Participants must be courteous and professional
   - Presentations must be factual
   - Opening arguments are four minutes for each side

- Each side presents, and then for three minutes each side is allowed to counter any fact
- Closing arguments are five minutes for each side

Have the class vote on which side was more persuasive.

3. In a medical law textbook or journal, research a malpractice case. Prepare a 10-minute presentation for the class in which you summarize both sides of the case (patient and caregiver). Include when and where the case took place. Explain how the case was settled and whether the settlement took place in a court of law or through arbitration. Close with your opinion about whether the case was settled fairly.

4. Research a piece of legislation on a health-care issue or practice, either a bill passed in the last 5 years or a bill currently being considered in Washington. What impact has this bill had or might this bill have on the medical assisting profession? Summarize your findings in a oneto two-page report.

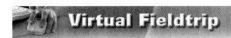

Virtual Fieldtrip

Visit the McGraw-Hill Higher Education Medical Assisting website at www.mhhe.com/medicalassisting4e to complete the following activity:

As a medical assistant, it is imperative to be knowledgeable about your state regulations regarding medical assisting practice. Research the scope of practice for the state where you will work. The AAMA and American Medical Technologists are good resources for this information. Prepare a one-page summary and share your research with your classmates.

Open the CD and complete this chapter's practice activities, play the games, listen to the key terms, and test yourself with the interactive review. E-mail, print, and/or save your results to document your proficiency.

Communication with Patients, Families, and Coworkers

MEDICAL ASSISTING COMPETENCIES

CAAHEP

Cognitive (Knowledge Base)

Concepts of Effective Communications

IV. C (1) Identify styles and types of verbal communication

IV. C (2) Identify nonverbal communication

IV. C (3) Recognize communication barriers

IV. C (4) Identify techniques for overcoming communication barriers

IV. C (7) Identify resources and adaptations that are required based on individual needs, i.e., culture and environment, developmental life stage, language, and physical threats to communication

IV. P (1) Use reflection, restatement, and clarification techniques to obtain a patient history

IV. P (2) Report relevant information to others succinctly and accurately

IV. P (12) Develop and maintain a current list of community resources related to patients' health-care needs

IV. P (13) Advocate on behalf of patients

IV. A (1) Demonstrate empathy in communicating with patients, family, and staff

IV. A (2) Apply active listening skills

IV. A (3) Use appropriate body language and other nonverbal skills in communicating with patients, family, and staff

(continued)

ABHES

5. Psychology of Human Relations

a. Define and understand abnormal behavior patterns

b. Identify and respond appropriately when working/caring for patients with special needs

c. Use empathy with treating terminally ill patients

d. Identify common stages that terminally ill patients go through and list organizations/support groups that can assist patients and family members of patients struggling with terminal illness

e. Advocate on behalf of family/patients, having ability to deal and communicate with family

f. Identify and discuss developmental stages of life

g. Analyze the effect of hereditary, cultural, and environmental influences

8. Medical Office Business Procedures Management

cc. Communicate on the recipient's level of comprehension

dd. Serve as liaison between physician and others

ii. Recognize and respond to verbal and non-verbal communication

LEARNING OUTCOMES

After completing Chapter 4, you will be able to:

4.1 Identify elements of the communication circle.

4.2 Describe and define the developmental stages of the life cycle.

4.3 Model examples of positive and negative communication.

4.4 Model ways to improve listening and interpersonal skills.

4.5 Model the difference between assertiveness and aggressiveness.

4.6 Model examples of effective communication strategies with patients in special circumstances.

4.7 Carry out ways to establish positive communication with coworkers and management.

(continued)

4.8 Describe how the office policy and procedures manual is used as a communication tool in the medical office.

4.9 Explain community resources and how they enhance the services provided by your office.

4.10 Differentiate how stress relates to communication and identify strategies to reduce stress.

MEDICAL ASSISTING COMPETENCIES *(concluded)*

CAAHEP	ABHES
IV. A (4) Demonstrate awareness of the territorial boundaries of the person with whom communicating **IV. A (7)** Demonstrate recognition of the patient's level of understanding in communications **IV. A (8)** Analyze communications in providing appropriate responses/feedback **VII. A (2)** Demonstrate sensitivity in communicating with both providers and patients **VII. A (3)** Communicate in language the patient can understand regarding managed care and insurance plans **IX. A (1)** Demonstrate sensitivity to patient rights **X. A (1)** Recognize the effects of stress on all persons involved in emergency situations **X. A (2)** Demonstrate self-awareness in responding to emergency situations	**9. Medical Office Clinical Procedures** 　p. Advise patients of office policies and procedures **11. Career Development** Demonstrate professionalism by: 2) Exhibiting a positive attitude and a sense of responsibility 3) Maintaining confidentiality at all times 4) Being cognizant of ethical boundaries 5) Exhibiting initiative 6) Adapting to change 7) Expressing a responsible attitude 8) Being courteous and diplomatic 9) Conducting work within scope of education, training, and ability

MEDICAL ASSISTING MEDIA

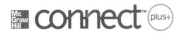 **Connect Plus+™**
connect.mcgraw-hill.com

- Elecronic Health Records (E.H.R.) SpringCharts®
- eBook

SpringCharts®
Electronic Health Records

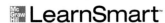 **LearnSmart™**

www.mhhe.com/learnsmart

Complete Learning Module: Communication with Patients, Families, and Coworkers

---

 Student CD-ROM

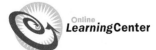 **Online Learning Center™**

www.mhhe.com/medicalassisting4e

KEY TERMS

active listening	burnout	hierarchy	passive listening
aggressive	closed posture	homeostasis	personal space
assertive	conflict	hospice	rapport
body language	empathy	interpersonal skills	
boundaries	feedback	open posture	

CHAPTER OUTLINE

- Communicating with Patients and Families
- The Communication Circle
- Understanding Human Behavior and How It Relates to the Provider-Patient Relationship
- Types of Communication
- Improving Your Communication Skills

- Communicating in Special Circumstances
- Communicating with Coworkers
- Written Communication Tools and Community Resources
- Personnel Management
- Managing Stress
- Preventing Burnout

PREPARATION FOR CERTIFICATION

RMA (AMT) Exam
- Interpersonal skills
- Cultural diversity
- Oral and written communication

CMA (AAMA) Exam
- Recognizing and responding to verbal and written communication
- Patient interviewing techniques
- Professional communication and behavior

CMAS Exam
- Communication
- Professionalism

Introduction

The ability to recognize human behaviors and the ability to communicate effectively are vital to a medical assistant and the pursuit for success. This chapter has taken a psychological approach to understanding human behavior and the challenges that influence therapeutic communication in a health-care setting. Patients will often have more interaction with the medical assistant than with any other health-care practitioner in the facility. It is important that patients develop a good rapport and feel confident in the care they are receiving from your office. The medical assistant sets the tone for the communication cycle and must be aware of all the obstacles that can affect human communication. As a medical assistant, you are often exposed to all kinds of patients. You will see patients from different cultures, socioeconomic backgrounds, educational levels, ages, and lifestyles. You must be able to communicate with each patient with professionalism and diplomacy.

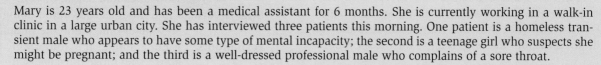

CASE STUDY

Mary is 23 years old and has been a medical assistant for 6 months. She is currently working in a walk-in clinic in a large urban city. She has interviewed three patients this morning. One patient is a homeless transient male who appears to have some type of mental incapacity; the second is a teenage girl who suspects she might be pregnant; and the third is a well-dressed professional male who complains of a sore throat.

As you read this chapter, consider how you would answer the following questions relative to each of the patients:

1. How will Mary adapt her communication style to communicate with each patient?
2. What types of communication roadblocks will she encounter with each one?
3. What types of communication techniques will she use for each patient?

Communicating with Patients and Families

Think about the last time you had a doctor's appointment. How well did the staff and physicians communicate with you? Were you greeted cordially and pleasantly invited to take a seat, or did someone thrust a clipboard at you and say, "Fill this out"? If you had a long wait in the reception area or examination room, did someone come in to explain the delay? Did you become frustrated and angry because nobody told you what was happening?

As a medical assistant, you are a key communicator between the office and patients and families. The way you greet patients, explain procedures, ask and answer questions, and attend to the individual needs of patients forms your communication style. Your interaction with the patient sets the tone for the office visit and can significantly influence how comfortable the patient feels in your practice. Developing strong communication skills in the medical office is just as important as mastering administrative and clinical tasks.

Customer service is the most important part of communication to families and patients. Your mastery of clinical and administrative skills is only a portion of your skills; customer service and communication skills are the other 70%.

A definition of customer service includes the following two points:

1. The patient comes first
2. Patient needs are satisfied

In today's health-care environment, patients are consumers and are more educated than ever before. Patients have more options in choosing a physician or a health-care facility. Patients who feel that they were not given exceptional customer service will choose another physician or facility to meet their needs. Another reason a facility must strive for exceptional customer service is that a medical facility grows rapidly from referral business. A medical facility that acquires a reputation for having an "unfriendly" staff will feel the negative impact from that reputation.

Listed here are some examples of customer service in the physician's office:

- Using proper telephone techniques
- Writing or responding to telephone messages
- Explaining procedures to patients
- Expediting insurance referral requests
- Assisting with billing issues
- Answering questions or finding answers to patient questions
- Ensuring that patients are comfortable in your office
- Creating a warm and reassuring environment

From a business perspective, exceptional customer service is vital to a medical facility's success. Any business that does not provide exceptional customer service will not grow and thrive in today's business economy.

The Communication Circle

As you interact with patients and their families, you will be responsible for giving information and ensuring that the patient understands what you, the doctor, and other members of the staff have communicated. You will also be responsible for receiving information from the patient. For example, patients will describe their symptoms. They may also discuss their feelings or ask questions about a treatment or procedure. The giving and receiving of information forms the communication circle.

Elements of the Communication Circle

The communication circle involves three elements: a message, a source, and a receiver. Messages are usually verbal

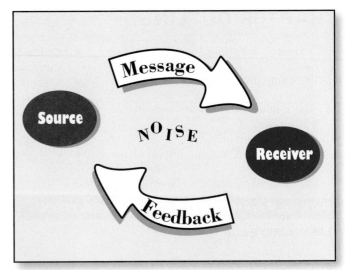

Figure 4-1. The process of communication involves an exchange of messages through verbal and nonverbal means.

or written. (As you will see later in the chapter, some messages are nonverbal.) The source sends the message, and the receiver receives it. The communication circle is formed as the source sends a message to the receiver and the receiver responds (Figure 4-1).

Consider this example, in which Fernando, a medical assistant who works in a physical therapy office, is speaking with Mrs. Riveria, a patient who is having therapy for a back injury. Watch the communication circle at work.

Fernando: The physical therapist says you're making great progress and that you can start on some simple back exercises at home. I'd like to go over them with you. Then I'll give you a sheet that illustrates the exercises. How does that sound to you?

Mrs. Riveria: I'm a little nervous about doing exercises. I still have some pain when I bend over.

Fernando: I understand. It's important, though, to start using those muscles again. Why don't you show me exactly where it hurts. Then we can go over proper body mechanics, such as bending down to pick something up and getting in and out of chairs, the car, and bed. Then we'll just start with one or two of the exercises and save the rest for next time, when you're feeling more ready.

Mrs. Riveria: Yes, I only feel up to doing a little bit today.

The medical assistant (the source) gives a verbal message (about back exercises) to the patient (the receiver). The patient responds by drawing attention to her pain and uneasiness about certain movements. The patient's response is also a message to the medical assistant, who responds in turn. The giving and receiving of information continues within the communication circle until the exchange is finished.

Feedback.   Another word for response is **feedback,** which is verbal or nonverbal evidence that the receiver got and understood the message. When you communicate information to a patient or ask a patient a question, always look for feedback. For example, if you calculate a pregnant patient's due date and tell her she's 12 weeks pregnant, look for a response. If she responds, "Oh, good, that means I'm out of danger of having a miscarriage," you would respond that whereas most miscarriages occur in the first 12 weeks, some risk of miscarriage remains throughout the pregnancy. If she responds, "I thought I was 14 weeks pregnant," you would need to clarify how you worked out your calculation and compare it with hers, to uncover any discrepancy. Good communication in the medical office requires patient feedback at every step.

Noise.   Anything that distorts the message in any way or interferes with the communication process can be referred to as noise. Noise refers not only to sounds, such as a siren or jackhammer on the street below the medical office suite. It also refers to room temperature and other types of physical comfort or discomfort, such as pain, and to emotions, such as fear or sadness. If patients are feeling uncomfortable in a chilly or hot room, upset about their illness, or in great pain, they may not pay close attention to what you are saying. Conversely, if you are feeling upset about a personal problem outside work or if you are unwell or preoccupied with all the things you have on your to-do list, you may not communicate well.

As you deal with each patient, try to screen out or eliminate both literal and figurative noise. For example, before you start a conversation with a patient in an examination room, you might ask, "Are you too chilly or too warm? Is the temperature in here comfortable for you?" If there is construction going on outside the building, see if there is a less noisy inner room or office that you might be able to use. If a patient seems nervous or upset, address those feelings before you launch into a factual discussion.

If you are feeling stressed or out of sorts, that feeling constitutes a type of noise. Try to take a "breather" between patients or a break from desk work—walk downstairs, get some fresh air, stretch your legs. Feeling dehydrated or hungry affects your communication efforts too. Limit your caffeine and sugar intake. Drink plenty of water and juice throughout the day. Eat a good lunch and healthful snacks. Leave your personal problems at home.

Humanizing the Communication Process in the Medical Office.   As highly structured managed care organizations and technological advances rapidly change the face of health care, many patients feel that health care is becoming impersonal. Every time you communicate with patients, you can counteract this perception by playing a humanistic role in the health-care process. Being humanistic means that you work to help patients feel attended to and respected as individuals, not just as descriptions in a chart. Good communication supports this patient-centered approach.

Make a point of developing and using strong communication skills to show patients that you, the doctors, and other staff members care about them and their feelings. Taking care to treat patients as people helps humanize the communication process in the medical office.

Understanding Human Behavior and How It Relates to the Provider-Patient Relationship

Understanding human behavior is important when you are communicating with patients. Medical assistants are exposed to many different personality types in addition to different illnesses. When you understand why a person is behaving in a certain way, you can adjust your communication style to adapt to that person.

The Developmental Stages of the Life Cycle

As a professional medical assistant, it is important to understand human growth and development. This understanding will enable you to enhance your communication skills, such as patient education, with patients of all age groups, cultures, and religions. Human growth is not only about the physical development of your patients, but about their psychological and emotional growth as well. Many scientists and behaviorists have studied and researched the developmental stages of human life and have developed guidelines to assist us in our patient communication skills. Table 4-1 is an example of a Lifespan Development model created by Erik Erikson (1902–1994). He is best known for his personality development research regarding children.

Maslow's Hierarchy of Human Needs

Abraham Maslow, a well-known human behaviorist, developed a model of human behavior known as the **hierarchy** (i.e., a classification) of needs (Figure 4-2). This hierarchy states that human beings are motivated by unsatisfied needs and that certain lower needs have to be satisfied before higher needs, like self-actualization, are met. Maslow felt that people are basically trustworthy, self-protecting, and self-governing and that humans tend toward growth and love. He believed that humans are not violent by nature, but are violent only when their needs are not being met.

Deficiency (Basic) Needs.   According to Maslow, there are general types of needs—physiological, safety, love/belonging, and esteem—that must be satisfied before a person can act unselfishly. He called these needs *deficiency (basic) needs*.

TABLE 4-1	Lifespan Development
Life Stage	**Expected Development**
I. Infant (years 0–1)	**Trust vs. Mistrust.** The newborn begins to experience a degree of familiarity and begins to trust the world around her. She also begins to trust her own body.
II. Toddler (years 2–3)	**Autonomy vs. Shame and Doubt.** The child will begin to explore the environment at home and everywhere else. He will begin to gain autonomy (independence) and develop self-control. He also can begin to feel shame and doubt in his abilities. Firm but tolerant parenting is the best practice during this stage.
III. Preschooler (years 3–6)	**Initiative vs. Guilt.** A child begins to learn new things, and has an active imagination and curiosity about everything. As she grows older, she begins to feel guilt for actions taken, which is a sign that she is developing the capacity for moral judgment.
IV. School Age (years 7–12)	**Industry vs. Inferiority.** The child becomes exposed to people other than family members, such as teachers and peers, who contribute to his development. He begins to experience feelings of success that can arise from sports, academics, or social acceptance. Failure to experience success at this stage can result in inferiority feelings.
V. Adolescence (years 12–18)	**Ego Identity vs. Role Confusion.** An adolescent begins to discover who she really is as a preadult human being. She begins to realize how she fits into society (ego identity). When an adolescent is confused about who she is and where she fits in society, role confusion results. Role confusion develops "follower" personality traits, which can lead to inappropriate decision making.
VI. Young Adult (20s)	**Intimacy vs. Isolation.** A young adult begins to think about marriage, family, and career responsibilities. These issues can come into conflict with the isolation that is an issue in modern society; careers often move people to different cities, and working at home has become more common.
VII. Middle Adult (late 20s to 50s)	**Generativity vs. Stagnation.** This stage is primarily devoted to raising children. Middle adults have a desire to help future generations and will often teach, write, or become involved in social activism.
VIII. Old Adult (60s and older)	**Integrity vs. Despair.** Older adults are usually retired and live without children in the house. They tend to question their usefulness at this stage. They begin to notice changes in their physical health and begin to become concerned about these changes. They begin to experience the deaths of relatives, friends, spouses, and, in some cases, their children.

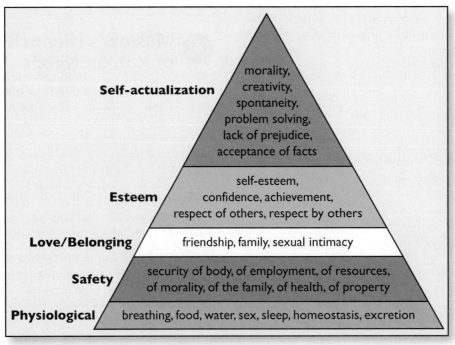

Figure 4-2. Maslow's hierarchy.

Physiological Needs.   Physiological needs are humans' very basic needs, such as air, water, food, sleep, and sex. When these needs are not satisfied, we may feel sickness, irritation, pain, and discomfort. These feelings motivate us to alleviate them as soon as possible to establish **homeostasis** (that is, a state of balance or equilibrium). Once those feelings are alleviated, we may think about other things.

Safety Needs.   People have the need and desire for establishing stability and consistency. These basic needs are security, shelter, and existing in a safe environment.

Love/Belonging Needs.   Humans have a desire to belong to groups: clubs, work groups, religious groups, family, and so on. We need to feel loved and accepted by others. Humans are like pack animals—we place great importance in belonging to society.

Esteem Needs.   Humans like to feel that they are important and have worthiness to society. There are two types of self-esteem. The first results from competence or mastery of a task, such as completing an educational program. The second is the attention and recognition that comes from others.

Self-Actualization.   The need for self-actualization is finding self-fulfillment and realizing one's own potential. To reach this level, a person utilizes many tools to maximize potential, such as education, a fulfilling career, and a balanced personal life.

When working and communicating with patients, remember this hierarchy of human needs and observe what need a patient is deficient in. For example, if an elderly patient has recently lost her husband, she may feel lonely and deficient in the love need. You may see homeless patients who are deficient in their physiological and safety needs. You may have a young girl as a patient who is overweight and has low self-esteem. On the other hand, you may have a high-level executive as a patient who has reached self-actualization. Each of these scenarios would require a communication style adjustment in order for you to effectively communicate with these patients.

Types of Communication

Communication can be positive or negative. It can also be verbal, nonverbal, or written. To help ensure effective communication with patients, familiarize yourself with these different types of communication. (Chapter 7 discusses written communication.)

Positive Verbal Communication

In the medical office, communication that promotes patients' comfort and well-being is essential. Treating patients brusquely or rudely is unacceptable in the health-care setting. It is your responsibility—not the patient's—to set the stage for positive communication.

When information—even bad news—is communicated with some positive aspect, patients are more likely to listen attentively and respond positively themselves. For example, you might explain to a patient who is about to get an injection, "This will sting, but only for a couple of seconds. When we're through, you're free to go." You would not just say, "This is going to hurt."

Other examples of positive communication are:

- Being friendly, warm, and attentive ("It's good to see you again, Mrs. Armstrong. I know you're on your lunch hour, so let's get started right away.")
- Verbalizing concern for patients ("Are you comfortable?" "I understand it hurts when I do this; I'll be gentle." "This paperwork won't take long at all.")
- Encouraging patients to ask questions ("I hope I've explained the procedure well. Do you have any questions, or are there any parts you would like to go over again?")
- Asking patients to repeat your instructions to make sure they understand
- Looking directly at patients when you speak to them
- Smiling (naturally, not in a forced way)
- Speaking slowly and clearly (enunciate). Be sure to pronounce words correctly.
- Listening carefully

Negative Verbal Communication

Most people do not purposely try to communicate negatively. Some people, however, may not realize that their communication style has a negative impact on others. Look for and ask for feedback to help you curb negative communication habits. Ask yourself, "Do the physicians and my other coworkers seem glad to speak with me? Are they open and responsive to me?" "Do patients seem at ease with me, or are they very quiet, turned off, or distant?" (Note that some patients may respond this way because of the way they feel, not because of the way you are communicating with them.) Here are some examples of negative communication:

- Mumbling
- Speaking brusquely or sharply
- Avoiding eye contact
- Interrupting patients as they are speaking
- Rushing through explanations or instructions
- Treating patients impersonally
- Making patients feel they are taking up too much of your time or asking too many questions
- Forgetting common courtesies, such as saying please and thank you
- Showing boredom

A good way to avoid negative communication is to open your eyes and ears to others in service-oriented workplace settings. The next time you buy something at a store, call a company for information over the phone, or eat out at a restaurant, take note of the way the staff treats you. Do they answer your questions courteously? Do they give you the information you ask for? Do they make you feel welcome? What specifically makes their communication style positive or negative? Remember, you can always improve your communication skills.

Nonverbal Communication

Verbal communication refers to communication that is spoken. Nonverbal communication is also known as **body language.** Body language includes facial expressions, eye contact, posture, touch, and attention to personal space. In many instances, people's body language conveys their true feelings, even when their words may say otherwise. A patient might say, "I'm OK about that," but if she is sitting with her arms folded tightly across her chest and avoids looking at you, she may not mean what she says.

Facial Expression. Your face is the most expressive part of your body. You can often tell whether someone has understood your message simply by his facial expression. For example, when you are explaining a procedure to a patient, look at his expression. Does he seem puzzled? Is his brow wrinkled? Does he look surprised? Facial expressions can give you clues about how to tailor your communication efforts. They also serve as a form of feedback.

Eye Contact. Eye contact is an important part of positive communication. Look directly at patients when speaking to them. Looking away or down communicates that you are not interested in the person or that you are avoiding her for some reason.

There may be cultural differences in the ways patients react to eye contact. In some cultures, for example, it is common to avoid eye contact out of respect for someone who is considered a superior. Thus, children may be taught not to look adults in the eye.

Posture. The way you hold or move your head, arms, hands, and the rest of your body can project strong nonverbal messages. During communication, posture can usually be described as open or closed.

Open Posture. A feeling of receptiveness and friendliness can be conveyed with an **open posture.** In this position, your arms lie comfortably at your sides or in your lap. You face the other person, and you may lean forward in your chair. This demonstrates that you are listening and are interested in what the other person has to say. Open posture is a form of positive communication.

Closed Posture. A **closed posture** conveys the opposite, a feeling of not being totally receptive to what is being said. It can also signal that someone is angry or upset. A person in a closed posture may hold his arms rigidly or fold them across his chest. He may lean back in his chair, away from the other person. He may turn away to avoid eye contact. Slouching is a kind of closed posture that can convey fatigue or lack of caring. Watch for patients with closed postures that may indicate tension or pain. Avoid closed postures yourself—they have a negative effect on your communication efforts.

Touch. Touch is a powerful form of nonverbal communication. A touch on the arm or a hug can be a means of saying hello, sharing condolences, or expressing congratulations. Family background, culture, age, and gender all influence people's perception of touch. Some people may welcome a touch or think nothing of it. Others may view touching as an invasion of their privacy. In general, in the medical setting, a touch on the shoulder, forearm, or back of the hand to express interest or concern is acceptable.

Personal Space. When communicating with others, it is important to be aware of the concept of personal space. **Personal space** is an area that surrounds an individual. By not intruding on patients' personal space, you show respect for their feelings of privacy.

In most social situations, it is common for people to stand 4 to 12 ft away from each other. For personal conversation, you would typically stand between 1½ and 4 ft away from a person. Some patients may feel uncomfortable—and may become anxious—when you stand or sit close to them. Others prefer the reassurance of having people close to them when they speak. Watch patients carefully. If they lean back when you lean forward or if they fold their arms or turn their head away, you may be invading their personal space. If they lean or step toward you, they may be seeking to close up the personal space.

Improving Your Communication Skills

Sharpening your communication skills should be an ongoing effort and will help you become a more effective communicator. Good communication skills can enhance the quality of your interaction with patients and coworkers alike. Among the skills involved in communication are listening skills, interpersonal skills, therapeutic communication skills, and assertiveness skills.

Listening Skills

Listening involves both hearing and interpreting a message. Listening requires you to pay close attention not only to what is being said but also to nonverbal cues, such as those communicated through body language.

Listening can be passive or active. **Passive listening** is simply hearing what someone has to say without the need for a reply. An example is listening to a news program on the radio; the communication is mainly one-way. **Active listening** involves two-way communication. You are actively involved in the process, offering feedback or asking questions. Active listening takes place, for example, when you interview a patient for her medical history. Active listening is an essential skill in the medical office.

There are several ways to improve your listening skills:

- Prepare to listen. Position yourself at the same level (sitting, standing) as the person who is speaking and assume an open posture (Figure 4-3).
- Relax and listen attentively. Do not simply pretend to listen to what is being said.
- Maintain eye contact.
- Maintain appropriate personal space.

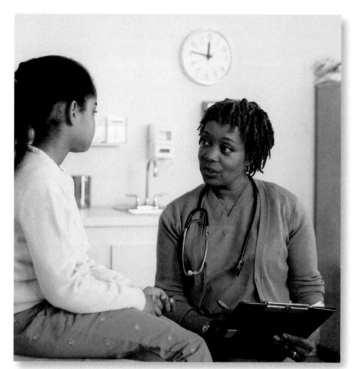

Figure 4-3. Active listening requires two-way communication and positive body language.

- Think before you respond.
- Provide feedback. Restate the speaker's message in your own words to show that you understand.
- If you do not understand something that was said, ask the person to repeat it.

Interpersonal Skills

When you interact with people, you use **interpersonal skills.** When you make a patient feel at ease by being warm and friendly, you are demonstrating good interpersonal skills. In addition to warmth and friendliness, valuable interpersonal skills include empathy, respect, genuineness, openness, and consideration and sensitivity.

Warmth and Friendliness. A friendly but professional approach, a pleasant greeting, and a smile get you off to a good start when communicating with patients. When your approach is sincere, patients will be more relaxed and open.

Empathy. The process of identifying with someone else's feelings is **empathy.** When you are empathetic, you are sensitive to the other person's feelings and problems. For example, if a patient is experiencing a migraine headache and you have never had one, you can still let her know you are trying to imagine, or relate to, her situation. In other words, you can acknowledge the severity of her pain and show support and care. You must, however, always remain objective in your interaction with patients.

Respect. Showing respect can mean using a title of courtesy such as "Mr." or "Mrs." when communicating

with patients. It can also mean acknowledging a patient's wishes or choices without passing judgment.

Genuineness. Being genuine in your interactions with patients means that you refrain from "putting on an act" or just going through the motions of your job. Patients like to know that their health-care providers are real people. In a medical setting, being genuine means caring for each patient on an individual basis, giving patients the full attention they deserve, and showing respect for them. Being genuine in your communication with patients encourages them to place trust in you and in what you say.

Openness. Openness means being willing to listen to and consider others' viewpoints and concerns and being receptive to their needs. An open individual is accepting of others and not biased for or against them.

Consideration and Sensitivity. You should always try to show consideration toward patients and act in a thoughtful, kind way. You must be sensitive to their individual concerns, fears, and needs.

 ## Therapeutic Communication Skills

Therapeutic communication is the ability to communicate with patients in terms that they can understand and, at the same time, feel at ease and comfortable in what you are saying. It is also the ability to communicate with other members of the health team in technical terms that are appropriate in a health-care setting. Therapeutic communication techniques are methodologies that can improve communication with patients.

Therapeutic communication involves the following communication skills:

- Being Silent. Silence allows the patient time to think without pressure.
- Accepting. This skill gives the patient an indication of reception. It shows that you have heard the patient and follow the patient's thought pattern. Some indicators of acceptance include nodding; saying "Yes," "I follow what you said," and other such phrases; and body language.
- Giving Recognition. Show patients that you are aware of them by stating their name in a greeting or by noticing positive changes. With this skill, you are recognizing the patient as a person or individual.
- Offering Self. Make yourself available to the needs of the patient.
- Giving a Broad Opening. Allow the patient to take the initiative in introducing the topic. Ask openended questions such as "Is there something you'd like to talk about?" or "Where would you like to begin?"
- Offering General Leads. Give the patient encouragement to continue by making comments such as "Go on" or "And then?"

- Making Observations. Make your perceptions known to the patient. Say things like "You appear tense today" or "Are you uncomfortable when you . . . ?" By calling patients' attention to what is happening to them, you encourage them to notice it for themselves so that they can describe it to you.
- Encouraging Communication. Ask patients to verbalize what they perceive. Make statements such as "Tell me when you feel anxious" or "What is happening?" Patients should feel free to describe their perceptions to you, and you must try to see things as they seem to the patients.
- Mirroring. Restate what the patient has said to demonstrate that you understand.
- Reflecting. Encourage patients to think through and answer their own questions. A reflecting dialogue may go like this:
  - Patient: Do you think I should tell the doctor?
  - Medical Assistant: Do you think you should?

  By reflecting patients' questions or statements back to them, you are helping patients feel that their opinions about their health are of value.
- Focusing. Focusing encourages the patient to stay on the topic.
- Exploring. Encourage patients to express themselves in more depth. Try to get as much detail as possible about a patent complaint, but avoid probing and prying if the patient does not wish to discuss it.
- Clarifying. Ask patients to explain themselves more clearly if they provide information that is vague or not meaningful.
- Summarizing. This skill involves organizing and summing up the important points of the discussion and gives the patient an awareness of the progress made toward greater understanding.

Ineffective Therapeutic Communication. In the previous section, the focus was on how to communicate effectively in a therapeutic environment. Oftentimes people think they are communicating thoroughly, but they are not. Here are some roadblocks that can interfere with your communication style:

- Reassuring. This type of communication indicates to the patient that there is no need for anxiety or worry. By doing this, you devalue the patient's feelings and give false hope if the outcome is not positive. The communication error here is a lack of understanding and empathy.
- Giving Approval. Giving approval is usually done by overtly approving of a patient's behavior. This may lead the patient to strive for praise rather than progress.
- Disapproving. Being disapproving is done by overtly disapproving of a patient's behavior. This implies that you have the right to pass judgment on the patient's thoughts and actions. Find an alternate attitude when dealing with patients. Adopting a moralistic attitude may take your attention away from the patient's needs and may direct it toward your own feelings.
- Agreeing/Disagreeing. Overtly agreeing or disagreeing with thoughts, perceptions, and ideas of patients is not an effective way to communicate. When you agree with patients, they will have the perception that they are right because you agree with them or because you share the same opinion. Opinions and conclusions should be the patient's, not yours. When disagreeing with patients, you become the opposition to them instead of their caregiver. Never place yourself in an argumentative situation regarding the opinions of a patient.
- Advising. If you tell the patient what you think should be done, you place yourself outside your scope of practice. You cannot advise patients.
- Probing. Probing is discussing a topic that the patient has no desire to discuss.
- Defending. Protecting yourself, the institution, and others from verbal attack is classified as defending. If you become defensive, the patient may feel the need to discontinue communication.
- Requesting an Explanation. This communication pattern involves asking patients to provide reasons for their behavior. Patients may not know why they behave in a certain manner. "Why" questions may have an intimidating effect on some patients.
- Minimizing Feelings. Never judge or make light of a patient's discomfort. It is important for you to perceive what is taking place from the patient's point of view, not your own.
- Making Stereotyped Comments. This type of communication involves using meaningless clichés when communicating with patients. An example of a stereotypical comment is "It's for your own good." These types of comments are given in an automatic, mechanical way as a substitute for a more reasonable and thoughtful explanation.

Defense Mechanisms. When working with patients, it is important to observe their communication behaviors. Patients often will develop defense mechanisms (also known as coping strategies), which are unconscious, to protect themselves from anxiety, guilt, and shame.

The following are some common defense mechanisms that a patient may display when communicating with the doctor, medical assistant, or other health-care team members. The mechanisms may be adaptive (ability to change or adjust) or nonadaptive (the inability to change or adjust).

- Compensation: Overemphasizing a trait to make up for a perceived or actual failing
- Denial: An unconscious attempt to reject unacceptable feelings, needs, thoughts, wishes, or external reality factors
- Displacement: The unconscious transfer of unacceptable thoughts, feelings, or desires from the self to a more acceptable external substitute

- Dissociation: Disconnecting emotional significance from specific ideas or events
- Identification: Mimicking the behavior of another to cope with feelings of inadequacy
- Introjection: Adopting the unacceptable thoughts or feelings of others
- Projection: Projecting onto another person one's own feelings, as if they had originated in the other person
- Rationalization: Justifying unacceptable behavior, thoughts, and feelings into tolerable behaviors
- Regression: Unconsciously returning to more infantile behaviors or thoughts
- Repression: Putting unpleasant thoughts, feelings, or events out of one's mind
- Substitution: Unconsciously replacing an unreachable or unacceptable goal with another, more acceptable one

Assertiveness Skills

As a professional, you need to be **assertive,** that is, to be firm and to stand by your principles while still showing respect for others. Being assertive means trusting your instincts, feelings, and opinions (not in terms of diagnosing, which only the doctor can do, but in terms of basic communication with patients), and acting on them. For example, when you see that a patient looks uneasy, speak up. You might say, "You look concerned. How can I help you feel more comfortable?" versus asking the patient "What is the matter with you?"

Being assertive is different from being aggressive. When people are **aggressive,** they try to impose their position on others or try to manipulate them. Aggressive people are bossy and can be quarrelsome. They do not appear to take into consideration others' feelings, needs, thoughts, ideas, and opinions before they act or speak.

To be assertive, you must be open, honest, and direct. Be aware of your body position: an open posture conveys the proper message. When you communicate, speak confidently and use "I" statements such as "I feel . . ." or "I think . . ." (Assertiveness is also discussed later in the chapter in the section on communicating with coworkers.)

Developing your assertiveness skills increases your sense of self-worth and your confidence as a professional. Being assertive will also help you prevent or resolve conflicts more peacefully and increase your leadership ability. People look up to and respect professionals who are assertive in the workplace. See Table 4-2 for a comparison of assertive, nonassertive, and aggressive behaviors.

TABLE 4-2	A Comparison of Nonassertive, Assertive, Aggressive, and Nonassertive Aggressive Behavior			
	Nonassertive Behavior	**Assertive Behavior**	**Aggressive Behavior**	**Nonassertive Aggressive Behavior (NAG)**
Characteristics of the Behavior	Emotionally dishonest, indirect, self-denying; allows others to choose for self; does not achieve desired goal	Emotionally honest, direct, self-enhancing, expressive; chooses for self; may achieve goal	Emotionally honest, direct, self-enhancing at the expense of another, expressive; chooses for others; may achieve goal at expense of others	Emotionally dishonest, indirect, self-denying; chooses for others; may achieve goal at expense of others
Your Feelings	Hurt, anxious, possibly angry later	Confident, self-respecting	Righteous, superior, derogative at the time and possibly guilty later	Defiance, anger, self-denying; sometimes anxious, possibly guilty later
The Other Person's Feelings Toward You	Irritated, pity, lack of respect	Generally respected	Angry, resentful	Angry, resentful, irritated, disgusted
The Other Person's Feelings About Her/Himself	Guilty or superior	Valued, respected	Hurt, embarrassed, defensive	Hurt, guilty or superior, humiliated

Source: Adapted from Alberti, Robert E., and Emmons, Michael, *Your Perfect Right: A Guide to Assertive Behavior,* San Luis Obispo, California: Impact, 1970.

Communicating in Special Circumstances

If you make an effort to develop good interpersonal skills, most patients will not be difficult to communicate with. You will, however, encounter patients in special circumstances, when they may be anxious or angry. These situations sometimes inhibit communication. Patients from different cultures may pose challenges to communication. Others may have some type of impairment or disability that makes communication difficult. Similarly, young patients, parents with children who are ill or injured, and patients with terminal illnesses may present communication difficulties. Learning about the special needs of these patients and polishing your own communication skills will help you become an effective communicator in any number of situations.

 ## The Anxious Patient

It is common for patients to be anxious in a doctor's office or other health-care setting. This reaction is commonly known as the "white-coat syndrome." There can be many reasons for anxiety. A patient can become anxious because she is ill and does not know what is wrong with her—she may fear the worst. A patient may have recently been diagnosed with an illness that he knows nothing about, which may necessitate a severe lifestyle change. Fear of bad news or fear that some procedure is going to be painful can create anxiety. Anxiety can interfere with the communication process. For example, because of anxiety a patient may not listen well or pay attention to what you are saying.

Some patients—particularly children—may be unable to verbalize their feelings of fear and anxiety. Watch for signs of anxiety. They may include a tense appearance, increased blood pressure and rates of breathing and pulse, sweaty palms, reported problems with sleep or appetite, irritability, and agitation. Procedure 4-1 will help you communicate with patients who are anxious.

The Angry Patient

In a medical setting, anger may occur for many reasons. Anger may be a mask for fear about an illness or the outcome of surgery. Anger may come from a patient's feeling of being treated unfairly or without compassion. Anger may stem from a patient's resentment about being ill or injured. Anger may be a reaction to frustration, rejection, disappointment, feelings of loss of control or self-esteem, or an invasion of privacy.

As a medical assistant, you will encounter angry patients and will need to help them express their anger constructively, for the sake of their health. At the same time, you must learn not to take expressions of anger personally; you may just be the unlucky target. The goal with angry patients is to help them refocus emotional energy toward solving the problem. Study the following steps in communicating with an angry patient:

1. Learn to recognize anger and its causes. Anger is easy to recognize in most people, but it can be subtle in others. Patients who speak in a tense tone, are stubborn, or appear to ignore your attempts at communication may be angry.

2. Remain calm and continue to demonstrate genuineness and respect. Communicate that you respect and care about the patient's feelings.

3. Focus on the patient's physical and medical needs.

4. Maintain adequate personal space. Place yourself on the same level as the patient. If the patient is standing, encourage him to sit down. Maintain an open posture to show that you are receptive to listening. Maintain eye contact, but avoid staring at the patient, which can make the person angrier.

5. Avoid the feeling that you need to defend yourself or to give reasons why the patient should not be angry. Instead, listen attentively and with an open mind to what the patient is saying. Most patients' anger will lessen if they know someone is really listening to them and showing an interest in their emotions and needs.

6. Encourage patients to be specific in describing the cause of their anger, their thoughts about it, and their feelings. Be empathic and acknowledge the patient's feelings and perceptions. Follow through with any promises you might make concerning correction of a problem, but avoid totally agreeing or disagreeing with the patient. State what you can and cannot do for the patient.

7. Present your point of view calmly and firmly to help the patient better understand the situation. If patients are receptive to your viewpoint, their perspective may change for the better.

8. Avoid a breakdown in communication. Allow the patient to voice anger. Trying to outtalk the patient or overexplain will only annoy and irritate him. You might also suggest that the patient spend a few moments alone to gather his thoughts or to cool off before continuing any type of communication.

9. If you feel threatened by a patient's anger or if it looks as if the patient's anger may become violent, leave the room and seek assistance from one of the physicians or other members of the office staff. Document any threats in the patient's chart.

Patients of Other Cultures

Our beliefs, attitudes, values, use of language, and views of the world are unique to us, but they are also shaped by our cultural background. In any health-care setting, you will most likely have contact with patients of diverse cultures and ethnic groups. Each culture and ethnic group has its own behaviors, traditions, and values. Rather than

PROCEDURE 4-1

Communicating with the Anxious Patient

Procedure Goal: To use communication and interpersonal skills to calm an anxious patient

Materials: None

Method:

1. Identify signs of anxiety in the patient.
2. Acknowledge the patient's anxiety. (Ignoring a patient's anxiety often makes it worse.)

   ### Rationale
   Good therapeutic communication techniques can help reduce patient anxiety.

3. Identify possible sources of anxiety, such as fear of a procedure or test result, along with supportive resources available to the patient, such as family members and friends. Understanding the source of anxiety in a patient and identifying the supportive resources available can help you communicate with the patient more effectively.
4. Do what you can to alleviate the patient's physical discomfort. For example, find a calm, quiet place for the patient to wait, a comfortable chair, a drink of water, or access to the bathroom (Figure 4-4).
5. Allow ample personal space for conversation. Note: You would normally allow a 1½- to 4-ft distance between yourself and the patient. Adjust this space as necessary.
6. Create a climate of warmth, acceptance, and trust.
   a. Recognize and control your own anxiety. Your air of calm can decrease the patient's anxiety.
   b. Provide reassurance by demonstrating genuine care, respect, and empathy.
   c. Act confidently and dependably, maintaining truthfulness and confidentiality at all times.
7. Using the appropriate communication skills, have the patient describe the experience that is causing anxiety, her thoughts about it, and her feelings. Proceeding in this order allows the patient to describe what is causing the anxiety and to clarify her thoughts and feelings about it.

   ### Rationale
   The use of open-ended questioning will result in more information about the patient's feelings of anxiety.

   a. Maintain an open posture.
   b. Maintain eye contact, if culturally appropriate.
   c. Use active listening skills.
   d. Listen without interrupting.
8. Do not belittle the patient's thoughts and feelings. This can cause a breakdown in communication, increase anxiety, and make the patient feel isolated.
9. Be empathic to the patient's concerns.
10. Help the patient recognize and cope with the anxiety.
    a. Provide information to the patient. Patients are often fearful of the unknown. Helping them understand their disease or the procedure they are about to undergo will help decrease their anxiety.
    b. Suggest coping behaviors, such as deep breathing or other relaxation exercises.
11. Notify the doctor of the patient's concerns.

    ### Rationale
    The physician must be aware of all aspects of the patient's health, including anxiety, to allow for optimal patient care. Part of your job as a medical assistant is to act as a liaison between the patient and the physician.

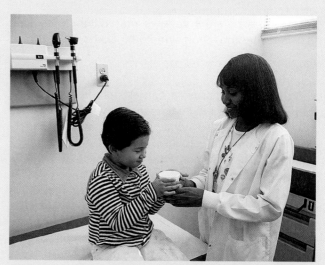

Figure 4-4. You can calm children's anxiety by spending time talking with them, playing a game, reading a story, or just offering a glass of water.

Reflecting On . . . Cultural Issues

Multicultural Attitudes About Modern Medicine

Patients' cultural backgrounds have a great effect on their attitudes toward health and illness. Patients from different cultural backgrounds often have beliefs about the causes of illness, what symptoms mean, and what to expect from health-care professionals that are different from those of modern medicine. Understanding some of these perceptions, behaviors, and expectations will help you communicate effectively with patients of different cultures.

Beliefs About Causes of Illness

Some cultures have beliefs about the causes of illness that differ sharply from accepted notions in the mainstream culture. As an example, many cultures believe that some illnesses are caused by hot or cold forces in the body. Some believe that winds and drafts cause illness or that illness can be caused by blood that is too thick or too thin. Others believe that having bad feelings toward others can create ill health.

Because of such beliefs, it may be hard to obtain information from patients about possible reasons for their medical problems. It may also be hard for some patients to realize the importance of taking medication to treat certain illnesses. In this case, you may have to be very persuasive and firm when giving the patient instructions for medication usage. It may be helpful or necessary to involve other family members in persuading the patient.

How Symptoms Are Presented and What They Mean

People from different cultures may differ in the way they perceive and report symptoms. Some may express pain very emotionally because their culture may feel that suppressing pain is harmful. In contrast, people from other cultures may not admit that they are in pain, thinking that acknowledging pain is a sign of weakness. People of all cultures may be more likely to report physical symptoms of illness than they are to report psychologic symptoms. Be aware of nonverbal indications of pain or other symptoms.

Treatment Expectations

Patients from other cultures may be totally unaccustomed to some of the practices of modern medicine. Patients of certain ethnic or cultural groups often consult other types of healers before seeing a doctor. They are likely to have different expectations of treatment from each.

Patients from other cultures may be wary of certain treatments because these treatments are so different from what they are accustomed to. This is especially true of some of the medical procedures and interventions considered to be state-of-the-art, such as laser surgery or diabetes management.

When dealing with patients of other cultures, keep in mind their perspectives on health care. Try to avoid generalizations and cultural stereotyping, however, because there can be a variation of attitudes within ethnic groups. Treat each patient as an individual, and you will be providing the best care possible.

viewing these differences as barriers to communication, strive to understand and be tolerant of them.

As a medical professional, it is important to understand the cultural differences of the patients who come to your medical office for care. Many medical facilities are located in heavily populated ethnic locations, and it is important that the medical staff understand the differences among patient cultures. A medical assistant who is employed in a medical facility in which the majority of its patients are Latino should learn as much as possible about the specific Latin culture in her area in order to provide good customer service. It is also important to understand the difference between stereotyping and generalizing. *Stereotyping* is a negative statement about the specific traits of a group that is applied unfairly to an entire population. A *generalization* is a statement about common trends within a group, but it is understood that further investigation is needed to determine if the trend applies to an individual.

Remember that the beliefs of other cultures are neither superior nor inferior to your own. They are simply different. Never allow yourself to make value judgments or to stereotype a patient, a culture, or an ethnic group. Each patient is an individual in her own right.

The Reflecting On . . . Cultural Issues box on this page discusses different cultural views of health care. You may research multicultural resources for health information at http://sis.nlm.nih.gov/outreach/multicultural.html and locate information on interpersonal communication at http://www.work911.com/communication/index.html.

Language Barriers. Patients who cannot speak or understand English may have difficulty expressing their needs or feelings effectively. One of the first things that you can do is use a family member who is present as an interpreter. However, federal policies require health-care providers who receive federal funds (i.e., Medicare) to make interpretive services available to their patients with limited English. The interpreter should be a medically trained interpreter, especially for patients having surgery or if a consent form needs to be signed.

If your medical office has a large number of non-English speakers, it is a good idea to have forms translated and available for use. Another great idea is to also have non-English videos available that educate the patient about different procedures or illnesses.

Translation services can be used for video and telephone translation as well. The services can be purchased from a number of vendors. Speakerphones provide another source of translation to the patient, while speaking to the medical interpreter.

Patients with Reading Problems. You will find on occasion that some of your patients are functionally illiterate. They may try to hide this by saying, "I didn't bring my glasses with me" or "this is too much to read right now." Be polite and go over the information with them and ask if they have any questions. Send the information home and have them further discuss it with a family member before requesting that they sign forms such as consent forms or before having surgery.

There are several vendors that will publish your patient education materials on a specific readability level (see www.wordswork.com). It is recommended that patient education brochures should not exceed fourth- to eighth-grade reading levels. If patients with higher reading levels want to know more about a specific topic, make sure your office has additional reading materials on hand.

Another tool for providing services to patients with reading problems is to have videos on hand concerning medical topics and procedures.

The Patient with a Visual Impairment

When communicating with a patient who has a visual impairment, be aware of what you say and how you say it. Since people with visual impairments cannot usually rely on nonverbal clues, your tone of voice, inflection, and speech volume take on greater importance.

Following are some suggestions for communicating with a patient who has a visual impairment.

- Use large-print materials whenever possible.
- Make sure there is adequate lighting in all patient areas.
- Be especially aware that you use a normal speaking voice.

- Talk directly and honestly. Explain instructions thoroughly.
- Don't talk down to the patient; preserve the patient's dignity.

The Patient with a Hearing Impairment

Hearing loss can range from mild to severe. How you communicate depends on the degree of impairment and on whether the patient has effective use of a hearing aid.

Following are some tips to help you communicate effectively with a hearing-impaired patient.

- Find a quiet area to talk, and try to minimize background noise.
- Position yourself close to and facing the patient. The patient will rely on visual clues such as the movement of your lips and mouth, your facial expression, and your body language (Figure 4-5).

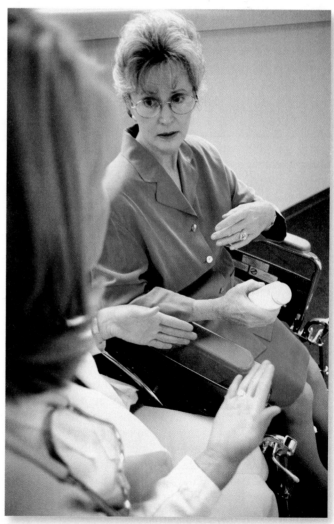

Figure 4-5. When communicating with a patient who has a hearing impairment, position yourself close to the patient and use gestures and effective body language.

- Speak slowly, so the patient can follow what you are saying.
- Remember that elderly patients lose the ability to hear high-pitched sounds first. Try speaking in lower tones.
- Speak in a clear, firm voice, but do not shout, especially if the patient wears a hearing aid.
- To verify understanding, ask questions that will encourage the patient to repeat what you said.
- Whenever possible, use written materials to reinforce verbal information.

The Patient Who Is Mentally or Emotionally Disturbed

There may be times when you will need to communicate with patients who are mentally or emotionally disturbed. When dealing with this type of patient, you need to determine what level of communication the patient can understand. Keep these suggestions in mind to improve communication.

- It is important to remain calm if the patient becomes agitated or confused.
- Avoid raising your voice or appearing impatient.
- If you do not understand what the patient said, ask him to repeat what he said.

The Elderly Patient

Medical assistants now spend at least 50% of their time caring for older patients. Be aware of the vast differences in the capabilities of people of this age group. Do not stereotype all elderly patients as frail or confused. Most are not, and each patient deserves to be treated according to her own individual abilities.

Always treat elderly patients with respect. Regardless of their physical or mental state, elderly patients are adults. Do not talk down to them. Use the title "Mrs." or "Mr." to address older people unless they ask you to call them by their first name.

Denial or Confusion. Some elderly patients deny that they are ill. For example, in a survey of elderly people, the majority of whom had at least one chronic condition, 85% reported that they were in good or excellent health (Bradley and Edinberg, 1990). Patients' perception of how they feel may be quite different from their actual state of health.

The reverse situation can also occur. Elderly patients may overreact to a problem and consider themselves sicker than they really are. They may become dependent, passive, or anxious. Elderly patients may also over- or underestimate their ability to perform certain tasks or to deal with certain limitations.

Elderly patients may be confused if they have some impairment in memory, judgment, or other mental abilities. Signs of confusion can occur with Alzheimer's disease, senility, depression, head injury, or misuse of medications or alcohol. Elderly patients may or may not be aware of their condition. They may have difficulty understanding instructions.

The Importance of Touch. Because they often live alone, many elderly patients experience a lack of physical touch. Using touch—offering to hold a patient's hand or placing an arm around his shoulder—communicates that you care about the patient's well-being.

Terminally Ill Patients

Terminally ill patients are often under extreme stress and can be a challenge to treat. It is important that health-care professionals respect the rights of terminal patients and treat them with dignity. It is also important that you communicate with the family and offer support and empathy as their loved one accepts her condition. You should also provide information on **hospice,** which is an area of medicine that works with terminally ill patients and their families. Hospice workers often go to the home of the terminally ill patient or work with patients in facilities. Hospice care is usually staffed with RNs and other health-care providers who have specialized training in issues related to death and dying. They work with the family and patient in the beginning, assisting with medications, comfort care and emotional support. If the patient dies at home they may end by making arrangements with the funeral home and coroner.

Elisabeth Kübler-Ross, a world-renowned authority in the areas of death and dying, developed a model of behavior that patients will experience on learning their condition. This is called the Stages of Dying or Stages of Grief. This model is widely used today in work with terminally ill patients.

Kübler-Ross's Stages of Dying include five stages, which usually—but not always—progress in the following order:

1. Denial. Patients are in direct denial or periods of disbelief. This defense is generally temporary.
2. Anger. Patients may suddenly realize what is really happening and respond with anger. They can become difficult patients in this stage and display temper tantrums and fits of rage.
3. Bargaining. Patients attempt to make deals with physicians, clergy, and family members. Patients at this stage may become more cooperative and congenial.
4. Depression. The patient will begin to show signs of depression, such as withdrawal, lethargy, and sobbing. The patient's body is beginning to deteriorate, and the patient may experience more pain and realize that relationships with family and friends will soon be gone.
5. Acceptance. Patients accept the fact that they are dying. They will begin arrangements for when they

Talking with the Geriatric Patients

If you work in a practice that specializes in geriatrics or in any practice with older patients, certain communication skills will help you in your job. You may find yourself in various situations in which knowing how to talk with the older patient will be a necessary skill. Taking a medical history and helping a patient describe her symptoms are two such situations. The following tips will help you and the patient communicate with each other more effectively.

1. Make sure you select a private setting for the patient interview.

2. Many older patients are hard of hearing, but *not deaf*. Speak slightly more slowly than you normally would. Speak clearly and loudly (but do not shout—shouting will insult and anger an older patient who does hear well). Enunciate well, and use a lower tone of voice (elderly people lose the ability to hear high-frequency sounds first). If the patient asks you to repeat a question, rephrase it instead of repeating it verbatim.

3. Look at the patient directly so that she knows you care about what she has to say and so that you can make sure she understands what you tell or ask her.

4. You can show respect for the patient's age by addressing the patient with Mr., Mrs., Ms., or Miss, unless the patient asks to be called by his or her first name.

5. Be patient. Some older patients live alone or in relative isolation and may be out of practice with the two-way communication skills that make a conversation or interview go smoothly. The simple act of being interviewed, even for what may seem to you a straightforward medical history, may unsettle the older patient. For example, he may need to stop and think

of a word here and there. Do not supply the word. Wait and let the patient think of it on his own. Also, do not rush through your questions. Rushing will only make the patient feel anxious and incompetent if he feels he cannot keep up with you.

6. Practice active listening skills. Pay attention to the patient's verbal and nonverbal cues. Do not interrupt the patient. After the patient finishes giving each answer, repeat it, to give her a chance to correct you if you misheard or misunderstood.

7. If you are interviewing the patient to obtain a medical history, explain before you begin the type of questions you will ask and how the information will be used.

8. If you need to use medical terminology, try also to express the same information in lay terms. For example, you might ask, "Do you use a diuretic or pill to help you eliminate fluids?"

9. Be cheerful and friendly but not sugary-sweet. Do not talk down to older patients; they are not stupid.

10. Avoid sounding surprised or excited by any answer to a question or to any information the patient gives.

11. Under no circumstances use endearments such as dear, honey, or sweetie.

12. Look for ways to make a connection so that the patient feels relaxed and comfortable. For example, in the course of taking a patient's history, you might find out that he enjoys swimming. Ask him to tell you about it.

13. Show an interest in the patient as a person. Ask about something she is interested in. For example, a patient might be wearing a piece of handmade jewelry. Ask where it came from. She might have a wonderful story to tell.

---

expire, making funeral or burial requests. The patient's family needs the most support at this stage.

Even though these stages have been generalized to dying, many experts have applied them to the grieving process as well.

The Young Patient

A doctor's office can be a frightening place for children. They often associate the doctor's office with getting a

shot or being sick. Sometimes parents have misled their children about what to expect from a visit to the doctor. When dealing with children, it is better to recognize and accept their fear and anxiety than to dismiss these emotions. When children realize that you take their feelings seriously, they are more apt to be receptive to your requests and suggestions.

Explain any procedure, no matter how basic (such as testing a reflex with a reflex hammer), in very simple terms. Let the child examine the instrument.

Other suggestions include using praise ("You were very brave") and always being truthful. Do not tell children that a procedure will not hurt if it will, or you will lose their trust.

As children get older, you can use more detailed descriptions when explaining procedures. Remember that after the age of 7 or 8, children can tell if they are being talked down to or treated like babies. Encourage them to participate actively in their care, and direct any questions or instructions to them, when appropriate. You should also respect the adolescent's request not to have a parent present during private conversations.

Parents

Parents are naturally concerned about their children and are likely to be worried or anxious when a child is ill. Children often react to a situation based on how they see their parents react. Reassuring parents and keeping them calm can also help children relax.

The Patient with AIDS and the Patient Who Is HIV-Positive

Patients with acquired immunodeficiency syndrome (AIDS) and patients who have the human immunodeficiency virus (HIV), the virus that causes AIDS, have a grave illness to deal with. They also face a society that often stigmatizes them, saying they have only themselves to blame. These patients often feel guilty, angry, and depressed.

To communicate effectively with these patients, you need accurate information about the disease and the risks involved. Take the initiative to educate yourself about AIDS and HIV. Patients will have many questions. Part of your role as a good communicator will be to answer as many questions as you can. If a patient asks a question you cannot answer, tell the physician so he can respond quickly.

Above all, remember that HIV is not transmitted through casual or common physical contact, such as brushing by a person in a crowded hall or shaking hands. It is transferred only through bodily fluids. Patients with AIDS and those who are HIV-positive need to know you are not afraid to be near them, to touch them, or to talk to them. Like any patient whose body is being ravaged by a serious illness, these patients need human contact (verbal and physical) and they need to be treated with dignity.

Patients' Families and Friends

Family members or friends sometimes accompany a patient to the office. These individuals can provide important emotional support to the patient. Always ask patients if they want a family member or friend to accompany them to the examination room, however. Do not just assume their preference. Acknowledge family members and friends, and communicate with them as you do with patients. They should be kept informed of the patient's progress, whenever possible, to avoid unnecessary anxiety on their part. You must always protect patient confidentiality, however. Too often, health-care workers think that it is acceptable to discuss patient cases in detail with family members, even without the consent of the patient.

Communicating with Coworkers

The quality of the communication you have with coworkers greatly influences the development of a positive or negative work climate and a team approach to patient care. In turn, the workplace atmosphere ultimately affects your communication with patients.

Positive Communication with Coworkers

In your interactions with coworkers, use the same skills and qualities that you use to communicate with patients. Have respect and empathy; be caring, thoughtful, and genuine; and use active listening skills. These skills will help you develop **rapport,** which is a harmonious, positive relationship, with your coworkers (Figure 4-6).

Following are some rules for communication in the medical office.

- Use proper channels of communication. For example, if you are having problems getting along with a coworker, try first to work it out with her. Do not go over her head and complain to her supervisor. Your coworker may not have realized the effect of her behavior and may wish to correct it without involving her supervisor. If you go to the supervisor right away, working relationships can become even more strained.

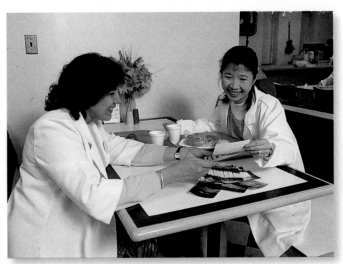

Figure 4-6. Rapport with coworkers is easy to build when you are open, friendly, and thoughtful.

- Have the proper attitude. You can avoid conflict and resolve most problems if you maintain a positive attitude. A friendly approach is much more effective than a hostile approach. Remember that many problems are simply the result of misinformation or lack of communication.
- Plan an appropriate time for communication. If you have something important to discuss, schedule a time to do so. For example, if you want to talk with the office manager about renewing the lease of a piece of office equipment, tell him you would like to discuss that topic and ask him to let you know a time that is convenient.

As an example of good communication with coworkers, consider this exchange between Mai Lee, a medical assistant, and Margot, a coworker in a pediatric practice. Note the way Mai Lee demonstrates assertiveness.

Mai Lee: I know you spent a lot of time choosing the new toys for the reception area. I love the wooden safari animal puzzles.

Margot: Thanks. I think the children really enjoy themselves now.

Mai Lee: I wanted to mention to you, though, that I'm concerned about the toy tea set with miniature cupcakes and sandwiches. Anything that's smaller than a golf ball is a choking hazard to infants and toddlers.

Margot: I don't think the little ones pay much attention to the tea set. It's mostly for older kids.

Mai Lee: Yes, but I'm still afraid that a baby could put one of those pieces in his mouth. What if we put up a little shelf in the play area that is low enough for kids 4 years old or more to reach but high enough to be out of reach of the babies. We could put the tea set on it in a clear plastic box and any other toys with small parts.

Margot: I see your point. Sounds like a good idea to me.

Mai Lee started with a statement that acknowledged the coworker's situation and feelings. Then she stated her own opinion. When her coworker disagreed, she repeated her concern, describing what might happen if the situation remained unchanged. Then she made a constructive suggestion for solving the problem without hurting the coworker's feelings. As you interact with coworkers, be sensitive to the timing of your conversations, the manner in which you present your ideas and thoughts, and your coworkers' feelings.

Communicating with Management

Positive or negative communication can affect the quality of your relationships with your supervisor or manager. For example, problems arise when communication about job responsibilities is unclear or when you feel that your supervisor does not trust or respect you, or vice versa.

Consider these suggestions when communicating with your direct supervisor:

- Keep your supervisor informed. If the office copier is not working properly, talk to your supervisor about it before a breakdown occurs that will hold everyone up. If several patients express the same types of complaint about the examination rooms, make sure the right people are told. If the doctor asks you to call a patient and you reach the patient, tell the doctor.
- Ask questions. If you are unsure about an administrative task or the meaning of a medical term, for example, do not hesitate to ask your supervisor. It is better to ask a question before acting than to make a mistake. It is also better to ask than to risk annoying someone because you carried out a task or wrote a term incorrectly. Asking your supervisor or manager a question means that you respect him or her professionally.
- Minimize interruptions. For example, before launching into a discussion, make sure your supervisor has time to talk. Opening with "Can I interrupt you for a moment, or should I come back?" or "Do you have a minute to talk?" goes a long way toward establishing good communication. It is also better to go to your supervisor when you have several questions to ask rather than to interrupt her repeatedly.
- Show initiative. Any manager or supervisor will greatly appreciate this quality. For example, if you think you can come up with a more efficient way to get the office newsletter written and distributed, write out a plan and show it to your supervisor. He or she is likely to welcome any ideas that improve office efficiency or patient satisfaction.

Dealing with Conflict

Conflict, or friction, in the workplace can result from opposition of opinions or ideas or even from a difference in personalities. Conflict can arise when the lines of communication break down or when a misunderstanding occurs. Conflict can also result from prejudices or preconceived notions about people or from lack of mutual respect or trust between a staff member and management. Whatever the cause, conflict is counterproductive to the efficiency of an office.

Following these suggestions can help prevent conflict in the office and improve communication among coworkers.

- Do not "feed into" other people's negative attitudes.
- For example, if a coworker is criticizing one of the doctors, change the subject or walk away.
- Try your best at all times to be personable and supportive of coworkers. For example, everyone has bad days. If a coworker is having a bad day, offer to pitch in and help or to run out and get her lunch if she is too busy to go out.

- Refrain from passing judgment on others or stereotyping them (women are bad at math, men don't know how to communicate, and so on). Coworkers should show respect for one another and try to be tolerant and nonjudgmental.
- Do not gossip. You are there to work. Act professionally at all times.
- Do not jump to conclusions. For example, if you get a memo about a change in your schedule that disturbs you, bring your concern to your supervisor. She may be able to be flexible on certain points. You do not know until you ask.

Set Boundaries in the Health-Care Environment. As a medical assistant, your professional behavior is extremely important. In many instances, when dealing with patients, physicians, and other staff members, you must set **boundaries,** whether physical or psychological. This will limit undesirable behavior.

If a patient, physician, or staff member is acting inappropriately toward you, you must take immediate action. Do not let the situation "fester." You must act tactfully, assertively, and diplomatically. Let the aggressor know that his actions or language is inappropriate, and that you are not obligated in any way to accept such behavior.

If none of the actions assist with stopping the unacceptable behavior, report the behavior to your immediate supervisor so she can assist you in identifying a solution to the behavior. If the aggressor is your immediate supervisor, follow the office policy and procedure (make sure you read your policy and procedure in detail before this type of situation arises).

Written Communication Tools and Community Resources

Communication is not effective if it is communicated incorrectly. It is important to be knowledgeable in the policies and procedures in your medical facility and the community resources that you have implemented into your facility. Many offices provide written documentation regarding the policies and procedures in their unique setting.

The Policy and Procedures Manual

The policy and procedures manual is a key written communication tool in the medical office. No discussion of communication in the medical office would be complete without a description of this important document. The manual is used by permanent employees as well as by temporary employees who may be hired when others are ill or on vacation, or when there is an unusually heavy workload. The manual covers all office policies and clinical procedures. It is usually developed as a joint effort by the physician (or physicians) and the staff (often the medical assistant).

Policies. Policies are rules or guidelines that dictate the day-to-day workings of an office. Although individual policies vary from office to office, most medical office manuals describe the following policy areas:

- Office purposes, objectives, and goals as set down by the physician(s)
- Rules and regulations
- Job descriptions and duties of staff personnel
- Office hours
- Dress code
- Insurance and other benefits
- Vacation, sick leave, and other time away from the office
- Salary and performance evaluations
- Maintenance of equipment and supplies
- Mailings
- Bookkeeping
- Scheduling of appointments and maintenance of patient records
- OSHA guidelines

The policy section of the manual also typically describes the chain of command for the office, or the person to whom each employee reports. This information is sometimes presented in chart form and called an organizational chart. For example, the receptionist, secretary, medical assistant, and billing person might report to the office manager. The office manager, in turn, might report directly to the physician or physicians. This chain of command varies from office to office, depending on the size and needs of the practice.

Procedures. Detailed instructions for specific procedures are covered in the procedures section of the manual (Figure 4-7). The areas discussed include clinical procedures and quality assurance programs.

Each clinical procedure should include instructions about the following:

- Purpose of the test, clinical application, and usefulness
- Specimen required and collection method; special patient preparation or restrictions
- Reagents, standards, controls, and media used; special supplies
- Instrumentation, including calibration and schedules
- Step-by-step directions

Community Resources

There are many community resources available in your local area that provide needed services to patients. The medical

SAMPLE POLICY AND PROCEDURE

GENERAL HOSPITAL & MEDICAL CENTER

POLICY AND PURPOSE

Subject: Competency of Staff   Policy # 1001
Date of Issue: Sept. 25, 200X   Effective Date: Oct. 18, 200X

I. **POLICY**
    It is the policy of General Hospital & Medical Center that all employees meet the standards of competency as defined by its various policies and the requirements of TJC and other regulatory and credentialing agencies.

II. **PURPOSE**
    The competence of staff members is (a) defined by job descriptions designed by the director; (b) assessed initially during the orientation process; (c) maintained through educational updates; and (d) evaluated periodically in conjunction with the performance appraisal process.

III. **IMPLEMENTATION**
    a. Job Descriptions
        i. The director/manager will write and/or review the job description annually. The job description will reflect the educational experience and training needed for the position and include competency-based performance standards.

Figure 4-7. Sample from a procedure manual.

facility often works with outside resources such as laboratories, home health-care agencies, and social service agencies. It is beneficial to the patient if the medical assistant is familiar with services that could assist with his or her care. Good customer service is founded on providing or researching services that can assist in the goal of patient health and well-being. Some community resources include:

- Alcoholics Anonymous
- Shelters for abused individuals
- Hospice care
- Mental health services
- Meals on Wheels
- PASSPORT
- Easter Seals
- Various state agencies, such as health insurance for the indigent; Women, Infants, and Children (WIC); etc.
- Support groups for grief, obesity, and various diseases

If a medical assistant discovers that an external community resource is needed for a patient, the medical assistant should first discuss with the physician the needs of the patient. If the physician is in agreement, then the medical assistant can arrange for services. The first step in developing a community resource library is to gather a listing of local agencies. You will need the correct name, address, phone number, contact person, and directions for submitting a referral for each resource listed. It may take some research on your part to locate and organize this information. The Internet and phone directory can be useful tools. Contact the community resource and request information, such as brochures, newsletters, and referral applications. Type up an inventory sheet of your resources and make sure that all appropriate departments have a copy. A filing drawer can be used to organize and maintain the informational material regarding each resource. See Procedure 4-2 about Identifying Community Resources.

PROCEDURE 4-2

Identifying Community Resources

Procedure Goal: To create a list of useful community resources for patient referrals

Materials: Computer with Internet access, phone directory, printer

Method:

1. Determine the needs of your medical office and formulate a list of community resources.

   Rationale

   It is important to understand the specific needs of your patients and be able to assist them with finding outside assistance when necessary.

2. Use the Internet to research the names, addresses, and phone numbers of local resources such as Meals on Wheels, state and federal agencies, home health-care agencies, long-term nursing facilities, mental health agencies, and local charities. Use the phone directory to assist in locating local agencies as well.

3. Contact each resource and request information such as business cards and brochures. Some agencies may send a representative to meet with you regarding their services.

   Rationale

   If patients can access information easily, they are more likely to avail themselves of the services available to them.

4. Compile a list of community resources with the proper name, address, phone number, e-mail address, and contact name. Include any information that may be helpful to the office.

5. Update and add to the information often because outdated information will only frustrate you and your patients, creating even more anxiety.

6. Post the information in a location where it is readily available.

Other Communication Resources

Often a medical office will work with an external business or facility to assist with the care of a patient. Such facilities can include reference laboratories, insurance companies, office equipment suppliers, and maintenance companies. It is efficient if you follow the protocol of each organization in order to maximize the level of service that you receive from them. For example, many reference laboratories, such as LabCorp, have reference manuals available to medical facilities. These manuals can provide answers to questions about the correct method to obtain a specimen and the amount of specimen required for testing. Insurance manuals such as the annual Medicare changes and coding reference books provide you with updated information. Insurance company manuals provide information regarding precertifying procedures or referrals. Even the office equipment can be repaired and maintained with little disruption to the daily office flow if protocol is followed. Make sure that you familiarize yourself with these important resources to assist in your daily communication interactions.

Personnel Management

Personnel management, also known as human resources, combines employee relations, benefits, employee performance, and a combination of other administrative tasks.

Medical facilities, whether they are hospitals or small medical practices, handle key functions through this department. Additionally, hiring, training, and compensation of employees also are handled in this area.

It is best to stress competencies such as teamwork, policies and procedures, and cross-training during the interview process as well as during orientation. Employee orientation is essential in the personnel management phase. During this process, the new hire gets to see and meet important people within the organization. He or she also gets to know what is expected of him or her, as well as gain information about company benefits.

The basics of hiring a successful employee are

- Always try to find the most qualified person for the job.
- Scrutinize and check references carefully.
- Have a salary range so that you can negotiate successfully and pay for the "most qualified" person.
- Discuss policies and procedures early.
- Train properly and retrain when new technology arrives.

Managing Stress

Stress can be a barrier to communication. For example, if you are feeling very pressured at work, you might snap at a coworker or patient, or you might forget to give the physician an important message.

Professionals in the health-care field may experience high levels of stress in their daily work environment. Stress can result from a feeling of being under pressure, or it can be a reaction to anger, frustration, or a change in your routine. Stress can increase your blood pressure, speed up your breathing and heart rate, and cause muscle tension. To minimize stress—for the sake of your health as well as for good communication in the office—it is helpful to understand some basic information about stress.

Stress—Good or Bad?

A certain amount of stress is normal. A little bit of stress—the kind that makes you feel excited or challenged by the task at hand—can motivate you to get things done and push you toward a higher level of productivity. Ongoing stress, however, can be overwhelming and affect you physically. For example, it can lower your resistance to colds and increase your risk for developing heart disease, diabetes, high blood pressure, ulcers, allergies, asthma, colitis, and cancer. It can also increase your risk for certain autoimmune diseases, which cause the body's immune system to attack normal tissue. The Points on Practice boxes list the potential causes of stress and ways to reduce stress.

Reducing Stress

Some stress at work is inevitable. An important goal is to learn how to manage or reduce stress. Take into account your strengths and limitations, and be realistic about how much you can handle at work and in your life outside work. Pushing yourself a certain amount can be motivating.

Pushing yourself too much is dangerous. The Points on Practice box lists tips for reducing stress.

Preventing Burnout

Burnout is the end result of prolonged periods of stress without relief. Burnout is an energy-depleting condition that will affect your health and career. Certain personality types are more prone to burnout than others. If you are a highly driven, perfectionist-type person, you will be more susceptible to burnout. Experts often refer to such a person as a characteristic Type A personality. A more relaxed, calm, laid-back individual is considered a Type B person. Type B personalities are less prone to burnout but have the potential to suffer from it, especially if they work in health care.

According to some experts on stress, there are five stages that lead to burnout (Miller and Smith). The road to burnout follows this path:

1. The Honeymoon Phase. During the honeymoon phase, your job is wonderful. You have boundless energy and enthusiasm, and all things seem possible. You love the job and the job loves you. You believe it will satisfy all your needs and desires and solve all your problems. You are delighted with your job, your coworkers, and the organization.

2. The Awakening Phase. The honeymoon wanes and the awakening stage starts with the realization that your initial expectations were unrealistic. The job isn't working out the way you thought it would. It doesn't satisfy all your needs, your coworkers and the organization are less than perfect, and rewards and recognition are scarce.

   As disillusionment and disappointment grow, you become confused. Something is wrong, but you can't quite put your finger on it. Typically, you work harder to make your dreams come true. But working harder doesn't change anything and you become increasingly tired, bored, and frustrated. You question your

---

Points on Practice

Potential Causes of Stress

- Death of a spouse or family member
- Divorce or separation
- Hospitalization (yours or a family member's) due to injury or illness
- Marriage or reconciliation from a separation
- Loss of a job or retirement
- Sexual problems
- Having a new baby
- Significant change in your financial status (for better or worse)

- Job change
- Children leaving or returning home
- Significant personal success, such as a promotion at work
- Moving or remodeling your home
- Problems at work, such as your boss's retiring, that may put your job at risk
- Substantial debt, such as a mortgage or overspending on credit cards

Points on Practice

Tips for Reducing Stress

- Maintain a healthy balance in your life among work, family, and leisure activities.
- Exercise regularly.
- Eat balanced, nutritious meals and healthful snacks.
- Avoid foods high in caffeine, salt, sugar, and fat.
- Get enough sleep.
- Allow time for yourself, and plan time to relax.
- Rely on the support that family, friends, and coworkers have to offer. Don't be afraid to share your feelings.
- Try to be realistic about what you can and cannot do. Do not be afraid to admit that you cannot take on another responsibility.
- Try to set realistic goals for yourself. Remember that there are always choices, even when there appear to be none.
- Be organized. Good planning can help you manage your workload.
- Redirect excess energy constructively—clean your closet, work in the garden, do volunteer work, have friends over for dinner, exercise.
- Change some of the things you have control over. Keep yourself focused. Focus your full energy on one thing at a time, and finish one project before starting another.
- Identify sources of conflict, and try to resolve them.
- Learn and use relaxation techniques, such as deep breathing, meditation, or imagining yourself in a quiet, peaceful place. Choose what works for you.
- Maintain a healthy sense of humor. Laughter can help relieve stress. Joke with friends after work. Go see a funny movie.
- Try not to overreact. Ask yourself if a situation is really worth getting upset or worried about.
- Seek help from social or professional support groups, if necessary.

competence and ability, and start losing your self-confidence.

3. The Brownout Phase. As brownout begins, your early enthusiasm and energy give way to chronic fatigue and irritability. Your eating and sleeping patterns change, and you indulge in escapist behaviors such as partying, overeating, recreational drugs, alcoholism, and binge shopping. You become indecisive and your productivity drops. Your work deteriorates. Coworkers and managers may comment on it.

Unless interrupted, brownout slides into later stages. You become increasingly frustrated and angry and project the blame for your difficulties onto others. You are cynical, detached, and openly critical of the organization, superiors, and coworkers. You are beset with depression, anxiety, and physical illness.

4. The Full-Scale Burnout Phase. Unless you wake up and interrupt the process or someone intervenes, brownout drifts remorselessly into full-scale burnout. Despair is the dominant feature of this final stage. It may take several months to get to this phase, but in most cases it takes three to four years. You experience an overwhelming sense of failure and a devastating loss of self-esteem and self-confidence. You become depressed and feel lonely and empty.

Life seems pointless, and there is a paralyzing, "what's the use" pessimism about the future. You talk about "just quitting and getting away." You are exhausted physically and mentally. Physical and mental breakdowns are likely. Suicide, stroke, or heart attack is not unusual as you complete the final stage of what all started with such high hopes, energy, optimism, and enthusiasm.

5. The Phoenix Phenomenon. You can arise from the ashes of burnout (like a phoenix), but it takes time.

First, you need to rest and relax. Don't take work home. If you're like many people, the work won't get done and you'll only feel guilty for being "lazy."

Second, be realistic in your job expectations as well as your aspirations and goals. Whoever you're talking to about your feelings can help you, but be careful. Your readjusted aspirations and goals must be yours and not those of someone else. Trying to be and do what someone else wants you to be or do is a surefire recipe for continued frustration and burnout.

Third, create balance in your life. Invest more of yourself in family and other personal relationships, social activities, and hobbies. Spread yourself out so that your job doesn't have such an overpowering influence on your self-esteem and self-confidence.

Scope of Practice

A medical assistant is a representative of the physician. Patients often will view you as a health-care practitioner with medical decision-making ability. The physician will diagnose and prescribe treatment to a patient based on his or her examination and diagnostic test results. A medical assistant is not allowed to give his or her opinions on the decisions that are made by the physician. By doing so, a medical assistant will find him- or herself in an "advising" position, which could cause legal complications for the practice or physician. "Advising" is out of the scope of practice for a medical assistant and could be considered practicing medicine, which is illegal in most states.

Summary

4.1 The communication circle involves a message being sent, a source, and a receiver that responds.

4.2 The development of the life cycle is important for the medical assistant to understand. Understanding the various stages of human life assists us in our communication skills with patients. The lifespan developmental stages start in infancy and extend until patients reach 60 years old and older.

4.3 Communication that promotes comfort and well-being is considered positive communication. Negative communication can be a turn-off. Medical assistants may not be aware of some of the signs of negative communication they display. Lack of eye contact with patients or speaking sharply to a patient is considered negative communication. To assist in avoiding this type of communication, ask yourself, "Does this make me feel good?" or "Do I feel welcome?"

4.4 Listening and other interpersonal skills can be improved by becoming more involved in the communication process by offering feedback or asking questions of the patient.

4.5 Assertive medical professionals trust their instincts. They respect their self-worth, while still making the patient feel comfortable and important. Aggressive medical professionals try to impose their positions through manipulation techniques.

4.6 Learning about the special needs of patients and polishing your communication skills will help you become an effective communicator. This will assist you with handling diversity in the workplace, handling anxious and annoyed patients, as well as dealing with others who may have language barriers.

4.7 The quality of communication you have with your coworkers and your supervisor greatly influences the development of a positive or negative work climate. Use proper channels of communication. Be open-minded. Keep supervisors informed of office problems as they arise and show initiative in your work habits.

4.8 The policy and procedures manual is a key communication tool. It is used for a variety of issues such as how to schedule appointments properly, the purpose of a clinical test, as well as office hours and the dress code.

4.9 Community resources are available in your local area. Medical assistants should be assertive in providing information to patients who may need additional outside resources, such as support groups for new mothers. Community resources in your area can be searched on the Internet. Key in "community resources in 'Anytown, Anystate.'"

4.10 Stress can be good or bad. However, it is how we handle stress that makes the difference. Stress can be reduced by exercising regularly, eating properly, and learning relaxation techniques.

REVIEW

CHAPTER 4

CASE STUDY QUESTIONS

Now that you have completed this chapter, review the case study at the beginning of the chapter and answer the following questions:

1. How will Mary adapt her communication style to communicate with each patient?
2. What types of communication roadblocks will she encounter with each one?
3. What types of communication techniques will she use for each patient?

Multiple-Choice Questions

1. The main elements in the communication cycle include
   a. a message (verbal and nonverbal), a source, and a receiver.
   b. a message and a receiver.
   c. a receiver, feedback, a sender, and a source.
   d. a source, feedback, and a receiver (verbal and nonverbal).
2. Personal space in a health-care environment is approximately
   a. 7–18 feet.
   b. 1–2 feet.
   c. 3–6 feet.
   d. 4–12 feet.
3. Which is an example of negative communication?
   a. Speaking sharply to the patient
   b. Listening carefully
   c. Being friendly and warm
   d. Looking directly at the patient
4. One suggestion for communicating with visually impaired patients is to
   a. speak very loudly so they can hear.
   b. use large-print materials whenever possible.
   c. make patients accept you as a health-care provider.
   d. deny that they are visually impaired to make them feel better.
5. Burnout from jobs and other conditions tends to build up stress. To avoid burnout, the medical assistant should
   a. be realistic about his or her expectations and have balance in his or her life.
   b. feel good by spending more time on what he or she likes.

c. discuss problems with patients and anyone who will listen.
d. become aggressive and stand up for himself/herself.

Discussion Questions

1. Discuss the difference between verbal and nonverbal communication. Give examples of each.
2. Suggest some of the communication problems that can arise with patients from other cultures. How might you deal with these problems?
3. Discuss defense mechanisms and apply them to everyday communication with friends, family, and classmates.

Critical Thinking Questions

1. You notice that you have not been feeling well lately, and you suspect that it is job-related stress. What kinds of activities can you take part in to help reduce stress and prevent job burnout?
2. How does learning about the cultural differences related to ethnic groups enhance a medical assistant's professional development?
3. An established patient has just recently lost her husband of 56 years and is very depressed. Which stage of the Kübler-Ross model best describes this patient?

Application Activities

1. With a partner or group, take turns using body language to indicate a variety of emotions and see if the others can correctly guess what message you are sending.
2. With a group of classmates, create an outline for an office policy and procedures manual. Identify sections that might need updating on an ongoing basis and why the updating might be necessary.

3. With a partner, take turns being blindfolded and communicate a list of activities each of you wants the other person to do. For example:
   - Walk to the bathroom
   - Purchase a candy bar out of the vending machine
   - Find the light switch
   - Turn on a computer

This activity will teach you how to communicate with someone who depends on you and allows the partner to feel what it is like to depend on someone.

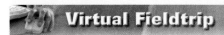

Virtual Fieldtrip

Visit the McGraw-Hill Higher Education Medical Assisting website at www.mhhe.com/medicalassisting4e to complete the following activity:

Research the predominant ethnic group in your location and write a one-page report on the perspectives members of various cultures may have on their attitudes about health care.

Open the CD and complete this chapter's practice activities, play the games, listen to the key terms, and test yourself with the interactive review. E-mail, print, and/or save your results to document your proficiency.

PART

Two

Administrative Medical Assisting

"In my 15 years as a medical assistant and transcriptionist in a large cardiology practice, I have gained invaluable experience that enhances the care of our patients. Cardiology patients require complex care. State-of-the-art equipment, pleasant office surroundings, and a well-educated, warm, and caring staff are key elements in helping patients feel at ease. As I work with patients, I do everything I can to help them feel comfortable in the office. Using reassuring words and good listening skills helps them overcome the anxieties they may have about their illness or a test they are about to have performed.

"Administrative duties are as important as clinical duties. For example, make sure the medical transcription work space is quiet and comfortable. Transcription requires intense concentration to ensure accuracy. Accuracy in all administrative tasks contributes to the success of each patient's treatment plan."

Kaye H. Listug
Medical Assistant, La Mesa, California

SECTION ONE
Office Work

Chapter 5 Using and Maintaining Office Equipment
Chapter 6 Using Computers in the Office
Chapter 7 Managing Correspondence and Mail
Chapter 8 Managing Office Supplies
Chapter 9 Maintaining Patient Records
Chapter 10 Managing the Office Medical Records

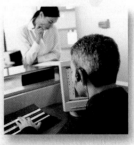

SECTION TWO
Interacting with Patients

Chapter 11 Telephone Techniques
Chapter 12 Scheduling Appointments and Maintaining
the Physician's Schedule
Chapter 13 Patient Reception
Chapter 14 Patient Education

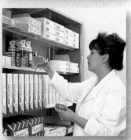

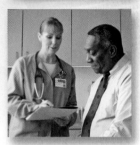

SECTION THREE
Financial Responsibilities

Chapter 15 Health Insurance Billing Procedures
Chapter 16 Medical Coding
Chapter 17 Patient Billing and Collections
Chapter 18 Accounting for the Medical Office

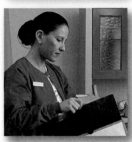

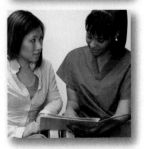

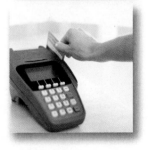

SECTION 1

OFFICE WORK

CHAPTER 5
Using and Maintaining Office Equipment

CHAPTER 6
Using Computers in the Office

CHAPTER 7
Managing Correspondence and Mail

CHAPTER 8
Managing Office Supplies

CHAPTER 9
Maintaining Patient Records

CHAPTER 10
Managing the Office Medical Records

Using and Maintaining Office Equipment

MEDICAL ASSISTING COMPETENCIES

CAAHEP

V.C. (14) Discuss the importance of routine maintenance of office equipment

V.P. (9) Perform routine maintenance of office equipment with documentation

V.P. (10) Perform an office inventory

ABHES

8. **Medical Office Business Procedures Management**
   y. Perform routine maintenance of administrative and clinical equipment

11. **Career Development**
   Demonstrate professionalism by:
   5) Exhibiting initiative
   9) Conducting work within scope of education, training, and ability

LEARNING OUTCOMES

After completing Chapter 5, you will be able to:

5.1 Describe the types of office equipment used in a medical practice.

5.2 Explain how each piece of office equipment is used.

5.3 Explain the steps in making purchasing decisions for office equipment.

5.4 Compare and contrast leasing and buying.

5.5 Explain a warranty, a maintenance contract, and a service contract, and discuss the importance of each.

5.6 Explain when troubleshooting is appropriate and what actions may be taken.

5.7 Explain the information included in an equipment inventory.

5.8 Explain how HIPAA law applies to faxing confidential patient information.

5.9 Explain how HIPAA law applies to telephone conversations and conversations with patients.

MEDICAL ASSISTING MEDIA

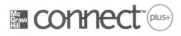 **Connect Plus+™**
connect.mcgraw-hill.com

- Electronic Health Records (E.H.R.) SpringCharts®
- eBook

SPRINGCHARTS
Electronic Health Records

 LearnSmart **LearnSmart™**

www.mhhe.com/learnsmart

Complete Learning Module: Using and Maintaining Office Equipment

 Student CD-ROM

Online **LearningCenter** **Online Learning Center™**

www.mhhe.com/medicalassisting4e

KEY TERMS

abuse	electronic media	microfiche	voice mail
cover sheet	interactive pager	microfilm	warranty
covered entity	lease	service contract	
disclaimer	maintenance contract	troubleshooting	

CHAPTER OUTLINE

- Office Communication Equipment
- Office Automation Equipment
- Purchasing Decisions
- Maintaining Office Equipment

PREPARATION FOR CERTIFICATION

RMA (AMT) Exam
- Supply and equipment management

CMA (AAMA)
- Equipment operation
- Maintenance and repair
- Equipment and supply inventory

CMAS Exam
- Supplies and equipment

Introduction

Today's medical office requires many different types of clerical equipment in order to function effectively and smoothly. The role of the medical assistant includes learning how to evaluate, purchase or lease, operate, and maintain this essential equipment.

Think how difficult it would be to communicate with others outside the office without the use of a communication system, which could include office telephones, cell phones, e-mail, beepers or pagers, interactive pagers, text messaging, answering machines, and fax machines. How limited would a medical practice become if the recording of the care given to a patient had to be done *without* the use of a computer? What if all patient billing, bank deposits, and payroll management had to be done *without* the use of a calculator or business accounting software? Without a paper shredder, each piece of confidential paper would have to be torn many times before discarding. Possibly the most difficult of all tasks would be the duplication of endless documents by hand instead of using a copy machine!

In this chapter you will be learning about the use and maintenance of many important pieces of administrative medical office equipment. Additionally, you just might come away with a new appreciation of the importance they play in the function of the efficient medical practice.

Meg is a CMA (AAMA) and is the first to arrive each morning at the busy medical practice where she works. As she unlocks the back door, she is thinking about the entry process. She knows she will set off an alarm as she enters and that she must go immediately to the security alarm box on the nearby wall and type in her security code number to turn off the system.

Meg walks through the office to the administrative section of the practice. As she walks, she notices the fire extinguisher hanging on the wall. She makes a note to herself to call the maintenance company today to notify them that the expiration date on the extinguisher is this month. They will replace the old one with a new extinguisher.

Meg next turns on all the lights in the administrative and clinical areas. As she walks through the quiet office, she sees three messages in the fax machine that have come in overnight. She picks them up and scans them quickly before she places them in the center of her desk. She notices that the late-night pick-up specimen boxes are empty. She now knows that all items placed there last evening at the close of the day were picked up by the lab.

She switches on the copy machines. On the top display is a four-digit number that indicates the number of copies each machine has made this month. Because it is the first of the month, she will call the leasing company today to report that number. Her office is billed based on how many copies are made each month.

Sitting at her desk, Meg turns off the telephone answering machine, which has been in operation throughout the night. There are four messages. As she listens, she makes careful notes before she discards each message and turns off the system. She knows that the phone will start ringing soon.

Meg turns on her computer and reviews all the tasks ahead of her today as a CMA (AAMA) in a busy medical practice. She has received e-mail from another doctor's office asking her to call about a new referral. Another e-mail is requesting medical records. Meg prints out two computer lists of appointments scheduled for the day, placing one in the front office and one in the back office for easy reference.

Next, she moves to the patient medical charts already pulled from the medical chart area the night before. She makes sure they are in chronological order. Comparing the charts against the computer list of appointments, she makes sure she has a chart for every name on the list.

A quick look around the administrative office helps her to identify items that need to be restocked. She checks and restocks the supply of pens and forms, and makes sure the copier tray is filled with paper. Making her way into the patient reception area, she turns on the soft lighting and music, tidies the magazines, feeds the fish in the fish tank, picks up the physician's morning newspaper at the front door, and unlocks the front door.

There is one more thing Meg must check before she settles in to her day's work. She makes her way to the break room and makes a big pot of coffee for all the staff. With a steaming coffee mug in hand, Meg walks back to her desk. Let the day begin!

As you read this chapter, consider the following questions:

1. What factors might go into the choice of an answering machine over the use of an answering service?
2. What backups for system failure might be important for the equipment in a medical office?
3. How could a misdialed phone number on the fax machine impact the life of a patient?
4. Why is routine maintenance of all office equipment important?

Office Communication Equipment

When you think of equipment for a medical office, you probably imagine x-ray machines, blood pressure monitors, and stethoscopes. You will, however, find many other kinds of equipment in a medical practice. Medical offices also use business communication equipment, including telephones, facsimile machines, computers, and photocopiers. Part of your responsibilities as a medical assistant is maintaining and operating the medical office's communication equipment.

Just as medical equipment has evolved over the years, so has office equipment. The office communication equipment available not so many years ago handled only the most basic tasks. Today's technology allows almost instantaneous communication of information throughout the world. This instant communication can be critical for the fast-paced medical profession, where information often translates to the need for immediate treatment, sometimes in life-threatening situations. Communicating effectively within a medical office can be as vital as providing the correct treatment to patients—and often ensures that they receive such treatment (Figure 5-1).

Telephone Systems and Call Handling

The telephone is one of the most important pieces of communication equipment in a medical practice. Not only is it the primary instrument patients use to communicate

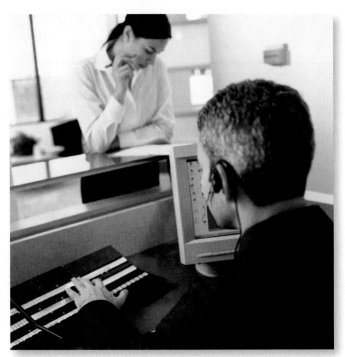

Figure 5-1. Most medical offices today rely on many up-to-date pieces of communication equipment.

with the office, but it is also the primary means of communication with other doctors, hospitals, laboratories, and other businesses important to the practice.

Multiple Lines. Few practices can function with just one or two telephone lines because if those lines are in use, no other calls can be placed or received. Most medical offices have a telephone system that includes several telephones and telephone lines. The key telephone system with multiple buttons is a traditional choice in medical practices. This system has multiple lines for incoming or outgoing calls, an intercom line, and a button for putting a call on hold. The larger a practice becomes, the greater will be the demand on the phone system. Larger practices may need complex communications systems to handle all their needs.

A telephone system can be set up so that all incoming calls ring on all the telephones in the office. A more common setup in busy practices is to use a switchboard, a device that receives all calls. The receptionist then routes calls to the appropriate telephone extensions.

An alternative to the use of a switchboard and receptionist is an automated voice response unit. This unit will automatically answer all calls. A recorded voice offers the caller various options for routing of the call. Once the caller selects an option, the system automatically routes the call to another detailed menu or to the designated department. The use of automated voice response units can provide greater flexibility for the medical staff, as well as enhanced service to the patient. However, the use of more than three menu levels may be frustrating to callers.

Advances in technology and the advent of the Internet is dramatically changing voice communications. Technologies such as Voice over Internet Protocol (VoIP), also known as Internet Voice, allow the integration of voice and data communication through the computer and Internet service. This means that medical practices have the option of using the computer for Internet access and telephone conversations.

Voice Mail. An automated menu is often used in conjunction with **voice mail,** which is a form of an answering machine. If the office is closed or the person the patient is calling is on the phone or away from her desk, the call is answered by voice mail, and the caller can leave a message. The advantage of a voice-mail system is that the caller never receives a busy signal. Another advantage to voice mail is that it is a more secure system, in that each person on a voice mail system has a unique password to retrieve only her messages.

Patient Courtesy Phone. Some offices have a patient courtesy phone, which provides an outside local phone line strictly for the use of patients. Long-distance calls can be blocked from this phone. The addition of such a line leaves office lines free for business calls. The patient courtesy phone is usually located in the reception area. A patient courtesy phone provides a line of communication for patients to call for transportation or to contact work or family as needed. It is helpful to post a sign near the phone to indicate guidelines for its use. Calls are usually limited to three minutes.

Cellular (Cell) Phones—Personal and Business Use. The use of cell phones has become widespread. Today, physicians, medical practice employees, and patients may all be carrying their own personal cell phones into the medical office. With all that technology available at the touch of a button, it is important to address cell phone etiquette. Generally, it is appropriate to turn off all personal cell phones inside a physician's office. The patient should be shown this consideration by the physician and staff, and the physician and staff deserve the same consideration from the patient. Many medical facilities post signs near their doors to ask the public to turn off all cell phones before entering. Cell phone calls from outside the practice are usually an interruption to the communication among the physician, the staff, and the patient. More importantly, the use of personal cell phones can interfere with other electronic equipment that may be functioning inside the medical practice.

However, cell phones do play an important part in the business functioning of the medical office. Physicians may use a cell phone to respond quickly to a message from staff or a hospital. Office staff may use personal cell phones in the case of emergency, when traditional phone systems fail. Some medical practices will even issue a cell phone to key employees who conduct business for the practice outside the office. In addition, patients may use their cell phones to call for a taxi after a doctor's appointment. If your medical office allows staff and patients to use cell phones, make sure that it is clearly noted in which areas cell phone use is permitted and for employees, when use of personal cell phones is permitted. In most offices personal cell phone usage is only permitted during break times. At other times the phones are to be turned off or left in vibrate mode.

Reflecting On . . . HIPAA

Avoiding Abuse of Patient Confidentiality

HIPAA law describes **abuse** as a practice or behavior that is not indicative of sound medical or fiscal activity. Improper or careless use of a patient's answering system or fax machine can be viewed as abusive behavior in the eyes of the law. It is imperative that the patient's right to privacy be carefully guarded at all times. If in doubt that the patient's privacy might be violated by leaving a verbal or written message on a machine, it is best to leave no message at all.

Leaving a Message on an Answering Machine or Fax Machine. On occasion, it is also important to leave a message on a patient's answering machine or to send a message to a patient's fax machine. It is now required by HIPAA law that you use these pieces of equipment correctly and confidentially. The goal in calling a patient's home is to speak directly to the patient or to leave a message with enough information to get the patient to call back. It is unlawful to disclose confidential patient information to anyone but the patient. The law requires that you guard the patient's private medical information. HIPAA requires that you *never* leave any information if unsure of the phone number dialed. As a medical assistant, you cannot ensure that only the intended patient will receive any message left on an answering machine or sent to a fax machine. To guard the patient's privacy, *state only the following information:*

- The name of the individual for whom the message is intended
- The date and time of the call
- The name of your office or practice
- Your name as the contact person in the office
- The phone number of your office or practice
- The hours the office is open for a return call
- A request for a return call

A word of caution: leave the name of the practice only if it does not reveal the purpose of the call. For instance, you would not state, "Please call Tiffany Heath from the STD Clinic." An example of an appropriate substitute would be, "Please call Tiffany Heath from Dr. Greene's office at 413-788-0001, Monday through Friday between 8 AM and 5 PM."

Alternatively, when patients sign the Office Privacy Agreement, a release may be added inquiring if messages may be left on an answering machine and if there are any restrictions to that permission. A second release may also be added asking if there is anyone at the home number to whom the office may speak and the relationship of that person to the patient. Each release should be signed and dated by the patient. Be especially careful of the hasty and indiscriminate use of fax machines. HIPAA law states that the best format for the use of fax machines involves the use of a locked mailbox at the receiver's end of the transmission.

Further information regarding this topic can be accessed on the HIPAA website, www.hipaa.org. Most in-home users, however, will not have this feature. It is always best to simply fax a request containing only the same information that was recommended for answering machines.

Answering Machine. Many offices use a telephone answering machine or voice mail system to answer calls after office hours, on weekends and holidays, and when the office is closed for any reason. A typical recorded message announces that the office is closed and states when it will reopen. The message must always indicate how the caller can reach the doctor or the covering physician in an emergency.

An answering machine may be programmed simply to play a taped message from the office, or it may also record messages from callers. If callers can leave messages, you have a responsibility to check the answering machine to retrieve them at the start of each day and after the lunch break. Do not use the speaker phone setting when retrieving messages from an answering machine, as you won't know what personal information a patient will leave in a message that might be heard by others in the office.

Answering Service. Instead of, or in addition to, an answering machine, many medical offices use an answering service. Unlike answering machines, answering services provide people to answer the telephone. They take messages and communicate them to the physician on call. The doctor on call is responsible for handling emergencies that may occur when the office is closed, such as at night or on weekends or holidays. Upon receiving a message from the answering service, the doctor calls the patient.

Answering services can be used in a number of ways. The doctor's office may use an answering machine to record calls of a routine nature and give the number of the answering service to call in emergencies. Alternatively, the answering service may have a direct connection to the doctor's office, picking up calls after a certain number of rings day or night or during specific hours.

Although most answering services provide satisfactory, sometimes even outstanding, service, it is good practice to check up on the service every so often by calling it during its coverage hours. This quality check ensures that the service meets office standards and expectations.

Routing Calls Through an Automated Menu

An automated menu system answers calls for you and separates requests into categories so that you can deal with them efficiently. You may already be familiar with automated menus, which are widely used by many large businesses. Someone who calls an automated system hears a recorded message identifying the business. The message gives the caller a list of options from which to choose to identify the purpose of the call. The caller selects an option by pressing the corresponding button on her push-button telephone. If she does not have a push-button telephone, her call is automatically routed so that she can talk to a person or leave a voice-mail message. For example, the voice response may say, "Press or say 1 for appointments. Press or say 2 for prescription renewals. Press or say 3 for referrals."

How does an automated menu system save time and effort in a medical office? You don't have to answer calls as they come in but can instead reserve a block of time in which to listen and respond to messages. This system allows you to complete other work without interruption. Though this practice is efficient, this is a policy that needs to be approved by the office manager and physicians within the practice before it is implemented. Some medical offices maintain a philosophy that places the importance of a patient's call above all other office tasks. Always ask the supervisor

in charge of the office how you should use the automated system.

To set up an automated system, you need to plan specific categories from which patients can choose. Categories may include but are not limited to (1) making and changing appointments, (2) asking billing questions, (3) asking medical questions of the doctors or nurses, (4) reporting patient emergencies, and (5) receiving calls from another doctor's office.

When the caller presses the code for a patient emergency, the call rings in the office because it needs to be answered immediately. You or other staff members can respond to calls in the other categories in a timely fashion. Questions for doctors or nurses can be routed immediately to the appropriate voice mail, bypassing the front office lines.

Automated menu systems can be set up by telephone vendors listed in the Yellow Pages. When choosing an automated telephone system, be careful that callers do not become lost in the process. It is a good idea to set up a system that allows callers to return easily to the main menu. Be sure to build in an option for rotary dial telephones as well. Following up on messages promptly also will help callers feel comfortable with your voice-mail system, so you should check for messages at least once every hour.

Some answering services specialize in medical practices. These medical specialty services will ask the medical practice to give specific directives for the triage of calls. Always ask any service for references before signing a contract for service.

Pagers (Beepers)

Physicians often need to be reached when they are out of the office, so many carry pagers. Pagers or beepers are small electronic devices that give a signal to indicate that someone is trying to reach the physician. Today, this is considered an outdated technology, but it is still used in some areas.

Technology of Paging. Each paging device is assigned a telephone number. When someone calls that number, the pager picks up the signal and beeps, buzzes, or vibrates to indicate that a call has been made. Most pagers have a window that displays the caller's telephone number so that the person who has been paged can return the call promptly. Certain models display a short message. Some pagers store telephone numbers so that the receiver can return several calls without having to write down the numbers.

Paging a Physician. Many telephone messages can wait until the physician returns to the office or calls in for messages. When a message needs to be delivered immediately, however, paging is an efficient response. The paging process is as simple as making a telephone call.

1. A list of pager numbers for each physician in the practice should be kept in a prominent place in the office, such as by the main switchboard. Make sure you know where these numbers are kept. Look up the telephone number for the pager of the physician you need to contact.

2. Dial the telephone number for the pager.

3. You will hear the telephone ringing and the call picked up. Listen for a high-pitched tone, which signals the connection between the telephone and the pager.

4. To operate most pagers, you need to dial the telephone number you wish the physician to call, followed by the pound sign (#), located below the number 9 on a push-button telephone. (Some pager services have an operator and work much like an answering service. Give the operator a message, and the operator will contact the physician.)

HIPAA and Faxing

Faxed material may include protected health information. For this reason, fax machines should never be placed in patient examination rooms or reception areas where unauthorized persons may be able to view incoming or outgoing documents. Only staff members with a "need to know" should have access to faxed and other confidential information.

5. Listen for a beep or a series of beeps signaling that the page has been transmitted. Then hang up the phone. The physician will call the number at his earliest convenience.

Interactive Pagers (I-Pagers)

Interactive pagers (I-pagers) are designed for two-way communication. The individual carrying the pager is paged in much the same way as the traditional pager. The pager can be set on "Audio" or "Vibrate" to alert the carrier that a message is coming in. However, the interactive pager screen displays a printed message and allows the physician to respond by way of a mini keyboard.

The physician can respond to the printed page by typing a return message (done by typing with the thumbs). The physician can respond back in real time to the office. The office computer and the physician enter into a conversation much like e-mail or an Internet chat room. Many problems can be handled quickly and efficiently in this manner. Additionally, because the I-pager can function silently, the physician can communicate with her office while in a meeting without disturbing others.

Each interactive pager has its own wireless Internet address. The user types in the receiving party's e-mail address and creates a message on a monitor screen. The interactive pager will give the sender the status of his message by indicating on the screen when the message has been sent, received, or read.

I-pagers can communicate with other I-pagers as well. I-pagers also have broadcast capability, meaning the sender can send to more than one receiver at a time. For this reason, practices with multiple physicians may find them very helpful.

Interactive pagers can also send messages to traditional telephones. The message is typed into the pager, and the system "calls" the telephone number. When answered, an electronic-type voice reads the message to the individual who has answered.

Facsimile Machines

Critical documents, such as laboratory reports or patient records, often need to be sent immediately to locations outside the office. Documents can be sent by means of a facsimile machine, or fax machine. A fax machine scans each page, translates it into electronic impulses, and transmits those impulses over the telephone line. When they are received by another fax machine, they are converted into an exact copy of the original document.

A fax machine in a medical office should have its own telephone line. A separate line ensures that transmission of incoming and outgoing faxes will not be interrupted and that the machine will not tie up a needed telephone line when sending or receiving information.

Benefits of Faxing. A fax machine can send an exact copy of a document within minutes. The cost for sending a fax is the same as for making a telephone call to that location. For a short document, this is usually less expensive than an overnight mail service.

When faxing documents such as ultrasounds and other types of documents that are heat-sensitive, it is appropriate to copy them on separate sheets of paper and then fax them to the appropriate persons. These documents can be easily destroyed with the use of a fax machine.

Many fax machines have a copier function and can be used as an extra copy machine. This function may only be useful, however, if the machine uses plain paper. The telephone for the fax may also be used as an extra extension for outgoing calls, if needed. Procedure 5-1 details the correct steps for using a facsimile (fax) machine.

Thermal Paper versus Plain Paper. Older fax machines print on rolls of specially treated paper called electrothermal, or thermal, paper, which reacts to heat and electricity. Thermal paper tends to fade over time, so documents received on this type of paper may need to be photocopied. Most models of fax machines use plain copy paper instead of thermal paper, avoiding the need for making copies. Information is transferred to the plain paper by either a carbon ribbon or a laser beam.

Receiving a Fax. Faxes can be received 24 hours a day if the fax machine is turned on and has an adequate supply of paper (Figure 5-3). Newer-model fax machines have memories and can store and receive documents. If the fax machine is not already sending or receiving a fax, the fax telephone rings, or the machine buzzes briefly, signaling the start of a transmission. The transmission begins shortly thereafter, with the machine printing out the document as it is sent. When completed, the

Using a Facsimile (Fax) Machine

Procedure Goal: To correctly prepare and send a fax document, while following all HIPAA guidelines to guard patient confidentiality

Materials: Fax machine, fax line, cover sheet with statement of disclaimer, area code and phone number of fax recipient, document to be faxed, telephone line, and telephone

Method:

1. Prepare a **cover sheet,** which provides information about the transmission. Cover sheets can vary in appearance but usually include the name, telephone number, and fax number of the sender and the receiver; the number of pages being transmitted; and the date of the transmission. Preprinted cover sheets can be used.

   Rationale

   The fax should clearly identify where it originated and to whom it is being sent. If another recipient receives the fax in error, they will know who to notify regarding the error.

2. All cover sheets must carry a statement of disclaimer to guard the privacy of the patient. A **disclaimer** is a statement of denial of legal liability. (A sample cover sheet is shown in Figure 5-2.) A disclaimer should be included on the cover sheet and may read something like the following:

   This fax contains confidential or proprietary information that may be legally privileged. It is intended only for the named recipient(s). If an addressing or transmission error has misdirected the fax, please notify the author by replying to this message. If you are not the named recipient, you are not authorized to use, disclose, distribute, copy, print, or rely on this fax and should immediately shred it.

   Rationale

   This step helps guard the privacy of the patient.

3. Place all pages of the document, including the cover sheet, either facedown or faceup in the fax machine's sending tray, depending on the directions stamped on the sending tray.

4. If the documents are placed facedown, write the area code and fax number on the back of the last page.

5. Dial the telephone number of the receiving fax machine, using either the telephone attached to the fax machine or the numbers on the fax keyboard. Include the area code for long-distance calls.

6. When using a fax telephone, listen for a high-pitched tone. Then press the "Send" or "Start" button, and hang up the telephone. This step completes the call circuit in older-model fax machines. Your fax is now being sent. Newer fax machines do not require this step.

   Rationale

   This step completes the call circuit in older-model fax machines.

7. If you use the fax keyboard, press the "Send" or "Start" button after dialing the telephone number. This button will start the call.

8. Watch for the fax machine to make a connection. Often a green light appears as the document feeds through the machine.

9. If the fax machine is not able to make a connection, as when the receiving fax line is busy, it may have a feature that automatically redials the number every few minutes for a specified number of attempts.

10. When a fax has been successfully sent, most fax machines print a confirmation message. When a fax has not been sent, the machine either prints an error message or indicates on the screen that the transmission was unsuccessful.

    Rationale

    This message confirms to the sender that the fax has been sent or indicates that the fax needs to be sent again.

11. Attach the confirmation or error message to the documents faxed. File appropriately.

    Rationale

    This step ensures thorough documentation related to the fax.

12. If required by office policy, the sender should call the recipient to confirm the fax was received.

continued ⟶

Using a Facsimile (Fax) Machine *(concluded)*

City Medical Associates

555 London Street Strathspey, PA 19919

Janet Michaels, MD   INTERNAL MEDICINE   Scott J. Michaels, MD

FACSIMILE COVER SHEET

Date: _____

To: _____   From: _____

Fax #: _____   Fax #: _____

# of pages (including this cover sheet): _____

Message: _____

_____

_____

_____

_____

The information contained in this transmission is privileged and confidential, intended only for the use of the individual or entity named above. If the reader of this message is not the intended recipient, you are hereby notified that any dissemination, distribution, or copying of this communication is strictly prohibited. If you have received this transmission in error, do not read. Please immediately respond to the sender that you have received this communication in error and then destroy or delete it. Thank you.

Figure 5-2. Every document that is sent by fax transmission should include a cover sheet, which provides details about the transmission. A disclaimer should be included on the cover sheet.

machine may print a transmission report that includes the number of pages, the date and time, and the originating fax number. Chapter 6 discusses sending and receiving faxes via computers, scanners, servers, and the Internet.

Typewriters

Typewriters are used very little in a medical practice. They may still be used to complete medical forms brought in by patients or sent from an insurance company. These forms

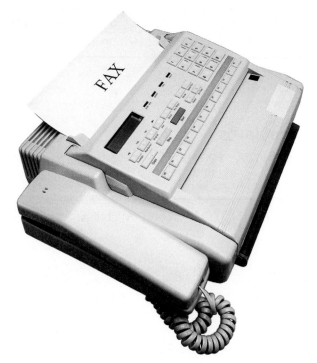

Figure 5-3. A fax machine scans a document, translates it into electronic impulses, and then transmits those impulses over the telephone line.

can be completed more clearly when the information is typed instead of handwritten.

Models and Features. Although typewriter models differ in features, all use a standard keyboard. Most typewriters have replaceable cartridge ribbons for printing and a second correction ribbon for corrections.

A wide variety of electric and electronic typewriter models are available. Although both are powered by electricity, they differ in their ability to perform certain functions. Electronic typewriters can store limited amounts of information for further use, but electric typewriters cannot. Both electric and electronic typewriters provide a selection of features, including, but not limited to, automatic carriage return, automatic centering, self-correction, and changeable typefaces or fonts. Today, most medical practices use computers with word processing software and scanners to create and manipulate word documents.

Office Automation Equipment

Using automated equipment enables you to perform a task more easily and quickly than doing it manually. For example, adding numbers on a calculator is a much faster process than doing it on paper. Many of the administrative tasks in a medical practice can be accomplished with the assistance of automated equipment, allowing you more time to perform other tasks.

Photocopiers

A photocopier, also called a copier or copy machine, instantly reproduces office correspondence, forms, bills, patient records, and other documents. Before photocopiers were available, offices used carbon paper to reproduce documents as they were being typed. The number of copies that could be made was limited.

A photocopier takes a picture of the document it is to reproduce and prints it on plain paper using a heat process. Photocopiers use either liquid or dry toner, a form of ink. Photocopiers do not require treated or otherwise special paper. Various kinds of paper can be used in the machine, including office stationery and colored paper. Many photocopiers accept different sizes of paper, from the standard 8½- by 11-inch paper to 8½- by 14-inch legal paper and even larger.

Photocopiers come in many models, from desktop machines for limited use to industrial models for continual heavy use. The machines vary in features and speed. All styles of machines are available through purchase or lease. Procedure 5-2 describes the correct method for using a photocopier machine.

Special Features. Copiers offer a wide range of special features. They may collate (assemble sets of multiple pages in order) and staple pages, punch holes, enlarge or reduce images, and produce double-sided copies (print on both sides of the page). Some also can adjust contrast and even track the cost of a job via a specific code input into the machine. Some photocopiers produce black-and-white copies as well as color copies. Some copiers can make transparencies (text and images printed on clear acetate), which physicians often use for presentations. Copiers can even be configured to electronically scan documents for electronic communications, and to send and receive facsimiles.

One of the more useful features of photocopiers is the help function. Selecting this function displays directions in plain English that explain how to fix a paper jam or deal with other routine copier problems. Some copiers are even programmed to indicate that service is needed.

Adding Machines and Calculators

For handling tasks such as patient billing, bank deposits, and payroll, many medical practices depend on adding machines and calculators. The difference between the two types of machines is minimal. Adding machines typically plug into an outlet and produce a paper tape on which calculations are printed. Calculators are more often battery or solar powered, with memory to store figures. Calculators are portable and usually do not produce a paper tape.

Routine Calculations. Both adding machines and calculators are sufficient for most routine office calculations. These machines perform basic arithmetic functions, such as addition, subtraction, multiplication, and division. Many of today's models perform such specialized functions as computing percentages and storing data. Some are even computerized.

Checking Your Work. It is easy to hit an incorrect key or to key in a number twice when using an adding machine or a calculator. Therefore, check all mathematical computations.

PROCEDURE 5-2

Using a Photocopier Machine

Procedure Goal: To produce copies of documents

Materials: Copier machine, copy paper, documents to be copied

Method:

1. Make sure the machine is turned on and warmed up. It will display a signal when it is ready for copying.

2. Assemble and prepare your materials, removing paper clips, staples, and self-adhesive flags.

   Rationale

   This step helps avoid loose items getting caught in the copier and provides for optimum efficiency.

3. Place the document to be copied in the automatic feeder tray as directed, or upside down directly on the glass. The feeder tray can accommodate many pages; you may place only one page at a time on the glass. Automatic feeding is a faster process, and you should use it when you wish to collate or staple packets. Page-by-page copying is best if you need to copy a single sheet or to enlarge or reduce the image. To use any special features, such as making double-sided copies or stapling

the copies, press a designated button on the machine.

4. Set the machine for the desired paper size.

   Rationale

   The copier will select the paper size automatically if the size is not selected. This could result in a waste of paper.

5. Key in the number of copies you want to make, and press the "Start" button. The copies are made automatically.

6. Press the "Clear" or "Reset" button when your job is finished.

   Rationale

   The machine is now ready for the next user and will not perform unwanted functions on the next document.

7. If the copier becomes jammed, follow the directions on the machine to locate the problem (for example, there may be multiple pieces of paper stuck inside the printer), and dislodge the jammed paper. Most copy machines will show a diagram of the printer and the location of the problem.

If the machine produces a paper tape, check the numbers on the tape against the numbers you are adding. The paper tape is especially useful when adding a long series of numbers. Without a printed record, you must perform the same calculations again to make sure the total is correct.

Folding and Inserting Machines

Letter-folding equipment can help minimize the amount of time staff spends preparing large volumes of outgoing mail. Letter folders are also used for creating folded brochures. A medical practice may use folding and inserting machines for a variety of items, including invoices, newsletters, checks, statements, letters, and flyers.

Lower-end folding equipment requires letters to be fed manually. The speed of this machine is limited to the speed an individual can feed in letters, which is typically about 200 pieces per hour. An automatic feeder is required for faster folding. Letter-folding machines can make many different types of folds, including standard business letter folds (c-fold), accordion folds (z-fold), single folds, right-angle folds, and brochure folds (Figure 5-4). Most machines can fold more than one sheet of paper together, but do not allow stapled pages to be fed and folded.

Many special features are available that may help the processing of mail and brochures. Batch counters and stackers help to prevent a letter folding machine from folding more sheets than desired. A jogger helps align stacks of paper and dissipates static electricity. Some machines are better designed for certain types of paper, such as glossy or carbonless paper. Inserters are used to insert a folded document into an envelope.

Postage Meters

Every medical office uses the U.S. Postal Service. Patient bills, routine correspondence, purchase orders, and payments are just some of the items typically sent by mail. (See Chapter 7 for additional information on mailing correspondence.)

Although some medical offices use stamps, most use a postage meter. A postage meter is a machine that applies postage to an envelope or package, eliminating the need for postage stamps (Figure 5-5). There are often two parts to a postage meter: the meter, which belongs to the post office, and the mailing machine, which the practice can own. The meter actually applies the postage, and the mailing machine (if available) seals the envelope.

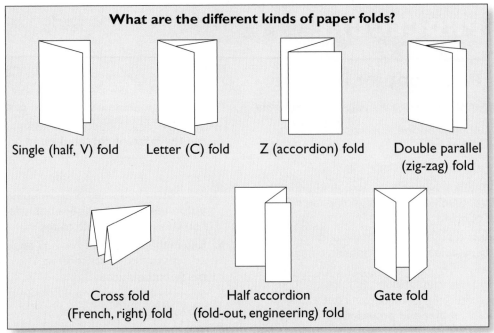

What are the different kinds of paper folds?

Single (half, V) fold

Letter (C) fold

Z (accordion) fold

Double parallel
(zig-zag) fold

Cross fold
(French, right) fold

Half accordion
(fold-out, engineering) fold

Gate fold

Figure 5-4. Folding machines can make many different kinds of paper folds.

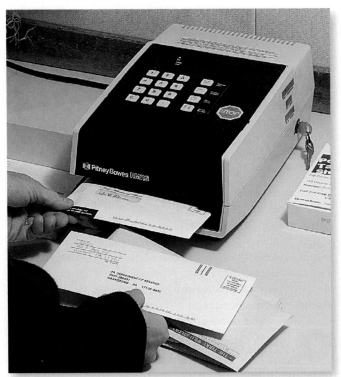

Figure 5-5. The postage meter is a convenient and cost-effective way to apply postage to office correspondence and packages.

Benefits of Using a Postage Meter. There are several advantages to using a postage meter instead of purchasing stamps. It saves frequent trips to the post office. It also saves money for the office by providing the exact amount of postage needed for each item. When you have to use a combination of stamps, you may exceed the minimum required postage. It is unlikely as well as

impractical for a practice to keep every denomination of stamps on hand.

Some postage meters can imprint envelopes with the name of your medical practice or with a message at the same time postage is applied. The message appears immediately to the left of the postal mark, at the top of the envelope.

Many types of postage meters are available, from basic models for a small office to advanced models for large businesses. The latest machines include automatic date setting, memory to program a large mailing, and display alerts for low postage or the need for ribbon replacement. Some models can apply postage to parcels without the use of labels or tape. Procedure 5-3 describes how to use a postage meter.

Prepaying for Postage. To use a postage meter, you must prepay the postage. You can take your meter to the post office to add postage, or you can use a postage meter service. A service maintains the postal account for you. Although the money in each account is the property of the U.S. Postal Service, the provider manages the account and adds postage to the meter. Postage can also be added to the meter by telephone or by modem, with data sent directly to the meter over the telephone line. The process takes only a few minutes, and the call is often toll-free. Before postage can be added, however, money must be deposited into an account. Keeping the postage account current ensures that all mail is sent on a timely basis. This task may be one of your responsibilities.

On any meter, you can check the amount of postage used and the amount remaining with the touch of a button. On some models, the meter must have $10 or more for the machine to apply postage to an envelope or package.

PROCEDURE 5-3

Using a Postage Meter

Procedure Goal: To correctly apply postage to an envelope or package for mailing, according to U.S. Postal Service guidelines

Materials: Postage meter, addressed envelope or package, postal scale

Method:

1. Check that there is postage available in the postage meter.

   Rationale

   For the postage meter to function, there must be money in your postal account. Contact the company that is managing your account or your local post office for more information.

2. Verify the day's date.

   Rationale

   U.S. Postal Service guidelines prohibit mailing envelopes and packages that are postmarked with an incorrect date.

3. Check that the postage meter is plugged in and switched on before you proceed

4. Locate the area where the meter registers the date. Many machines have a lid that can be flipped up, with rows of numbers underneath. Months are represented numerically, with the number "1" indicating the month of January, "2" indicating February, and so on. Check that the date is correct. If it is incorrect, change the numbers to the correct date.

5. Make sure that all materials have been included in the envelope or package. Weigh the envelope or package on a postal scale. Standard business envelopes weighing up to 1 oz require the minimum postage (the equivalent of one firstclass stamp). Oversize envelopes and packages require additional postage. A postal scale will indicate the amount of postage required.

6. Key in the postage amount on the meter, and press the button that enters the amount. For amounts over $1, press the "$" sign or the "Enter" button twice.

   Rationale

   This feature verifies large amounts, catching errors in case you mistakenly press too many keys.

7. Check that the amount you typed is the correct amount. Envelopes and packages with too little postage will be returned by the U.S. Postal Service. Sending an envelope or package with too much postage is wasteful to the practice.

8. While applying postage to an envelope, hold it flat and right side up (so that you can read the address). Seal the envelope (unless the meter seals it for you). Locate the plate or area where the envelope slides through. This feature is usually near the bottom of the meter. Place the envelope on the left side, and give it a gentle push toward the right. Some models hold the envelope in a stationary position. (If the meter seals the envelope for you, it is especially important that you insert it correctly to allow for sealing.) The meter will grab the envelope and pull it through quickly.

9. For packages, create a postage label to affix to the package. Follow the same procedure for a label as for an envelope. Affix the postmarked label on the package in the upper-right corner.

10. Check that the printed postmark has the correct date and amount and that everything written or stamped on the envelope or package is legible.

Postal Scales

Besides the postage meter, a medical practice also needs a postal scale. Postal scales are a good investment because they show both the weight and the amount of postage required. Some postage meters include an electronic scale. If you need a postal scale but one is not available, you can use any scale that weighs in ounces. When using a simple scale, you can then translate the weight into the correct postage by using a current postal rate chart, available from the U.S. Postal Service which cuts down on mail being returned for inadequate postage.

Posting Mail

Before you begin posting mail, make sure the envelope or package is complete, with all materials included. After applying the proper postage, place the postmarked envelope or package in the area of your office designated for mail pickup.

Dictation-Transcription Equipment

Physicians usually do not type their own correspondence, patient records, or other documents. Medical assistants, although not professional medical transcriptionists, may be asked to transcribe recorded words into written text. Using dictation-transcription equipment is the most efficient way to complete this task. *Dictation* is another word for speaking; *transcription* is another word for writing. Together they mean to transform spoken words into written form.

Dictation-transcription equipment has greatly advanced. There are now "starter kits" that are generally for smaller medical offices, as well as more advanced digital dictation and transcription kits. Speechmikes are great for the physicians. They are lightweight and when the physician speaks, the sounds are more audible to the transcriber. The standard functions of transcription equipment include controls for starting, stopping, reversing and fast-forwarding, volume, tone and speed control, headphones, and a counter.

Larger medical facilities may provide call-in transcription services for the physician. This type of service makes it easy to link to external databases. Doctors can dictate from remote locations and the information can be uploaded to the computer so that the medical assistant can transcribe it.

Voice recognition software is available to provide help to the physician when he or she wants to set up dictation via the computer. There are specialized programs that are provided for medical specialties.

Dictating. Quite often, the physician's handwriting can be confusing. Dictation is a wonderful tool that not only assists the medical assistant, but, frankly, keeps the physician out of trouble (see Figure 5-6). Using these steps can make transcribing much easier. Ask the physician to

1. Indicate the date and the type of document being dictated and provide explicit instructions about the document. For example, it is helpful to indicate that the document is a letter and that it is to be produced on office stationery and mailed to a patient.
2. Spell out all names and addresses as well as any unfamiliar terms.
3. Indicate punctuation by saying, for example, "comma" or "begin new paragraph."
4. Speak clearly and slowly. Neither eat while dictating nor record in a noisy environment, if at all possible.

Procedure 5-4 shows you how to operate a dictation-transcription machine. Chapter 9 describes the medical transcription process in greater detail.

Check Writers

Medical practice personnel need to write checks to pay for equipment, supplies, and payroll. This common office procedure can be automated by using a check writer, which is a machine that imprints checks. Procedure 5-5 details the correct steps for operating a check-writing machine.

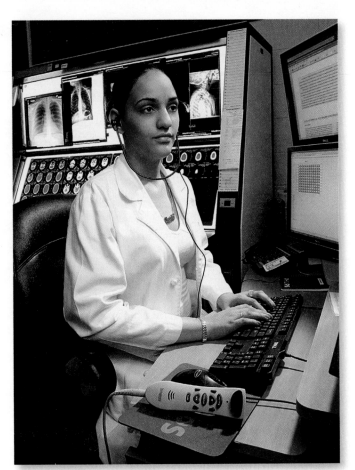

Figure 5-6. One of the responsibilities of a medical assistant may be to use dictation-transcription equipment.

The safety advantage of using such a machine is that the name of the payee (the person receiving the check) and the amount of the check, once imprinted, cannot be altered. There are numerous check-writing software packages that can assist you, such as QuickBooks, Checksoft, and VersaCheck.

Voiding a Check. If the information on an imprinted check is incorrect, it cannot be changed. Therefore, you must issue a new check and void the previous one. To void the check, write "VOID" in clear letters across it, or use a VOID stamp with red ink. Then file the check with the office bank records so that the practice's money manager is aware that it has been voided.

Paper Shredders

Paper shredders are quite common in medical practices. A paper shredder, such as the one shown in Figure 5-7, is often used when confidential documents, such as patient records, need to be destroyed. Paper shredders cut documents into tiny pieces to make them unreadable.

The most common type of shredder cuts paper into ribbonlike strips, which differ in width, depending on the

PROCEDURE 5-4

Using a Dictation-Transcription Machine

Procedure Goal: To correctly use a dictation transcription-machine to convert verbal communication into the written word

Materials: Dictation-transcription machine, audiocassette or magnetic tape or disk with the recorded dictation, word processor or computer, and printer

Method:

1. Assemble all the necessary equipment.
2. Select a transcription tape, cassette, or disk for dictation. Select any transcriptions marked "Urgent" first. If there are none, select the oldest-dated transcription first.

   Rationale
   The items marked "urgent" are needed as soon as possible. The other items need to be completed in the order in which they were received for the smoothest flow of work within the office.

3. Turn on all equipment and adjust it according to personal preference.

Rationale
Making adjustments for comfort and proper body alignment will help you avoid injury and strain.

4. Prepare the format and style for the selected letter or form.
5. Insert the tape or cassette and rewind.

   Rationale
   The tape or cassette will be positioned at the end of the transcription.

6. While listening to the transcription tape, cassette, or disk, key in the text.
7. Adjust the speed and volume controls as needed.
8. Proofread and spell-check final document, making any corrections.

   Rationale
   This step ensures a professional and accurate document.

9. Print the document for approval and signature.
10. Turn off all equipment. Place the transcription tape, cassette, or disk in the proper storage area.

PROCEDURE 5-5

Using a Check-Writing Machine

Procedure Goal: To produce a check using a check-writing machine

Materials: Check-writing machine, blank checks, office checkbook or accounting system

Method:

1. Assemble all equipment.
2. Turn on the check-writing machine.
3. Place a blank check or a sheet of blank checks into the machine.
4. Key in the date, the payee's name, and the payment amount. The check-writing machine imprints the check with this information, perforating it with the payee's name. The perforations are actual little holes in the paper, which prevent anyone from changing the name on the check.

5. Turn off the check-writing machine.
6. A doctor or another authorized person then signs the check.

   Rationale
   The check is not valid without the proper signature.

7. To complete the process, record the check in the office checkbook or accounting system.

   Rationale
   To maintain accurate records, all financial transactions must be promptly and accurately recorded.

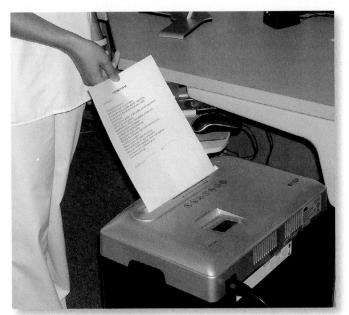

Figure 5-7. As a medical assistant, you may be asked to use a paper shredder to destroy confidential documents that are no longer needed by the practice.

model. Other shredders cut the paper in two directions, forming small pieces. Some paper shredders offer additional options, such as an electronic eye that automatically starts the machine when paper is inserted and stops when it is done. Other features available are paper jam detection, automatic reverse, and automatic shutdown when the machine gets too hot.

How to Shred Materials. A paper shredder is ready to use when it is turned on. To shred a document, insert it into the feed tray at the top of the shredder. The machine feeds the paper through hundreds of knifelike cutters, instantaneously shredding the paper. A basket attached beneath the shredder catches the bits of paper. Different models can accommodate different amounts of paper through the cutters. Shredder baskets must be emptied periodically to allow room for additional shredded paper. Some shredders signal when the basket is full. It is very important not to wear loose-fitting clothing while operating a shredder to avoid accident and personal injury.

When to Shred Materials. Medical practices need to eliminate old patient records or other sensitive materials. These items cannot simply be thrown into the trash because of confidentiality problems. The shredder is an effective disposal solution. If records have incorrect information that has been corrected on subsequent documents, the old records are shredded so that the incorrect information is not mistakenly placed in the patient's folder. A document that has been shredded cannot be put back together. Therefore, do not decide on your own to shred a document. The physician or office manager will set guidelines regarding when a document should be shredded. If you are not sure whether to shred a document, check with a senior staff member before beginning the process. Note that external shredding companies should be used for medical facilities because they have the ability and capacity to make sure shredding is done properly. Use a reputable vendor.

Microfilm and Microfiche Readers

Microfilm is a roll of film imprinted with information and stored on a reel. Film also can be stored in cartridges to protect the film from being touched. **Microfiche** is film imprinted with information and stored in rectangular sheets. See Figures 5-8 and 5-9.

Although considered to be old technology, the use of microfilm and microfiche is still in use in many medical practices today. Even if your office does not store records on microfilm or microfiche, you may still need to have a reader because back issues of medical journals and other publications are often available only in these formats.

Purchasing Decisions

As a medical assistant, you may be involved in making purchasing decisions for office equipment. For example, the physician or office manager may ask you to investigate whether the practice needs a certain piece of equipment, such as a new photocopier or microfiche reader. To make a sound decision about whether the office will benefit from such a purchase, you will need to conduct thorough research.

Reflecting On . . . HIPAA

HIPAA and Shredding

Shredding is an important way to responsibly handle confidential information that is no longer needed. Many medical practices contract with a shredding company to come into the practice, remove, and shred designated materials. Using another company for this task does not relieve the medical practice of the responsibility for the confidential materials. The healthcare provider is still considered the **covered entity** and must comply with HIPAA law. It is important to contract only with companies that also abide by HIPAA law.

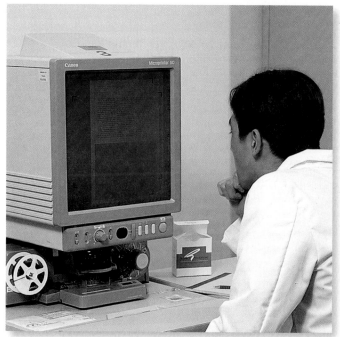
Figure 5-8. Storing information on microfilm helps reduce the amount of storage space needed by the practice.

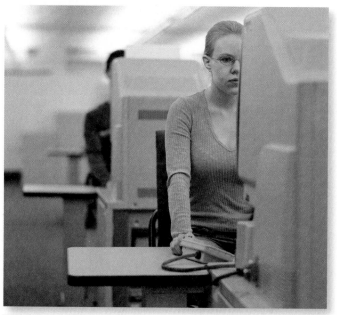
Figure 5-9. Special equipment must be used to read text that has been converted to microfiche.

Evaluating Office Needs

The first step in evaluating the equipment needs of a health-care office is the research process. Make note of the equipment that is already available and consider the different tasks the equipment can perform. To obtain a complete list of office needs, consult other staff members for their ideas.

When considering replacing an old piece of equipment, ask what advantages the new piece of equipment offers over the current one. Create a list of equipment on hand, and a list of any new products the office staff recommends. Compare the benefits offered by the new product to the capability of the currently used equipment. Many medical magazines review medical office equipment periodically and are good resources to consult in making your purchasing decisions. Go online to shop and compare products, features, and prices. Discuss with the office manager the budget for the equipment under consideration. Consider calling a supplier for more detailed information.

Contacting Suppliers. Put together a list of the features you would like in your machine. Then contact suppliers who sell models that offer those features. You can call or e-mail the manufacturer directly to find out the name of a local vendor. Many manufacturers prepare brochures giving information about their products. Request that this information be sent to you.

Go online or look in the Yellow Pages for office supply stores and other companies that sell office equipment. Obtain product and pricing information on each model. For certain equipment, such as photocopiers, a sales representative will come to your office to demonstrate and discuss the product.

Evaluating Warranty Options. Most products come with a warranty. A **warranty** is a contract that guarantees free service and replacement of parts for a certain period, usually 1 year. Warranties are valid only for specified service and repairs. They usually do not cover accidents, vandalism, acts of God (such as damage caused by floods or earthquakes), or mistreatment of the machine. In most cases, warranty repairs must be made at an authorized service center.

Reflecting On . . . HIPAA

HIPAA and Electronic Media

According to HIPAA law, transmissions that are physically moved from one location to another using magnetic tape, disk, or compact disk media are considered **electronic media**. This form of patient information must be handled in the same confidential manner as patient records. All patient information, regardless of the form, is required by HIPAA law to be guarded by the health-care provider.

Metropolitan Office Systems

Lease Agreement

Customer (Location)

Standard Education Corporation
Full Legal Name (Please Print)

119 Washington Blvd.
Address

Spokane,   *WA*   *98548*
City   County   State   Zip

Billing Contact

Dealer:

Customer (Billing address, if different)

Full Legal Name (Please Print)

Address

City   County   State   Zip

Phone

Quantity	Description: Make, Model, and Serial Number	Quantity	Description: Make, Model, and Serial Number
1	*FT 6655 Copier AA3365430358*		
1	*Sorter A337502010902*		
1	*Document Feeder A338506*		
1	*RT 314 Large-capacity Tray*		

Minimum Lease Term:	Payment Due:	Amount of Monthly Payment With Sales, Use, and Property Tax:	Advance Payment of *$965.56* (Tax Included) by Check #_____	Documentation Fee
60 Months	_X_ Monthly ___ Quarterly ___ Annually ___ Other: *$455.46*	*$482.78*	___ First Month's Rent _X_ First and Last ___ Security Deposit (Without Tax) ___ Other _____	$ _—0—_

Figure 5-10. Read lease agreements carefully.

If you want more coverage than the warranty allows, consider buying an extended warranty. Extended warranties increase the amount of time that equipment is covered. For expensive pieces of equipment or parts, the additional cost of an extended warranty may be justified.

After you purchase a product, you must fill out the warranty card and mail it to the manufacturer. File the receipt in a safe place in the office where it can easily be retrieved.

Preparing a Recommendation. After you have obtained all the information, you are ready to evaluate it. To compare and contrast the different models, construct a chart. Place the product model names in columns across the top. Down the left side, list factors that will influence the purchase decision: cost, warranty options (including the length of the warranty and the price of an extended warranty), special features, and delivery time. Then fill in the information. This chart will provide an easy-to-use summary of your research.

Finally, analyze the list, and choose the product that will best meet the needs of the office. Meet with the physician or office manager to discuss your recommendation.

Leasing versus Buying Equipment

Once the product has been selected, there is one more decision to make: whether to lease or to buy the item. When buying a product, the purchaser becomes the owner of the product. Owners are free to do with the product anything they choose, which may include selling it to someone else.

For most large pieces of office equipment, such as photocopiers, there is also an option to **lease** the equipment. Leasing, or renting, usually involves an initial charge and a monthly fee. On average, the initial charge is equal to about two monthly payments. The ownership of a leased piece of equipment is retained by the leasing company.

Lease Agreement. A lease is for a specified time, after which time the equipment is returned to the seller (Figure 5-10). Some leases allow purchase of the equipment at the end of the rental period for an additional payment. The details of the purchase option are covered in the lease agreement.

Advantages of Leasing. When you lease a product, your office does not own it, but you have several advantages.

1. Leasing allows purchasers to keep more of their money. The initial cost of obtaining the machine is a fraction of the full cost of purchasing it. Therefore, the remainder of the money can earn interest in the bank or be used for other expenses. Leasing is advantageous when you do not have enough money to buy the equipment but need the services it provides. In

addition, leasing allows businesses to update equipment every few years at the end of each lease period. Updating may not be as affordable if you buy equipment.

2. Often the company that leases the product is also responsible for servicing it.

3. In most cases, businesses are able to take lease payments as a tax deduction each year.

Leasing is not always the best solution. It is important to weigh the advantages of leasing against the advantages of buying equipment for your medical practice.

Negotiating. Whether you decide to lease or buy equipment, always ask whether the price is firm or if there is room for negotiation. Many discounted rates are never extended to the customer simply because the customer did not ask. Although some equipment prices are nonnegotiable, terms can sometimes be negotiated on more expensive pieces of equipment. Companies that lease office equipment are often flexible in determining the monthly payment. Equipment companies may accept smaller payments in the beginning of the rental or purchase agreement period, and require larger payments near the end.

In a competitive market, some suppliers may match their competitors' prices. When purchasing several pieces of equipment at the same time, a supplier may be able to offer some savings on the total cost of the purchase or provide some service, such as delivery, free of charge.

Maintaining Office Equipment

Office equipment must be regularly maintained to provide high-quality service. Daily or weekly maintenance, such as cleaning the glass on the photocopier or replacing toner, can be performed by the office staff. However, more extensive maintenance should be done by the equipment supplier. Consult the equipment manual for details about the care of each piece of equipment.

Equipment Manuals

The best source of information about maintaining a piece of equipment is the manual that comes with it. This booklet gives basic information about the equipment, including how to set it up, how it works, special features, and problems you may encounter. The information in an equipment manual is extremely valuable. If the manual is lost, call the manufacturer to obtain another one. Equipment manuals should be stored where they can be retrieved easily. Some large pieces of office equipment provide racks or slots on the side of the equipment for storage of the manual.

Maintenance and Service Contracts

Equipment suppliers provide standard maintenance contracts when office equipment is purchased. A **maintenance contract** specifies when the equipment will be cleaned, checked for worn parts, and repaired. A standard maintenance contract may include regular checkups as well as emergency repairs.

In addition, some suppliers offer a **service contract,** which covers services that are not included under the standard maintenance agreement. A service contract may cover emergency repairs not covered under standard maintenance. In some cases, service contracts are combined with maintenance contracts in one document.

It is important to keep track of all maintenance performed on your equipment. Many offices keep a maintenance log, where staff members record the date and purpose of each service call. This log is helpful in identifying whether equipment should be replaced because of the need for frequent servicing.

Troubleshooting

When a piece of equipment stops functioning properly, what is the correct course of action? One option is to call a service supplier. However, you can also take steps to determine and correct the problem yourself. This process is called **troubleshooting.** Resolving the problem can save you the cost of a service call that may not be covered by the standard agreement.

The first step in troubleshooting is to eliminate possible simple causes of a problem. For example, if the equipment is powered by electricity, make sure that it is plugged into a functioning outlet and that it is turned on. Are all doors and other openings in their correct positions? Are all machine connections firmly in place?

Points on Practice

Equipment Manual Tips

It is helpful to write the following information on the inside front cover of the equipment manual upon initial setup. If there is a problem with the equipment that requires a maintenance call, this valuable information will be quick and easy to retrieve.

1. The date of purchase or lease
2. The serial number of the equipment
3. The phone number of the company contracted to repair the equipment

If you cannot discover a simple cause for the problem, it is time to test the machine to determine what it is failing to do. In the case of a malfunctioning photocopier, for example, try making a copy and note the response. Write down any error messages the machine provides.

Next, consult the equipment manual. Many manuals devote a section to troubleshooting. If you cannot find the solution after reading the manual, call the manufacturer or the place of purchase for additional assistance. Be prepared to explain the steps you have already taken toward resolving the problem.

Backup Systems

Occasionally, more than one piece of equipment can be affected by a single problem. For example, if the electricity goes off, all electrical equipment will go out at once. To avoid losing important information and records, it is important to have backup systems in place.

Computers. Computers should be placed on a backup system. The company that services the computer system usually sets this up. Computer backup may occur either automatically off-site over the phone lines or on-site, which may require that a staff member manually plug in a backup tape every night before going home. Computer backup usually occurs at midnight, when the office is not using the system. Computer backup ensures that all information will be retrievable even if the computers suffer a catastrophic failure.

Telephones. The use of cell phones in addition to traditional phones offers a backup to communication in the event that phone service is interrupted. Cell phones are also helpful during emergency weather conditions.

Electricity. An emergency generator may supply emergency power for lighting in key hallways and exam rooms. Interior rooms and halls can quickly become very dark and hazardous when the electricity is unexpectedly cut off.

Battery Power. Battery power backup is a key component of security and warning system backups. Audio warning signals sound when it is time to replace the batteries in smoke and security detectors. All batteries should routinely be replaced every six months.

Fire Extinguishers. Fire extinguishers need to be serviced or replaced once a year to ensure maximum performance. The office may choose to contract with a local company to provide this annual maintenance evaluation.

Equipment Inventory

Each piece of equipment is an asset of a business. It is part of the business's net worth and should be listed on the medical practice's balance sheet. Therefore, taking inventory of office equipment provides relevant information for the practice's money manager. It may also indicate whether old equipment is due for replacement.

There are many different ways to take an office equipment inventory. Figure 5-11 shows one example. Many offices use a master inventory sheet to survey all equipment at a glance. The master sheet usually includes such general information as equipment name and purchase price, and the quantity of each type of equipment.

Many offices also keep more detailed information about each individual piece of equipment in files or on a single sheet of paper. Detailed information may include the following:

- Name of the equipment, including the brand name
- Brief description of the equipment
- Model number and registration number
- Date of purchase
- Place of purchase, including contact information
- Estimated life of the product
- Product warranty
- Maintenance and service contracts

EQUIPMENT INVENTORY

ITEM	PURCHASE DATE	PURCHASE PRICE
1. TotalOffice oak desk	07/25/10	$295.00
2. TotalOffice rolling desk chair	02/19/10	$119.00
3. TotalOffice 4-drawer file cabinet	12/21/11	$150.00
4. TotalOffice 2-drawer file cabinet	08/05/11	$100.00
5. HYtech Pentium 100 computer	03/10/12	$1150.00
6. HYtech 14-inch monitor	03/10/12	$200.00

Figure 5-11. An equipment inventory sheet includes equipment names and the quantity of each type of equipment.

All equipment inventories should be updated periodically. Inventory software packages are becoming more effective in managing your equipment and supplies. Make sure you choose an inventory software package that best fits your needs.

Summary

5.1 The types of office equipment used in a medical office practice are fax machines, computers, photocopiers, postage meters, paper shredders, dictation-transcription machines, scanners, and all-in-one equipment (printer, fax, copier).

5.2 Telephone systems are the primary communication tool in a medical office. Answering machines and answering services provide messages to be left for medical office staff by either recorded message or being routed to a "live" individual. Fax machines are used to send documents via electronic transmission. Computers are used to compose written correspondence and other documents. Transcription equipment is essential in the medical office for dictated notes from the physician.

5.3 In order to effectively establish your medical office's needs and supplies, you must first evaluate the needs. Next, decide whether you want to purchase or lease major equipment, then prepare a recommendation and negotiate for best pricing.

5.4 After you select the equipment you need, the decision to buy or lease is critical. Buying a product means that it belongs to the office. However, leasing has its advantages. Leasing allows you to keep more of your money, and is tax deductible for business owners.

5.5 A maintenance contract differs from a service contract. A service contract covers services that are not usually included in the standard maintenance agreement. A maintenance contract generally includes regular checkpoint reports. A warranty is a contract that guarantees free service and replacement of parts for a certain period.

5.6 Troubleshooting is appropriate when a piece of equipment stops functioning properly. Many times a problem can be solved by taking steps to determine and correct the problem yourself. You may have to use your equipment manual. If the problem persists, contacting your service agent is the next step. There may be a fee involved.

5.7 The information that is located in the equipment inventory is (1) the name of the equipment, (2) a description of the equipment, (3) the model and registration numbers, (4) the date and place of purchase, and (5) the product warranty and maintenance and service contracts.

5.8 Protected health information may periodically have to be faxed. HIPAA states that the medical staff use confidentiality at all times by placing fax machines in locations where unauthorized persons may not view documents. Also, only staff members with need-to-know capabilities should have access to information that is being faxed.

5.9 It is imperative that the medical staff abide by the HIPAA laws when it pertains to a patient's privacy on the telephone. If you are in doubt about a violation when handling telephone messages and leaving messages via the answering machine, it is best not to leave one at all.

REVIEW

CHAPTER 5

CASE STUDY QUESTIONS

Now that you have completed this chapter, review the case study at the beginning of the chapter and answer the following questions:

1. What factors might go into the choice of an answering machine over the use of an answering service?

2. What backups for system failure might be important for the equipment in a medical office?
3. How could a misdialed phone number on the fax machine impact the life of a patient?
4. Why is routine maintenance of all office equipment important?

Multiple-Choice Questions

1. Faxes can be received ____ hours a day.
   a. 2   c. 12
   b. 8   d. 24
2. A caller listening to a recorded menu and, in response, pressing a number on his telephone keypad is an example of
   a. multiple telephone lines.
   b. a pager.
   c. an answering machine.
   d. an automated menu.
3. Which of the following answers calls after office hours and on weekends and holidays?
   a. Automated menu
   b. Multiple phone lines
   c. Pagers
   d. Answering machine
4. The advantage of using plain paper instead of thermal paper in a fax machine is to
   a. provide a softer and thinner paper.
   b. eliminate the need to make copies.
   c. reduce the heat sensitivity of the paper.
   d. protect the original document from damage during the fax.
5. Medical assistants may be asked to transcribe recorded words into written text by using
   a. an answering machine.
   b. voice mail.
   c. dictation-transcription equipment.
   d. microfiche.

Discussion Questions

1. Why is office equipment important to the medical office? Give at least three examples of pieces of typical office equipment, and describe their use in the medical office.
2. Compare and contrast the advantages and disadvantages of buying and leasing equipment.
3. What are some features of a standard product warranty?
4. Describe a scenario in which an interactive pager might be helpful in a medical office.

Critical Thinking Questions

1. Imagine that you are responsible for the maintenance of the office equipment in a busy medical practice. What weekly, monthly, and yearly checks might you perform? How would you document these checks?
2. You think that your office needs a new photocopier. Explain how you would justify this need to the office manager.
3. You have been asked to fax confidential patient information to another medical office. What precautions will you take to protect this information?
4. The fax machine in your office is malfunctioning. Explain the steps you might take to troubleshoot the problem.
5. Typewriters and microfiche machines are not commonly used in medical offices today. What technology has replaced them?

Application Activities

1. Your office frequently uses temporary employees to help with copying. The office manager asks you to write directions for the use of the photocopier, to be posted near the machine. Using the computer, create a sign suitable for posting.
2. Your office is moving soon, and you have been asked to assist in the design of a new communication system for the practice. What features would you include in the new system?
3. You have been asked to design a cover sheet for the fax machine for your office. Using the computer, design a cover sheet with a disclaimer.
4. Go online and research three different types of photocopiers. Write a report describing each. Be sure to include the equipment name, manufacturer, warranty options, price, advantages to buying or leasing, features, and recommendations for use.

Virtual Fieldtrip

Visit the McGraw-Hill Higher Education Medical Assisting website at www.mhhe.com/medicalassisting4e to complete the following activity:

Use the American Association of Medical Assistants and the U.S. Department of Health and Human Services websites. Prepare an oral presentation about one of the following topics:

- HIPAA law and the use of fax machines
- HIPAA law and the use of answering machines
- The advantages and disadvantages of an automated phone system
- The appropriate use of a cell phone while on the job

Ask your instructor how many references and citations you should minimally include in your research. Present your report to the class, using all available multimedia, including PowerPoint slides or an overhead projector if possible.

Open the CD and complete this chapter's practice activities, play the games, listen to the key terms, and test yourself with the interactive review. E-mail, print, and/or save your results to document your proficiency.

CHAPTER 6

Using Computers in the Office

MEDICAL ASSISTING COMPETENCIES

CAAHEP

IV. C (9) Discuss applications of electronic technology in effective communication

V. P (6) Use office hardware and software to maintain office systems

V. P (7) Use the Internet to access information related to the medical office

ABHES

4. Basic Computer Keyboarding/Computer Concepts
   b. Identify and properly utilize office machines, computerized systems and medical software

8. Medical Office Business Procedures Management
   kk. Adapt to individualized needs
   ll. Apply electronic technology

11. Career Development
   Demonstrate professionalism by:
   1) Exhibiting dependability, punctuality, and a positive work ethic
   2) Exhibiting a positive attitude and a sense of responsibility
   5) Exhibiting initiative
   6) Adapting to change
   7) Expressing a responsible attitude
   9) Conducting work within scope of education, training, and ability

LEARNING OUTCOMES

After completing Chapter 6, you will be able to:

6.1 Identify common types of computers.

6.2 Describe computer hardware and software components and explain the functions of each.

6.3 Describe the types of computer software commonly used in the medical office.

6.4 Explain how to select computer equipment for the medical office.

6.5 Execute security measures for computerized medical records, including HIPAA compliance.

6.6 Execute the basic care and maintenance of computer equipment.

6.7 Distinguish advances in computer technology and explain their importance to the medical office.

MEDICAL ASSISTING MEDIA

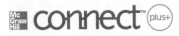 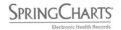

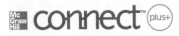 **Connect Plus+™** connect.mcgraw-hill.com	• Electronic Health Records (E.H.R.) SpringCharts® • eBook	**SpringCharts** Electronic Health Records
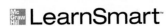 **LearnSmart™**	www.mhhe.com/learnsmart	Complete Learning Module: Using Computers in the Office
Student CD-ROM		
Online Learning Center™	www.mhhe.com/medicalassisting4e	

KEY TERMS

antivirus software	firewalls	multimedia	tablet PC
bandwidth	hard copy	multitasking	touch pad
CD-ROM	hardware	netbook	touch screen
central processing unit (CPU)	icon	network	tower case
clock speed	ink-jet printer	optical character	trackball
cursor	instruction set	recognition (OCR)	tutorial
database	Internet	random-access memory	VPN
disk cleanup	LAN	(RAM)	WAN
disk defragmentation	laser printer	read-only memory (ROM)	zip drive
dot matrix printer	modem	scanner	
digital subscriber line (DSL)	motherboard	screen saver	
electronic mail (e-mail)	mouse	software	

CHAPTER OUTLINE

- The Computer Revolution
- Types of Computers
- Components of the Computer
- Using Application Software
- Selecting Computer Equipment
- Medical Practice Websites
- Security in the Computerized Office
- Computer System Care and Maintenance
- Computers of the Future

PREPARATION FOR CERTIFICATION

RMA (AMT) Exam
- Medical office computer application

CMA (AAMA) Exam
- Computer components
- Computer applications

CMAS Exam
- Fundamentals of computing
- Medical office computer applications

Introduction

The practice of medicine has grown to be increasingly complex:

- Never before has so much medical information been available for the physician.
- Never before has the practice of billing and collecting for medical services rendered and also the scheduling and coordinating of services among multiple providers been so complicated.
- Never before has a "super computer" been more needed to assist with all aspects of a busy practice. We

live in the age of information. The need for a device to organize and correlate all this information has never been greater.

The computer has become an integral tool of the medical office. It is used to organize and categorize thousands of bits of information required to accurately record patient care, transmit information to others at distant points, and maintain an orderly record of all the activities of the business.

In this chapter you will learn about the many aspects of using a computer in a medical practice. Regardless of your past experience with computers, after you complete this chapter, you will have a growing awareness and respect for the marvelous technology it represents. You may even become enthusiastic about the possibilities of its many uses.

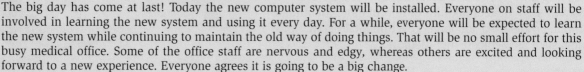

CASE STUDY

The big day has come at last! Today the new computer system will be installed. Everyone on staff will be involved in learning the new system and using it every day. For a while, everyone will be expected to learn the new system while continuing to maintain the old way of doing things. That will be no small effort for this busy medical office. Some of the office staff are nervous and edgy, whereas others are excited and looking forward to a new experience. Everyone agrees it is going to be a big change.

Chris is a medical assistant and is excited and eager to get started. She has been waiting for this day ever since she studied the use of computers in medical assisting school. She knows the next few weeks are going to be full of training and building data sets. She knows she is going to be an integral part of the creation of a new way of getting things done. Chris is excited.

Alicia, a medical assistant who works with Chris, thinks that life would be much easier if the administration had just chosen to leave things the way they were. Alicia is not alone in thinking that computers are just an unnecessary inconvenience. The truth is, Alicia is a little afraid that she will not be able to learn the new system. She has tried to ask questions and express her concerns about the new computer system. But each time she tried to talk to one of the computer specialists, she felt stupid and clumsy. They spoke in a language she didn't understand, and she was too intimidated to tell them she didn't understand what they were talking about. Alicia will go along with this new system just to keep her job. But she has decided that she is definitely not going to waste her time learning anything more than she absolutely has to.

As you read this chapter, consider the following questions:

1. Are you more like Chris or Alicia? What background do you bring to the study of computers that makes you feel the way you do?
2. Why is it important for an office to continue to use the manual system at the same time that it converts to a computerized system?
3. Who should be trained in the use of a new computer system in a medical practice? Why?
4. Which group do you think would be the most difficult to train in an average medical practice?
   a. Those who think like Chris?
   b. Those who think like Alicia?
   c. The physicians?
5. What would be the best way to approach the group you just identified?

The Computer Revolution

Over the past decade computers have revolutionized the way we live and work. Computers make many tasks easier because they process information with great speed and accuracy. They are also capable of storing vast amounts of information in a small space.

In today's world, computer skills are essential for most career choices, and medical assisting is no exception. As a medical assistant, you need to understand the fundamentals of computers and their uses. This knowledge will enable you to perform many office tasks with ease.

In addition, the more you know about computers, the more easily you will be able to solve or avoid computer problems.

Types of Computers

Four basic types of computers are used today: supercomputers, mainframe computers, minicomputers, and personal computers. Each type of computer is suitable for a certain type of work in a particular kind of workplace.

Supercomputers

Supercomputers are the biggest, fastest, and most complex computers in use. They are primarily used in research medicine and are considered to be the hope of the medicine of tomorrow. They are used for genetic coding and for DNA and cancer research. The IBM Roadrunner located at Los Alamos National Laboratory (2009) is currently the fastest supercomputer, and can perform at 1000 trillion operations per second.

Mainframe Computers

Often used by government facilities and large institutions, including universities and hospitals, mainframes can process and store huge quantities of information. Mainframe computers are used for large governmental service programs such as Medicare and Medicaid.

Minicomputers

Minicomputers are smaller than mainframes but larger than personal computers. Minicomputers have traditionally been used in network settings. A **network** is a system that links several computers together. In this environment a minicomputer typically functions as a server, which is a computer used as a centralized storage location for shared information. However, personal computers are becoming as powerful as minicomputers and may eventually replace them.

Personal Computers

Also called microcomputers, personal computers can be found in homes, offices, and schools. They are ideal for these settings because they are small, self-contained units. Because users have different needs, personal computers are available in three different types: desktop, notebook, and subnotebook.

Desktop. The most common type of personal computer, a desktop model fits easily on a desk or other flat surface. The system unit of many newer desktop models is housed in a **tower case,** which extends vertically instead of horizontally. A tower case—often placed on the floor next to the desk—allows more surface area at the workstation (Figure 6-1). Both large and small medical offices commonly use desktop computers. Information is displayed on a monitor screen. Monitors may be flat, resembling a framed picture. In many health-care facilities, these flat-screen monitors are commonly LCD (liquid crystal diode) monitors. Monitors may also resemble a standard television screen. LCD screens provide for better privacy because they can't be seen from the side. They also generate less heat.

Laptop and Notebook. A laptop computer is small—about the size of a magazine—and weighs only a few pounds. Laptops operate either on battery power or on an AC adapter. As advances in technology make laptops smaller, more powerful, and less expensive, they are becoming increasingly popular. Their portability makes them

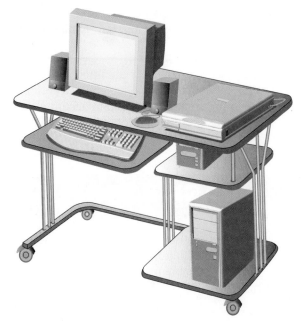

Figure 6-1. Offices can free up much-needed desktop space by using computers in tower cases, which can be kept on the floor.

especially convenient for students, for those who travel, and for anyone who desires fast and easy access to the Internet. Using laptops and their smaller counterparts, notebook computers, physicians and other health-care professionals can instantly communicate with the medical office computer, accessing data and information from other locations.

Subnotebook. Subnotebooks are smaller than laptops but larger than handheld computers. They often have screens that are 14 inches or less. In 2007, a new subnotebook was released, known as the **netbook.** These devices were based around the Internet. They are designed for accessing Web applications. Another new type of subnotebook is the **tablet PC.** It is a laptop or a slate-shaped mobile computer. It is equipped with a touchscreen or graphics table technology. This allows users to operate the computer with a stylus or a digital pen instead of a keyboard or mouse.

Personal Digital Assistant (PDA). PDAs, sometimes called palmtops, are common in medical offices and other health-care facilities. Doctors often use them to look up medications and other reference information (Figure 6-2). They may also enter data that is transferred into a patient's chart.

Cell Phones and the Internet Cell phones are now most often used personally and not professionally, but for research purposes the capabilities of cell phones have increased exponentially in the last several years and will continue to expand. Phones such as BlackBerry® and Apple's iPhone allow users to access the Internet and perform multiple applications in addition to simply making phone calls and sending text messages. Many "techies" believe that cell phones are the "computers of the future."

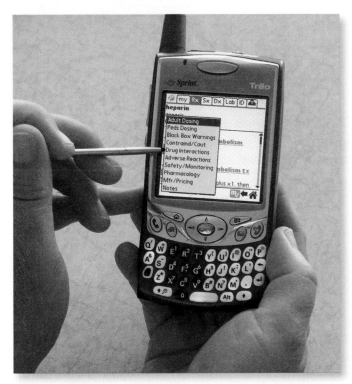

Figure 6-2. A handheld computer or PDA like this one can be used as a handy reference to look up medications or perform calculations in the medical office. Handheld computers are also used as part of a sophisticated computer network for the physician to enter and receive patient data.

Components of the Computer

Computer components are divided into hardware and software. **Hardware** comprises the physical components of a computer system, including the monitor, keyboard, and printer. **Software** is a program or set of instructions that tells the computer what to do. Software includes both the operating system and applications that run on the operating system.

 Hardware

The computer's hardware serves four main functions: inputting data, processing data, storing data, and outputting data. Various hardware components are needed to perform each of these functions (Figure 6-3). In order to work, hardware devices must be connected by a cable, such as a USB or serial cable.

Input Devices. For a computer to handle information, such as patient records, the data must first be entered, or input. Several types of input devices may be used to enter data into the computer. Keyboards, pointing devices, modems, and scanners are input devices. After information is entered into the computer, it can be displayed on the monitor, processed, or stored.

Keyboard. The keyboard is the most common input device. The main part of a keyboard resembles a typewriter. Most keyboards have several additional keys, however. A typical keyboard contains the following:

- Standard typewriter keys to enter letters, numbers, symbols, and punctuation marks
- Separate numerical keypad for entering numbers faster and more easily
- Arrow keys to move the **cursor,** a blinking line or cube on the computer screen showing where the next character that is keyed will appear
- Function keys to perform such tasks as saving and printing files

When you use the keyboard, it is important to position your hands properly to avoid injury. The Caution: Handle with Care section provides tips for preventing and coping with carpal tunnel syndrome, a condition resulting from repetitive motion.

Pointing Device. Many sophisticated software programs need not only a keyboard but also a pointing device to enter information into the computer. When you move the pointing device, an arrow appears. You can point and click the arrow on various buttons that appear on the screen. The four common types of pointing devices are the mouse, the trackball, the touch pad, and the touch screen.

1. A **mouse,** the most common pointing device, has two or three buttons on top and sometimes a rolling ball on the bottom. A laser mouse detects movement through a laser and does not have a ball. As you move the mouse across a flat surface or mouse pad, you cause a light-sensing device on the bottom to move. This controls an arrow on the screen that points at the desired button or object on the screen. Then, as shown in Figure 6-4, you push one of the buttons on the mouse to access a function, such as opening a file.
2. A **trackball** is similar to a mouse except that the rolling ball is on the top of the device instead of on the bottom. Rather than pushing a trackball across a pad, you roll the ball with your fingers while the trackball remains stationary.
3. A **touch pad** is a form of pointing device and is common on laptop and notebook computers. It is a small, flat device that is highly sensitive to the touch. To move the arrow on the screen, you simply slide your finger across the touch pad. To click on an item, you push a button similar to that on a mouse or trackball, or you tap your finger on the touch pad.
4. A **touch screen** is a monitor screen that is illuminated at the touch of a pen, wand, or finger. When an object is touched on the screen, the touch itself acts as a pointing device and conveys information to the computer. Touch screens are increasingly being used in clinical and hospital settings.

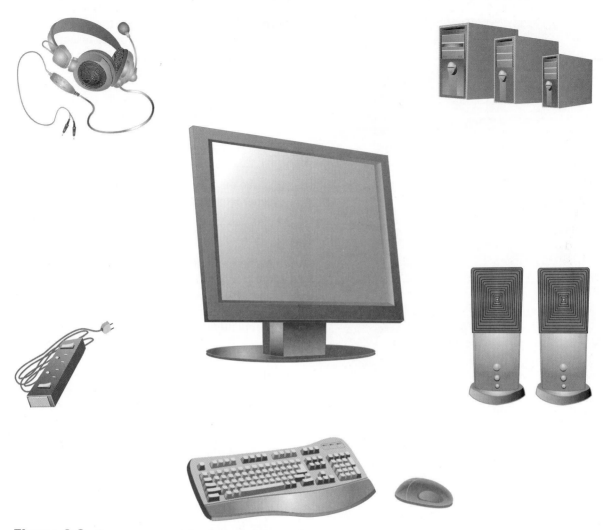

Figure 6-3. Some components of a computer system.

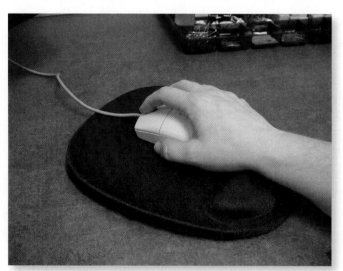

Figure 6-4. Using a mouse, you can point and click to access a variety of functions.

Modem. This term **modem** is a shortened form of the words *modulator-demodulator*. A modem is used to transfer information from one computer to another over telephone lines. Because modems allow information to be transferred both to and from a computer, they are considered input/output devices. The speed at which a modem transfers data is called the bit rate. Modem speeds are continually being improved. Modems are essential for any medical office that needs to transfer files electronically, as when submitting insurance claim forms. Modems can be internal or external, as well as wireless.

A cable modem is a modem that operates over cable television lines to provide fast Internet access. **DSL (digital subscriber line)** modems operate over telephone lines but use a different frequency than a telephone frequency. This type of modem allows computer Internet access and telephone use at the same time.

An advanced type of modem is a fax modem. This device allows the computer to send and receive files much as a fax machine does. A fax modem is not quite as versatile as a regular fax machine, however. The information being sent must first be input into the computer. In addition, without the use of a scanner, you cannot use a fax modem to send a patient record with handwritten notes on it.

Carpal Tunnel Syndrome

As the number of computers used in the home and workplace has escalated in recent years, the number of cases of carpal tunnel syndrome has also risen dramatically. Carpal tunnel syndrome is a hand disorder that is often associated with computer use. The term for this condition comes from the name for a canal (the carpal tunnel) located in the wrist. Several tendons pass through this tunnel, allowing the hand to open and close.

Carpal tunnel syndrome results from repetitive motion, such as keyboarding, for hours at a time. This motion may cause swelling to develop around the tendons and carpal tunnel. The swelling compresses the nerve. The people most likely to develop carpal tunnel syndrome are workers whose jobs require them to perform repetitive hand and finger motions.

Symptoms

The symptoms associated with carpal tunnel syndrome include the following:

- Tingling or burning in the hands or fingers
- Weakness or numbness in the hands or fingers
- Hands that go to sleep frequently
- Difficulty opening or closing the hands
- Pain that stems from the wrist and travels up the arm

Tips for Prevention

If you use a keyboard for extended periods, you should practice proper techniques to prevent carpal tunnel syndrome (Figure 6-5).

- While seated, hold your arms relaxed at your sides, and check to make sure that your keyboard is positioned slightly higher than your elbows. As you input, keep your elbows at your sides, and relax your shoulders (see Figure 6-5).
- Use only your fingers to press keys, and do not use more pressure than necessary. Use a wrist rest, and keep your wrists relaxed and straight.

- When you need to strike difficult-to-reach keys, move your whole hand rather than stretching your fingers. When you need to press two keys at the same time, such as "Control" and "F1," use two hands.
- Try to break up long periods of keyboard work with other tasks that do not require computer use.

Tips for Relieving Symptoms

If you have symptoms of carpal tunnel syndrome, try these suggestions for relief.

- Elevate your arms.
- Wear a splint on the hand and forearm.
- Discuss your symptoms with a physician, who may prescribe medication.

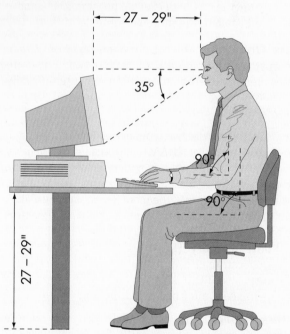

Figure 6-5. Maintaining proper posture and hand positions helps to avoid strain or injury of the back, eyes, neck, or wrist when keyboarding.

Scanner. A **scanner** is a device used to input printed matter and convert it into a format that can be read by the computer. Scanners are useful in the medical office because patient reports from another doctor, a hospital, or another outside source can be easily entered into the computer. Scanners are also making it possible to move into a paperless medical system. Using a scanner is much faster than keying, or inputting the information with a keyboard. Three types of scanners are available:

1. Handheld scanners are generally the least expensive but are more difficult to use and produce lower-quality results than the other two types.
2. A single-sheet scanner feeds one sheet of paper through at a time and looks similar to a single-sheet printer.
3. A flatbed scanner is the most expensive type of scanner but is the easiest to use and produces the highestquality input. It works much like a small photocopier: the paper lies flat and still on a glass surface while the

machine scans it. Today many photocopiers are configured with a scanning capability and can transmit the images of scanned documents directly into computers.

Processing Devices. There are two major processing components inside the system unit, or computer cabinet. The **motherboard** is the main circuit board that controls the other components in the system. The **central processing unit (CPU),** or microprocessor, is the primary computer chip responsible for interpreting and executing programs. The CPU is considered the most important piece of hardware in a computer system. It interprets instructions from software programs.

CPUs have three central elements that define their function: bandwidth, clock speed, and instruction set. **Bandwidth** is a measurement of how much information can be sent or processed with one single instruction, and is calculated in bits or bytes. **Clock speed** is a measurement of how many instructions per second the CPU can process. Clock speed is measured in megahertz (MHz) or gigahertz (GHz). An **instruction set** includes the groups of instructions from installed programming that a CPU can employ. The greater the bandwidth and clock speed, the faster and more powerfully the CPU can execute programs. The more programs are installed, the more versatile the CPU is.

Storage Devices. One of the main tasks of a computer is to store information for later retrieval. The computer uses memory to store information either temporarily or permanently. Several types of drives are used for permanent information storage.

Memory. Computers use two types of memory to store data: **random-access memory (RAM)** and read-only memory (ROM). RAM is temporary, or programmable, memory. While you are working on a software program, the computer is accessing RAM. In general, the more RAM that is available, the faster the computer will perform. As software programs become more sophisticated, they require more RAM.

Read-only memory (ROM) is permanent memory. The computer can read it, but you cannot make changes to it. The purpose of ROM is to provide the basic operating instructions the computer needs to function.

Hard Disk Drive. The hard disk drive is where information is stored permanently for later retrieval. Software programs and important data are usually stored on the hard disk for quick and easy access. The amount of hard disk space needed to store software programs is increasing rapidly. The more software programs you want to store, the larger the hard disk you will need.

Diskette Drive. A diskette drive can read from and write to diskettes (also called disks). Rigid 3.5-inch disks were once commonly used but they are now considered outdated technology. The use of CDs, jump drives, and DVDs has quickly taken the place of disks because they all have a much greater storage capacity.

CD-ROM Drive. CD-ROMs look just like audio compact discs, but they contain software programs. The term

CD-ROM stands for "compact disc—read-only memory." The main advantage of a CD-ROM over a diskette is its ability to store large amounts of data. CD-ROMs can be used to back up information from the hard drive.

CD-ROM drives have become standard equipment on most personal computers. Although many software packages are available on both CD-ROM and diskettes, some large programs are available only on CD-ROM. These programs include multimedia applications such as medical encyclopedias. **Multimedia** refers to software that uses more than one medium—such as graphics, sound, and text—to convey information (Figure 6-6).

Some computers have a CD burner or recorder (CD-R), which allows information to be taken from one CD (or any other source) and "burned" to a CD. CD-Rs work when software to operate the burner is installed in the computer. This software provides instruction for the burner operation.

Tape Drive. This storage device is used to back up (make a copy of) the files on the hard disk. The information is copied onto magnetic tapes that resemble audiotapes. If the hard drive malfunctions, you will have a copy of the information on these tapes.

It is possible to back up information onto diskettes. Most hard disks, however, contain so much information that a large number of diskettes would be required to back up all the data. With most tape drives, the entire contents of the hard disk can be stored on one or two tapes. Store these tapes at night in a fireproof container.

Jump Drive. A jump drive is an externally attached drive that is small enough to be carried on a key chain, yet holds 16 gigabytes or more of data. (Gigabytes are a measurement of memory space.) It also may be called a flash drive, a pen drive, a key drive, a memory key, a flash key, or simply a USB drive. It provides easy portability for large bodies of data. It may be used for backup operations in a medical practice when stored off-premise.

Zip Drive. A **zip drive** is a high-capacity floppy disk drive developed by Iomega®. Zip disks are slightly larger and about twice as thick as a conventional floppy disk. Zip disks can hold up to 750 MB of data. They are durable and relatively inexpensive. They may be used for backing up hard disks and transporting large files.

DVD. DVD (digital video disc) is optical disc storage technology. It is similar to CD technology except it is bigger and faster. It can hold movie-like video, including audio, photos, and computer data. One double-sided, dual-layer disk can store about eight hours of high-quality video.

Output Devices. Output devices are used to display information after it has been processed. A monitor and a printer are two output devices needed in the medical office.

Monitor. A standard computer monitor looks like a television screen or may be an LCD flat screen. It displays the information that is currently active, such as a word processing document, an Internet link, or e-mail. Monitors are available in color and a variety of sizes. They also

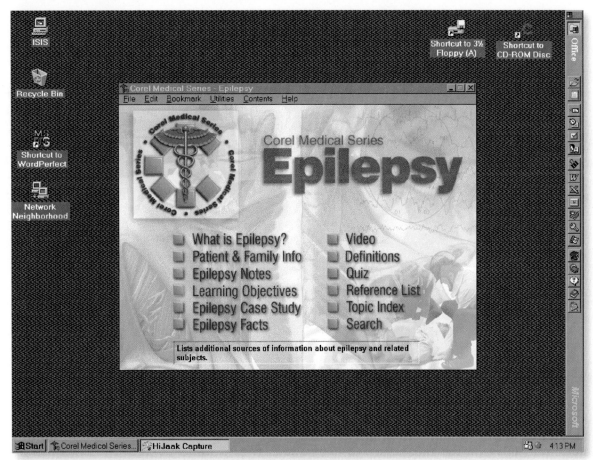

Figure 6-6. A CD-ROM provides features, such as video and sound, that are not possible in a standard printed book.

come in a flat-screen model that conserves desk space. All of the software programs that are used today, including multimedia applications, require a color monitor to run.

Color monitors vary in the number of colors they can display and in the resolution of the images. *Resolution* refers to the crispness of the images and is measured in dot pitch. The lower the dot pitch, the higher the resolution. For example, a monitor with a 0.26 dot pitch displays sharper images than a monitor with a 0.39 dot pitch. Using a high-resolution monitor can help you avoid eye strain.

Printer. A printer is required to produce a **hard copy**, which is a readable paper copy or printout of information (Figure 6-7). You will need a printer to print out correspondence, patient reports, bills, insurance claims, and other documents. Printer resolution is noted in terms of dots per inch (dpi). The higher the dpi, the better the print quality. Printer output varies, depending on the type of printer and the model. The three most commonly used printers are dot matrix, ink-jet, and laser.

1. **Laser printers** are high-resolution printers that use a technology similar to that of photocopiers. Laser printers are the fastest and produce the highest-quality

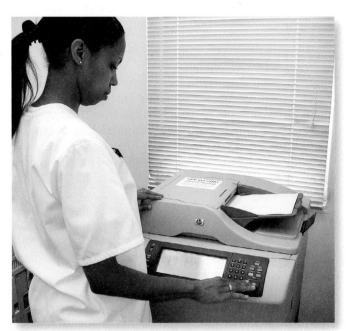

Figure 6-7. You may need to print out hard copies of documents to send to patients, vendors, insurance companies, or other doctors' offices.

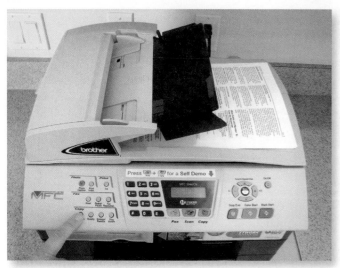

Figure 6-8. An "all-in-one" printer can send and receive faxes, print, and copy. Some models like this one can be networked to more than one computer in the medical office.

output. Laser printers are more expensive than dot matrix or ink-jet printers.

2. **Ink-jet printers** form characters using a series of dots. They are nonimpact printers in which the dots are created by tiny drops of ink. Many ink-jet printers are capable of printing in both black and color. Because of their high-quality output and affordable prices, ink-jet printers are popular for home and small-office use.

3. At one time, **dot matrix printers** were commonly used in medical offices. However, they are rarely used today except in instances where lab reports or other types of reports are used. With the advancement in technology printers, quieter and faster printers are used.

Because each type of printer has advantages and disadvantages, some medical offices may purchase more than one type. For example, a medical office may have a dot matrix printer for creating internal memos and multipage insurance forms and a laser printer for creating documents whose quality resembles that of typeset documents.

A current trend in printers is the "all-in-one" model (Figure 6-8), which functions not only as an ink-jet printer but also as a fax machine, scanner, and photocopier. This type of machine may be convenient for a small medical office that requires each of these functions but does not have space for four separate devices. In addition, purchasing an all-in-one unit is usually more economical than purchasing the machines separately.

Software

Computer software is generally divided into two categories: operating system and application software. The operating system controls the computer's operation. Application software allows you to perform specific tasks, such as scheduling appointments.

Operating System. When you turn on a computer, the operating system starts working, providing instructions that the computer needs to function. Examples of operating system software include Microsoft Windows XP and Vista, and Linux. Most computers come pre-installed with Windows XP or Vista.

Operating system software is sometimes referred to as the platform for the system. Most medical practices use IBM-compatible personal computers, which are most suitable for businesses that use computers primarily to manipulate words. Apple computers are used by businesses such as advertising agencies or design firms that are extensively involved in graphics, visual images, or desktop publishing.

Windows. This operating system employs a graphical user interface (GUI). With a GUI, menu choices are identified by icons, or graphic symbols (Figure 6-9). For example, the "Print" command is usually identified by a button with a tiny illustration of a printer on it. To print a document, you move the pointing device until the arrow is on the printer icon and then click the button.

Windows operating systems are easy to learn because you do not have to remember commands, you simply need to recognize the icon to know what command will be performed if the icon is clicked with the mouse. Another benefit of Windows is that it is a **multitasking** system—users can run two or more software programs simultaneously. You could, for example, enter patient information into a **database,** a collection of records created and stored on the computer, while a word processing program is running in the background.

Windows XP. Windows XP is a Windows operating system that is reliable and versatile. In most businesses, Windows XP has become the standard operating system for IBM and IBM-compatible computers. Some new computers are shipped with Windows XP preinstalled, and many software programs are being written to run exclusively under this operating system.

Windows Vista includes built-in accessibility settings and programs that make it easier for you to see, hear, and use your computer. The accessibility settings and programs in Windows Vista are great for people with visual difficulties, hearing loss, problems with their hands or arms, or reasoning and cognitive issues.

Major accessibility improvements in Windows Vista include:

- Settings and tools that make it easier for you to see, hear, and use your computer.
- Improved magnification capabilities.
- Improved text-to-speech capabilities.
- Speech recognition that lets you interact with your computer by voice.

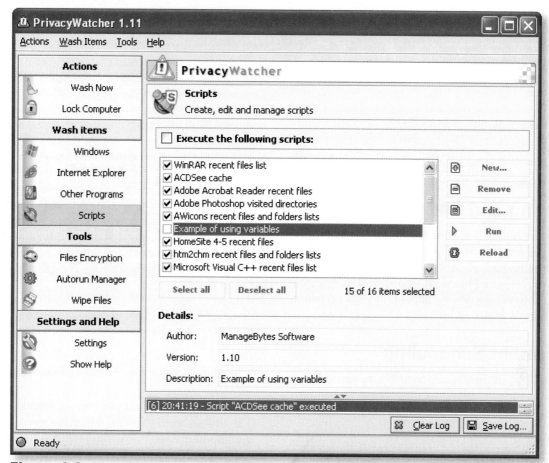

Figure 6-9. An online help system allows you to access helpful information when you are using a software program, while protecting the privacy of the patient.

Applications. Most of the software sold in stores is application software. An example of application software is Microsoft® Office. Microsoft® Office includes word processing (Word), presentation software (Power-Point), spreadsheets (Excel), database management (Access), and desktop publishing (Publisher). Medical Manager®, Medware®, Medasis, and MediSoft™ are practice management applications. These software packages are specifically designed to meet the needs of a medical practice. Standard computer practice management software packages can be purchased. In addition, custom-made computer practice management software can be designed to meet the needs of a particular practice. Word processing, database, and accounting software are just a few examples of the wide variety of applications available.

Optical Character Recognition. **Optical character recognition** or **OCR** software enables the conversion of images to text so they can be treated like any other type of word processing document. An OCR system includes an optical scanner for reading text and state-of-the-art software for analyzing images. An OCR system enables an article or patient file to be fed into an optical scanner,

where it is transferred into an electronic computer file. It is then possible to manipulate and edit the file using a word processor.

Using Application Software

Computer software has been developed for nearly every office function imaginable. Using software, you can complete tasks with greater speed, accuracy, and ease than with a manual system. Learning how to use the software correctly, however, is the key to getting the most out of your computer system.

Word Processing

In the medical office, as in any office, word processing is a common computer application. It has replaced the typewriter for writing correspondence and reports, transcribing physicians' notes, and performing many other functions. Correcting errors is easy on a word processor, and you can save documents for later retrieval and modification. With word processing, a form letter can be merged with a patient mailing list to create letters that are personalized with patients' names.

Database Management

A database is a collection of records created and stored on a computer. In a medical office, databases are used to store patient records such as billing information, medical chart data, and insurance company facts. These records can be sorted and retrieved in many ways and for a variety of purposes. You may be asked to find, add to, or modify information in a database. For example, you might use a database to determine all the patients covered by a particular insurance company.

Accounting and Billing

Accounting and billing software is extremely useful in an office environment. It enables you to perform many tasks, including keeping track of patients' accounts, creating billing statements, preparing financial reports, and maintaining tax records. (You will learn more about billing and accounting functions in Chapters 17 and 18.)

Appointment Scheduling

Instead of writing in an appointment book, you can use software to schedule appointments. Some scheduling packages allow you to enter patient preferences, such as day of the week and time, and then to list available appointments based on that information. If the office system is on a network, scheduling software is particularly valuable because more than one user can access the appointment schedule at a time.

Electronic Transactions

Using a computer equipped with a modem and communications software, you can perform several types of electronic transactions. This technology enables you to send and receive information instantaneously rather than waiting the days or weeks required for regular mail. Common electronic transactions include sending insurance claims and communicating with other computer users. Electronic medical records can easily be sent anywhere in seconds.

Sending Insurance Claims. Today, except in the smallest of medical offices, insurance claims are submitted electronically directly from the medical office to an insurance company. This procedure enables claims to be processed quickly and efficiently. (Chapter 15 discusses health insurance billing procedures.)

Communicating. The ability to communicate and share information with other computer users and systems is important in many medical offices. This communication may take place through electronic mail, online services, and the Internet. The Points on Practice section gives valuable ideas for saving time online.

Electronic Mail. Commonly known as e-mail, **electronic mail** is a method of sending and receiving messages almost instantly through a network. Through e-mail, it is possible to communicate with computer users in your own office, across town, or on the other side of the world. Unlike regular mail, e-mail operates in real time.

As the use of e-mail has increased, e-mail etiquette rules designed especially for Internet use have become important. By requiring employees to use appropriate, professional language in all electronic communications, employers limit their liability risk and maintain their professional image. E-mail etiquette is established when a practice creates a written e-mail policy spelling out the "dos" and "don'ts" concerning the use of the company's e-mail system. The implementation of e-mail etiquette rules can be monitored by using e-mail management software and response tools. Professional organizations such as the American Medical Informatics Association and Health E-mail (a nonprofit physician outreach program) have established policies relating to e-mail.

Managing E-mail. E-mail management can be helpful in a medical office. Here are several management tools that you can use:

- Regularly check your e-mail and empty any unwanted e-mails.
- If there is e-mail that you cannot identify, do not open it unless you have an antivirus protector on your computer. Even then, be very careful of unsolicited e-mails.
- Set up subfolders for e-mails that have to be kept for an indefinite period of time.
- Set time limits for deleting or retaining messages.
- Save all e-mail responses that contain personal health information (PHI).

Online Services. These services, known as servers, provide a means for health-care professionals to communicate with one another. Most online services contain forums that offer information and discussion groups focusing on a wide range of medical topics. Health-care workers can learn about the latest medical research and technology or exchange ideas with others in their field. In addition, some online services provide access to medical databases such as MEDLINE®, created by the National Library of Medicine. Users can search MEDLINE® for records and abstracts from thousands of medical journals from around the world.

Internet. The **Internet** is a global network of computers. Through the Internet, you can communicate with millions of computer users around the world. E-health or medical information and products are easy to access worldwide through the use of the Internet. Many large medical facilities, universities, and other organizations—such as the National Institutes of Health (NIH) and the Centers for Disease Control and Prevention (CDC)—provide medical resources, databases, and other information on the Internet. Users can visit Internet sites to find multimedia textbooks, presentations, and links to other related sites

PROCEDURE 6-1

Creating a Form Letter

Procedure Goal: To use a word processing program to create a form letter

Materials: Computer equipped with a word processing program, printer, form letter to be created, 8½- by 11-inch paper.

Method:

1. Turn on the computer. Select the word processing program.

2. Use the keyboard to begin entering text into a new document.

3. To edit text, press the arrow keys to move the cursor to the position at which you want to insert or delete characters, and enter the text. Either type directly or use the "Insert" mode to type over and replace existing text.

4. To delete text, position the cursor to the left of the characters to be deleted and press the "Delete" key. Alternatively, place the cursor to the right of the characters to be deleted and press the "Backspace" key (the left-pointing arrow usually found at the top right corner of the keyboard).

5. If you need to move an entire block of text, you must begin by highlighting it. In most Windows-based programs, you first click the mouse at the beginning of the text to be highlighted. Then you hold down the left mouse button, drag the mouse to the end of the block of text, and release your finger from the mouse. The text should now be highlighted. Right click the mouse and choose the button or command for cutting text. Then move the cursor to the place where you want to insert the text, right click the mouse again, and select the button or command for retrieving or pasting text.

6. As you input the letter, it is important to save your work every 15 minutes or so. Some programs do this automatically. If yours does not, use the "Save" command or button to save the file. Be sure to save the file again when you have completed the letter.

Rationale
The document must be saved periodically so that if power is lost or if part of the document is accidentally deleted, at least part of the document is still retrievable.

7. Carefully proofread the document and use the spell checker, correcting any errors in spelling or formatting.

Rationale
Your documents should contain no spelling or grammatical errors and should be professional in appearance.

8. Print the letter using the "Print" command or button.

Reflecting On . . . HIPAA

HIPAA and E-mail

HIPAA law requires that all transactions containing patient health information be protected. Consider the following guidelines when sending e-mail within a medical practice:

1. Do not send e-mail containing protected health information without specific written authorization from the patient.

2. Always check the patient's medical record and the computer system for any special instructions for contacting the patient through e-mail. Follow all patient requests. When in doubt, do not send an e-mail. Check with the office manager or supervisor.

3. Maintain virus protection to guard your computer system against viruses, which commonly infect a computer system through e-mail.

TABLE 6-1　Medical Resources on the Internet

Organization	Web Address	Description
American Medical Association	www.ama-assn.org	News announcements and press releases; articles from *JAMA* and other AMA journals; links to other medicine-related Internet sites
eMedicineHealth	www.emedicinehealth.com	Health resource center where you can learn about health issues and the latest treatments available
MedlinePlus®	http://medlineplus.gov	A service of the U.S. National Library of Medicine and NIH; site includes current health news, medical encyclopedia, and directories for doctors, dentists, and hospitals
National Institutes of Health	www.nih.gov	Medical news and current events; press releases; biomedical information about health issues; scientific resources; links to Internet sites of related government agencies
National Library of Medicine	www.nlm.nih.gov	Internet site for world's largest biomedical library; research and development activities; connections to online medical information services
New England Journal of Medicine	http://content.nejm.org	Articles and abstracts; archives of past issues
Virtual Hospital	http://radiology.uiowa.edu	Information on a variety of health issues, medical resources, tutorials, and multimedia textbooks
WebMD Health®	www.webmd.com	Trustworthy, credible, and timely health information written by experts in medicine, journalism, and health communications

on the Internet. Table 6-1 describes some popular medical resources available on the Internet.

Search engines are specialized websites that search other websites for information. The user connects with the search engine and indicates a topic of interest. Typically, a box is provided for the topic and then the user selects a box marked "Go." The search engine electronically searches for the information requested and lists many different website link options for the user. Examples of popular search engines include Google™ and Yahoo!®.

Research

The advent of CD-ROM technology has revolutionized the world of research and education. Not only can an immense amount of information be contained on one compact disc, but the CD-ROM usually provides additional information in the form of videos and sound (see Figure 6-6). A CD-ROM encyclopedia, for example, might also provide spoken pronunciations of medical terms. This type of software may help patients—especially children—understand the human body as well as various medical conditions.

Software Training

Software programs may seem quite complex. Most people need a period of training before they feel comfortable using the application. Several methods of training—some from outside sources and some provided by the software manufacturer—are available.

Classes. Many computer vendors offer training classes for the software packages they sell. In addition, community

Working Efficiently Online

If the medical office where you work is computerized, the system most likely has a modem for sending e-mail and transferring files electronically. The modem may also be used to access various online services and the Internet, a global network of computers. If this access is not currently available in the medical office, it probably will be in the near future. You may even be asked to help choose an online service or Internet provider for the office.

These services, known as *Internet service providers (ISPs),* allow access to a network of servers that provides a means for health-care professionals to communicate with one another.

Choosing an Online Service

Compare several services for the following features:

- The speed and accessibility of services. A cable modem or DSL through the phone line has faster speeds for communicating information than a regular phone line service. Plus these services are always on and do not interfere with the telephone service at the facility.

- Free trial membership. Many services offer a free 1-month membership to try out the service. The trial periods enable office staff members to test several services to determine which one best suits their needs.

- Local access telephone number. Make sure the service provides an access number within the local dialing area of the office. If it does not, the office will be charged long-distance telephone rates each time someone goes online. These fees are separate from the online service's rates and can add up quickly.

- Extra fees. Although access to most of the information found in online services is included in the membership fee, some providers charge extra for premium or extended services. If you want to read or print out the full text of an article in a medical journal, for example, some providers charge an additional fee. Make sure you consider these extra fees when comparing costs of online services.

- Availability of health-care information. Some online services provide discussion groups (commonly known as chat rooms) and resources that would be useful to the medical office. Other services may not offer as much relevant information. By comparing several services, you can determine which service best meets the needs of the practice.

Sending and Receiving E-Mail

When using e-mail, follow these guidelines to manage your online time efficiently.

- Use computerized address books. As part of the e-mail system, most services provide an online address book in which you can store frequently used e-mail addresses. Instead of wasting time searching for an e-mail address in a standard card file, you simply click on the person's name in the address book and the mail is automatically sent to that person. You can also use the address book to send the same e-mail message to several people at once. If one message is being sent to several people, you can bcc (blind copy) the other recipients. By using bcc (blind copy), you are protecting the privacy of other recipients' e-mail addresses.

  To use bcc (blind copy) effectively, insert your own e-mail address in the TO box. In the BCC box, enter the e-mail addresses of the people you wish to receive the e-mail. Each recipient will see only your name and e-mail address and no one else's, thus protecting the privacy of each person's e-mail address.

- After sending an e-mail, watch for any alert that the message did not go through. If an alert appears, check the address again and resend the e-mail.

Doing Research

Although a great deal of valuable information can be found through online services and the Internet, searching for this information can be time-consuming. The following tips are provided to make the most of your online time.

- Use the favorite places feature. Keep a list of favorite places, or sites that you visit frequently.

- Refine your searches. Searching for *arthritis,* for example, might produce hundreds of references that you would have to read through to determine their relevance. Narrowing your search to *juvenile rheumatoid arthritis,* on the other hand, would produce fewer references but would provide more exact matches.

- Download files. *Download* means to transfer a file to the hard disk. Instead of reading through information while you are online, download the files and later retrieve them or print them to read later.

colleges and high schools sometimes offer adult education classes for a variety of applications, including word processing and communications. These classes may be at the beginner, intermediate, or advanced level.

Tutorials. Many software packages come with a **tutorial,** which is a small program designed to give users an overall picture of the product and its functions. The tutorial usually provides a step-by-step walk-through and exercises in which you can try out your newly acquired knowledge.

Documentation. Nearly all software manufacturers provide some type of documentation with their programs. Documentation is usually in the form of written instruction manuals or online help that is accessed from within the program.

Manuals. Some manuals provide detailed information on software operation and may include an index and sections on troubleshooting and commonly asked questions. Other manuals may simply give installation instructions and brief information on program basics. This type of manual may refer users to the software's online help.

Online Help. In most software applications, users access the online help screen by clicking on a "Help" button or by pressing a certain function key, such as "F1." The online help usually provides a "Contents" section (see Figure 6-9), in which you can browse for topics. An index, in which you can search for key words, is also provided.

Technical Support. A software company's technical support service is designed to assist you with problems that go beyond the scope of the user's guide or manual. A call to technical support is important when you encounter a problem that cannot be solved by simple problem-solving techniques. By calling a toll-free number, you can access a knowledgeable team who will listen to the description of the problem and suggest solutions over the phone.

Before calling technical support:

- Check the system for errors to the best of your ability.
- Check your manual for answers. Ask your supervisor for assistance.
- Have the software registration number available.
- Be prepared to follow the instructions of the technical support personnel.
- Allow uninterrupted time to spend on the phone with the technical support person.
- Plan to call from a location that gives ready access to the computer with the problem.

Technical support is also helpful when you are upgrading software. Some software companies automatically notify their customers of available upgrades. The technical support service is always a good source of information regarding the latest products and their applications.

Selecting Computer Equipment

Most medical offices are computerized. If the decision is made to upgrade the system, you may be a part of the decision-making process in selecting equipment. As a medical assistant who will be using the system, you may be asked for your input in selecting software, adding a network, or choosing a vendor.

The first step for helping in the selection process is to learn as much as you can about hardware and software. You can get information by taking an introductory computer class at an adult school or community college; by reading computer magazines or books; or by talking to friends, relatives, or coworkers who use computers.

Upgrading the Office System

Computer hardware is changing and improving at such a rapid pace that a system seems to become outdated almost as soon as it is purchased. In addition, more advanced software is introduced every day, and this software requires more advanced hardware to run. Consequently, an office system purchased only a year or two ago may need to be upgraded. Sometimes an upgrade simply requires replacement or addition of certain components. For instance, a laser printer can take the place of a dot matrix printer, or a CD-ROM drive can be added. In other cases, such a solution is not possible or cost-effective, so an entirely new system must be purchased.

Selecting Software

After a decision is made regarding the type of software needed, such as an accounting program, a specific product must be chosen. To make an informed decision, you can read software reviews in computer magazines or trade publications. Check with other medical offices to get opinions on software packages. A crucial step in selecting software is to make sure the office computer system meets the minimum system requirements listed on the software box.

Adding a Network

There are several advantages to adding a network to the computer system in a medical office. A computer network enables users to share software programs and files and allows more than one person to work on the same patient's information at one time. While you are working on a patient's insurance claim, for example, another medical assistant might be inputting billing information. Some medical offices are virtually paperless. They use a highly sophisticated network with a notebook or desktop computer in every examination room. Doctors input information into patients' computerized charts. If a doctor is in her office and a patient is waiting, a staff member at the front desk sends an e-mail message to the doctor's desktop computer, and a beep sounds as an alert. Networks also allow large medical facilities to communicate with employees via e-mail. For instance, an internal memo about changes in office policies may be sent by e-mail to all employees. For networks to operate, the computer must have either a network interface card or wireless connection to the network. Networks can be run with Windows®, Novell®, or Unix® network operating systems.

Virtual Private Networks

When a group of two or more computer systems are linked together, it is known as a network system. Local-area networks are called **LAN**s. The computers in this system are geographically close together (for example, in the same building). Wide-area networks are known as **WAN**s. The computers in this network are farther apart and are connected by telephone lines. Virtual private networks, known as **VPN**s, are used to connect two or more computer systems. They are also constructed using public telephone lines. They use the Internet as the medium for transporting data. VPNs use encryption and other security methods to ensure that only authorized users can access the network. This type of network makes it possible for physicians to access patient records in a secure manner from a variety of locations.

Choosing a Vendor

When purchasing computer equipment, you should look for a reputable vendor who not only offers a reasonable price but also provides training, service, and technical support. A first step might be to check with personnel in other medical offices that use a computer system. Find out which dealer they use and if they are satisfied with the system, salespeople, and support. You can also ask dealers for names of references—medical offices that have purchased systems from them. It is a good idea to get cost estimates from at least three vendors, and it is preferable to buy all hardware components from the same vendor.

Medical Practice Websites

The Internet has become a profitable marketing tool. Medical websites can generate more new patients than paper advertising. Within the website, doctors can include patient education, newsletters, referring provider forms, and other patient-related information.

Additionally, patients can e-mail the medical office personnel to ask questions and find out other pertinent non-PHI (protected health information).

Security in the Computerized Office

Although security measures are important in any office, they are especially important in a computerized medical office. Great care must be taken to safeguard confidential files, make backup copies on a regular basis, and prevent system contamination. HIPAA law requires that privacy and security procedures are in place to prevent the misuse of health information. These procedures also must ensure confidentiality.

Safeguarding Confidential Files

Much of the information collected in a medical office is confidential. Just as with paper records, confidential information stored on the computer should be accessible only to authorized personnel. Two common ways to provide security in a computerized office are to employ passwords and to install an activity-monitoring system.

Passwords. In many hospitals and physicians' offices, each employee who is allowed access to computerized patient files is given a password. The employee must enter the password into the computer when using the files. Access codes or passwords only allow the user into approved areas according to the individual's job description. If you are given a password, do not divulge it to anyone else unless your office manager asks you to do so. If an employee leaves or is fired, the user account should be deleted. When you choose a password, do not use common ones such as your birthday.

Activity-Monitoring Systems. In conjunction with passwords, some health-care facilities use a computer system that monitors user activity. Whenever someone accesses computer records, the system automatically keeps track of the user's name and the files that have been viewed or modified. In this way, problems or security breaches can be traced back to specific employees.

Making and Storing Backup Files

For securing important computer files, it is essential to routinely make diskette or tape backups of them (Figure 6-10). How often backups are made varies among medical offices; your supervisor will tell you the policy for your office. Just as important as making the backups is storing them properly. Backup files should not be stored near the

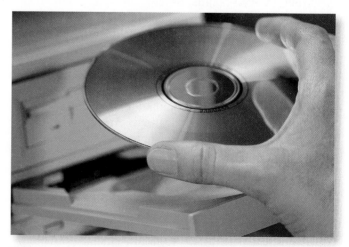

Figure 6-10. It is important to back up computer files and store them properly.

Guidelines for HIPAA Privacy Compliance and the Computer

The use of computers is widespread within the typical medical practice. Though the computer is valuable for many administrative functions, it also can be a risk in terms of patient privacy and HIPAA compliance. You must follow special safeguards for computers in order to protect the patient's privacy.

1. Computers are typically placed in or near the patient reception area. Keep the computer screen positioned so that it is not visible to unauthorized personnel or patients. Screensavers can be used to minimize the amount of time any information is visible on the screen.

2. All computers should automatically log the user off after a period of no activity. The computer should require that all users must reenter their password to regain access after an idle period.

3. Always keep your computer username and password confidential. Change your password often, using a variety of numbers, symbols, and both lower- and uppercase letters.

4. Consider the use of practice management software, which can track users and follow their activity within a computer system.

5. Formal policies should be developed for every practice regarding the transfer and acceptance of outside protected health information. When using any computer system, always follow practice policy to assure that protected health information is being transferred in a secure and compliant manner.

---

original files. Ideally, they should be kept outside the medical office—perhaps at the physician's home—so that they will be secure in case of fire, burglary, or other catastrophe at the office.

Preventing System Contamination

Another important security issue in the computerized medical office is computer viruses. Computer viruses are programs written specifically to contaminate the hard disk by damaging or destroying data.

Viruses can be passed from computer to computer through shared diskettes that have been infected. Computer viruses can also be spread through infected files retrieved from online services, the Internet, e-mails, and electronic bulletin boards. Several software programs are available to detect and correct computer viruses. Most are fairly inexpensive but provide an invaluable service.

Antivirus Software and Firewalls. Chances are there are hundreds of security vulnerabilities awaiting your computer's system. You need to be concerned about everything on your computer from the operating system to the software applications. **Antivirus software** provides protection for your computer. It scans your system for viruses automatically and manually. If it finds a virus, it either destroys it automatically or alerts the user to respond by "cleaning" the file, thus destroying it. Antivirus software responds to spammers (persons that abuse e-mails by sending them in mass without permission). Many times they send malicious e-mails and files. If you do not know who sent you the e-mail, it is best not to open the file.

Firewalls (barriers to keep destructive forces away from your computer) also are called security protection. Firewalls are helpful in putting a stop to offensive Internet sites and potential computer hackers (a person that can get inside of a computer—legally or illegally—and do anything) who are trying to gain access to your computer.

Computer System Care and Maintenance

Like a car, a computer needs routine care and maintenance to stay in sound condition. The computer user's manual outlines the steps required. Also, a good general rule is not to eat or drink near the computer. Crumbs and spilled liquids can damage the system components and storage devices.

Disk Cleanup and Disk Defragmentation

Disk cleanup is a computer maintenance utility designed to free up space on your computer by getting rid of unnecessary files that are on your hard drive. It compresses old files, deletes temporary Internet files, and sends some files to the recycle bin. Microsoft Windows already has this capability included in its package.

Disk defragmentation physically organizes the contents of your hard disk drive to store pieces of each file closely. This also frees up space on your computer as well. Fragmentation occurs when the operating system cannot or will not allocate contiguous (adjacent) space to store a complete file as a unit.

System Unit

The system unit should be placed in a well-ventilated location, with nothing blocking the fan in the back of the cabinet. To keep the system's delicate circuitry from being damaged by an electrical power surge, you should use a power strip with a surge protector. You plug the computer into the power strip and then plug the power strip into the electrical outlet (see Figure 6-3).

Monitor

A **screen saver** automatically changes the monitor display at short intervals or constantly shows moving images on the computer monitor or screen. All Windows® operating systems come equipped with screen savers. A wide variety of screen savers are also available as separate software packages. Adding a screen cover to a monitor will protect the monitor.

To protect their screens, many monitors "power down" after a certain period of inactivity. If no one uses the computer for 30 minutes, for example, the monitor screen goes blank. To resume using the computer after the screen saver has been activated or the monitor has powered down, simply touch any key or move the mouse.

In addition, the computer monitor power settings can be set to meet the needs of the health-care facility. Powering down can also be adjusted to suit the facility's needs.

Printer

Maintenance of a printer generally consists of replacing the ink cartridge, or toner cartridge. When the cartridge needs to be changed, the ink on your printouts becomes very light and colors become faded. Some integrated computer and printer systems automatically provide a "Low Ink" message on the screen when printer cartridges need replacing. The message appears when the "Print" command is given. A graph indicates the amount of ink left in the cartridge. Ink can be ordered online through a link provided with the printer program. Replacement is usually a simple process, described in the printer manual.

Information Storage Devices

Jump drives, CD-ROMs, diskettes, and magnetic tapes are highly sensitive devices. Even a small scratch may cause permanent damage or make it impossible to retrieve data. To avoid problems, handle and store disks and tapes properly.

Jump Drives. Jump drives are connected to the computer through a USB port (Figure 6-11). This port should be protected when the drive is not attached to the computer, so be certain to put the cap back on the drive when you are transporting the drive to another location.

CD-ROMs. Figure 6-12 shows the proper way to handle a CD-ROM. When you pick it up, touch only the edges or the edge and the hole in the center. CD-ROMs should be stored in the clear plastic case in which they are packaged,

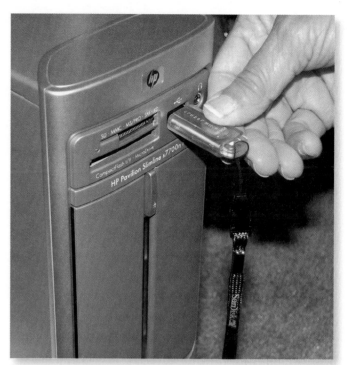

Figure 6-11. A jump drive is a small portable storage device that attaches to the USB port and can store and move 16 gigabytes or more of electronic data.

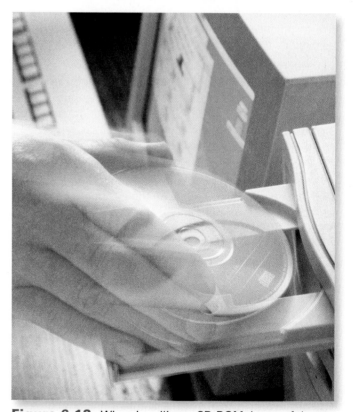

Figure 6-12. When handling a CD-ROM, be careful not to touch the flat surface of the disc.

sometimes called a jewel case. If a CD-ROM becomes dusty or smudged with fingerprints, clean it by rubbing it gently with a soft cloth. Always rub from the center to the outside. *Never* rub in a circular motion.

Diskettes. Diskettes should be kept away from magnetic fields, such as a paper clip holder that has a magnet in it. They should also be kept out of direct sunlight and away from extreme temperatures. Although 3.5-inch disks are sturdy, they should be handled with care. They should be labeled appropriately and stored in a durable storage case.

Magnetic Tapes. Magnetic tapes should be treated much the same as you would treat audiotapes. They should be stored in a relatively cool, dry place, away from magnetic fields.

Computer Disaster Recovery Plan

When any business is dependent on computer technology for daily functioning, a computer disaster recovery plan for the business must be in place. A recovery plan offers a possible solution if the primary computer system should fail or "crash," making all information on the hard drive unavailable.

In a medical practice, it is important to discuss the computer disaster recovery plan with the staff so that everyone knows the part they will play if the computer system fails. As devices, systems, and networks become more complex, there are simply more things that can go wrong. As a result, computer disaster recovery plans have become more important and more sophisticated.

A computer disaster recovery plan will vary from practice to practice. However, all plans should include these elements:

1. Minimizing damage to equipment. Automatic warnings are built into computer systems to indicate when a fatal error has occurred. Warnings also provide direction to help prevent loss of information and minimize damage to the computer equipment.

2. Retrieving information. A backup computer system should copy all of the information in the primary computer system every day. If the main system fails, this backup system will allow all the information to be retrieved and not permanently lost.

   This backup system can either be automated or manual. An example of an automated system is a second computer, networked to the first, to which information is regularly backed up in the event the primary computer system fails. With this type of backup, the operation of the office can continue while the primary system is repaired or replaced. An example of a manual backup system, which is less useful, is a handwritten list of patients and the procedures performed each day.

3. Protecting protected health information. Even during an office emergency, such as a computer failure, healthcare professionals are still required to carefully guard the privacy of the patient records. If an electronic or manual backup system is implemented, safeguards to protect patient information must still be observed.

Disaster recovery planning can be purchased as a software application or a service, or it can be developed within an organization.

Computers of the Future

Computers are evolving at such a rapid pace that it is virtually impossible to predict the changes that will take place even in the next few years. Some important new technologies, however, have already been introduced in the medical office and will be improved in the near future. Telemedicine, CD-R technology, and speech recognition technology are only three examples of new computer technologies. Undoubtedly, more will be explored and developed every year.

Telemedicine

Telemedicine refers to the use of telecommunications to transmit video images of patient information. These images are already used to provide medical support to physicians caring for patients in rural areas. The use of telemedicine and advancements in computer technology allow medical practices to quickly access vast amounts of current medical information.

CD-R and DVD-R Technology

While CD-ROMs and DVDs can only be *read* by the computer, CD-R (compact disc–recordable) media and DVD-Rs can be read *and* written to. CD-R and DVD-R technology allows you to use compact discs like diskettes—to store data and information. Recordable CDs and DVDs, however, can store much more information than diskettes can.

Speech Recognition Technology

Speech recognition technology enables the computer to comprehend and interpret spoken words through the use of a specialty software program. The user simply speaks into a microphone instead of inputting information with a keyboard or a scanner. Because every human voice is different, however, and the English language is vast and complex, this technology is difficult to perfect. As speech recognition technology becomes more advanced, more accurate, and less expensive, it will most likely gain widespread acceptance. It has a great deal of potential, including the ability to virtually eliminate the need for medical assistants to transcribe physicians' notes. There are a variety of speech recognition software applications available for use.

Summary

6.1 The supercomputer is the fastest and largest computer and is used for research in medicine and other complex uses. The mainframe computer is normally used by organizations such as government services (Medicaid and Medicare). They process huge quantities of information. Minicomputers are smaller than mainframes but are larger than personal computers. Personal computers are also called microcomputers. They are available as desktops, notebooks, and subnotebooks.

6.2 Hardware comprises the physical components of a computer system, which includes the monitor, keyboard, CPU, and printer. Software is a set of instructions, or a program that tells the computer what to do.

6.3 There are various kinds of computer software for the medical office. Word processing is the most common application. Medical offices also use software for database management, accounting and billing, scheduling, and electronic transfer and research.

6.4 The first step in selecting computer equipment for the medical office is to learn as much as you can about hardware and software. Find a reputable vendor that has reasonable costs and make sure you choose software that meets the medical office's needs and the system requirements of the computer.

6.5 Security measures are extremely important in the medical office. Law requires that privacy and security procedures are in place to prevent the misuse of health information.

6.6 A computer needs routine care and maintenance to stay in good condition. The system should be in a well-ventilated area. Use a power surge protector. Your computer monitor's power setting can be set to meet the needs of the health-care facility. Replace printer cartridges as needed. Information storage devices are very sensitive, so be sure to safeguard them.

6.7 Computers are evolving rapidly. New medical technology is introduced at a fast pace. Your office computer system should be as up-to-date as possible so that the advances in the medical field can be easily accessed.

REVIEW

CHAPTER 6

CASE STUDY *QUESTIONS*

Now that you have completed this chapter, review the case study at the beginning of the chapter and answer the following questions:

1. Are you more like Chris or Alicia? What background do you bring to the study of computers that makes you feel the way you do?
2. Why is it important for an office to continue to use the manual system at the same time that it converts to a computerized system?
3. Who should be trained in the use of a new computer system in a medical practice? Why?
4. Which group do you think would be the most difficult to train in an average medical practice?
   a. Those who think like Chris?
   b. Those who think like Alicia?
   c. The physicians?
5. What would be the best way to approach the group you just identified?

Multiple-Choice Questions

1. How many "basic" types of computers are there?
   a. 3   c. 4
   b. 1   d. 8
2. Which of the following comprises the physical components of a computer system, including the monitor, keyboard, and printer?
   a. Mouse   c. Cursor
   b. Hardware   d. Trackball
3. PDAs are used to look up what kind of information?
   a. Age   c. Address
   b. Medication   d. Your favorite kind of ice cream
4. A _____ is a form of pointing device and is common on laptop and notebook computers.
   a. touch pad   c. cursor
   b. touch screen   d. mouse
5. When a group of two or more computer systems are linked together, it is known as a network system. A Local-area network is also called a
   a. VPN   c. ROM
   b. WAN   d. LAN

Discussion Questions

1. Compare and contrast the three kinds of printers. What are the advantages of each?
2. What do you think is in the future in the development of computers? Describe your vision of the typical medical office and its use of computers 25 years from now.
3. A new computer system has just been installed at your office. How would you encourage and assist a fellow employee in learning the new system?
4. Compare and contrast bandwidth, clock speed, and instruction set.
5. Though the computer is valuable for many administrative functions, it also can be a risk in terms of patient privacy and HIPAA compliance. Describe some special computer safeguards that protect the patient's privacy.
6. Describe optical character recognition (OCR) software and how it is useful.

Critical Thinking Questions

1. A computer virus has attached itself to your computer. What would you do? Explain in detail.
2. A fellow employee asks to use your password to the computer because she has forgotten hers. How do you respond and why?
3. Summarize the proper care and maintenance of computer diskettes and CDs. How does proper care reduce problems?
4. Which do you think is a better choice for a medical practice: a LAN, WAN, or VPN system?
5. Think about the future. What do you think the future holds for computers in the medical office?

Application Activities

1. Go online and research the purchase of a new software package for a medical encyclopedia. Which would you recommend for purchase by your office and why?
2. Look through computer magazines or trade journals for descriptions or reviews of the latest software upgrades for your computer system. Describe what new benefits the upgrades offer and how each feature would benefit a medical practice.

3. Research one of the technological advances mentioned in this chapter—telemedicine, CD-R technology, or speech recognition technology—to learn more about it. Find out how the technology benefits the medical office. Write and present a full report on your topic.
4. Review Table 6-1. Research medical resources on the Internet and find three additional organizations, giving their websites and a brief description of each site.

Virtual Fieldtrip

Visit the McGraw-Hill Higher Education Medical Assisting website at www.mhhe.com/medicalassisting4e to complete the following activity:

Use the American Association of Medical Assistants and the U.S. Department of Health and Human Services websites as well as websites about wireless technology. Prepare a onepage report about one of the following topics:

- The future use of laptop, notebook, and palmtop computers in a medical practice
- The increasing use of wireless configuration for computer access and what it could mean to a medical practice
- An overview of pointer devices used today and what might be used in the future
- HIPAA laws and their application to electronic mail

Ask your instructor how many references and citations you should minimally include in your paper.

Open the CD and complete this chapter's practice activities, play the games, listen to the key terms, and test yourself with the interactive review. E-mail, print, and/or save your results to document your proficiency.

Managing Correspondence and Mail

MEDICAL ASSISTING COMPETENCIES

CAAHEP

IV. C (8) Recognize elements of fundamental writing skills

IV. P (10) Compose professional/business letters

ABHES

7. Basic Keyboarding/Computer Concepts

a. Perform basic keyboarding skills including:
   1. Locating the keys on a keyboard
   2. Typing medical correspondence and basic reports

b. Identify and properly utilize office machines, computerized systems, and medical software such as:
   1. Efficiently maintain and understand different types of medical correspondence and medical reports
   2. Apply computer application skills using a variety of different electronic programs including both practice management software and EMR software

8. Medical Office Business Procedures Management

a. Perform basic clerical duties

d. Apply concepts for office procedures

y. Perform routine maintenance of administrative and clinical equipment

jj. Perform fundamental writing skills including correct grammar, spelling, and formatting techniques when writing prescriptions, documenting medical records, etc.

11. Career Development

Demonstrate professionalism by:
1) Exhibiting dependability, punctuality, and a positive work ethic
2) Exhibiting a positive attitude and a sense of responsibility
3) Maintaining confidentiality at all times
7) Expressing a responsible attitude
8) Being courteous and diplomatic
9) Conducting work within scope of education, training, and ability

LEARNING OUTCOMES

After completing Chapter 7, you will be able to:

7.1 Identify the supplies necessary for creating and mailing professional-looking correspondence.

7.2 Identify the types of correspondence used in medical office communications.

7.3 Describe the parts of a letter and the different letter and punctuation styles.

7.4 Carry out a business letter.

7.5 Explain the tasks involved in editing and proofreading.

7.6 Explain the process of handling incoming and outgoing mail.

7.7 Differentiate between the services provided by the U.S. Postal Service and other delivery services.

MEDICAL ASSISTING MEDIA

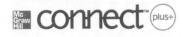 **Connect Plus+™**
connect.mcgraw-hill.com
- Elecronic Health Records (E.H.R.) SpringCharts®
- eBook

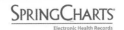

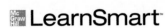 **LearnSmart™**
www.mhhe.com/learnsmart
Complete Learning Module: Managing Correspondence and Mail

 Student CD-ROM

 Online Learning Center™
www.mhhe.com/medicalassisting4e

KEY TERMS

annotate	dateline	key	proofreading
body	editing	letterhead	salutation
clarity	enclosure	modified-block letter style	signature block
complimentary closing	full-block letter style	notations	simplified letter style
concise	identification line	optical character reader (OCR)	subject line
courtesy title	inside address		template

CHAPTER OUTLINE

- Correspondence and Professionalism
- Choosing Correspondence Supplies
- Written Correspondence
- Effective Writing
- Interoffice Memorandum (Memo)
- Editing and Proofreading
- Preparing Outgoing Mail
- Mailing Equipment and Supplies
- U.S. Postal Service Delivery
- Other Delivery Services
- Processing Incoming Mail

Introduction

Communication skills are important in every profession. Written materials are tangible demonstrations of an office staff's ability to communicate and conduct business.

Others often evaluate the entire medical practice by the work of one employee. When a letter, form, or document is carelessly prepared and sent into the community, the physician may be judged as "careless." However, when a letter or general business correspondence is constructed in a neat, concise, and well-organized fashion, the physician is often judged to be organized and competent. The skill demonstrated in the creation of a simple business letter reflects on the medical skills of the physician and the practice. Professional image is conveyed in written correspondence.

Because written documents also serve as legal records, all documents must be prepared with great care and attention to detail. The administrative role of the medical assistant includes the creation of documents that are consistently accurate and clear.

In this chapter you will learn how to write effectively. You will develop skills in composing a business letter. You will learn different styles and formats of writing and will learn how to professionally manage all forms of correspondence commonly used in an ambulatory care setting.

Paula and Tom are medical assistants whose duties include making sure the daily correspondence is created and on the physician's desk before they go home at the end of the day. Today, they are working together to complete these tasks.

Paula will key into the computer letters of referral to other physicians. She is using a template saved within the computer to easily and quickly turn out many different letters. She is simply keying in different fields of information with the specifics for each patient referral. She then prints out a draft copy for proofreading and review by the physician or office manager. Once reviewed, corrected, and approved, she will print out the final letters onto the more expensive letterhead of the office. She will also copy the address from the letters and complete a mailing envelope for each letter.

Tom is assisting as he takes each completed letter and attaches all materials noted as enclosures to each letter. He then folds each letter and its enclosures carefully and inserts them into the properly addressed envelope. Next, he determines the weight of each envelope and the best choice for mailing it. He sorts the mailing into separate piles for different mail handling. The routine mailing is run through the stamp machine. The appropriate forms for the specialty mailing are created and attached. Tom makes sure copies of all mailings are carefully placed in the patient's chart. Both Paula and Tom know the importance of careful and accurate handling of all patient correspondence.

As you read this chapter, consider the following questions:

1. Why is it important to accurately and carefully prepare correspondence for an ambulatory setting? What could the poor management of documents and correspondence mean to a medical practice?
2. What are the differences between the language used in an informal or casual letter and that used in a formal or professional business letter?
3. What are some appropriate shortcuts that can assist in the daily management of correspondence and mailing?
4. What are some factors to consider in choosing the best mode of delivery for letters and parcels?

Correspondence and Professionalism

As in any business, correspondence from health-care professionals to patients and colleagues must be handled carefully, with appropriate attention to content and presentation. By learning how to create, send, and receive correspondence and other types of mail, you can ensure positive, effective communication between your office and others. Well-written, neatly prepared correspondence is one of the most important means of communicating a professional image for the medical office (Figure 7-1).

Choosing Correspondence Supplies

The first step in preparing professional-looking correspondence is choosing the right supplies. Many offices already have most of these supplies on hand. However, you may be responsible for choosing and ordering such supplies. You may need to make decisions about letterhead paper, envelopes, labels, invoices, and statements.

Letterhead Paper

Letterhead refers to formal business stationery on which the doctor's (or office's) name and address are printed at

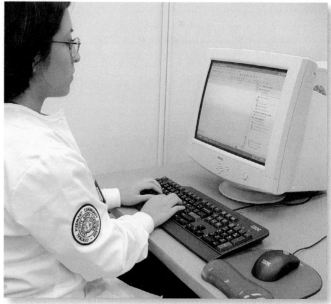

Figure 7-1. The correspondence that goes out of and comes into a medical office is vital to a well-run practice.

the top. In most cases, the office phone number is listed, along with the names of all the associates in the practice. Letterhead is used for correspondence with patients, colleagues, and vendors. Letterhead is used only for the first page of a letter. If a letter is more than one page, all additional pages of the letter are printed on a plain paper (the same color and bond as the letterhead).

Letterhead paper can be cotton fiber bond (sometimes called rag bond) or sulfite bond. Cotton fiber bond is usually more expensive than other types of paper. Cotton bond contains a watermark, which is an impression or pattern that can be seen when the paper is held up to the light. A watermark indicates that the paper is of high quality. The most popular cotton bond used for letterhead is 25% cotton because it is economical, but all higher grades can be used. Sulfite bond paper begins as wood pulp which is treated with peroxide or hypochlorite bleaching it to a paler color. Further chemical processes give sulfite paper a brilliant white appearance, making it a favorite for producing photographs. Businesses use sulfite paper for portfolios, folders, and other items that need a durable paper that is beautiful in appearance.

The two most common sizes of letterhead paper are standard and legal. Standard or letter-size paper is 8½ × 11 inches. Legal size is 8½ × 14 inches. Most general business correspondence is done on standard size. Legal size paper, as the name indicates, is used for legal documents, especially very lengthy documents.

A formal invitation or announcement may be engraved or embossed. Embossing involves a process where the letters are pressed into the paper. The letters are often set in black, gold, or silver.

Envelopes

Envelopes are used for correspondence, invoices, and statements. Typically, business letterhead, matching envelopes, and sometimes invoice and statement letterhead are printed together.

Familiarize yourself with the several types of envelopes used in the medical office.

- The most common envelope size used for correspondence is the No. 10 envelope (also called business size). It measures 4⅛ by 9½ inches.
- Envelopes used for invoices and statements can range from No. 6 (3⅝ by 6½ inches) to No. 10. These envelopes commonly have a transparent window that allows the address on the invoice or statement to show through, saving time and reducing the potential for errors involved in retyping the address.
- Smaller payment-return envelopes—preaddressed to the doctor's office—are often included along with a bill, for the patient's convenience.
- Tan Kraft envelopes, also called clasp envelopes, are available in many sizes and are used to send large or bulky documents.
- Padded envelopes are used to send documents or materials, such as slides, that may be damaged in the normal course of mail handling.
- The stock and quality of the envelope should always match the stationery. An office typically has two grades of envelopes with a return address. One is a less expensive stock and quality of paper with a block format return address printed in black. The second is a more expensive stock and quality of paper with a block format return address printed in black or a dark color.
- Data mailers are produced by a computer and are used by larger businesses and hospitals for batch mailings for items such as paychecks, appointment reminders, and some invoices. The envelopes are opened by tearing off perforated sides, peeling the envelope apart, or by a pull tab.

Labels

Address labels, printed from a computerized mailing list, can greatly speed the process of addressing envelopes for bulk mailings. For example, you may have to send a notice of a change in office hours or a quarterly office newsletter to a large number of patients in a practice.

You may choose to set up a system for frequently used labels. Many practices write referrals and other business letters to the same addresses again and again. For fast and easy access, it is helpful to print out labels a full page at a time of the same address. Pages of labels can then be stored in alphabetized folders near the transcription desk. Excel databases can also be set up to print labels and to insert names and addresses in standardized **templates.**

Invoices and Statements

There are several different types of invoices and statements in use today. They include:

- Preprinted invoices (used to send an original bill)
- Preprinted statements (used to send a reminder when an account is 30 or more days past due)
- Computer-generated invoices and statements
- Superbills (discussed in Chapter 17)

Written Correspondence

A letter is a form of communication—much like holding a conversation in person. The recipient will form an impression of the physician or the office based on the letter. Therefore, letters must be clear and well written and must politely convey the appropriate information.

Commonly used paragraphs and even entire letter formats, or templates, are used repeatedly in some practices. It is handy to save these bodies of text in the computer for quick and easy repeated access. With very few keystrokes, the material can be selected and displayed quickly. Then minor changes specific to the letter or document can be added.

It is also helpful to use the cut, paste, and copy features in word processing software to quickly piece together a correspondence that uses sentences or paragraphs from other documents. Large and small bodies of text can easily be moved or copied from document to document, saving time for the medical assistant.

Types of Correspondence in the Medical Office

As a medical assistant, you will be responsible for preparing routine letters at the doctor's request. You may transcribe some letters from the doctor's dictation and compose others from notes.

The purpose of most letters is to explain, clarify, or give instructions or other information. Correspondence includes letters of referral; letters about scheduling, canceling, or rescheduling appointments; patient reports for insurance companies; instructions for examinations or laboratory tests; answers to insurance or billing questions; and cover letters or form letters to order supplies, equipment, or magazine subscriptions.

Parts of a Business Letter

Figure 7-2 illustrates the parts of a typical business letter. Details about format may vary from office to office.

Letterhead. The letterhead is the preprinted portion of formal business stationery.

Dateline. The **dateline** consists of the month, day, and year. It should begin about three lines below the preprinted letterhead text on approximately line 15. The month should always be spelled out, and there should be a comma after the day.

Inside Address. The **inside address** contains all the necessary information for correct delivery of the letter. The inside address spells out the name and address of the person to whom the letter is being sent. In general, you should:

- **Key,** or type, the inside address on the left margin, two to four spaces down from the date. It should be two, three, or four lines in length.
- Include a **courtesy title** (Dr., Mr., Mrs., and so on) and the intended receiver's full name. Note: If Dr. is used, it is not followed by MD after the name. For example, either of these forms is acceptable: Dr. John Smith; John Smith, MD. This form is not acceptable: Dr. John Smith, MD. Generally the John Smith, MD format is used for the inside address and Dear Dr. Smith format is used for the salutation.

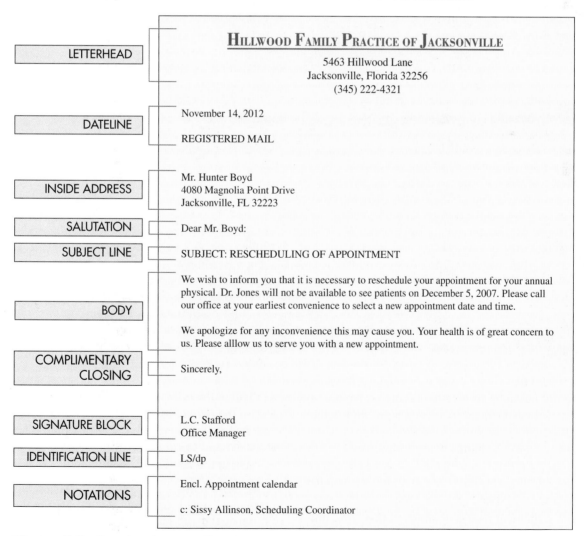

LETTERHEAD	**HILLWOOD FAMILY PRACTICE OF JACKSONVILLE**
	5463 Hillwood Lane
	Jacksonville, Florida 32256
	(345) 222-4321

DATELINE — November 14, 2012

REGISTERED MAIL

INSIDE ADDRESS —
Mr. Hunter Boyd
4080 Magnolia Point Drive
Jacksonville, FL 32223

SALUTATION — Dear Mr. Boyd:

SUBJECT LINE — SUBJECT: RESCHEDULING OF APPOINTMENT

BODY —
We wish to inform you that it is necessary to reschedule your appointment for your annual physical. Dr. Jones will not be available to see patients on December 5, 2007. Please call our office at your earliest convenience to select a new appointment date and time.

We apologize for any inconvenience this may cause you. Your health is of great concern to us. Please alllow us to serve you with a new appointment.

COMPLIMENTARY CLOSING — Sincerely,

SIGNATURE BLOCK —
L.C. Stafford
Office Manager

IDENTIFICATION LINE — LS/dp

NOTATIONS —
Encl. Appointment calendar

c: Sissy Allinson, Scheduling Coordinator

Figure 7-2. Knowing the parts of a typical business letter enables medical assistants to create written communications that reflect well on the office.

TABLE 7-1　USPS State Abbreviations

State	Abbreviation	State	Abbreviation
Alabama	AL	Montana	MT
Alaska	AK	Nebraska	NE
Arizona	AZ	Nevada	NV
Arkansas	AR	New Hampshire	NH
California	CA	New Jersey	NJ
Colorado	CO	New Mexico	NM
Connecticut	CT	New York	NY
Delaware	DE	North Carolina	NC
District of Columbia	DC	North Dakota	ND
Florida	FL	Ohio	OH
Georgia	GA	Oklahoma	OK
Hawaii	HI	Oregon	OR
Idaho	ID	Pennsylvania	PA
Illinois	IL	Puerto Rico	PR
Indiana	IN	Rhode Island	RI
Iowa	IA	South Carolina	SC
Kansas	KS	South Dakota	SD
Kentucky	KY	Tennessee	TN
Louisiana	LA	Texas	TX
Maine	ME	Utah	UT
Maryland	MD	Vermont	VT
Massachusetts	MA	Virginia	VA
Michigan	MI	Washington	WA
Minnesota	MN	West Virginia	WV
Mississippi	MS	Wisconsin	WI
Missouri	MO	Wyoming	WY

- Include the intended receiver's title on the same line with the name, separated by a comma, or on the line below it.
- Include the company name, if applicable.
- Use numerals for the street address, except the single numbers one through nine, which should be spelled out—for example, Two Markham Place.
- Spell out numerical names of streets if they are numbers less than ten.
- Spell out the words *Street, Drive,* and so on.

- Include the full city name; do not abbreviate.
- Use the two-letter state abbreviation recommended by the U.S. Postal Service (USPS) (Table 7-1).
- Leave one space between the state and the zip code; include the zip + 4 code, if known.

Attention Line.　An attention line is used when a letter is addressed to a company but sent to the attention of a particular individual. If you do not know the name of the individual, call the company directly to inquire the name of the appropriate contact person. A colon between the word *Attention* and the person's name is optional.

Salutation.   When addressing a person by name, use a **salutation,** a written greeting such as "Dear," followed by Mr., Mrs., or Ms., and the person's last name. The salutation should be keyed at the left margin on the second line below the inside address. A colon should follow. When you do not know the name, it is becoming common practice to use the business title or department in the salutation, as in "Dear Sir," "Dear Laboratory Director," or "Dear Claims Representative." This also avoids confusion if you do not know the gender of a person with a name such as Pat or Chris.

Subject Line.   A **subject line** is sometimes used to bring the subject of the letter to the reader's attention. The subject line is not required. However, if it is used, it should be keyed on the second line below the salutation. The subject line may be flush with the left margin, indented five spaces, or centered to the page. The subject line should be limited to two to three words and should be keyed in all capital letters to capture the attention of the reader. Some offices use "RE:" (short for regarding) instead of the word Subject.

Body.   The **body** of the letter begins two lines below the salutation or subject line. The text is single-spaced with double-spacing between paragraphs.

If the body contains a list, set the list apart from the rest of the text. Leave an extra line of space above and below the list. For each item in the list, indent five to ten spaces from each margin. Single-space within items, but leave an extra line between items. A bulleted list has a small, solid, round circle before each item.

Complimentary Closing.   The **complimentary closing** is placed two lines below the last line of the body. Capitalize only the first word of the closing. "Sincerely" is a common closing. "Very truly yours" and "Best regards" are also acceptable closings in business correspondence. A comma is placed after the complimentary closing.

Signature Block.   The **signature block** contains the writer's name on the first line and the writer's business title on the second line. The block is aligned with the complimentary closing and typed three to four lines below it, to allow space for the signature.

Identification Line.   The letter writer's initials followed by a colon or slash and the typist's initials are sometimes included in the letter. These initials are called the **identification line.** This line is typed flush left, two lines below the signature block.

Notations.   **Notations** include information such as the number of **enclosures** (make sure the typist notes what is enclosed) that are included with the letter and the names of other people who will be receiving copies of the letter (sometimes referred to as c:). If there are enclosures, a notation should appear flush left, one or two lines below the identification line (or one or two lines below the signature

block, if no identification line is present). You may abbreviate the word *Enclosure* by typing "Enc," "Encl," or "Encs" (with or without punctuation, depending on the style of the letter you are writing). The copy notation, "c," appears after the enclosure notation and includes one or more names or initials.

Punctuation Styles

Two different styles of punctuation are used in correspondence: open punctuation and mixed punctuation. A writer should use one punctuation style consistently throughout a letter.

Open Punctuation.   This style uses no punctuation after the following items when they appear in a letter:

- The word *Attention* in the attention line
- The salutation
- The complimentary closing
- The signature block
- The enclosure and copy notations

Mixed Punctuation.   This style includes the following punctuation marks used in specific instances:

- A colon after *Attention* in the attention line
- A colon after the salutation
- A comma after the complimentary closing
- A colon or period after the enclosure notation
- A colon after the copy notation

Letter Format

Follow these general formatting guidelines for all letters.

- The margin is the space around the edges of a form or letter that is left blank. The standard setting for margins in business correspondence is one inch (left and right margins) for 8½-inch-wide paper.
- Roughly center the letter on the page according to the length of the letter. For shorter letters, you can use wider margins and start the address farther down the page. For longer letters, use standard margins but start higher up on the page.
- Single-space the body of the letter. Double-space between paragraphs or parts of the letter.
- Use short sentences (no more than 20 words on average).
- Include at least two to three sentences in each paragraph.
- Divide long paragraphs—more than 10 lines of type— into shorter ones.

For multipage letters, use letterhead for the first page and matching plain bond paper for the subsequent pages. (When you order letterhead, be sure to order plain paper of the same texture and color as the letterhead for subsequent sheets.) Using a 1-inch margin at the top, include a heading with the addressee, date, and page number on all pages following the first one. Resume typing or printing the text about three lines below the heading.

Letter Styles

Different letter styles are used for different purposes. Your office is likely to have a preferred style in place. The four most common letter styles are full-block, modified-block, modified-block with indented paragraphs, and simplified.

Full-Block Style. The **full-block letter style,** also called block style, is typed with all lines flush left. Figure 7-3 shows an example of the block letter style. This style may include a subject line two lines below the salutation. Block-style letters are quick and easy to write because there are no indented paragraphs to slow the typist. Block style is one of the most common formats used in the medical office.

Modified-Block Style. The **modified-block letter style** is similar to full block but differs in that the dateline, complimentary closing, signature block, and notations are aligned and begin at the center of the page or slightly to the right (Figure 7-4). This type of letter has a traditional, balanced appearance.

Modified-Block Style with Indented Paragraphs. This style is identical to the modified-block

style except that the paragraphs are indented one-half inch (Figure 7-5).

Simplified Style. The **simplified letter style** is a modification of the full-block style. Figure 7-6 shows an example of the simplified letter style. The salutation is omitted, eliminating the need for a courtesy title. A subject line in all-capital letters is placed between the address and the body of the letter. The subject line summarizes the main point of the letter but does not actually use the word *subject*. All text is typed flush left. The complimentary closing is omitted, and the sender's name and title are typed in capital letters in a single line at the end of the letter. Note that this letter style always uses open punctuation, so it is both easy to read and quick to type. In most situations in a medical office, however, the simplified letter style may be too informal.

Effective Writing

To create effective, professional correspondence that reflects well on the practice, be sure that you use an appropriate style, clear and **concise** language, and the active voice. Though there are many forms of written communication other than a business letter, all of them must be written in such as way as to convey information clearly. Most medical practices make use of internal memos and external forms of communication, including all types of

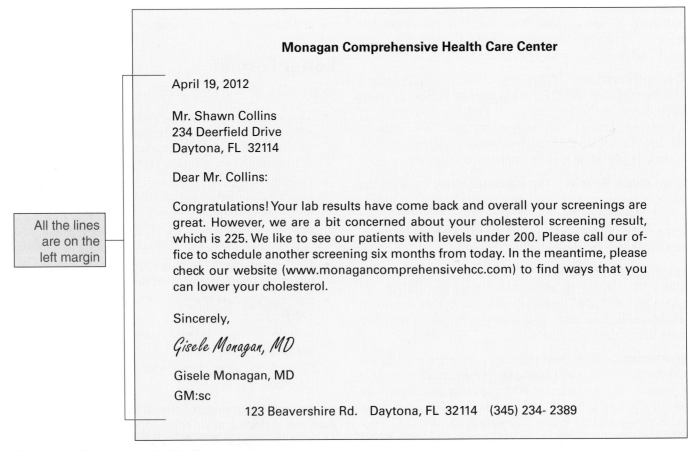

Figure 7-3. Example of a block style letter.

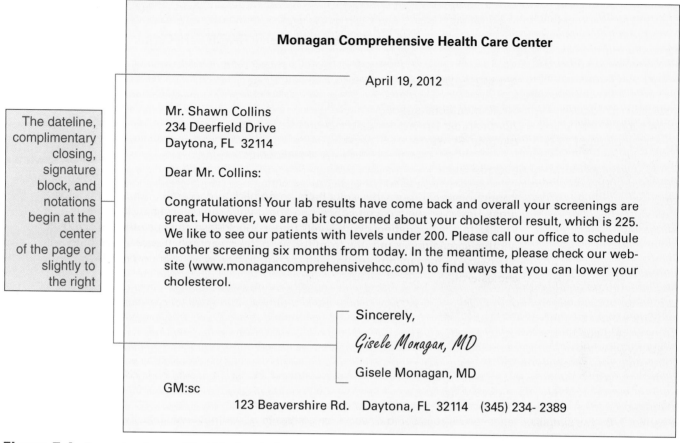

The dateline, complimentary closing, signature block, and notations begin at the center of the page or slightly to the right

Monagan Comprehensive Health Care Center

April 19, 2012

Mr. Shawn Collins
234 Deerfield Drive
Daytona, FL 32114

Dear Mr. Collins:

Congratulations! Your lab results have come back and overall your screenings are great. However, we are a bit concerned about your cholesterol result, which is 225. We like to see our patients with levels under 200. Please call our office to schedule another screening six months from today. In the meantime, please check our website (www.monagancomprehensivehcc.com) to find ways that you can lower your cholesterol.

Sincerely,

Gisele Monagan, MD

Gisele Monagan, MD

GM:sc

123 Beavershire Rd.   Daytona, FL 32114   (345) 234- 2389

Figure 7-4. Example of a modified-block style letter.

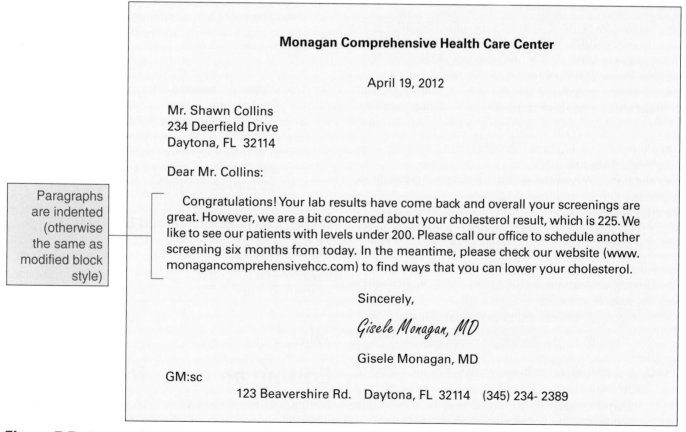

Paragraphs are indented (otherwise the same as modified block style)

Monagan Comprehensive Health Care Center

April 19, 2012

Mr. Shawn Collins
234 Deerfield Drive
Daytona, FL 32114

Dear Mr. Collins:

   Congratulations! Your lab results have come back and overall your screenings are great. However, we are a bit concerned about your cholesterol result, which is 225. We like to see our patients with levels under 200. Please call our office to schedule another screening six months from today. In the meantime, please check our website (www. monagancomprehensivehcc.com) to find ways that you can lower your cholesterol.

Sincerely,

Gisele Monagan, MD

Gisele Monagan, MD

GM:sc

123 Beavershire Rd.   Daytona, FL 32114   (345) 234- 2389

Figure 7-5. An example of the modified-block style letter with indented paragraphs.

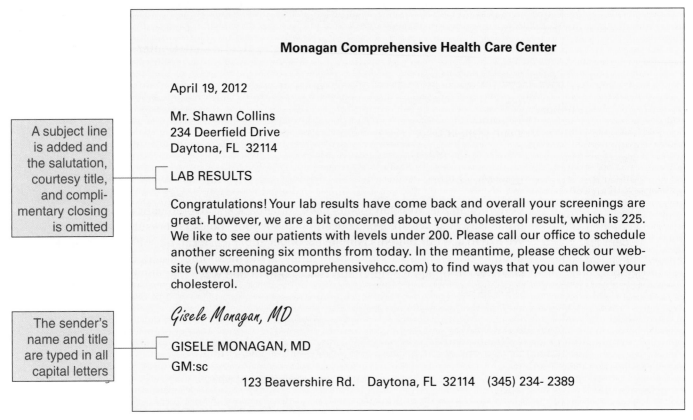

Monagan Comprehensive Health Care Center

April 19, 2012

Mr. Shawn Collins
234 Deerfield Drive
Daytona, FL 32114

A subject line is added and the salutation, courtesy title, and complimentary closing is omitted

LAB RESULTS

Congratulations! Your lab results have come back and overall your screenings are great. However, we are a bit concerned about your cholesterol result, which is 225. We like to see our patients with levels under 200. Please call our office to schedule another screening six months from today. In the meantime, please check our website (www.monagancomprehensivehcc.com) to find ways that you can lower your cholesterol.

Gisele Monagan, MD

The sender's name and title are typed in all capital letters

GISELE MONAGAN, MD
GM:sc

123 Beavershire Rd.   Daytona, FL 32114   (345) 234- 2389

Figure 7-6. The simplified letter style is considered by some executives to be the most readable style for correspondence.

business letters. Following are some general tips to help you write more effectively.

- Before you write, know the type of person to whom you are writing. Is the letter to a physician, a patient, a vendor, or fellow staff members? Decide if the tone should be formal or more relaxed.
- Know the purpose of the letter before you begin, and make sure your letter accurately conveys that purpose.
- Be concise. Use short sentences. Be brief. Be specific.
- Do not use unnecessary words. Use the simplest way to say what you mean.
- Show **clarity** in your writing; state your message so that it can be understood easily.
- Use the active voice whenever possible. Voice shows whether the subject of a sentence is acting or is being acted upon. Here is an example of the active voice:

  "Dr. Huang is seeing 18 patients today."

  Here is an example of the same sentence, written in the passive voice:

  "Eighteen patients will be seen by Dr. Huang today."

  Note that the active voice is more direct and livelier to read.
- Use the passive voice, however, to soften the impact of negative news:

  "Your account will be turned over to a collection agency if we do not receive payment promptly."

  It would sound harsher to say:

  "We will turn over your account to a collection agency if we do not receive payment promptly."

- Always be polite and courteous.
- Always check spelling and the accuracy of dates and monetary figures.
- Always check your grammar. Do not use slang.
- Avoid leaving "widows and orphans" or dangling words and phrases. These are words and short phrases at the end or beginning of paragraphs that are left to sit alone at the top or bottom of a page or column or separated from the rest of the thought. Do not start a paragraph at the bottom of a page if the rest of the sentence must be continued on the next page.

Interoffice Memorandums (Memos)

Interoffice memorandums (memos) are periodically used by medical offices, clinics, and hospitals. Most word processing software have templates that can be used to format an interoffice memo. Memos generally facilitate informal written communication within an office (Figure 7-7).

Editing and Proofreading

Editing and proofreading take place after you create the first draft of a letter. **Editing** involves checking a document for factual accuracy, logical flow, conciseness, clarity,

```
┌──────────────────────────────────────────────────────────────────┐
│                                                                    │
│  ═══════════════════════════════════════════════════════════════  │
│                         INTEROFFICE MEMO                           │
│  ═══════════════════════════════════════════════════════════════  │
│                                                                    │
│    DATE:    2/24/200X                                              │
│                                                                    │
│    TO:      K. SHERE HALL, VANESSA VAUGHN                          │
│                                                                    │
│    CC:      FILE                                                   │
│                                                                    │
│    FROM:    DREW MCGHEE, MD                                        │
│                                                                    │
│    RE:      PATIENT CHARTS                                         │
│  ────────────────────────────────────────────────────────────────│
│                                                                    │
│       It has come to my attention that a patient's chart was left  │
│    in a location where other patients and visitors could view it.  │
│    This is unacceptable.                                           │
│                                                                    │
│       Please be sure that all staff members understand that it is  │
│    imperative that patient charts are kept in the patient charting │
│    area. All staff should be reminded that patient charts are      │
│    highly confidential. HIPAA law states that the information      │
│    within a patient chart is protected health information and      │
│    should only be seen by members of our staff on a "business      │
│    need to know basis."                                            │
│                                                                    │
│    DM/IM                                                           │
│                                                                    │
└──────────────────────────────────────────────────────────────────┘
```

Figure 7-7. Example of an interoffice memo.

and tone. **Proofreading** involves checking a document for grammatical, spelling, and formatting errors. When possible, ask another person to proofread your work as well. *Never* skip over the very important steps of editing and proofreading! Spell check alone is not enough. It will not catch correctly spelled words used in the incorrect manner.

Tools for Editing and Proofreading

Reference books can help you prepare letters that appear professional. Keep the following tools available.

Dictionary. An up-to-date dictionary gives you more than definitions of words. A dictionary tells you how to spell, divide, and pronounce a word and what part of speech it is, such as a noun or adjective. A dictionary can be accessed on the Internet or in book form.

Medical Dictionary. It is nearly impossible for even the most experienced health-care professional to be familiar with every medical term and its correct spelling. A medical dictionary will serve as a handy reference for terms with which you are unfamiliar or about which you would like more information. Like a regular dictionary, a medical dictionary can also be accessed on the Internet or in book form. However, a medical dictionary in book form may not have the most updated terms. Like other medical reference books, a medical dictionary needs to be replaced periodically.

Becoming familiar with some of the prefixes and suffixes commonly used in medical terms can help you understand the meanings of many words. Appendix IV at the back of the book lists some common medical prefixes and suffixes.

Thesaurus. A thesaurus provides synonyms or similar words to a word you are using. It helps you avoid repetition in your writing and helps you find a word for an idea you have in mind. A thesaurus can be found in word processing programs, in print, and online.

Physicians' Desk Reference (PDR). The *PDR* is a dictionary of medications. Published yearly, it provides up-to-date information on both prescription and nonprescription drugs. Consult the *PDR* for the correct spelling of a particular drug or for other information about its usage, side effects, contraindications, and so on.

English Grammar and Usage Manuals. These manuals answer questions concerning grammar and word usage. They usually contain sections on punctuation, capitalization, and other details of written communication.

Word Processing Spelling Checkers. Most word processing programs used in medical offices have built-in spelling checkers. There are also programs designed specifically to check spelling in medical documents. These spelling checkers include most common medical terms that would not be found in a regular software program.

Spelling checkers pick up many spelling errors and often give suggestions for correct spellings. If you indicate the choice you meant to input, the program automatically replaces the misspelled word. These programs may not detect all spelling errors, however. They should not be relied on as the only means of checking a document. For example, spelling checkers cannot tell you that you used the wrong word if you type the word *form* instead of *from* because *form* is also a correctly spelled word.

You may be able to add words that are not currently recognized by the spelling checker in your computer. Use this feature to add medical terms. A word of caution is important here! Before you add the word to the computer's dictionary, be sure to look up the exact spelling in a medical dictionary. The computer will recognize only the spelling you add. If you place the *wrong* spelling in the computer, your spelling checker will not correct it.

When you type e-mails, take special care to use correct grammar and punctuation. Spelling checkers are available in most e-mail programs and should be used at the completion of the e-mail. The e-mail spelling checker does not automatically point out mistakes as you type.

Some software packages offer grammar-checking and style-checking features. These programs can identify certain problems, but the person using them still needs to know basic rules of grammar and style to correct errors.

Editing

The editing process ensures that a document is accurate, clear, and complete; free of grammatical errors; organized logically; and written in an appropriate style. It is a good idea to leave some time between the writing and editing stages so that you can look at the document in a fresh light. As you edit, you must examine language usage, content, and style.

Language Usage.   Learn basic grammar rules. When in doubt, refer to a grammar handbook or reference manual. Make sure all sentences are complete. Continually ask yourself, "Is this the best way to convey what I want to say? Do my word choices reflect the overall tone of the document?" For example, in a business letter, you would avoid choosing phrases that are too casual such as, "Thanks a million" or "Take it easy." These expressions are inappropriate for a business letter.

Content.   A business letter should contain all the necessary information the writer intends to convey. If you are editing someone else's letter and something appears to be missing, check with the writer. She or he may have omitted information by mistake.

The content of a letter should follow a logical thought pattern. Create a clean, concise letter by:

- Stating the purpose of the letter in the first sentence
- Discussing one topic at a time
- Changing paragraphs when you change topics

- Listing events in chronological order
- Sticking to the subject
- Selecting words carefully
- Reading over what you have written before printing

Style.   Use a writing style that is appropriate to the reader. A letter written to a patient is likely to require a different style than one written to a physician.

Proofreading

Proofreading means thoroughly checking a document for errors. After editing a document, put it aside for a short time before proofreading it. Ideally, have a coworker proofread your work. Someone else will often notice errors that you may miss. There are three types of errors that can occur when preparing a document: formatting, data, and mechanical.

Formatting Errors.   These errors involve the positioning of the various parts of a letter. They may include errors in indenting, line length, or line spacing. To avoid these errors, take the following two steps:

1. Scan the letter to make sure that the indentions are consistent, that the spacing is correct, and that the text is centered from left to right and top to bottom.
2. Follow the office style.

Data Errors.   Data errors involve mistyping monetary figures, such as a balance on a patient statement. Verify the accuracy of all figures by checking them twice or by having another coworker check them.

Mechanical Errors.   Mechanical errors are errors in spelling, punctuation, spacing between words, and division of words. Make sure that your word processing spell-checker has medical terminology included; otherwise, medical terms may be overlooked. Mechanical errors also include reversing words or characters, typing them twice, or omitting them altogether. Here are some tips to help you avoid mechanical errors.

- Learn basic spelling, punctuation, and word division rules. When in doubt, be sure to check a manual on English usage. Table 7-2 presents some basic rules concerning the mechanics of writing. Table 7-3 lists some of the most commonly misspelled medical terms and other words.
- Check carefully for transposed characters or words.
- Avoid dividing words at the end of a line. Most word processing programs automatically wrap words to the next line, so if you are writing on a computer, word division should not present a problem.

Creating a business letter involves many steps. Procedure 7-1 organizes these steps for you.

TABLE 7-2   Basic Rules of Writing

Word Division	Divide: • According to pronunciation • Compound words between the two words from which they derive • Hyphenated compound words at the hyphen • After a prefix • Before a suffix • Between two consonants that appear between vowels • Before *-ing* unless the last consonant is doubled; in that case, divide before the second consonant Do not divide: • Such suffixes as *-sion, -tial,* and *-gion* • A word so that only one letter is left on a line
Capitalization	Capitalize: • All proper names • All titles, positions, or indications of family relation when preceding a proper name or in place of a proper noun (not when used alone or with possessive pronouns or articles) • Days of the week, months, and holidays • Names of organizations and membership designations • Racial, religious, and political designations • Adjectives, nouns, and verbs that are derived from proper nouns (including currently copyrighted trade names) • Specific addresses and geographic locations • Sums of money written in legal or business documents • Titles, headings of books, magazines, and newspapers

Plurals	• Add *s* or *es* to most singular nouns (plural forms of most medical terms do not follow this rule)
	• With medical terms ending in *is,* drop the *is* and add *es:*
	    metastasis/metastases
	    epiphysis/epiphyses
	• With terms ending in *um,* drop the *um* and add *a:*
	    diverticulum/diverticula
	    atrium/atria
	• With terms ending in *us,* drop the *us* and add *i:*
	    calculus/calculi
	    bronchus/bronchi
	    (Two exceptions to this are virus/viruses and sinus/sinuses.)
	• With terms ending in *a,* keep the *a* and add *e:*
	    vertebra/vertebrae

Possessives	To show ownership or relation to another noun: • For singular nouns, add an apostrophe and an *s* • For plural nouns that do not end in an *s,* add an apostrophe and an *s* • For plural nouns that end in an *s,* just add an apostrophe
Numbers	Use numerals: • In general writing, when the number is 11 or greater • With abbreviations and symbols • When discussing laboratory results or statistics • When referring to specific sums of money • When using a series of numbers in a sentence Tips: • Use commas when numerals have more than three digits • Do not use commas when referring to account numbers, page numbers, or policy numbers • Use a hyphen with numerals to indicate a range

TABLE 7-3 Commonly Misspelled Medical Terms and Other Words

Medical Terms

abscess	dissect	leukemia	pneumonia
aerobic	eosinophil	leukocyte	polyp
anergic	epididymis	malaise	prescription
anesthetic	epistaxis	menstruation	prophylaxis
aneurysm	erythema	metastasis	prostate
anteflexion	eustachian	muscle	prosthesis
arrhythmia	fissure	neuron	pruritus
asepsis	flexure	nosocomial	psoriasis
asthma	fomites	occlusion	psychiatrist
auricle	glaucoma	ophthalmology	pyrexia
benign	glomerular	oscilloscope	respiration
bilirubin	gonorrhea	osseous	rheumatism
bronchial	hemocytometer	palliative	roentgenology
calcaneus	hemorrhage	parasite	scirrhous
capillary	hemorrhoids	parenteral	serous
cervical	homeostasis	parietal	specimen
chancre	humerus	paroxysm	sphincter
choroid	ileum	pericardium	sphygmomanometer
chromosome	ilium	perineum	squamous
cirrhosis	infarction	peristalsis	staphylococcus
clavicle	inoculate	peritoneum	surgeon
curettage	intussusception	pharynx	vaccine
cyanosis	ischemia	pituitary	vein
defibrillator	ischium	plantar	venous
desiccation	larynx	pleurisy	wheal
diluent			

Other Words

absence	believe	dilemma	fluorescent
accept	benefited	disappear	forty
accessible	brochure	disappoint	grammar
accommodate	bulletin	disapprove	grievance
accumulate	business	disastrous	guarantee
achieve	category	discreet	handkerchief
acquire	changeable	discrete	height
adequate	characteristic	discrimination	humorous
advantageous	cigarette	dissatisfied	hygiene
affect	circumstance	dissipate	incidentally
aggravate	clientele	earnest	indispensable
all right	committee	ecstasy	inimitable
a lot	comparative	effect	insistent
already	complement	eligible	irrelevant
altogether	compliment	embarrass	irresistible
analysis	concede	emphasis	irritable
analyze	conscientious	entrepreneur	its
apparatus	conscious	envelope	it's
apparent	controversy	environment	labeled
appearance	corroborate	exceed	laboratory
appropriate	counsel	except	led
approximate	courtesy	exercise	leisure
argument	defendant	exhibit	liable
assistance	definite	exhilaration	liaison
associate	dependent	existence	license
auxiliary	description	fantasy	liquefy
balloon	desirable	fascinate	maintenance
bankruptcy	development	February	maneuver

miscellaneous	pleasant	recede	supersede
misspelled	possession	receive	surprise
necessary	precede	recommend	tariff
noticeable	precedent	referral	technique
occasion	predictable	relieve	temperament
occurrence	predominant	repetition	temperature
offense	prejudice	rescind	thorough
oscillate	preparation	résumé	transferred
paid	prerogative	rhythm	truly
pamphlet	prevalent	ridiculous	tyrannize
panicky	principal	schedule	unnecessary
paradigm	principle	secretary	until
parallel	privilege	seize	vacillate
paralyze	procedure	separate	vacuum
pastime	proceed	similar	vegetable
persevere	professor	sizable	vicious
persistent	pronunciation	stationary	warrant
personal	psychiatry	stationery	Wednesday
personnel	psychology	stomach	weird
persuade	pursue	subpoena	
phenomenon	questionnaire	succeed	
plagiarism	rearrange	suddenness	

PROCEDURE 7-1

Creating a Letter

Procedure Goal: To follow standard procedure for constructing a business letter

Materials: Word processor or personal computer, letterhead paper, dictionaries or other sources

Method:

1. Format the letter according to the office's standard procedure. Use the same punctuation and style throughout.

   Rationale
   Consistency in format creates a professional-looking document.

2. Start the dateline three lines below the last line of the printed letterhead. (Note: Depending on the length of the letter, it is acceptable to start between two and six lines below the letterhead.)

   Rationale
   The letter should be centered both vertically and horizontally on the page for visual appeal.

3. Two lines below the dateline, type in any special mailing instructions (such as REGISTERED MAIL, CERTIFIED MAIL, and so on).

4. Three lines below any special instructions, begin the inside address.

Type the addressee's courtesy title (Mr., Mrs., Ms.) and full name on the first line. If a professional title is given (M.D., RN, Ph.D.), type this title after the addressee's name instead of using a courtesy title.

   Rationale
   A professional title is used when available in professional correspondence. Never use both a courtesy title and professional title at the same time.

5. Type the addressee's business title, if applicable, on the second line.

   Type the company name on the third line. Type the street address on the fourth line, including the apartment or suite number.

   Type the city, state, and zip code on the fifth line. Use the standard two-letter abbreviation for the state, followed by one space and the zip code.

6. Two lines below the inside address, type the salutation, using the appropriate courtesy title (Mr., Mrs., Ms., Dr.) prior to typing the addressee's last name.

continued ⟶

Creating a Letter (concluded)

Rationale

The salutation uses a courtesy title. Do not include the professional title or the addressee's first name in the salutation.

7. Two lines below the salutation, type the subject line, if applicable.

8. Two lines below the subject line, begin the body of the letter. Single-space between lines. Double-space between paragraphs.

9. Two lines below the body of the letter, type the complimentary closing.

10. Leave three blank lines (return four times), and begin the signature block. (Enough space must be left to allow for the signature.) Type the sender's name on the first line. Type the sender's title on the second line.

Rationale

Adequate space must be left for the signature. If the signer has a long signature, more than three blank lines may be left. Typing the name allows the addressee to understand who sent the letter if the sender's signature is not legible.

11. Two lines below the sender's title, type the identification line. Type the sender's initials in all capitals and your initials in lowercase letters, separating the two sets of initials with a colon or a forward slash.

12. One or two lines below the identification line, type the enclosure notation, if applicable.

13. Two lines below the enclosure notation, type the copy notation, if applicable.

14. Edit the letter.

Rationale

Make appropriate changes to clarify the meaning of the letter.

15. Proofread and spell-check the letter.

Rationale

Every letter must be read again to assure there are no errors.

Preparing Outgoing Mail

After you have created, edited, and proofread a letter, you need to prepare it for mailing. This preparation includes having the letter signed, preparing the envelope, and folding and inserting the letter into the envelope (Figure 7-8). It will then be ready for postage to be calculated and affixed.

Two Delivery Addresses

Sometimes mail may have two delivery addresses, a post office box and a street address. The mail is delivered to the address that appears directly above the city-state-zip. If the two addresses have different zip codes, the zip must be the one of the actual delivery point (Figure 7-9).

Signing Letters

After the letter is complete—it has been proofread and the envelope and enclosures have been prepared—it is ready for signing. Some doctors authorize other staff members to sign for them. If you have been authorized to sign letters, you should sign the doctor's name and place your initials after the doctor's signature.

If the doctor prefers to sign all letters, you should place the letter on the doctor's desk in a file folder marked "For Your Signature." If the letter is of an urgent nature, give it to the doctor as soon as possible. Otherwise, you can collect several letters in the folder and present the entire group for signing at one time. However, all prepared work should be given to the physician at the end of the day.

Preparing the Envelope

To ensure the quickest delivery of mail, the USPS has issued several guidelines for preparing envelopes. The USPS uses electronic **optical character readers (OCRs)** to help speed mail processing. OCRs read the last two lines of an address and sort the mail accordingly. To take advantage of this technology, envelopes must be no smaller than 3½ by 5 inches and no larger than 6 by 11½ inches. They must be addressed in a specific format that can be read by the OCR. Use USPS guidelines for addressing envelopes.

Address Placement. The address must be placed in a certain location on the envelope for reading by the OCR (Figure 7-10). The area the OCR can read has the following characteristics:

- It is bordered by a 1-inch margin on both the left and right sides of the envelope.
- It has a ⅝-inch margin on the bottom. The top of the city/state/zip code line (the last line in the address block) must be no higher than 2¼ inches from the bottom edge of the envelope.

How to Fold a Standard Letter

A business letter is folded twice into horizontal thirds and placed into an envelope. This insures a little privacy in the letter. The letter is also easy to unfold after opening the envelope. The following diagram shows how a letter is normally folded. This type of fold is used regardless of letter style.

If the letter needs to have the address face out an envelope window, make the second fold in the same location but opposite direction. The letter will then be folded in a Z shape and the address can be positioned to face out the window of the envelope.

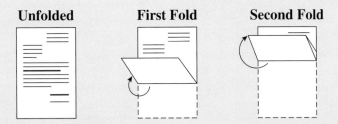

Unfolded   **First Fold**   **Second Fold**

Make a second horizontal crease one third from the top of the letter where the bottom of the letter had been folded to. Tuck the bottom into this crease and fold the top over it. The letter will be folded into thirds. It will fit any standard envelope.

If you are folding the letter so the address faces out the envelope window, fold the letter toward the back instead of the front. The letter address will appear through the envelope window, but it will still be folded in thirds.

Figure 7-8. It is important to fold a business letter correctly.

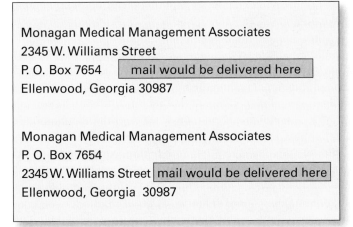

Figure 7-9. An example of two delivery addresses.

- An area 4½ inches wide in the bottom right corner of the envelope should be left clear. The OCR reads the address and prints a bar code that corresponds to the zip code in this area.

Address Format.   When you type an address, follow these format guidelines:

- Type or machine-print (for example, by computer) the address. (The OCR cannot read handwriting.) The OCR cannot read fancy script fonts.

- Single-space the lines and use the block format. Use only one or two spaces between numbers and words in the address. Do not punctuate because it is difficult for scanners to read.

- Use only USPS-approved abbreviations for location designations, as presented in Table 7-4.

- Put the addressee's name on the first line of the address block, the department (if any) on the second line, and the company name on the third line. If the letter is to go to someone's attention at a company, put the company name on the first line and "Attention:" before the address begins.

- The line above the city, state, and zip code should contain the street address or post office box number. Include suite or apartment numbers on the same line as the street address.

- The last line of the address must include the city, state, and zip code. Use the zip + 4 code whenever possible.

- Include the hyphen in the zip + 4 code, for example, 08520-6142. Obtain current zip codes by logging on to the USPS Web page at http://zip4.usps.com.

- Type any special notations (such as SPECIAL DELIVERY, CERTIFIED, or REGISTERED) two lines below the postage in all-capital letters. This information should appear outside the area the OCR can read.

- Type any handling instructions (such as PERSONAL or CONFIDENTIAL) three lines below the return address.

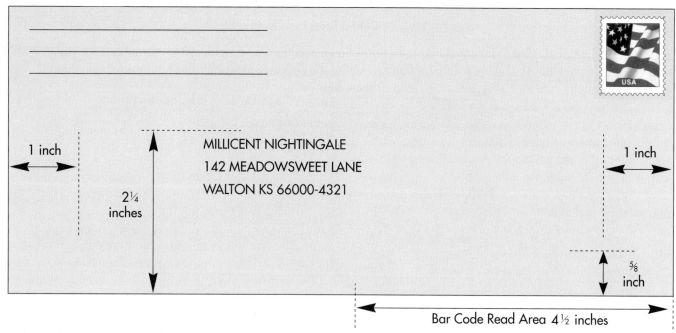

Figure 7-10. Following this format for typing an envelope ensures that it can be processed by USPS electronic equipment. Many software applications have envelope templates that are already formatted.

TABLE 7-4	USPS Abbreviations		
Word	**Abbreviation**	**Word**	**Abbreviation**
Avenue	AVE	Junction	JCT
Boulevard	BLVD	Lane	LN
Center	CTR	North	N
Circle	CIR	Parkway	PKY
Corner	COR	Place	PL
Court	CT	Plaza	PLZ
Drive	DR	South	S
East	E	Street	ST
Expressway	EXPY	West	W
Highway	HWY		

This information should also be outside the area the OCR can read.

- Letters going to foreign countries should have the name of the country on the last line of the address block in all-capital letters.
- Some letters may be appropriate for interoffice or company mail systems. These letters are usually placed in a large envelope with multiple address lines. The envelope can be reused many times by crossing out the previous name and address and using the next line. Place interoffice mail in a specially designated area or basket for pickup. Be sure not to mix it with outgoing mail.

Folding and Inserting Mail

Letters and invoices must be folded neatly before they are inserted into the envelopes. The proper way to fold a letter depends on the type of envelope into which the letter will fit.

- With a small envelope, fold the enclosure in half lengthwise, and insert it.
- With a regular business-size envelope, fold the letter in thirds. Fold the bottom third up first, then the top third down, and insert the letter.
- With a window envelope, use an accordion fold. Fold the bottom third up. Then, fold the top third back so

that the address appears in the window and insert the enclosure.

Before folding the letter, double-check that it has been signed, that all enclosures are included, and that the address on the letter matches the one on the envelope. Any enclosures that are not attached to the letter should be placed inside the folds so that they will be removed from the envelope along with the letter. (See Chapter 5 for information about folding and inserting machines.)

Mailing Equipment and Supplies

The proper equipment and supplies will help you handle the mail efficiently and cost-effectively. In addition to letterhead, blank stationery for multipage letters, and envelopes, you will need some standard supplies. The USPS provides forms, labels, and packaging for items that need special attention, such as airmail, Priority Mail, Express Mail, certified mail, or registered mail. Private delivery companies, such as United Parcel Service (UPS) and Federal Express (FedEx), also provide shipping supplies to their customers.

Airmail Supplies

In the past, any piece of mail that was transported by air was designated as airmail. Today nearly all first-class mail outside a local area is routinely sent by air. However, airmail services are still available for some packages and for most mail going to foreign countries.

If you are sending an item by airmail, attach special airmail stickers, available from the post office, on all sides. (The word *AIRMAIL* can also be neatly written on all sides.) Special airmail envelopes for letters can be purchased from the USPS.

Envelopes for Overnight Delivery Services

For correspondence or packages that must be delivered by the next day, a number of overnight delivery services are available through the USPS and private companies. Most companies require the use of their own envelopes and mailing materials. Make sure you keep adequate supplies on hand.

Postal Rates, Scales, and Meters

Postal rates and regulations change periodically, and every medical office should have a copy of the latest guidelines. These guidelines are available from the USPS. Chapter 5 describes postal scales and meters.

U.S. Postal Service Delivery

The USPS offers a variety of domestic and international delivery services for letters and packages. As a result of a comprehensive USPS Transformation Plan in 2002, many new services were added to the post office. As a result, the post office became much better able to compete with other mail and package delivery services. Following are some of the services you will be most likely to use in a medical office setting.

Regular Mail Service

Regular mail delivery includes several classes of mail as well as other designations such as Priority Mail and Express Mail. The class or designation determines how quickly a piece of mail is delivered.

First-Class Mail. Most correspondence generated in a medical office—letters, postcards, and invoices—is sent by first-class mail. Items must weigh 11 ounces or less to be considered first-class. (An item over 11 ounces that requires quick delivery must be sent by Priority Mail, which is discussed later in the chapter.) The cost of mailing a first-class item is based on its weight. The standard rate is for items 1 ounce or less that are not larger than 6⅛ inches high, 11½ inches wide, and ¼ inch thick. Additional postage is required for items that are heavier or larger. Postage for postcards is less than the letter rate. First-class mail is forwarded at no additional cost.

Second-Class Mail. Second-class mail is not used by most medical offices. This class of mail is designed for the delivery of newspapers and periodicals only.

Media Mail (Third-Class Mail). Media mail is also known as book rate mail. It is not often used in medical offices. Media mail is used for the mailing of books, catalogs, and other printed material that weighs less than 16 ounces. This class of mailing is available only to authorized mailers. Media mail is not forwarded unless it contains a special endorsement.

Parcel Post. This type of mail was formerly called Fourth-Class Mail. It is used for items that weigh at least one pound but not more than 70 pounds and that do not require speedy delivery. Rates are based on weight and distance. There is a special fourth-class rate for mailing books, manuscripts, and some types of medical information.

Bound Printed Matter. Formerly called Special Fourth-Class Mail, this is a rate applied to promotional advertising, directories, and other types of advertisements. No personal correspondence is allowed. Bulk rates are available for a minimum of 300 pieces.

Priority Mail. Priority class is useful for heavier items that require quicker delivery than is available for Fourth-Class Mail. Any first-class item that weighs between 11 ounces and 70 pounds requires Priority Mail service. Although the rate for Priority Mail varies with the weight of the item and the distance it must travel, the USPS offers a flat rate for all material that can fit into its special Priority Mail envelope. The USPS guarantees delivery of Priority Mail items in 2 to 3 days.

Express Mail. Express Mail is the quickest USPS service. Different types are available, including next-day and second-day delivery. Express Mail deliveries are made 365 days a year. Rates vary, depending on the weight and the specific service. A special flat-rate envelope is also available. Items sent by Express Mail are automatically insured against loss or damage. You can drop off packages at the post office or arrange for pickup service.

Special Postal Services

The USPS offers a variety of special mail delivery services in addition to the regular classes of mail. These services may require an additional fee above and beyond the cost of postage.

Online Postage

Postage can now be purchased online by using software that has been approved by the USPS. By using this software, customers are able to purchase products via the Internet. Pitney Bowes has software called ShipStream™; however, you may search the Internet for other USPS-approved software. USPS.com also sells postage online as well as other shipping and mailing supplies.

Special Delivery. Use special delivery if you want an item delivered as soon as it reaches the recipient's post office. Delivery of the item is typically made before the regularly scheduled mail delivery. Special delivery service is available within certain distance limits and during certain hours.

Certified Mail. Certified mail offers a guarantee that the item has been received. The item is marked as certified mail and requires the postal carrier to obtain a signature on delivery (Figure 7-11). The signature card is then returned to the sender. The card should be added to the patient's file. This documentation is evidence that the document was not only mailed but also received. The receiver's name is clearly printed along with the signature. The certified mail signature card becomes a legal document, which may be important in court.

Return Receipt Requested. You may request a return receipt (for a small additional fee) to obtain proof that an item was delivered. The receipt indicates who received the item and when. This type of mail service is very important when a medical practice requires proof that a letter was received. When returned to the office, the return receipt should be carefully added to the patient's record. It may become an important legal document and may be required at a later date in a court of law.

Registered Mail. Use registered mail to send items that are valuable, irreplaceable, or otherwise important. Registered mail provides the sender with evidence of mailing and delivery. It also provides the security that an item is being tracked as it is transported through the postal

system. Because of this tracking process, delivery may be slightly delayed.

To register a piece of mail, take it to the post office and indicate the full value of the item. Both first-class mail and Priority Mail can be registered.

Delivery Confirmation. Delivery confirmation is a service that tracks your mail with a tracking number by the delivery date and signature. There is an added fee involved.

International Mail

The USPS offers both surface (via ship) and airmail service to most foreign countries. Information on rates and fees is available from the post office.

There are various types of international mail, which are similar to the domestic classes. The USPS also provides international Express Mail and Priority Mail services, along with special mail delivery services such as registered mail, certified mail, and special delivery.

Tracing Mail

If a piece of registered or certified mail does not reach its destination by the expected time, you can ask the post office to trace it (Figure 7-12). You will need to present your original receipt for the item. You can also trace mail on the Internet through a UPC symbol that is scanned at the post office.

Other Delivery Services

In addition to the USPS, other companies provide mail and package delivery services across the world. UPS, FedEx, and DHL are three of the largest and most popular of these companies. DHL is one of the newest companies. The costs and types of services vary.

United Parcel Service

United Parcel Service (UPS) delivers packages and provides overnight letter and express services. You can either drop off packages at a UPS location or have them picked up at your office. Fees vary with the services provided, such as ground or air. Packages are automatically insured against theft or damage.

Express Delivery Services

Companies such as Federal Express and DHL provide several types of quick delivery services for letters and packages. Rates vary according to weight, time of delivery, and, in some cases, whether you have the package picked up at your office or drop it off at one of the company's local branches.

Back side of signature card

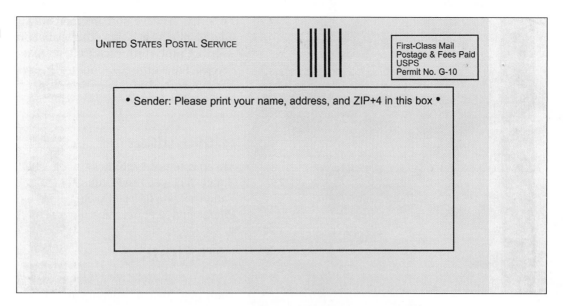

UNITED STATES POSTAL SERVICE

First-Class Mail
Postage & Fees Paid
USPS
Permit No. G-10

• Sender: Please print your name, address, and ZIP+4 in this box •

Front side of signature card

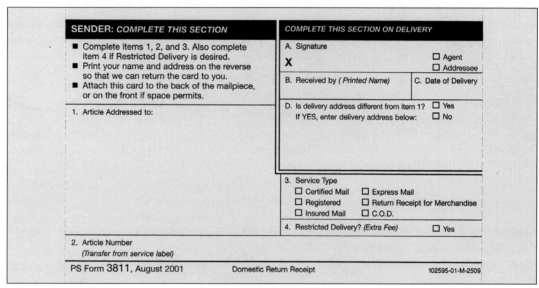

SENDER: *COMPLETE THIS SECTION*

- Complete items 1, 2, and 3. Also complete item 4 if Restricted Delivery is desired.
- Print your name and address on the reverse so that we can return the card to you.
- Attach this card to the back of the mailpiece, or on the front if space permits.

1. Article Addressed to:

COMPLETE THIS SECTION ON DELIVERY

A. Signature

X
☐ Agent
☐ Addressee

B. Received by (*Printed Name*) | C. Date of Delivery

D. Is delivery address different from item 1? ☐ Yes
If YES, enter delivery address below: ☐ No

3. Service Type
☐ Certified Mail   ☐ Express Mail
☐ Registered   ☐ Return Receipt for Merchandise
☐ Insured Mail   ☐ C.O.D.

4. Restricted Delivery? *(Extra Fee)*   ☐ Yes

2. Article Number
(Transfer from service label)

PS Form 3811, August 2001   Domestic Return Receipt   102595-01-M-2509

Certified mail receipt

U.S. Postal Service
CERTIFIED MAIL RECEIPT
(Domestic Mail Only; No Insurance Coverage Provided)

O F F I C I A L   U S E

Postage $

Certified Fee

Return Receipt Fee
(Endorsement Required)

Restricted Delivery Fee
(Endorsement Required)

Total Postage & Fees $

Postmark
Here

Sent To

Street, Apt. No.;
or PO Box No.

City, State, ZIP+ 4

PS Form 3800, January 2001   See Reverse for Instructions

7001 1140 0000 7637 2652

PLACE STICKER AT TOP OF ENVELOPE TO THE RIGHT
OF THE RETURN ADDRESS, FOLD AT DOTTED LINE

CERTIFIED MAIL

Figure 7-11. Certified mail offers a guarantee that the item has been received. The item is marked as certified mail and requires the postal carrier to obtain a signature on delivery. Registered mail provides the sender with evidence of mailing and delivery.

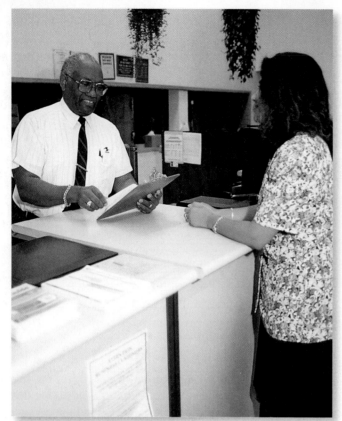

Figure 7-12. Tracing an item is a service that post offices perform when important items are delayed or do not reach their destinations.

Messengers or Couriers

When items must be delivered within the local area on the same day, local messenger services are an option. Many messenger companies are listed in the Yellow Pages of the telephone book.

Processing Incoming Mail

Mail is an important connection between the office and other professionals and patients. Often an office has an established procedure for handling the mail. It is best to set aside a specific time of the day to process all the incoming mail at once rather than trying to do a little bit at a time.

Although it sounds simple, processing mail involves more than merely opening envelopes. In general, it involves the following steps: sorting, opening, recording, annotating, and distributing.

Sorting and Opening

The first step in processing mail is to sort it. Always place any personal or confidential mail aside. Unless you have special permission never open personal mail addressed to another person. Carefully lay it on the desk of the addressee, unopened. Sort remaining mail according to

priority. Always sort all mail in an uncluttered area to avoid mixing it with other paperwork. Follow a regular sorting procedure each time so that you do not miss any steps. Procedure 7-2 outlines suggested steps for sorting and opening the mail. The Points on Practice section discusses how to recognize urgent incoming mail.

Recording

Keep a log of each day's mail. This daily record lists the mail received and indicates follow-up correspondence and the date it is completed. This method helps in tracing items and keeping track of correspondence.

Annotating

Because you will be reading much of the incoming mail, you may also be encouraged to annotate it. To **annotate** means to underline or highlight key points of the letter or to write reminders, comments, or suggested actions in the margins or on self-adhesive notes. An example of annotating is including "please sign here" next to where a signature should be. Annotating may involve pulling a patient's chart or any previous related correspondence from a file and attaching it to the letter.

Distributing

Sort letters into separate batches for distribution. These batches might include correspondence that requires the physician's attention, payments to be directed to the person in charge of billing, and correspondence that requires your attention. Each batch should be presented to the appropriate person in a file folder or arranged with the highest-priority items on top. You may be given specific instructions on how to distribute magazines, newspapers, and advertising circulars.

Handling Drug and Product Samples

Many physicians receive a number of drug and product samples in the mail. Handling procedures vary from office to office. Samples of nonprescription products, such as hand creams or cough drops, may be placed in the patient treatment area for patient distribution as directed by the physician.

The physician may ask that you put samples of any new prescription drugs in the consultation room for him to evaluate. Store all other drug samples in a locked cabinet reserved solely for such samples. Sort and label the samples by category, such as antibiotics, sedatives, painkillers, and so on. Never give samples to patients or use them yourself unless directed by the physician. If the doctor directs you to give samples to a patient, make sure to write this information in the patient's chart and date the entry.

PROCEDURE 7-2

Sorting and Opening Mail

Procedure Goal: To follow a standard procedure for sorting, opening, and processing incoming office mail

Materials: Letter opener, date and time stamp (manual or automatic), stapler, paper clips, adhesive notes

Method:

1. Check the address on each letter or package to be sure that it has been delivered to the correct location.
2. Sort the mail into piles according to priority and type of mail. Your system may include the following:
   - Top priority. This pile will contain any items that were sent by overnight mail delivery in addition to items sent by registered mail, certified mail, or special delivery. (Faxes and e-mail messages are also top priority.)
   - Second priority. This pile will include personal or confidential mail.
   - Third priority. This pile will contain all firstclass mail, airmail, and Priority Mail items. These items should be divided into payments received, insurance forms, reports, and other correspondence.
   - Fourth priority. This pile will consist of packages.
   - Fifth priority. This pile will contain magazines and newspapers.
   - Sixth priority. This last pile will include advertisements and catalogs.
3. Set aside all letters labeled "Personal" or "Confidential." Unless you have permission to open these letters, only the addressee should open them.
4. Arrange all the envelopes with the flaps facing up and away from you.
5. Tap the lower edge of the envelope to shift the contents to the bottom. This step helps to prevent cutting any of the contents when you open the envelope.
6. Open all the envelopes.

Rationale
It is more efficient to open all the envelopes first and then remove the contents.

7. Remove and unfold the contents, making sure that nothing remains in the envelope.
8. Review each document, and check the sender's name and address.
   - If the letter has no return address, save the envelope, or cut the address off the envelope, and tape it to the letter.
   - Check to see if the address matches the one on the envelope. If there is a difference, staple the envelope to the letter, and make a note to verify the correct address with the sender.
9. Compare the enclosure notation on the letter with the actual enclosures to make sure that all items are included. Make a note to contact the sender if anything is missing.
10. Clip together each letter and its enclosures.
11. Check the date of the letter. If there is a significant delay between the date of the letter and the postmark, keep the envelope.

Rationale
It may be necessary to refer to the postmark in legal matters or cases of collection.

12. If all contents appear to be in order, you can discard the envelope.
13. Review all bills and statements.
    - Make sure the amount enclosed is the same as the amount listed on the statement.
    - Make a note of any discrepancies.
14. Stamp each piece of correspondence with the date (and sometimes the time) to record its receipt. If possible, stamp each item in the same location—such as the upper-right corner.

Rationale
It may be necessary to refer to the date in legal matters or in cases of collection.

When a box of samples is outdated, you should properly dispose of them, following all state and DEA regulations. (See Chapter 3.) You will most likely use the disposal company that handles your biomedical waste to dispose of unused, outdated sample medications. Flushing samples down the sink or toilet is no longer allowed because of the possibility of polluting the environment. Samples should not be placed in the trash where unauthorized individuals could take the medications. Your local pharmacy may also have a program for disposing of outdated medications.

How to Spot Urgent Incoming Mail

How can you tell if a piece of incoming mail is urgent? First-class mail marked "Urgent" tells you that it requires immediate attention. Here are some other signals to look for (Figure 7-13).

Overnight Mail

Any package that has been sent by an overnight carrier or by USPS Express Mail should be considered urgent and should be opened immediately.

Certified Mail

Certified mail requires your signature on delivery. The sender used certified mail to be sure that the item would be sent to the proper person.

Registered Mail

Items sent by registered mail typically are valuable, irreplaceable, or otherwise important. Registered mail provides the sender with evidence of mailing and delivery.

Special Delivery

An item sent by special delivery is likely to be delivered sometime before the normal mail delivery—possibly even on a Sunday or holiday. The sender requested special delivery to ensure that the item would be delivered promptly after it was received at the addressee's post office.

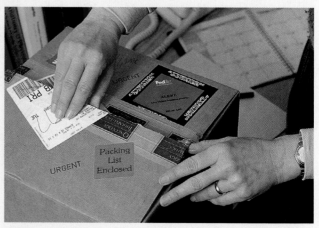

Figure 7-13. Urgent materials receive top priority upon arrival at an office.

Summary

7.1 Choose the right supplies for professional-looking office correspondence. Letterhead should be formal with the physician's or medical practice's name and address printed on the top. Envelopes, labels, and invoices are generally ordered together. There are several types you can choose from. Spreadsheets can be customized to print labels as well.

7.2 As a medical assistant you may be responsible for preparing correspondence. Routine letters as well as transcription may be part of your duties. Other correspondence includes letters of referral, scheduling letters, reports to insurance companies, and instructions for exams and lab reports.

7.3 The parts of the business letter are the dateline, the subject line (sometimes used to bring the subject to the reader's attention), the attention line, the body of the letter, the complimentary closing, the signature block, the identification line, and notations (for enclosures and attachments). Letter styles for correspondence include full-block style (typed flush left), modified-block style (similar to block; however, the dateline, signature block, and notation are aligned and begin at the center of the paper); modified block with indented paragraphs (identical to modified block except paragraphs are indented five spaces to the right); and simplified, which is a modification of the full block (the salutation is omitted). There are two different styles of punctuation used in correspondence. They are open punctuation and mixed punctuation. Be consistent in your choice throughout the letter.

7.4 Medical assistants should proofread and edit correspondence they create. Editing involves checking a document for accuracy, flow, conciseness, clarity, and tone. Proofreading involves checking a document for grammatical, spelling, and formatting errors.

7.5 When editing and proofreading, keep available tools such as a medical dictionary, thesaurus, *Physician's Desk Reference (PDR)*, and English grammar manuals.

7.6 The process of handling incoming and outgoing mail includes properly sorting, opening, recording, annotating, and distributing the mail.

7.7 The U.S. Postal Service offers a variety of services for letters and packages. It now has the ability to compete with other mail and package delivery services such as Federal Express and United Parcel Service (UPS).

REVIEW

CHAPTER 7

CASE STUDY QUESTIONS

Now that you have completed this chapter, review the case study at the beginning of the chapter and answer the following questions:

1. Why is it important to accurately and carefully prepare correspondence for an ambulatory setting? What could the poor management of documents and correspondence mean to a medical practice?

2. What are the differences between the language used in an informal or casual letter and that used in a formal or professional business letter?

3. What are some appropriate shortcuts that can assist in the daily management of correspondence and mailing?

4. What are some factors to consider in choosing the best mode of delivery for letters and parcels?

Multiple-Choice Questions

1. The _____ is the space around the edges of a form or letter that is left blank.
   a. dateline   **c.** letterhead
   b. courtesy title   **d.** margin
2. The complimentary closing is placed how many lines below the last line of the body?
   a. 2   **c.** 4
   b. 6   **d.** 3
3. What type of mail is required for sending items that are valuable, irreplaceable, or otherwise important?
   a. Certified   **c.** Registered
   b. Special delivery   **d.** Return receipt requested
4. Which of the following is spelled correctly?
   a. professor   **c.** profesur
   b. proffessur   **d.** profesor
5. Notations include information such as the number of _____ that are included with the letter and the names of other people who will be receiving copies of the letter.
   a. salutations   **c.** subject lines
   b. enclosures   **d.** complimentary closings

Discussion Questions

1. Why is it important to closely follow the basic rules of writing when creating a business letter?
2. Name and describe the five steps involved in processing incoming mail.
3. You have been asked to create a basic business letter format for use within a medical practice. Summarize the format, describing the placement of each part of the letter.
4. Name and describe the different types of invoices and statements and their use in a medical practice.

Critical Thinking Questions

1. You have been asked to mail a letter to a patient, withdrawing the services of the practice. What type of mail service would you use and why?
2. The physician tells you to make sure that all patient letters that address withdrawing the services of the practice are "well documented." What does the physician mean? What would you do?
3. Imagine that your coworker is out sick. You must make sure all the work is handled. Which is more important—typing referral letters or sorting the mail? Why? How might you proceed if you are responsible for both but don't have the time to complete both?
4. You need a quick and easy way to remember the parts of a business letter and how they are placed. How are you going to remember them?

Application Activities

1. You are employed in Dr. Angelo Carillo's office. A young patient of yours, Rodney Sills, has broken his wrist, and Dr. Carillo says that Rodney will be unable to participate in gym class for 10 weeks. Create a letter notifying his gym instructor of the situation.

2. Prepare a No. 10 business envelope using the USPS guidelines for addressing envelopes. Include the following information.

Return address:
Dr. Angelo Carillo, 123 Winding Way, Suite 2, Rockland, NJ 09876

Mailing address:
ABC Insurance, 987 Hill Street, Marrakesh, CA 01234

Attention:
Susan Jones, Claims Department

Special Instructions:
Certified Mail

3. Using proper letter formatting technique and the basic rules of writing reviewed in this chapter, correct the following letter:

September 18th, 2011

Mountainside Hospital
Samuel Adams, Educational Coordinator
1 Mountainside Lane
San Francisco, California, 94112

Dear mr. Adams:

I am writing in response to your letter of the 10th. I am very interested in presenting a talk at your Health Fare in February. I am avialable to speak on either the 20th or the 21st.

If there is any flexibility in scheduling, I would prefer to present my talk in the afternoon. Also, please let me know how long I should prepare to speak. I am including a copy of an article I recently wrote on the same subject for the local paper.

I am looking forward to hearing from you.

Sincerly,
Enclosure
Dr. Angelo Carillo AC/SCB

4. Create flashcards for use in class and for individual study. Use all the key terms and definitions in this chapter, 20 commonly misspelled words from Table 7-3, and 10 common USPS abbreviations from Table 7-4.

Virtual Fieldtrip

Visit the McGraw-Hill Higher Education Medical Assisting website at www.mhhe.com/medicalassistin4e to complete the following activity:

Use the American Association of Medical Assistants and other websites related to effective writing. Prepare an oral presentation about one of the following topics:

- The parts of a business letter and why each part is important
- Styles of business letters and the circumstances for using each type
- Techniques for becoming an effective writer
- Tools for editing and proofreading
- The process of preparing an envelope and mailing

Ask your instructor how many references and citations you should minimally include in your research. Present your report to the class, using all available multimedia, including PowerPoint slides or an overhead projector if possible.

Use the Internet to search for different types of approved USPS online postage software. Present to class as a report.

Open the CD and complete this chapter's practice activities, play the games, listen to the key terms, and test yourself with the interactive review. E-mail, print, and/or save your results to document your proficiency.

Managing Office Supplies

MEDICAL ASSISTING COMPETENCIES

CAAHEP

Identify both equipment and supplies needed for filing medical records

Perform an office inventory

ABHES

8. Medical Office Business Procedures Management
- d. Apply concepts for office procedures
- z. Maintain medical office equipment and supplies

11. Career Development
Demonstrate professionalism by:
- 1) Exhibiting dependability, punctuality, and a positive work ethic
- 2) Exhibiting a positive attitude and a sense of responsibility
- 5) Exhibiting initiative
- 7) Expressing a responsible attitude
- 9) Conducting work within scope of education, training, and ability

LEARNING OUTCOMES

After completing Chapter 8, you will be able to:

8.1 Identify examples of vital, incidental, and periodic supplies used in a typical medical office.

8.2 Describe how to store administrative and clinical supplies.

8.3 Implement a system for tracking the inventory of supplies.

8.4 Carry out inventories and ordering times to maximize office efficiency.

8.5 Select and evaluate supply sources.

8.6 Use strategies to obtain the best-quality supplies while controlling costs.

8.7 Implement procedures for ordering supplies.

8.8 Carry out a supply order and pay for the supplies.

MEDICAL ASSISTING MEDIA

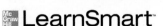 **Connect Plus+™**
connect.mcgraw-hill.com

- Electronic Health Records (E.H.R.) SpringCharts®
- eBook

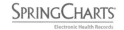

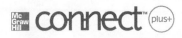 **LearnSmart™**

www.mhhe.com/learnsmart

Complete Learning Module: Managing Office Supplies

 Student CD-ROM

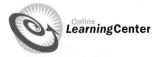 **Online Learning Center™**

www.mhhe.com/medicalassisting4e

KEY TERMS

disbursement
durable item
efficiency
expendable item

inventory
invoice
Material Safety Data Sheet (MSDS)

purchase order
purchasing groups
reputable

requisition
unit price

CHAPTER OUTLINE

- Organizing Medical Office Supplies
- Taking Inventory of Medical Office Supplies

- Ordering Supplies

PREPARATION FOR CERTIFICATION

RMA (AMT) Exam
- Supplies and equipment management

CMA (AAMA) Exam
- Inventory control
- Time management
- Purchasing

CMAS Exam
- Supplies and equipment
- Patient information and community resources

Introduction

The purpose of a medical office or clinic is to deliver appropriate care to those in need. However, no medical office can function without adequate supplies. It is therefore essential that the medical assistant routinely evaluate and replenish the office's supplies before a shortage is noted.

In this chapter, you will focus on the importance of adequate administrative and clinical supplies in the daily operation of a typical medical practice. You will learn to evaluate, replace, organize, and pay for expendable items used routinely in a practice.

The administration of the hospital where you are employed has made the decision to open a series of clinics across the city to provide ambulatory care to patients in their neighborhoods. As an experienced medical assistant, you have been asked to plan for the purchase of expendable items for stocking in the new clinics. What a task! How will you determine what items to provide for each clinic and the amount to order? Do you know where to go to get the best price for the best products? Who is the best vendor in each area? What about discounts for volume buying? Where do you start? You need a plan or a system to help organize your thoughts and then your actions.

As you read this chapter, consider the following questions:

1. What is an *expendable* item? What items would you list on the expendable administrative supply list? The clinical supply list? The general supply list?
2. What factors would you consider about each office as you determine the appropriate supplies?
3. How would you recommend that the supplies be stored with inventory management in mind?

Organizing Medical Office Supplies

Purchasing and maintaining administrative and medical supplies are essential skills that you will use in managing the office. You will be responsible for taking inventory of equipment and supplies, evaluating and recommending equipment and supplies, and negotiating prices with suppliers. When managing office supplies, your goal is to achieve **efficiency,** which is the ability to produce the desired result with the least effort, expense, and waste.

The word *supply* refers to an **expendable item,** or an item that is used and then must be restocked, such as prescription pads (Figure 8-1). Ideally, office supplies are stored on labeled shelves. More **durable items,** or pieces of equipment that are used indefinitely—such as telephones, computers, and examination tables—are not considered supplies. Also included in the category of durable items is medical equipment, such as stethoscopes and reflex hammers. Chapter 5 discusses ordering durable administrative items.

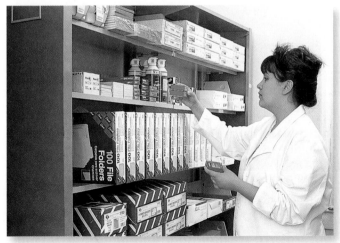

Figure 8-1. Making sure that supplies are in order is a continuous process that ensures an efficient, well-prepared office.

Determining Responsibility for Organizing Supplies

It is recommended that the responsibility for organizing office supplies lie with one to two individuals. Often this responsibility is given to the medical assistant. In a small practice, one medical assistant may be able to handle this responsibility. A practice with several physicians may require more help to manage supplies. When two medical assistants handle this responsibility, one is often assigned to handle administrative items and the other to handle clinical (medical) supplies. In a very large practice, a third assistant might handle computer, copier, and fax supplies.

 ## Categorizing Supplies

Most supplies in the medical office fall into two main categories: administrative and clinical. Examples of administrative supplies include items that are used in the office portion of the practice, such as stationery, insurance forms, pens, pencils, and clipboards. Clinical supplies are medically related and include alcohol swabs, tongue depressors, disposable tips for otoscopes, and disposable sheaths for thermometers.

General supplies are used by both patients and staff. Examples of general supplies include paper towels, liquid hypoallergenic soap, and facial and toilet tissue.

The Supply List. You will need to determine what items in your office are used routinely and reordered systematically. Keep a list of these items, and update it as needed. This master supply list is usually kept in the office procedures manual. Appropriate sections of this list may be posted on the cabinets where the items are stored.

One good way to help keep track of supplies is to categorize them according to their importance within the practice. Although all supplies in your office are necessary, some supplies are more important than others. You may find it helpful to identify an item in one of three categories: vital, incidental, and periodic use. Table 8-1 will help you determine vital, incidental, and periodic supplies for your office.

TABLE 8-1 — Typical Supplies in a Medical Office

Administrative Supplies

Appointment books, daybooks (still used in noncomputerized offices)
Back-to-school/back-to-work slips
Clipboards
Computer supplies
Copy and facsimile (fax) machine paper
File folders, coding tabs
HIPAA forms (Notice of Privacy Practices, authorization forms, disclosure logs, request to inspect/copy medical record forms, request for amendment forms, acknowledgment of request for amendment forms)
History and physical examination sheets/cards
Insurance forms: disability, HMO and other third-party payers, life insurance examinations, Veterans Administration, workers' compensation
Insurance manuals
Local welfare department forms
Patient education materials
Pens, pencils, erasers
Prescription pads
Rubber bands, paper clips
Registration forms
Social Security forms
Stamps
Stationery: appointment cards, bookkeeping supplies (ledgers, statements, billing forms), letterhead, second sheets, envelopes, business cards, prescription pads, notebooks, notepads, telephone memo pads

Clinical Supplies

Alcohol swabs
Applicators
Bandaging materials: adhesive tape, gauze pads, gauze sponges, elastic bandages, adhesive bandages, roller bandages (gauze and elastic)
Cloth or paper gowns and drapes
Cotton, cotton swabs
Culture tubes
50% dextrose solution
Disposable sheaths for thermometers
Disposable tips for otoscopes
Gloves: sterile, examination
Hemoccult test kits
Iodine or Betadine pads
Lancets
Lubricating jelly
Microscopic slides and fixative
Needles, syringes
Nitroglycerin tablets
Safety pins
Silver nitrate sticks
Suture removal kits
Sutures
Table covers (examination)
Tongue depressors
Topical skin freeze
Urinalysis test sticks
Urine containers
Injectable medications: diazepam (Valium), diphenhydramine hydrochloride (Benadryl), epinephrine (Adrenalin), furosemide (Lasix), isoproterenol (Isuprel), lidocaine (Xylocaine: 1%, 2%, and plain), meperidine hydrochloride (Demerol), morphine, phenobarbital, sodium bicarbonate, sterile saline, sterile water
Other medicines, chemicals, solutions, ointments, lotions, and disinfectants, as needed

General Supplies

Liquid hypoallergenic soap
Paper cups
Paper towels
Tampons and sanitary pads
Tissues: facial, toilet

Vital Supplies. These items are absolutely essential for the functioning of the practice. They include paper examination table covers and prescription pads. Without these items, the physician would be unable to work in a clean examination environment or to readily prescribe medication for patients during office visits. Another type of vital supply is an item that requires a special order, such as a printed form. Special orders take time to obtain, so they must be ordered well before supplies run low.

Incidental Supplies. These supplies are needed in the office but do not threaten the efficiency of the office if the supply runs low. Incidental supplies include staples and rubber bands, which can be purchased quickly and easily at a local stationery store.

Periodic Supplies. These supplies require ordering only occasionally. For example, if your office uses appointment books, you will order them only once or twice a year, probably in small numbers. The urgency of ordering some periodic items can depend on the size of the office. A multiphysician office, for example, would require more appointment books than a single-physician office. Another example of a periodic item might be holiday cards to send to the physician's colleagues and patients.

Storing Office Supplies

Storing office supplies requires good organizational skills and attention to detail. Many people in an office use these supplies, so the items should be stored neatly and in an orderly way. In addition, it is important to store supplies safely to prevent loss or theft, damage, or deterioration.

Location. In a small medical office, supplies are generally kept near the areas of the office where they are used. Administrative supplies are usually stored behind or adjacent to the reception area, with clinical supplies stored near the examination rooms. If the practice has a laboratory, pertinent supplies are stored in or near the laboratory. Offices that have separate supply rooms offer more storage space.

Small medical offices may not have ample space for storage. It may be tempting to store boxes on the floor behind the air-conditioning unit, stacked up close to the ceiling, or in potentially hazardous locations, such as near a source of heat. It is essential that supplies be stored according to the guidelines described by TJC (The Joint Commission).

Items may not be stored on the floor; instead, they must be raised off the floor, as on a crate or shelf, to avoid contamination by water. Items stored close to the ceiling are considered a fire hazard. TJC standards require that supplies stored on the top shelf of a closet or storage area be at least 18 inches below the ceiling.

Avoid storing any boxes or supplies near a water heater, air-conditioning unit, heater, or stove. Many expendable items and their packaging are combustible and can quickly become a fire hazard. Air-conditioning units may drip water on the floor. If boxes of expensive forms are stored nearby, they can quickly become ruined as water seeps unnoticed into the packaging.

Storage Cabinets. Each storage cabinet should be labeled with a list of its contents. Keep all stock of one item together.

Finding supplies is easier if you keep small items at eye level. Put large, bulky goods, such as reams of stationery, on lower shelves. Label boxes and containers clearly so that all employees can readily find what they need and so that the inventory process is easier.

As you initially arrange items on storage shelves, label the shelves. Reserve enough space to completely stock each item. Do not put anything but the appropriate item in each designated space. This easy system allows for a quick review when you reorder supplies.

To reduce the risk of errors on reorders, keep each item's original label attached to it. Cover the label with clear tape, if necessary. If you must replace a worn label, do it immediately when needed, making sure the new label has the same detailed information as the old one. Bottles with pouring spouts should be labeled on the side opposite the spout to prevent the liquid from dripping onto the label. Use a laundry marking pen to label linens with the name of your office. Linen services usually premark linens with the name of the company or the practice.

Many items have a shelf life after which they are no longer usable. By not over-ordering and by rotating supplies—using older ones first—your office will be able to use items during their shelf life. This is true not only for perishable items such as medications, but also for linens and paper, which can deteriorate. Keep in mind when stocking medications or chemicals that a more recent shipment may have an earlier expiration date than a previous shipment. Always check expiration dates when storing supplies.

Store all items based on the expiration date for the items. The oldest items should be stored in the front and the newer items stored in the rear of the cabinet. Be sure to rotate the inventory every time you add new stock, placing the newly received stock at the back of each shelf. Sometimes items expire before they are used. Check every item for the expiration date before use. Discard all expired items carefully and appropriately according to TJC and OSHA standards.

Administrative Supplies. In addition to such expendable items as pens, pencils, and paper clips, paper products are important to a medical office. In general, paper products should be stored flat in their original boxes or wrappings to prevent pages from bending or curling. Information booklets may be stored upright to save space. Envelopes and other paper goods with gummed surfaces must be kept dry to prevent them from sticking together.

Clinical Supplies. The rules of good housekeeping and asepsis apply to storage areas for clinical supplies. These areas must be kept clean and protected from damage and exposure to the elements.

All dressings and most bandaging materials must be kept sterile. For example, gauze that may be used to bandage an open wound must be sterile. Elastic rolled bandages, which do not touch open wounds, must be clean but not necessarily sterile.

Chemicals, drugs, and solutions should be kept in a cool, dark place because light and heat cause some substances to deteriorate. Refer to the **Material Safety Data Sheet (MSDS)** provided by each manufacturer for proper storage instructions. The importance of MSDS is discussed in further detail later in this chapter. Store all liquids in their original containers. Line cabinets with plastic-coated shelf paper, and wipe it frequently with a damp cloth. Do not store liquids above dry supplies.

Store all poisons and narcotics separately from each other and from all other products. Narcotics must be stored securely out of sight in a locked cabinet. Never store strong acids near alkaline solutions or flammable items near sources of heat. Solutions that will be stored for a considerable length of time should have a small amount of space at the top of the bottle to allow for heat expansion.

Some liquids should be stored in the refrigerator. Check each item for specific storage instructions. If storage space is limited, consider eliminating some items—especially bulky ones that are rarely used or items that a patient can purchase at surgical supply stores.

Clinical refrigerators may be needed to store certain clinical supplies that require refrigeration. Never store food items and clinical items in the same refrigerator. A clinical refrigerator must be kept at a constant temperature to properly maintain the chemical integrity of lab supplies. Monitoring and recording the date and temperature of the clinical refrigerator should be completed once a week or per office protocol. Refer to each MSDS for storage details on each substance.

Taking Inventory of Medical Office Supplies

The list of supplies your office uses regularly and the quantities you have in storage constitute the office **inventory.** Keeping track of the office's inventory is a job that requires careful planning, attention to detail, and basic math skills. Accurate inventory activity ensures that the office never runs out of much-needed supplies.

Understanding Your Responsibilities

It is important to have an understanding with the doctor or doctors in the practice about the extent of your responsibilities for maintaining supplies. Some doctors are more involved with the details of running an office than others. Your responsibilities may grow as you become more experienced. The doctor, however, usually takes care of certain duties, such as meeting with pharmaceutical representatives or authorizing large purchases.

Generally you will be responsible for overseeing the flow of supplies bought and used, calculating the budget for supplies, selecting supplies and vendors, following correct purchasing and payment procedures, and storing the goods properly.

All efficient offices will have a process for everyone within the practice to record their supply needs. The process may be as simple as a notebook stored at the front desk or a supply list positioned in a key location. As a supply need in the office is noted, it can be recorded on the supply list by anyone for the next order. It is then important that the medical assistant who is compiling the order check all the inventory cards, reorder reminder cards, and supply lists before ordering.

The Inventory Filing System. To oversee the flow of inventory efficiently, you will need a filing system (see Procedure 8-1). This system consists of several elements:

- The list of supplies (discussed earlier in the chapter)
- An itemized inventory

PROCEDURE 8-1 [WORK // PRODUCT]

Step-by-Step Overview of Inventory Procedures

Procedure Goal: To set up an effective inventory program for a medical office

Materials: Pen, paper, file folders, vendor catalogs, index cards or loose-leaf binder and blank pages, reorder reminder cards, vendor order forms

Method:

1. Discuss and define with your physician/employer the extent of your responsibility in managing supplies. Know whether the physician's approval or supervision is required for certain procedures, whether any systems have already been established, and if the physician has any preference for a particular vendor or trade-name item. If your medical practice is large, determine which medical assistant is responsible for each aspect of supply management.

2. Know what administrative and clinical supplies should be stocked in your office. Create a formal supply list of vital, incidental, and periodic items, and keep a copy in the office's procedures manual.

3. Start a file containing a list of current vendors with copies of their catalogs.

4. Create a wish list of brands or products the office does not currently use but might like to try. Inform other staff members of the list so that they can make entries.

5. Make a file for supply invoices and completed order forms. (Keep these documents on file for at least 3 years.)

Rationale
Keep completed documents for future reference as well as for legal protection, if needed.

6. Devise an inventory system of index cards, loose-leaf pages, or a computer spreadsheet for each item. List the following data for each item on its card:

   - Date and quantity of each order
   - Name and contact information for the vendor and sales representative

continued ⟶

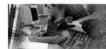
Step-by-Step Overview of Inventory Procedures *(concluded)*

- Date each shipment was received
- Total cost and unit cost, or price per piece for the item
- Payment method used
- Results of periodic counts of the item
- Quantity expected to cover the office for a given period of time
- Reorder quantity (the quantity remaining on the shelf that indicates when reorder should be made)

7. Have a system for flagging items that need to be ordered and those that are already on order. For example, mark their cards or pages with a self-adhesive tab or note. Make or buy reorder reminder cards to put into the stock of each item at the reorder quantity level.

Rationale
Having a system in place makes your job easier and will also make it easier for anyone else taking over the task at a later date.

8. Establish with the physician a regular schedule for taking inventory. Every 1 to 2 weeks is usually sufficient. As a backup system for remembering to check stock and reorder, estimate the times for these activities. Mark them on your calendar, or create a tickler file on your computer.

Rationale
A regular schedule means inventory and ordering will not be forgotten.

9. Order at the same times each week or month, after inventory is taken. However, if there is an unexpected shortage of an item, and more than a week or so remains before the regular ordering time, place the order immediately.

10. Fill in the vendor's order form (or type a letter of request). Order by telephone, fax, e-mail, or online. Online ordering will expedite the order. Follow procedures that have been approved by the physician or office manager. When placing an order, have all the necessary information at hand, including the correct name of the item and the order and account numbers. Record the order information in the inventory file for that item. Be sure to obtain from the vendor an estimated arrival time for the order, and mark that date and order number on your calendar.

11. When ordering online, save the website to "Favorites" for easy, one-click future access.

Select the website and establish an account with the company. To establish an account, you will need to give information about your office practice, including the name of the practice, contact name, the address, the phone number, an e-mail address, and a payment source. Ask about adding the practice to any special contact lists for promotional materials and discounts.

12. When you receive the shipment, record the date and the amount received on the item's inventory card or record page. Check the shipment against the original order and the packing slip inside the package to ensure that the right items, sizes, styles, packaging, and amounts have arrived. Initial each item on the packing slip as a record that the correct item and amount was received. If there is any error, immediately call or e-mail the vendor, with the catalog page and the inventory card or record page at hand.

Rationale
Items should be unpacked and checked immediately so that if a problem is discovered, it will be relatively easy to prove that the error or problem is with the shipment and not caused by office personnel.

13. Check the invoice carefully against the original order and the packing slip, making sure that the amount of the bill matches the items listed on the invoice and packing list, and to ensure that the bill has not already been paid. Sign or stamp the invoice to show that the order was received.

14. Write a check to the vendor to be signed by the physician. (Check writing procedures are described in Chapter 18.) Be sure to show the physician the original order, packing slip, and invoice. Record the check number, date, and amount of payment on the invoice, and initial it or have the physician do so. Write the invoice number on the front of the check.

Rationale
Writing the invoice number on the check will ensure that the payment is posted to the correct account. Writing the check number and date on the invoice will be useful for future reference if there is a payment dispute.

15. Mail the check and the vendor's copy of the invoice to the vendor within 30 days, and file the office copy of the invoice with the original order and packing slip. Complete the Application exercise in the *Student Workbook*.

- An inventory card or record page for each item
- A list of the names and addresses of current vendors
- A file of current catalogs from vendors (including some vendors not currently used, for comparison shopping)
- A want list of brands or items that the office does not currently use but may want to try in the future
- Files for **invoices,** or bills from vendors, and completed order forms
- Reorder reminder cards to indicate when an in-stock item should be reordered
- Color-coded, removable self-adhesive flags to indicate "Need to Order" or "On Order"
- An inventory and ordering schedule
- Order forms for each vendor (may be multicopy forms, fax forms, electronic forms, or e-mail forms)

The Inventory Card or Record Page. The inventory card or record page for each item or category of items may be a 4-by-6-inch index card, a page in a loose leaf binder, or a spreadsheet stored in the computer system (Figure 8-2). These methods make it easy to group together the items that need to be ordered at any given time. Records help you monitor how quickly items are used and how much should be ordered each time.

Some information may change. As you become more proficient at monitoring inventory or as the practice grows or diminishes in size, you may find that quantities, vendors, or reorder quantities need to be adjusted. With the help of the doctor or office manager, you will be able to determine the ideal quantity of each item to have on hand, depending on the size of the practice, the available storage space, and the ordering schedule.

It is important to check the storage areas regularly, preferably at specific times, and to count the items on hand. When the supply of an item begins to run low, you (or another staff member) should flag the inventory card or record page to indicate the need to reorder it at the next regular ordering time.

Color-coded, removable self-adhesive flags on the inventory card or record page are an efficient way to track inventory. A red flag, for example, might indicate that a supply needs to be ordered. A yellow flag might be substituted when the item has been ordered.

Reorder Reminder Cards. Reorder reminder cards (Figure 8-3) are usually brightly colored cards inserted directly into stock on the supply shelf to indicate when it is time to reorder an item. For example, if you have determined that four boxes of staples is a sufficient quantity

(ITEM NAME) Exam Table Paper 21"

ORDER QUANTITY 12 REORDER POINT 4

ORDER	QTY	REC'D	UNIT COST	PRICE	PREPAID	ON ACCT.	ORDER	QTY	REC'D	UNIT COST	PRICE	PREPAID	ON ACCT.
1/4	12	1/8	$12.25	$147.00	Check 1214	X							
2/5	12	2/9	$12.25	$147.00	Check 2110	X							

INVENTORY COUNT

	JAN.	FEB.	MAR.	APR.	MAY	JUNE	JULY	AUG.	SEPT.	OCT.	NOV.	DEC.
DATE ____	7	10										
DATE ____												

ORDER SOURCE

Smith Physician's Supply Co.
493 Carlton Avenue
South Union, NJ 07422
908-899-6123 Contact: Martin Kohn

UNIT PRICE

12 - $147.00
36 - $441.00

Figure 8-2. The inventory card, record page, or computer spreadsheet is the primary inventory-tracking tool in managing medical office supplies.

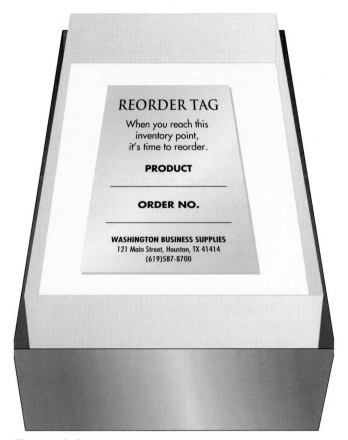

Figure 8-3. Reorder reminder cards are usually brightly colored cards inserted directly into the spare stock of an item on the supply shelf to indicate when it is time to reorder the item.

to keep on hand and your office supply orders are filled in 2 business days, you might place the reorder reminder card between the third and fourth boxes of staples. The reorder quantity on the inventory card or record page for staples would indicate "four boxes."

The reorder reminder cards also remind other staff members to tell you when an item is in short supply. In some offices, the medical assistant labels the reminder card with the name and bar code number of the supply item, such as "staples 002345." This method allows any staff member to pull the card when the last box of staples before the reminder card is taken from the supply shelf. The staff member can then place the card in a "To Be Ordered" envelope. Some offices can reorder simply by scanning the bar code. Staff members in some offices request supplies by writing them in an order book or on an order list.

Inventory Reminder Kits. Some mail-order supply vendors sell inventory kits, complete with cards and tabs or flags. Computerized inventory systems are also available. Shelves still need to be checked and counts logged on to the computer, however. Therefore, smaller offices generally do not benefit as much as larger ones from a computerized inventory system.

Scheduling Inventory and Ordering

Establish a regular schedule for counting the supplies in the office. Taking inventory every 1 or 2 weeks is usually sufficient. Estimating when you will probably need to reorder a particular item—and putting that date on your calendar or in your appointment book—is also helpful. You and the physician can determine how often storage areas should be checked.

Established Ordering Times. You should have established ordering times, such as the same day each week or month, after inventory is taken. For example, you might take inventory the first Tuesday of every month and order supplies the first Thursday of every month.

A regular schedule for taking inventory and ordering helps all staff members remember when they must give their requests to you. Although you may need to adjust the ordering time occasionally, try to adhere to the schedule to avoid the expense and inconvenience of rush orders.

When to Order Ahead of Schedule

When you take inventory, and the spare supply of an item has not been reached but is close to the placement of the reorder reminder card, you must decide whether you should reorder then or wait until the next regular ordering time. You will probably find it is more efficient to go ahead and order rather than wait. Ordering early assures you that the supply will not be depleted before the next regular ordering time. Make sure you consider your storage capacity; this could limit your purchases.

Ordering ahead of schedule can be especially important if there is a large demand for a particular product and manufacturers' production levels have not caught up with that demand. This situation can occur if there has been an outbreak of a particular flu or virus, or if the Food and Drug Administration has determined that a certain product is harmful, resulting in higher demand for an alternative product.

Unanticipated Shortage of a Supply Item. If the supply of an item reaches the reorder reminder card, and there is still a long time before the next regular ordering time, place the order immediately so that you do not risk running out of the item.

To help you oversee inventory effectively, finish one container before opening a new one. Keep all stock of the same item in one place. The need to count inventory of an item in more than one location or container increases the likelihood of errors. If an item is kept in more than one location, as in the case of multiple exam rooms, inventory is best maintained per room.

As a medical assistant, you want to be sure that there are always sufficient quantities of supplies to keep the office running efficiently. It is unwise to stock spare supplies in too great a quantity, however, because the administrative budget is not likely to support such expenditures. In addition, spare quantities of supplies can be a storage problem.

Ordering Supplies

Ordering supplies requires a procedure to deal with vendors and to order and check supplies. You can avoid common purchasing mistakes by understanding the most efficient way to order supplies for your office.

Locating and Evaluating Supply Vendors

A vendor will most likely already be in place when you join a practice. You should, however, be aware of competitors' prices, services, and other incentives intended to attract your office as a customer. Sometimes the incentives—such as bonus supplies with certain purchases—can represent sizable savings. Remember also that your time has a dollar value to the practice, and services that save you time are worth comparing when evaluating vendors.

Obtaining recommendations from other medical offices is a good way to locate office-supply dealers who sell items at reasonable prices and are also reputable. **Reputable** vendors fulfill orders accurately with quality items, deliver products in good condition, and charge fair prices. Keep in mind when evaluating vendors that the physician may have preferences for certain trade names or vendors.

Gathering Competitive Prices. The costs of maintaining a medical practice are continually rising. Saving money on supplies through careful purchasing strategies is one way to help your physician/employer reduce spending. The medical assistant is often largely responsible for comparison pricing, ordering, and establishing and maintaining relationships with vendors. Your awareness of the most up-to-date information about vendors and supplies is valuable to your physician/employer. Discuss prices with the physician, who in turn may want to discuss them with an accountant.

Setting Up a Supply Budget. The average medical practice spends 4% to 6% of its annual gross income on administrative, clinical, and general supplies. If an office is spending more than 6%, it may be time to reevaluate the office's spending practices. Remember, though, that any budget is only a guide. A budget is meant to serve your office, not the reverse. You and your physician/employer may need to adjust the supply budget based on prices and discounts available from vendors.

Comparing Vendors. To collect competitive data from vendors, contact them by telephone or in writing to request catalogs and other forms of product information. If you are not in charge of routing mail, make sure that supply-related mail, such as product catalogs and sale notices, is routed to you. Catalogs usually include basic information, such as the dealer's name, address, and telephone number, order numbers for items, and vendor policy (Figure 8-4). When investigating a vendor, obtain the following information:

- Prices—costs for supplies, delivery, and any other services; special discounts; minimum quantities applicable; bonus supplies with purchases
- Quality—product descriptions, illustrations, trade names, recommendations for use, durability, guarantees
- Service—availability of products, delivery time and procedures, sales representative availability, damaged-goods policy
- Payment policies

Competitive Pricing and Quality

Part of your responsibility in managing office supplies is to stay informed about the pricing and quality of competitors to your vendors. Savings can add up quickly, and ongoing comparison pricing can save the practice hundreds of dollars a year.

Unit Pricing. Because many medical items come in a variety of package sizes, you need to be aware of how much the office is actually paying per item. To calculate an item's **unit price,** divide the total price of the package by the quantity, or number of items. For example, if a package of 12 pens costs $12, the unit price, or price per pen, is $1 ($12 divided by 12 pens). If another vendor provides the same type of pen in a package of 18 for $17.10, the unit price is 95 cents ($17.10 divided by 18 pens). The second set of pens is the better buy.

Unit prices are generally lower at larger quantities. Therefore, it makes sense to place one large order for a nonperishable item to cover the office until the next ordering time. Generally, however, you should not order more than a year's supply of any one item, particularly if the item is custom-printed. Addresses, insurance codes, or additions to medical staff can change. When placing quantity discount orders, always consider the following factors: whether the supply can be used within a reasonable time, the possibility of spoilage or deterioration, the amount of storage space in the office, and whether the doctor will continue to use the item. Avoid overspending by not ordering more of an item than is reasonable or necessary.

Rush Orders. Unexpected rush orders usually cost the office more money than regularly scheduled orders. (In some cases, a vendor may not charge extra to a steady customer, but these cases would be exceptions.) To avoid rush orders, be aware of approximately how long the vendor takes to deliver an order. You can obtain this information from the vendor policy and by keeping accurate records of your own experience with deliveries.

Mail-Order Companies. Using large, established mail-order companies often saves money for the medical office, but there may be less control over orders and a greater potential for hidden costs. The neighborhood pharmacy may also offer discounts, but ordering from wholesalers or directly from the manufacturer is usually more economical. The Points on Practice section provides helpful information about cost-efficient ordering by telephone or fax or through an online service.

BY PHONE

Call our toll-free number:
(800) BIBBERO
(800-242-2376)
Monday through Friday,
6:00 a.m. – 5:00 p.m. (PT)

BY WEB

www.bibbero.com
email:info@bibbero.com

BY MAIL

Complete order
form and mail to:
Bibbero Systems, Inc.
1300 N. McDowell Blvd.
Petaluma, CA 94954-1180

BY FAX

Complete enclosed
order form and
transmit via fax to:
(800) 242-9330.
Our fax line is open 24 hours a day.

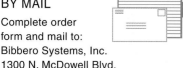

SHIPPING POLICY

Most in-stock items normally ship the same day (exclusive of file cabinets, file storage, office accessories and furnishings).

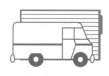

FREE DELIVERY

Free delivery on pre-paid orders totaling $300.00 or more, shipping within the Continental U.S.

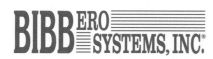

Thank you for reviewing our catalog. We are confident that you will be pleased with both our products and our service. If you are in a hurry for product or samples, CALL us toll-free at (800) BIBBERO, FAX us at (800) 242-9330, or visit our web site: www.bibbero.com Our Customer Service Department is always happy to assist you.

If ordering by mail or fax, fill out the enclosed order form located at the back of this catalog. Either return it in the enclosed postage-paid envelope or fax it to us.

For items requiring custom imprinting, please include the following information, either typed or hand printed: name, specialty, address, city/state/zip, telephone number, and state license number (when required).

Don't see what you are looking for in our catalog? Submit a sample or provide specifications for any folder, divider, patient registration form, clinical form, health history questionnaire, etc., and we will promptly provide you with a quote. We can print single or multiple part forms, custom imprint folders, and manufacture a wide range of chart dividers.

Please Note: All custom printed orders are subject to an overrun or underrun variance of 10%.

Most orders for in-stock items received by 2:00 p.m. (PT) are normally shipped the same day (excluding cabinets, file storage, office accessories and furnishings). Out-of-stock items are automatically backordered. Personalized stationery items normally ship in 5–7 working days, after proof approval. Custom printed orders normally leave our plant within 7–10 working days, after proof approval. If certain items require an extended ship time, such as those listed above, delivery time will be quoted when order is received.

Custom printing or personalization on a rush basis is available on most products for an additional charge.

Some combined stock and custom printed items can be shipped together if requested in advance. All orders are shipped via the most economical, expeditious method to your locale. Items ordered together may not ship from the same locations or be received at the same time.

Common carriers are used for large volume orders. Overnight, 2nd and 3rd Day delivery services are available upon request.

All orders prepaid by check, Visa, MasterCard or American Express totaling $300.00 or more will be shipped freight free via surface transport within the Continental U.S. This offer excludes file cabinets, file storage, office accessories and furnishings and special order items. We regret that the high cost of shipping outside the contiguous 48 states prohibits us from extending our freight free policy; however, we will use the most economical shipping methods available to your location.

TERMS

Full payment is due upon receipt of merchandise. Accounts are considered overdue after thirty (30) days and are subject to a 1% monthly service charge. A service charge of $10.00 will be applied to all returned checks. For information regarding special financial arrangements, please contact our Credit Department at (800) 242-2376.

GUARANTEE!

Your satisfaction
Guaranteed!

We guarantee our stock products. If you wish to return something, call to obtain a return authorization number and return shipment instructions. Most of our stock items can be returned within 60 days of purchase for full credit, exchange or a refund of your purchase price, with prior return authorization. After 60 days, your return is subject to a 20% restocking charge. Call our Customer Service Department at (800) 242-2376 for your return authorization number. Dymo® Products can be returned within 30 days of receipt with prior return authorization. Opened or unpackaged items are subject to a 15% or $15.00 restocking charge, which ever is greater. For disposable products located in our Clinical Supplies section, opened packages are subject to a 15% re-stocking charge with prior return authorization. Personalized items, custom printed items, custom manufactured or special order items, file cabinets, high density filing systems and opened and unlocked software are not returnable.

Items damaged in transit will be replaced as quickly as possible. Note any visible damage to the cartons on the bill of lading or delivery receipt and keep the original packaging in case items within are damaged.

Please Note: Self-adhesive products have a limited shelf life. Store in a cool, dry place.

Please Note: All custom printed orders are subject to an overrun or underrun variance of 10%.

We accept Visa, MasterCard and American Express for all your purchases.

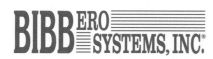

Figure 8-4. Examine supply catalogs and websites carefully to find out vendors' company policies.

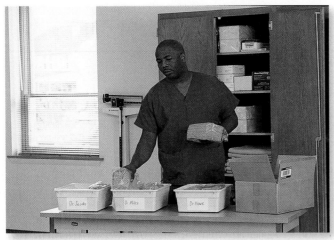

Figure 8-5. Ordering jointly with other offices can cut expenses for everyone.

Purchasing Groups. **Purchasing groups** are groups of physicians that order supplies together to obtain a quantity discount. For example, several medical offices associated with a nearby hospital may order through the hospital. In return for this convenience, the physicians pay dues and guarantee the vendors a certain amount of business. Some programs require members to spend a certain percentage of their supply budget through the group. Groups may also require that members not disclose the group's prices to other physicians. Large medical practices that participate in these groups usually save an average of 20% on supplies. The savings are not usually significant for small offices.

Group Buying Pools. If a medical office wants to use local vendors instead of, or in addition to, a purchasing group or if it is too small to benefit from a purchasing group, it can still pool resources with other area offices to qualify for quantity discounts. Even if the offices are ordering different items, discounts are based on the total order and savings can range from 10% to 20%. Under this arrangement the offices must usually take responsibility for distributing the items among themselves. A buying pool is convenient for medical practices that are in the same building or office complex (Figure 8-5).

Cost Controls. Medical practices are increasingly interested in saving money and controlling costs in general. Physician reimbursement is constantly being reevaluated. As a result, more than ever, physicians are interested in controlling the operating costs of their practices. Managing expenses within the practice is a very important responsibility for the medical assistant. What may seem to be just a small reduction in cost to the practice can actually result in a substantial reduction to office expenses over the course of a year. As a medical assistant, it is your job to constantly look for ways to reduce costs within the practice without sacrificing quality.

Benefits of Using Local Vendors

There are many potential vendors, including local dealers, mail-order companies, and nearby pharmacies. Try to establish good credit and business relationships with reputable local vendors. These companies often charge a little more than mail-order companies. Still, spending most of the office's supply budget through one favored local dealer often results in discounts, special service in the event of an emergency, and information about upcoming sales and specials. Local dealers may also offer more personal assistance, perhaps even a salesperson's help with taking inventory, to compete with larger vendors whose business is based primarily on catalog sales. The extra service may be worth the higher cost.

Buying from local vendors can also provide a public relations benefit for physicians; it means keeping business in the community. However, specialty items may need to be ordered from other vendors. For example, letterhead should be ordered from a reliable printer, whether that printer is located in the community or out of state.

Payment Schedules

Another factor that affects the cost of supplies is the payment schedule. Many vendors do not charge for handling if an order is prepaid. Others offer a discount for enclosing a check with an order. Some delay billing for 30 to 90 days, allowing the physician to keep the money in the bank, collecting interest for a longer period.

The vendor's invoice usually describes payment terms. Two examples of payment terms are:

1. If the invoice says "Net 30," you have 30 days in which to pay the total amount.
2. "1% 10 Days Net 30" means that you will get a savings of 1% of the total price by paying within 10 days.

Copies of all bills and order forms for supplies should be kept on file for at least 7 years in case the practice is audited by the Internal Revenue Service (IRS).

Ordering Procedures

Ordering procedures for supplies vary from office to office but always involve these tasks: completing paperwork, checking orders received, correcting errors in shipments, and making payment.

Order Forms. Before ordering merchandise, you should inquire about a vendor's ordering options, discuss them with the physician, and determine which method is best for the office. Many vendors now have ordering capability through telephone, fax, e-mail, and online as well as traditional written order forms. Always be sure to keep a copy of each order you submit.

Before you place an order, gather all the necessary information, such as correct names of items, item numbers, and order and account numbers. This information helps ensure the accuracy of the order. Immediately after placing the order, note all order information on the inventory card or record page for that item.

Purchase Requisitions. You will need to follow any special ordering procedures established in your medical

Points on Practice

Ordering by Telephone or Fax or Online

You may occasionally purchase office supplies at a local office supply store, but most often you will order them without leaving your office. Three common ways to do so are by telephone, by facsimile (or fax) machine, and through an online service. Here are tips to help make sure every order—no matter which option you choose—is successfully placed.

Ordering by Telephone

1. Clear communication is a must when ordering by telephone. Speak slowly, and enunciate your words carefully to make sure you are understood. It is also a good idea to spell each word of the practice's name and the address to ensure proper delivery. Use expressions like "S as in Sam, P as in people" to clarify your spelling.

2. Ask the representative taking your order to repeat the order. Check that every item is included with the appropriate price, quantity, style, and color.

3. Confirm the expected delivery date so that you will know if something is late. Also confirm how payment will be made, to prevent unexpected delays.

4. Record the name and telephone number of the person who takes the order in case there is a problem with the order. Get an order number (sometimes called a confirmation number) in case you have to call back with a question or a change in your order.

5. If possible, avoid placing telephone orders on Mondays and Fridays, when call volume is typically high.

Ordering by Fax

1. When ordering by fax, use the form provided by the vendor if one is available. This form uses the format to which the supply company is accustomed and will speed the processing of your order.

2. Type your order, or write it neatly and legibly, to prevent miscommunication. Fill out the form completely. Make sure you indicate quantities, descriptions, and prices (including shipping) for each item you order.

3. Proofread your order before you send it. Checking the accuracy of the order now will save time later.

4. Follow up by telephone to make sure your order was received and understood and to confirm the delivery date and payment requirements.

Ordering Online

1. Ordering online requires a computer and a modem connection to the Internet or to an online service. Before ordering online, make sure you are fully familiar with the equipment and the process, or have your supervisor or the supply company's sales representative oversee your initial orders.

2. Type your name and address accurately.

3. If pictures of supplies are not available online, consult the company's printed catalog or CD-ROM catalog. If you do not have access to a catalog, read the online text descriptions carefully, checking trade names and specifications, to select the appropriate merchandise (Figure 8-6). If you have questions, consult the supply company by telephone.

4. When you have completed the selections, the online service will display your order so that you can confirm it. Check that all the information is accurate, including your name, address, and telephone number.

5. If you have an account with the company, you may type in your account number to place the order. Otherwise, you may wish to arrange to make payment on delivery. If you prefer to pay by credit card, first make sure that the company is reputable and that it uses a security system that prevents your number from being read by anyone unauthorized to do so.

If, despite your best efforts, your order is processed incorrectly, take appropriate action immediately. Although ordering by telephone or fax or online is convenient, it still requires additional time to package items that must be returned.

By law, orders that you place must be fulfilled within a reasonable time. The Federal Trade Commission (FTC) monitors purchases by telephone, fax, and online services to protect consumers. The FTC requires supply companies to provide merchandise within 30 days or to give you the option of canceling the order and receiving a full refund.

continued ⟶

Ordering by Telephone or Fax or Online *(concluded)*

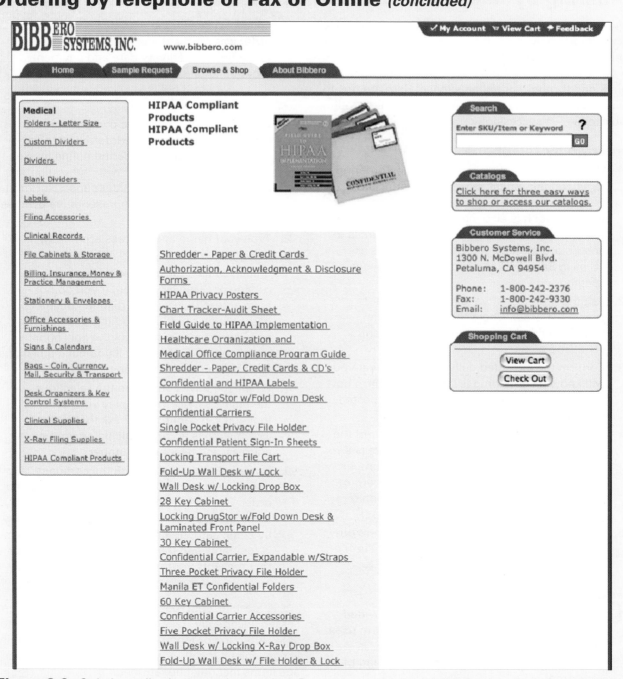

Figure 8-6. Ordering online is easy and convenient. Be certain to read the details of your order before sending the order.

office. The specific procedures and the medical assistant's level of authority vary from one office to another. Sometimes placing an order requires a **requisition** (a formal request from a staff member or doctor), which is given to the medical assistant who does the actual ordering. The doctor's approval may be necessary for large purchases—for example,

for orders that total more than $300. Recurring orders may not require the doctor's approval, but you may need to get approval before ordering a new brand or quantities of a particular item over a certain amount.

In a group practice where doctors order different items and several staffers are in charge of ordering, procedures

PURCHASE ORDER #2532

Submitted by: _____

Order Number: _____

Date Ordered: _____

Date Required: _____

SHIP TO: Dr. Carlotta Montoni

201 Oak Walk, Suite 32

Gilead, PA 19034

PHONE: 215-610-4120

	ITEM	DESCRIPTION/MODEL	COLOR	SIZE	QUANTITY	PRICE EACH	TOTAL
1.							
2.							
3.							
4.							
5.							
6.							
7.							
8.							
						TOTAL	

Approved: _____ Date: _____

Figure 8-7. A purchase order, when approved by the physician or office manager, is an authorization from the practice for a purchase.

for ordering can be complicated. One common way to simplify matters is to use **purchase orders,** forms that authorize a purchase for the practice. Figure 8-7 shows a sample purchase order. Purchase orders are usually pre-printed with consecutive numbers. The medical assistant submits approved purchase orders to the vendor for fulfillment. This method is most often used for expensive items, such as office equipment, but some large practices also use purchase orders for supplies.

Checking Orders Received.   When the shipment of supplies arrives, record on the inventory card or record page the date received as well as the quantity of each item. Check the shipment against the order form to make sure the correct items—in the correct sizes, styles, packaging, and quantity—have been delivered.

Then check the contents against the packing slip (a description of the package contents) enclosed in the package. This checking takes time, but catching even one error is worth the time taken. If several people on a staff have ordering responsibility, they can share the task. The employee should write on the package slip the date items were received; check off each item as you verify and initial.

Material Safety Data Sheets.   Every chemical item ordered in a medical practice must have a Material Safety Data Sheet (MSDS) on file in the office. This sheet is provided by the manufacturer of the product and describes

the chemical breakdown of the product as well as safety cautions and procedures to follow in using it. Items that require MSDS include, but are not limited to, all soaps, cleansers, waxes, reagents, clinical testing products, inks, toners, and any product that can be splashed or rubbed on the skin or eyes. TJC, OSHA (Occupational Safety and Health Administration), and other surveying organizations will require MSDS on all products used in the medical practice. The purpose of the sheet is to provide important safety information about the item that may be critical in the event of unintended exposure or potentially dangerous reactions.

For fast and easy access, organize these sheets in a binder in alphabetical order. As new items are ordered and delivered, add the MSDS into the master binder. As a medical assistant, you must always check the MSDS binder when stocking the supply shelves to ensure that all items stocked are included in the binder. If MSDS information is not included with the item, either immediately request the information from the vendor or go online to print information directly from the product manufacturer.

Correcting Errors.   All errors in a shipment should be reported immediately to the vendor so that the records can be corrected and missing supplies can be delivered. When you call to report errors, be sure you have all the paperwork in front of you. You will need the invoice number, order date, name of the person who placed the order,

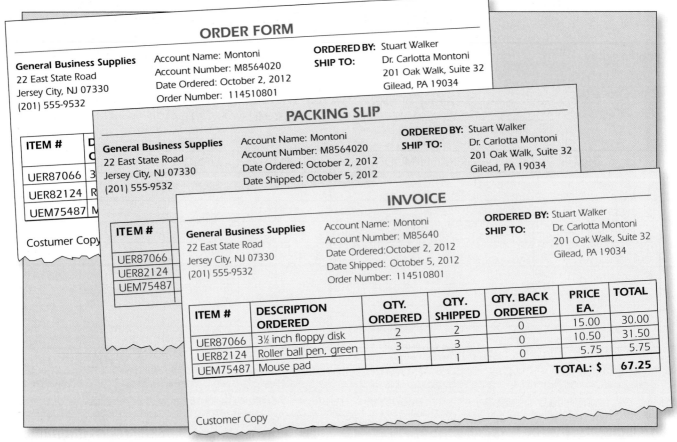

ORDER FORM

General Business Supplies
22 East State Road
Jersey City, NJ 07330
(201) 555-9532

Account Name: Montoni
Account Number: M8564020
Date Ordered: October 2, 2012
Order Number: 114510801

ORDERED BY: Stuart Walker
SHIP TO: Dr. Carlotta Montoni
            201 Oak Walk, Suite 32
            Gilead, PA 19034

ITEM #	D...
UER87066	3
UER82124	R
UEM75487	M

Costumer Copy

PACKING SLIP

General Business Supplies
22 East State Road
Jersey City, NJ 07330
(201) 555-9532

Account Name: Montoni
Account Number: M8564020
Date Ordered: October 2, 2012
Date Shipped: October 5, 2012

ORDERED BY: Stuart Walker
SHIP TO: Dr. Carlotta Montoni
            201 Oak Walk, Suite 32
            Gilead, PA 19034

ITEM #
UER87066
UER82124
UEM75487

INVOICE

General Business Supplies
22 East State Road
Jersey City, NJ 07330
(201) 555-9532

Account Name: Montoni
Account Number: M85640
Date Ordered:October 2, 2012
Date Shipped: October 5, 2012
Order Number: 114510801

ORDERED BY: Stuart Walker
SHIP TO: Dr. Carlotta Montoni
            201 Oak Walk, Suite 32
            Gilead, PA 19034

ITEM #	DESCRIPTION ORDERED	QTY. ORDERED	QTY. SHIPPED	QTY. BACK ORDERED	PRICE EA.	TOTAL
UER87066	3½ inch floppy disk	2	2	0	15.00	30.00
UER82124	Roller ball pen, green	3	3	0	10.50	31.50
UEM75487	Mouse pad	1	1	0	5.75	5.75
					TOTAL: $	67.25

Customer Copy

Figure 8-8. Check the information on the vendor invoice against the original order and the packing slip to make sure there are no errors.

name of the person who took the order, and a list of questions or a description of the complaint. If a catalog was used in ordering, have it open to the appropriate page. Always record the name and title of the person you speak with when reporting the error.

Invoices. Typically the vendor sends an invoice to the medical office, either accompanying the merchandise or separately. This invoice also should be checked carefully against the original order and the packing slip. It is also a good idea to staple the order list, packing list, and a copy of the invoice together for the office records to verify all items were received. Be sure to check the arithmetic as well. Then sign or stamp the invoice to confirm that the order was received. If an item you order is temporarily out of stock, the vendor usually sends an invoice stamped "Back Ordered." Later, when the item is back in stock, the vendor will ship it to your office.

It is a good habit to record the check number, date, and amount of payment on the invoice. You may initial it or have the doctor initial it. By keeping a copy of the paid invoice with the attached order slip and packing slip in the office records, it will be easy to track the items included within each invoice. This step makes verifying payments easier and decreases the chance of inadvertently paying an invoice twice.

Disbursements. An invoice is paid with a **disbursement** (payment of funds) to a vendor. Disbursements may be made in cash or by check or money order. Usually you will write a check to the vendor and have the physician sign it. Be sure to show the physician the original order, packing slip, and invoice. On the front of the check, record the invoice number. Finally, mail the check to the vendor with the vendor's copy of the invoice. File the office copy of the invoice, along with the original order and the packing slip, according to your inventory filling system (Figure 8-8).

If you make a cash disbursement, obtain a receipt to keep on file. If you are the one responsible for maintaining the practice's financial records and presenting them to the accountant, you may also be responsible for recording the payment information in the office's accounting books.

Avoiding Common Purchasing Mistakes

Even the most watchful professional can make purchasing mistakes. The best you can do is to educate yourself about common mistakes and try to avoid them. For example, be aware of the possibility of dishonest telephone solicitations. A caller may claim to be a sales representative for the manufacturer of the office photocopier, offering bargains on paper or toner. The caller may require advance payment to be sent to a post office box. The bargains may never arrive.

The best way to deal with these solicitations is to tell the caller that your office does not purchase supplies by telephone. If a telephone offer appears to be legitimate and to offer substantial savings, ask for the name and telephone number of the firm so that you can return the call at a more convenient time. Then you can verify the number with the telephone company and check the firm's name with the Better Business Bureau.

Another disreputable tactic some vendors use is bait and switch: The price of one item is lowered to attract the customer, but that item is always "sold out" and the customer is encouraged to buy a more expensive one. A vendor may also mislead you by raising the price of an item you have been ordering without informing you. Always confirm the current price, check invoices as they come in, and record everything in the item's file. Having your inventory card or record page open while ordering will prompt you to notice and question price changes. If there is an honest error, a reputable firm will readily and courteously correct it.

Problems can also be avoided by carefully supervising a new vendor's sales representative until a comfortable, professional rapport has been established. Discuss your inventory system with representatives, and ask them questions about their procedures.

Summary

8.1 Vital supplies are essential for functioning within a medical office setting. They include such items as prescription pads and examination table covers. Incidental supplies are rubber bands or staples. These supplies can be purchased quickly. Periodic supplies require occasional ordering and include appointment books or holiday cards for patients and the physician's colleagues.

8.2 Storing administrative and clinical supplies requires good organizational skills. Administrative supplies should be stored flat in their original boxes to prevent bending or curling. When storing clinical supplies, make sure the area is clean and protected from damage and exposure to the elements. Always refer to the rules of asepsis and the product MSDS when storing clinical supplies.

8.3 Make sure you track your inventory properly by using reorder reminder cards or inventory cards, and a supply checklist.

8.4 Establish a regular inventory and ordering system so that supplies will not be depleted before the next ordering cycle.

8.5 Always locate and use reputable vendors when ordering supplies. Find vendors with competitive prices, and make comparisons.

8.6 Savings can add up by obtaining the best quality supplies while controlling costs. Purchasing in groups and sometimes using mail-order supplies will be beneficial in the long run.

8.7 Ordering procedures may vary from office to office. However, make sure that you complete the paperwork properly, check orders received, correct errors in shipment, and make payments on time.

8.8 When you receive your supplies, make sure you check for any errors such as missing products as well as incorrect sizes, styles, or damaged products. If there are errors, notify the supplier immediately.

REVIEW

CHAPTER 8

CASE STUDY QUESTIONS

Now that you have completed this chapter, review the case study at the beginning of the chapter and answer the following questions:

1. What is an *expendable* item? What items would you list on the expendable administrative supply list? The clinical supply list? The general supply list?
2. What factors would you consider about each office as you determine the appropriate supplies?
3. How would you recommend that the supplies be stored with inventory management in mind?

Multiple-Choice Questions

1. When managing office supplies, the goal is to achieve
   a. efficiency.
   b. organization.
   c. resourcefulness.
   d. independence.
2. Expendable items are those that are
   a. able to be thrown away.
   b. used and must be restocked.
   c. used indefinitely.
   d. restored and reused.

3. The responsibility of organizing office supplies lies with the
   a. physician.   c. nurse.
   b. medical assistant.   d. housekeeper.
4. Examples of clinical supplies are
   a. needles, syringes, and lubricating jelly.
   b. paper cups and toilet tissue.
   c. rubber bands, stamps, and file folders.
   d. patient education materials and insurance forms.
5. Incidental supplies are
   a. occasionally reordered.
   b. those that are needed in the office but that do not threaten the efficiency of the office.
   c. used only once and thrown away.
   d. items absolutely necessary to ensure the smooth running of the practice.

Discussion Questions

1. As a new employee, what questions would you want to ask about the process of ordering supplies within the office?
2. Describe some ways you can avoid common purchasing mistakes.

Critical Thinking Questions

1. During a routine inventory inspection, you notice that the supply of prescription pads is extremely low for typical office use. Could there be a problem within the office other than just the need to order more pads from the printer? What would you do?
2. You share the responsibility of ordering supplies with another medical assistant in the office. You are checking supplies and ordering regularly, but the other employee is allowing items to become completely depleted. What would you do?
3. You discover that an error has been made in a shipment from a vendor. What should you do?

Application Activities

1. Using vendor catalogs, make a list of 10 typical office supply items for a medical practice. Create a fictional office supply list and ordering schedule (including quantities and prices) for the practice.
2. Select a supply company catalog and become familiar with it. Imagine that you are a sales representative for that company, and make a presentation to your class as if it were a typical medical practice. Your goal is to have the medical office choose your company as its vendor. Be prepared to answer questions about how your company handles various customer concerns.
3. Make a diagram of an office supply cabinet, indicating how you would label and store items for maximum efficiency. Try to use several of the inventory elements discussed in the chapter.

Virtual Fieldtrip

Visit the McGraw-Hill Higher Education Medical Assisting website at www.mhhe.com/medicalassistin4e to complete the following activity:

Use the Sterling Medical Products website and the Lights and Sirens website to research and comparatively price any five items commonly used in a medical practice. Based on your research, which company would you recommend to the office manager and why?

Open the CD and complete this chapter's practice activities, play the games, listen to the key terms, and test yourself with the interactive review. E-mail, print, and/or save your results to document your proficiency.

Maintaining Patient Records

MEDICAL ASSISTING COMPETENCIES

CAAHEP

IV. P (1) Use reflection, restatement, and clarification techniques to obtain a patient history

IV. P (8) Document patient care

IV. P (9) Document patient education

V. C (6) Describe various types of content maintained in a patient's medical record

V. C (11) Discuss principles of using electronic medical records (EMR)

V. C (12) Identify types of records common to the health-care setting

V. P (3) Organize a patient's medical record

V. P (5) Execute data management using electronic health-care records such as the EMR

IX. C (14) Describe the process to follow if an error is made in patient care

IX. P (7) Document accurately in the patient record

ABHES

4. Medical Law and Ethics
  b. Institute federal and state guidelines when releasing medical records or information

7. Basic Keyboarding/Computer Concepts
  a. Typing medical correspondence and basic reports
  b. Identify and properly utilize office machines, computerized systems and medical software such as:
    1. Efficiently maintain and understand different types of medical correspondence and medical reports
    2. Apply computer application skills using variety of different electronic programs including both practice management software and EMR software

8. Medical Office Business Procedures Management
  a. Prepare and maintain medical records
  d. Apply concepts for office procedures

11. Career Development
  Demonstrate professionalism by:
    1) Exhibiting dependability, punctuality, and a positive work ethic
    2) Exhibiting a positive attitude and a sense of responsibility
    3) Maintaining confidentiality at all times
    9) Conducting work within scope of education, training, and ability

LEARNING OUTCOMES

After completing Chapter 9, you will be able to:

9.1 Describe the purpose of compiling patient medical records.

9.2 Identify the forms that initialize a patient record.

9.3 Explain how to create and maintain a patient record.

9.4 Explain common approaches to documenting information in medical records.

9.5 Describe the need for neatness, timeliness, accuracy, and professional tone in patient records.

9.6 Carry out accurate transcription.

9.7 Explain how to correct a medical record.

9.8 Explain how to update a medical record.

9.9 Differentiate when and how a medical record may be released.

9.10 Differentiate advantages and disadvantages of the electronic health record.

MEDICAL ASSISTING MEDIA

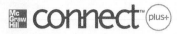 **Connect Plus+™**
connect.mcgraw-hill.com

- Electronic Health Records (E.H.R.) SpringCharts®
- eBook

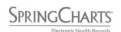

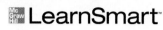 **LearnSmart™**

www.mhhe.com/learnsmart

Complete Learning Module: Managing Patient Records

 Student CD-ROM

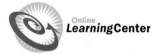 **Online Learning Center™**

www.mhhe.com/medicalassisting4e

KEY TERMS

audit
CHEDDAR
documentation
electronic health records (EHR)
electronic medical records (EMR)

individual identifiable health information (IIHI)
informed consent form
noncompliant
objective

patient record/chart
POMR
sign
SOAP
subjective

symptom
transcription
transfer

CHAPTER OUTLINE

- Importance of Patient Records
- Contents of Patient Charts
- Initiating and Maintaining Patient Records
- The Six Cs of Charting
- Types of Medical Records
- Appearance, Timeliness, and Accuracy of Records

- Electronic Health Records
- Medical Transcription
- Correcting and Updating Patient Records
- Release of Records

PREPARATION FOR CERTIFICATION

RMA (AMT) Exam

- Protect, store, and retain medical records according to HIPAA regulations
- Release of protected health information adhering to HIPAA regulations
- Charting guidelines and regulations

CMA (AAMA) Exam

- Patient interviewing techniques
- Legislation
- Medical records (paper/electronic)

CMAS Exam

- Procedures

Introduction

The medical assistant plays a major role in writing and maintaining patient records. These records document the evaluation and treatment given to the patient. Patient records are critical to the care of the patient. Without accurate and complete patient records, medical care could easily be compromised.

Patient records have many parts or sections that describe these facets of every patient:

- Personal information or data
- Physical and mental condition
- Medical history
- Medical care
- Medical future if the patient is referred to other physicians

In this chapter you will learn how to carefully manage the records of the patient. You will understand that if the medical care is not documented, in a legal sense, the medical care did not occur at all.

CASE STUDY

A man is waiting at the busy family practice door on Monday morning as Paul, the medical assistant, arrives to open the office. He instantly recognizes the man as Christopher Hansen, a patient of Dr. Jones's and the first scheduled patient of the day. Mr. Hansen states that he is very ill and needs to see a doctor as soon as possible. Paul assists Mr. Hansen to an examination room and picks up the patient chart from the rack that holds the charts for the day's patients.

As Paul begins to check the patient's vital signs, he asks Mr. Hansen what brings him to the doctor today. The patient grips his lower right side as he responds that his stomach hurts a lot. The patient also reports running a temperature between 100.5°F and 101.3°F for a full day and that he has not been able to eat in the last day because of his stomach pains. Paul knows that this information is important to chart in the permanent record as *subjective* information that has been stated by the patient.

Paul takes Mr. Hanson's vital signs, recording them as follows: T 100.8, P 86 and reg, R 20, BP 142/86. He carefully writes down the vital signs for inclusion in the patient chart. Paul knows that this information is important to chart in the permanent record as *objective* information that has been observed by the medical professional.

Paul is charting information in the patient record using the SOAP charting method:

- S for subjective
- O for objective
- A for assessment
- P for plan

Paul notifies the physician that the patient is ready for his exam. Dr. Jones completes the record after he evaluates the patient and makes entries to the chart for assessment and the plan for care. The medical record reflects the good clinical management that the patient receives.

As you read this chapter, consider the following questions:

1. Why is an accurate medical record important to the care of a patient?
2. Why is interviewing the patient important to the medical evaluation?
3. What are the six Cs of charting and what do they mean to you as a medical assistant?
4. What are the differences between the conventional and the POMR systems of keeping charts?
5. What are some helpful tips you might use as you perform transcription?

Importance of Patient Records

One of your most important duties as a medical assistant will be filling out and maintaining accurate and thorough patient records. **Patient records,** also known as **charts,** contain important information about a patient's medical history and present condition. Patient records serve as communication tools as well as legal documents. They also play a role in patient and staff education and may be used for quality control and research. Patient records may either be paper or electronic. The medical record is initiated by the medical assistant or another staff member and is consistently updated whenever the patient has contact with the office. The medical facility owns the physical record whether it is electronic or paper, but the patient owns the information contained within that record as his information.

Regardless of the type of record, the patient chart provides physicians and other medical care providers with all the important information, observations, and opinions that have been recorded about a patient. The health-care professional can read the complete patient medical history and information about treatment and outcomes. The information in the records can also be sent to other physicians or health-care specialists if the patient needs further treatment, changes physicians, or moves to a new location. The information recorded provides a "map" or plan to follow for the continuity of patient care. The medical chart also serves as supporting documentation for billing and coding purposes, and as a legal document that is admissible in a court of law. Medical records include the following general information about the patient:

- Address and phone number
- Occupation
- Medical history
- Current complaint or condition
- Health-care needs
- Medical treatment plan or services received
- Radiology and laboratory reports (sometimes)
- Response to care

Standard patient records are usually assembled for new patients well before their actual use. It is the medical assistant's responsibility to make sure there are adequate patient records prepared to meet the needs of the practice.

Legal Guidelines for Patient Records

Patient records are important for legal reasons. As a general rule, if information is not documented, no one can prove that an event or procedure took place. Medical records are used in lawsuits and malpractice cases to support a patient's claim of malpractice against a doctor and to support the doctor in defense against a claim. Medical records must be retained for 7 years; for pediatric records, the guideline is 7 years from the age of majority. Many legal experts suggest that medical records be kept for 10 years instead of the legally required 7 years.

All medical care, evaluation, and instruction given to the patient by the physician must be documented. Every chart entry must be clear, accurate, legible, dated, and per HIPAA guidelines, written in blue ink. The patient chart is a legal document. Always consider how the patient record would present if it was called into a court of law for review.

Additionally, it is very important to document when a patient is **noncompliant**. *Noncompliant* is a medical term used to describe a patient who does not follow the medical advice he or she is given. After a clear record has been made of the directions given to a patient for optimum health, it is essential to record the level of patient compliance. For example, after you have instructed a patient, you may write in her chart that "Patient stated she understood all directions. Written instruction given to patient." If it is determined that a patient did *not* follow the medical advice, it is then essential to chart this as well. The physician may wish to withdraw from the care of a patient because of the patient's noncompliance. Without a proper and accurate documentation of the patient's noncompliance, the physician may not be able to withdraw care without becoming legally liable. Additionally, documented noncompliance can be used in the physician's defense in a malpractice suit if it can be proven that, due to patient noncompliance, the physician was not solely responsible for inadequate medical care or result.

Standards for Records

Records that are complete, accurate, and well documented can be convincing evidence that a doctor provided appropriate care. On the other hand, altered, incomplete, inaccurate, or illegible records may imply that a doctor's entire medical practice is below standard.

It is important to understand that the physicians in a practice are not the only people who chart medical records within that practice. However, if an employee of the practice charts inappropriately or inaccurately in a patient's chart, in a court of law, the physician is held responsible for that action. All records, both medical and financial, are the responsibility of the physician. As a medical assistant, you are responsible to the patient and the physician for both the medical and administrative procedures you perform and the accurate recording of those procedures.

Additional Uses of Patient Records

Patient records serve as ongoing references about individual patients' medical care. They are also valuable for patient education, quality of treatment, and research.

Patient Education. Patient records can be used to educate patients about their own conditions and treatment plans. The physician can point out how test results have changed or how the patient's general health has improved or lessened. The physician can also emphasize the importance of following treatment instructions. The medical assistant in turn may use some of this information in educating the patient about his condition or its management. Records can also be used to educate the health-care staff about unusual medical conditions, patient progress, or results of treatment plans.

Quality of Treatment. Patient records may be used to evaluate the quality of treatment a facility or doctor's office provides. Auditing groups, such as peer review organizations or The Joint Commission (TJC), may review the charts to monitor whether the care provided and the fees charged meet accepted standards. Records also provide statistics for health-care analysis and future health-care plans and policy decisions.

Research. Patient records also play an important role in medical research. For example, a medical research team may be testing a new hypertension drug with volunteers who fit a certain medical category—perhaps men between the ages of 45 and 54 who have high blood pressure. Carefully kept records are valuable sources of data about patient responses, behavior, symptoms, side effects, and outcomes (Figure 9-1).

Information in charts may spur researchers to begin a study. For example, the records may show that 80% of all patients taking a particular heart medication experience dizziness. Researchers can investigate why this reaction might be happening.

Contents of Patient Charts

You will fill out a record for each new patient who comes to the office. Although each physician's office has its own forms and medical charts, in general, all records must contain certain standard information.

Standard Chart Information

Standard chart information covers a spectrum of different, carefully detailed notes and facts about a patient, from his

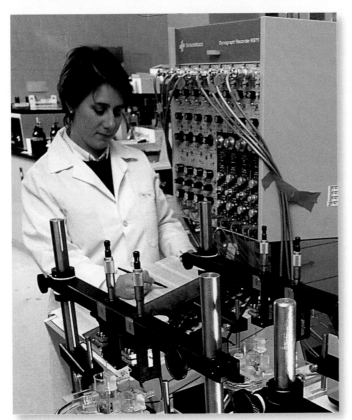

Figure 9-1. Medical researchers may rely on data gathered from patient records.

medical history to the doctor's diagnosis and comments on follow-up care. You must have an understanding of what each part means.

Patient Registration Form. Initial registration information includes the registration form and the patient medical history form (discussed below). Both forms are completed the by patient prior to, or collected at the beginning of the first patient visit. The patient registration form should list the date of the patient's current visit, the patient's age, address, Social Security number, DOB (date of birth), medical insurance information, occupation and employer, marital status, number of children, and the name of the person to contact in an emergency.

The completed registration form (with front and back copies of the patient's insurance card) is the base document for each patient's financial record. Patient financial and medical records are separated into two distinct records filed separately as well. Figure 9-2 is an example of a patient registration form.

Patient Medical History. The medical history form, the second part of the registration process, includes the patient's past medical history (including illnesses, surgeries, known allergies, and current medications), family medical history, and social and occupational history (including diet, exercise, smoking, and use of alcohol or drugs). Usually, the history form ends with a section for the patient to describe the condition or complaint that is

the reason for her visit. Medicare and managed care plans now require that the patient's complaint be entered into the medical record. Known as the chief complaint, this information should be recorded in the patient's own words if at all possible. The patient medical history form is used as the base for the patient's medical chart and is usually found on the left side of the chart.

Physical Examination Results. Sometimes a form is used to record the results of a general physical examination. Figure 9-3 shows a combination medical history and physical examination form.

Results of Laboratory and Other Tests. Test results include findings from tests performed in the office and those received from other doctors, hospitals, or independent laboratories or other outside sources. Some offices use a laboratory summary sheet to help the doctor detect significant changes more easily.

Test results received from sources outside the practice are best organized in sections within this part of the medical chart. Each section is determined by the source of the information. For example, all reports from a particular hospital may be grouped together in one section. Each section from outside sources should be arranged in chronological order, with the latest report on the top.

Records from Other Physicians or Hospitals. Incoming records from other sources must be entered into the patient's chart. A copy of the patient's written request authorizing release of the records from the other sources must also be included.

Doctor's Diagnosis and Treatment Plan. The doctor's diagnosis must be recorded, along with the treatment plan, which may consist of treatment options, the final treatment list, instructions to the patient, and any medications prescribed. The doctor may also put specific comments or impressions on record. All of this information is recorded with every patient visit (Figure 9-4).

Operative Reports, Follow-Up Visits, and Telephone Calls. Continuation of the record lasts as long as the patient is under the doctor's care. You should record and date all procedures, surgeries, follow-up care, and additional notes the doctor makes regarding the patient's case. You can use continuation forms to add more pages. In addition, you may keep a separate log of telephone calls to and from the patient.

Informed Consent Forms. Informed consent forms, such as the one shown in Figure 9-5, verify that a patient understands the treatment offered and the possible outcomes or side effects of the treatment. Consent forms should also specify what the outcome might be if the patient receives no treatment. They also describe alternative treatments and possible risks. The patient signs the consent form but may withdraw consent at any time.

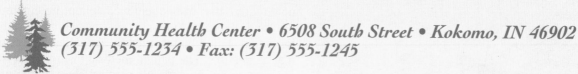

Community Health Center • 6508 South Street • Kokomo, IN 46902
(317) 555-1234 • Fax: (317) 555-1245

Patient Registration
Patient Information

Name: _____   Today's Date: _____

Address: _____

City: _____   State: _____   Zip Code: _____

Telephone (Home): _____   (Work): _____   (Cell): _____

Birthdate: _____   Age: _____   Sex: M F   No. of Children _____   Marital Status: M S W D

Social Security Number: _____   Employer: _____   Occupation: _____

Primary Physician: _____

Referred by: _____

Person to Contact in Emergency: _____

Emergency Telephone: _____

Special Needs: _____

Responsible Party

Party Responsible for Payment: Self   Spouse   Parent   Other

Name (If Other Than Self): _____

Address: _____

City: _____   State: _____   Zip Code: _____

Primary Insurance

Primary Medical Insurance: _____

Insured party: Self   Spouse   Parent   Other

ID#/Social Security No.: _____   Group/Plan No.: _____

Name (If Other Than Self): _____

Address: _____

City: _____   State: _____   Zip Code: _____

Secondary Insurance

Secondary Medical Insurance: _____

Insured party: Self   Spouse   Parent   Other

ID#/Social Security No.: _____   Group/Plan No.: _____

Name (If Other Than Self): _____

Address: _____

City: _____   State: _____   Zip Code: _____

Figure 9-2. The patient registration form is often the first document used in initiating a patient financial record.

The Medical Center at Springfield
Medical History

Name _____ Age _____ Sex _____ S M W D

Address _____ Phone _____ Date _____

Occupation _____ Ref. by _____

Chief Complaint _____

Present Illness _____

_____

_____

_____

History —Military _____
   —Social _____
   —Family _____
   —Marital _____
   —Menstrual _____ Menarche _____ Para. _____ LMP _____
   —Illness Measles Pert. Var. Pneu. Pleur. Typh. Mal. Rh. Fev. Sc. Fev. Diphth. Other
   —Surgery _____
   —Allergies _____
   —Current Medications _____

Physical Examination

Temp. _____ Pulse _____ Resp. _____ BP _____ Ht. _____ Wt. _____

General Appearance _____ Skin _____ Mucous Membrane _____

Eyes: _____ Vision _____ Pupil _____ Fundus _____

Ears: _____

Nose: _____

Throat: _____ Pharynx _____ Tonsils _____

Chest: _____ Breasts _____

Heart: _____

Lungs: _____

Abdomen: _____

Genitalia: _____

Rectum: _____

Pelvic: _____

Extremities: _____ Pulses: _____

Lymph Nodes: _____ Neck _____ Axilla _____ Inguinal _____ Abdominal

Neurological: _____

Diagnosis: _____

_____

_____

Treatment: _____

_____

_____

Laboratory Findings: _____

Date _____ Blood _____

_____

_____

_____

Date _____ Urine _____

_____

_____

_____

Figure 9-3. In some doctors' offices, the medical history form and the physical examination form are combined.

PROGRESS NOTES

11/11/12   10:30 am

S = patient states, "I have had a fever and a sore throat for the past two days"

O = Vital signs: T 101.1   P 96   R 24   BP 124/76   Weight: 155   Height: 5′ 7″

General: patient seems alert. HEENT: sclera clear. Pharynx red with pus pockets noted.   Heart: regular w/o murmur

Lungs: clear to auscultation and percussion. Abdomen: negative for tenderness

A = strep throat

P = 1. prescription for Amoxicillin, 1 tsp q8h for 10 days

2. schedule appointment for three weeks from today's date for repeat testing

Gregory Collins, MD — Attending Physician

E. James, RMA (AMT)   Date: November 11, 2012

Form OMB-1243

Figure 9-4. An example of progress notes.

THE OAK HILLS MEDICAL CENTER
Oak Hills, MA

CONSENT TO OPERATION, ADMINISTRATION OF ANESTHETICS,
AND RENDERING OF OTHER MEDICAL SERVICE

Patient: _____ Age: _____
Date: _____ Time: _____

1. I AUTHORIZE AND DIRECT _____ , with the associates
   and assistants of his/her choice, to perform upon myself the following operation
   _____
   _____
   _____

   If any unforeseen conditions arise in the course of the operation or in the postoperative period, calling in their judgment for other operations or procedures, I further request and authorize them to do whatever is deemed advisable for my health and well-being.

2. The positive and negative aspects of autologous blood transfusions (receiving my own blood donated prior to surgery), designated blood transfusions (donated in advance by family/friends for my use), or homologous blood transfusions (from general donor population) have been explained to me. I understand autologous and designated transfusions can be accommodated only for nonemergency surgery.

6. I certify that I understand the above consent to operation and that the explanations referred to have been made.

_____   _____
Witness (of signature only)   Signature

Figure 9-5. Patients are asked to sign informed consent forms to confirm that they understand the treatment offered.

Hospital Discharge Summary Forms. The discharge summary form generally includes information that summarizes the reason the patient entered the hospital; tests, procedures, or operations performed in the hospital; medications administered in the hospital; and the disposition, or outcome, of the case. Elements of the form may include the following:

- Date of admission
- Brief history
- Date of discharge
- Admitting diagnosis
- Operations and procedures or hospital course (course of action taken in the hospital)
- Complications
- Instructions to the patient for follow-up care after discharge from the hospital
- Physician's signature

Correspondence with or About the Patient. All written correspondence from the patient or from other doctors, laboratories, or independent health-care agencies must be kept in the patient's chart. Each piece of correspondence should be marked or stamped with the date the doctor's office received the document.

Information Received by Fax

Some information—such as laboratory results, physician comments, or correspondence—may be received by fax transmission. Always request that the original be mailed if possible.

Dating and Initialing

You must be careful not only to date everything you put into the patient chart but also to initial the entry. This

Guidelines for Handling Protected Health Information within the Medical Record

HIPAA (the Health Insurance Portability and Accountability Act) became law on August 21, 1996. This new law required that all health-care providers be in compliance by April 2003. HIPAA law states that all patients have rights regarding their health information, which is known as Protected Health Information (PHI). A patient's PHI is stored in the patient's medical chart. Federal law protects the individual's rights to know about how her or his PHI is used and disclosed.

The term *use* means the employment, application, utilization, sharing, examination or analysis of **individual identifiable health information (IIHI).** For example, when a medical assistant keys in a patient's health insurance number to determine the status of payment from the insurance company, the patient's PHI is being used. The term *disclosure* means the release or transfer in any way of patient IIHI beyond the confines of the health-care practice to which the information was given. For example, when a medical assistant gives patient information to another medical office to which the patient is being referred, PHI is being disclosed.

Patients have the following rights under HIPAA law:

1. *The right to notice of privacy practices.* Because it is unlikely that your patients will be reading federal laws, the law states it is your responsibility to give them a copy of the laws that protect them concerning their PHI. Patients must receive a written notice of privacy practices on their first visit to a health-care provider. They should sign a form stating they have received this information. This signed form must be carefully filed in the patients' medical record.

2. *The right to limit or request restriction on their PHI and its use and disclosure.* This means that patients can limit how your office uses their medical information, and how much of that information is shared. For example, a patient with a history of sexually transmitted disease may not wish to have that information released to the orthopedic physician who is setting his broken arm. It is not necessary. In general, only the minimal amount of patient information should be released to meet the current needs of the patient. This is called the "Need to Know" general rule.

3. *The right to confidential communications.* This means that patients can request to receive PHI in a manner other than during a medical appointment. For example, your patients may request that you call them at a variety of different numbers, including home, work, or cell phone number. The patient does not have to explain the request. The law says you must make a reasonable effort to communicate with the patient in a confidential manner as the patient requests.

4. *The right to inspect and obtain a copy of their PHI.* This means that patients have a right to request and receive a copy of their own medical records. There are a few exceptions to this rule; however, in general, the medical assistant receives and processes all patient requests for medical records. It is important to always follow the protocols established in your office for medical record copying. It is considered an acceptable practice to act on a request within 30 days of the request, and to charge a reasonable fee to cover the expense for copying supplies and labor.

5. *The right to request an amendment to their PHI.* Health-care providers have the right to require that a request to amend a record be made in writing. The request may be denied if the health-care provider receiving the request is not the original recorder of the PHI, or if the PHI is believed to be accurate and complete. All requests for amendment and response must be carefully documented and filed in the medical chart.

6. *The right to know if their PHI has been disclosed and why.* Providers are required to keep a written record of every disclosure made of a patient's PHI. You must also keep a written record of any request by the patient for this information and the response of the health-care provider. This information is usually filed in the patient's medical record. When making a disclosure of information, always record the date of the disclosure, the name and address of the person receiving the PHI, a brief summary of the information released, and the purpose of the disclosure.

system makes it easy to tell which items the assistant enters into the chart and which items others enter. In many practices the physician initials reports before they are filed to prove that he saw them.

Initiating and Maintaining Patient Records

Besides the receptionist, you will often be the first healthcare professional that new patients talk with when they visit a doctor's office. During your first contact with a patient, you will initiate a patient record. Recording information in the medical record is called **documentation.** Complete, thorough documentation ensures that the doctor will have detailed notes about each contact with the patient and about the treatment plan, patient responses and progress, and treatment outcomes.

Initial Interview

You usually perform the following tasks on your own, depending on the doctor's practice and your experience and background. Familiarize yourself with each task.

Completing Medical History Forms. You will help new patients fill out medical history forms or questionnaires. You may retrieve current patients' records from the files to update them. Type the patient's name and other identifying information on the first page and on all subsequent pages of the form.

You may interview patients to fill in some of the remaining blanks about medical history. Some doctors prefer to ask patients questions themselves. Others believe that people sometimes talk more freely with an assistant than they do with the doctor.

Documenting Patient Statements. You will record any signs, symptoms, or other information the patient wishes to share. Document this information in the patient's own words, not your interpretation of the words. Record these data in specific detail. For example, if the patient drinks alcohol, you should record the number of drinks per week, the type of liquor consumed, and whether the drinking has affected the patient's behavior and health. Chart this information by writing "Patient states that . . ." and then, whenever possible, complete the sentence with the exact words the patient used.

Conduct the interview in a private room or in a semiprivate office away from the reception area, as shown in Figure 9-6. Patients usually do not like to discuss their medical or personal problems in front of others. Your opinion of the patient, such as "the patient seems mentally unstable," is your own and should not be discussed or documented.

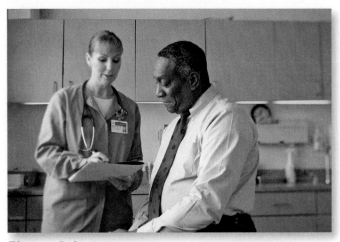

Figure 9-6. Conduct interviews with patients in a private or semiprivate room to make them feel more comfortable.

Documenting Test Results. Put a copy in the chart of any test results, x-ray reports, or other diagnostic results that the patient has brought with him. You may also record this information on a separate test summary sheet in the chart.

Examination Preparation and Vital Signs. In many instances, you will prepare patients for examination. You will record vital signs, medication the patient is currently taking, and any responses to treatment. Before you leave a patient, ask, "Is there anything else you would like the doctor to know?" The patient may be more comfortable sharing further information with you than with the doctor.

Follow-Up

After you record the initial interview and background information, the doctor decides what entries will be made regarding examinations, diagnosis, treatment options and plans, and comments or observations about each case. You will then maintain the patient record by performing some or all of the following duties:

- Transcribing notes the doctor dictates about the patient's progress, follow-up visits, procedures, current status, and other necessary information
  - Note that transcription by the medical assistant does not occur in all practices.
- Posting laboratory test results or results of examinations in the medical record or on the summary sheet
- Recording telephone calls from the patient and calls that the doctor or other office staff members make to the patient (Figure 9-7)
  - Telephone calls can be an important part of good follow-up care. Calls must be dated, and the content of the conversations must be documented.

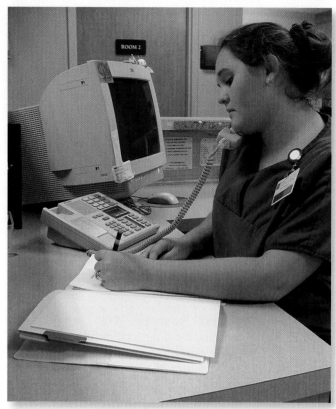

You must initial the entry. Even if the doctor did not reach the patient, the call should be recorded and dated. State whether the doctor got an answer, left a message on an answering machine or with a person, and so on. Legally, if an item is not in the record, it did not happen.

- Recording medical instructions or discharge instructions the doctor gives
  - At the doctor's request, you may counsel or educate the patient regarding the treatment regimen or home-care procedures the patient must follow. This information must be entered into the record, dated, and initialed. Some offices make carbon copies or photocopies of patient instructions.

Procedure 9-1 provides information about how to prepare a patient medical record/chart.

The Six Cs of Charting

To maintain accurate patient records, always keep these six Cs in mind when filling out and maintaining charts: Client's (patient's) words, Clarity, Completeness, Conciseness, Chronological order, and Confidentiality.

1. **Client's words.** Be careful to record the patient's exact words rather than your interpretation of them. For

Figure 9-7. All telephone conversations to and from the patient must be logged in the patient record.

PROCEDURE 9-1

Preparing a Patient Medical Record/Chart

Procedure Goal: To assemble new patient record/chart

Materials: File folder, labels as appropriate (alphabet, numbers, dates, insurance, allergies, etc.), forms (patient information, advance directives, physician progress notes, referrals, laboratory forms), hole punch

Method:
1. Carefully create a chart label according to practice policy. This label may include the patient's last name followed by the first name, or it may be a medical record number for those offices that utilize numeric or alphanumeric filing.

   Rationale
   The label must be correct to help avoid filing errors.

2. Place the chart label on the right edge of the folder, extending the label the length of the tab on the folder.

3. Place the date label on the top edge of the folder, updating the date according to the practice's policy. (The date is usually updated annually, provided the patient has come into the office within the last year.)

   Rationale
   It makes it easy to identify current patient records for retrieval as well as identify records for purging if the patient has not been seen for a specified amount of time (often, three years).

4. If alpha or numeric filing labels are utilized, place a patient name label on the chart according to the practice's policy.

5. Punch holes in the appropriate forms for placement within the patient's medical record/chart.

6. Place all the forms in appropriate sections of the patient's medical record/chart.

TABLE 9-1	Common Medical Abbreviations		
Abbreviation	Meaning	Abbreviation	Meaning
AIDS	acquired immunodeficiency syndrome	inj.	injection
a.m.a.	against medical advice	IV	intravenous
b.i.d./BID	twice a day	MI	myocardial infarction
BP	blood pressure	MM	mucous membrane
bpm	beats per minute	NPO	nothing by mouth
CBC	complete blood count	NYD	not yet diagnosed
C.C.	chief complaint	OOB	out of bed
CNS	central nervous system	OPD	outpatient department
CPE	complete physical examination	OR	operating room
CV	cardiovascular	PH	past history
D & C	dilation and curettage	PRN	as needed
Dx	diagnosis	PT	physical therapy
ECG/EKG	electrocardiogram	Pt	patient
ED/ER	emergency department/emergency room	q.i.d./QID	four times a day
FH	family history	ROS/SR	review of systems/systems review
Fl/fl	fluid	s.c./subq.	subcutaneously
F/U	follow up	SOB	shortness of breath
GBS	gallbladder series	S/R	suture removal
GI	gastrointestinal	stat	immediately
GU	genitourinary	t.i.d./TID	three times a day
GYN	gynecology	TPR	temperature, pulse, respiration
HEENT	head, ears, eyes, nose, throat	UCHD	usual childhood diseases
HIV	human immunodeficiency virus	VS	vital signs
I & D	incision and drainage	WNL	within normal limits
ICU	intensive care unit		

instance, if a client says, "My right knee feels like it's thick or full of fluid," write that down. Do not rephrase the sentence to say, "Client says he's got fluid on the knee." Often the patient's exact words, no matter how odd they may sound, provide important clues for the physician in making a diagnosis.

2. Clarity. Use precise descriptions and accepted medical terminology when describing a patient's condition. For instance, "Patient got out of bed and walked 20 feet without shortness of breath" is much clearer than "Patient got out of bed and felt fine."

3. Completeness. Fill out completely all the forms used in the patient record. Provide complete information

that is readily understandable to others whenever you make any notation in the patient chart.

4. Conciseness. While striving for clarity, also be concise, or brief and to the point. Abbreviations and specific medical terminology can often save time and space when recording information. For instance, you can write "Patient got OOB and walked 20 ft w/o SOB." OOB and SOB are standard abbreviations for "out of bed" and "shortness of breath," respectively. Every member of the office staff should use the same abbreviations to avoid misunderstandings. Table 9-1 lists some common medical abbreviations.

5. Chronological order. All entries in patient records must be dated to show the order in which they are

made. This factor is critical, not only for documenting patient care but also in case there is a legal question about the type and date of medical services.

6. Confidentiality. All the information in patient records and forms is confidential, to protect the patient's privacy. Only the patient, attending physicians, and the medical assistant (who needs the record to tend to the patient and/or to make entries into the record) are allowed to see the charts without the patient's written consent. Never discuss a patient's records, forward them to another office, fax them, or show them to anyone but the physician unless you have the patient's written permission to do so. (Review the section Reflecting On . . . HIPAA: Guidelines for Handling Protected Health Information Within the Medical Record.)

Types of Medical Records

You should be familiar with the different approaches to documenting patient information. The most common methods are conventional/source-oriented and problem-oriented medical records.

Conventional, or Source-Oriented, Records

In the conventional, or source-oriented, approach, patient information is arranged according to who supplied the data—the patient, doctor, specialist, or someone else. The medical form may have a space for patient remarks, followed by a section for the doctor's comments.

These records describe all problems and treatments on the same form in simple chronological order. For example, a patient's broken wrist would be recorded on the same form as her stomach ulcer. Although easy to initiate and maintain, this system presents some difficulty in tracking the progress of a specific ailment, such as the patient's ulcer. The doctor has to search the entire record to find information on that one problem.

Problem-Oriented Medical Records

One way to overcome the disadvantages of the conventional approach is to use the problem-oriented medical record (POMR) system of keeping charts. This approach, developed by Lawrence L. Weed, MD, makes it easier for the physician to keep track of a patient's progress. The information in a POMR includes the database; problem list; educational, diagnostic, and treatment plan; and progress notes.

Database. The database includes a record of the patient's history; information from the initial interview with the patient (for example, "Patient unemployed—second time in past 12 months"); all findings and results from physical examinations (such as "Pulse 105 bpm, BP 210/80"); and any tests, x-rays, and other procedures.

Problem List. Each problem a patient has is listed separately, given its own number, and dated. You then identify a problem by its number throughout the record. You can also list work-related, social, or family problems that may be affecting the patient's health. For instance, the problem list for the example patient who is unemployed might include "Severe stomach pain, worse at night and after eating."

You can alert the doctor to the fact that the patient has lost two jobs within 1 year. Such radical life changes can often provoke strong physical reactions. In this patient's case the elevated blood pressure may be related to the job losses, and stress may be causing the stomach pain.

When you document problems, be careful to distinguish between patient signs and symptoms. **Signs** are objective, or external, factors—such as blood pressure, rashes, or swelling—that can be seen or felt by the doctor or measured by an instrument. **Symptoms** are subjective, or internal, conditions felt by the patient, such as pain, headache, or nausea. Together, signs and symptoms help clarify a patient's problem.

Educational, Diagnostic, and Treatment Plan. Each problem should have a detailed educational, diagnostic, and treatment summary in the record. The summary contains diagnostic workups, treatment plans, and instructions for the patient. Here is an example.

Problem 2, Stomach Pain, 2/2/XX [date]
- *Upper GI exam negative, CBC normal.*
- *Prescribed over-the-counter antacid, 2 tablets by mouth t.i.d. after each meal.*
- *Set up appointment for patient with Dr. R. Neil at stress-management clinic (Broughten Professional Center) for Monday, February 4, at 4:30 p.m.*
- *Patient's anxiety is high. Recheck in 1 week.*

Progress Notes. Progress notes are entered for each problem listed in the initial record. The documentation always includes—in chronological order—the patient's condition, complaints, problems, treatment, and responses to care. Here is an example.

Problem 2, Stomach Pain, 2/9/XX. Patient enrolled in stress-reduction class. Reports stomach pain has diminished— "I can eat without pain; only a little discomfort at night." Vital signs improved: pulse 85 bpm, BP 115/70, respiration 20. Reduced antacid to one tablet by mouth two times daily after meals. Anxiety much reduced. Recheck anxiety level in 2 weeks.

SOAP Documentation

Many medical records, such as the POMR format, emphasize the **SOAP** approach to documentation, which provides an orderly series of steps for dealing with any medical case. SOAP documentation lists the patient's symptoms, the diagnosis, and the suggested treatment. Information is documented in the record in the following order.

1. S: **Subjective** data come from the patient; the patient describes his or her signs and symptoms and supplies any other opinions or comments.

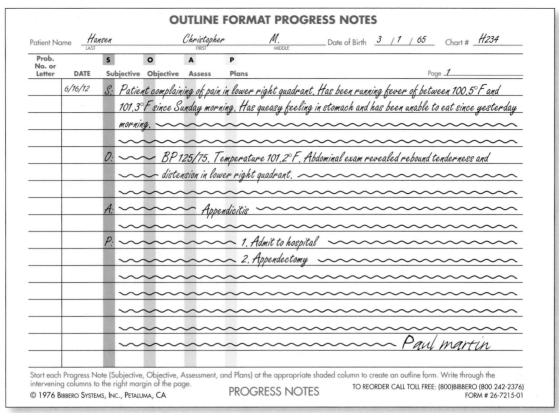

OUTLINE FORMAT PROGRESS NOTES

Patient Name: Hansen (LAST) Christopher (FIRST) M. (MIDDLE) Date of Birth 3 / 1 / 65 Chart # H234

Prob. No. or Letter	DATE	**S** Subjective	**O** Objective	**A** Assess	**P** Plans	Page 1
	6/16/12	S: Patient complaining of pain in lower right quadrant. Has been running fever of between 100.5°F and 101.3°F since Sunday morning. Has queasy feeling in stomach and has been unable to eat since yesterday morning.				
		O: BP 125/75. Temperature 101.2°F. Abdominal exam revealed rebound tenderness and distension in lower right quadrant.				
		A: Appendicitis				
		P: 1. Admit to hospital 2. Appendectomy				
					Paul Martin	

Start each Progress Note (Subjective, Objective, Assessment, and Plans) at the appropriate shaded column to create an outline form. Write through the intervening columns to the right margin of the page.

© 1976 BIBBERO SYSTEMS, INC., PETALUMA, CA   **PROGRESS NOTES**   TO REORDER CALL TOLL FREE: (800)BIBBERO (800 242-2376) FORM # 26-7215-01

Figure 9-8. The SOAP approach to documentation is one way to organize information in a patient record.

2. O: **Objective** data come from the physician and from examinations and test results.

3. A: *A*ssessment is the diagnosis or impression of a patient's problem.

4. P: *P*lan of action includes treatment options, chosen treatment, medications, tests, consultations, patient education, and follow-up.

Whether you keep conventional or POMR charts, you can include all these steps for each problem. Figure 9-8 shows an example of SOAP notes. If you abbreviate any term when entering data into the records, use only approved medical abbreviations. For example, use "5 g" instead of "5 grams." Several resources, including those published by TJC and the American Medical Association, list approved medical abbreviations for measurements, instructions for taking medication, and other topics. Keep these references readily available in the office.

CHEDDAR Format

The **CHEDDAR** format of medical records documentation takes the SOAP format further. CHEDDAR stands for

C: *C*hief complaint, presenting problems, subjective statements

H: *H*istory; social and physical history of presenting problem as well as contributing information

E: *E*xamination, including extent of body systems examined

D: *D*etails of problem and complaints

D: *D*rugs and dosage—for example, a list of current medications used with dosage and frequency

A: *A*ssessment of the diagnostic process and the impression (diagnosis) made by the physician

R: *R*eturn visit information or referral, if applicable

Appearance, Timeliness, and Accuracy of Records

You must ensure that the medical records are complete. They must also be written neatly and legibly, contain up-to-date information, and present an accurate, professional record of a patient's case.

Neatness and Legibility

A medical record is useless if the doctor or others have difficulty reading it. You should make sure that every word and number in the record is clear and legible. Follow these tips to keep charts neat and easy to read.

- Use a good-quality pen that will not smudge or smear.

- HIPAA requires that all original documents be maintained in the patient's medical record. Blue ink is considered the best choice for charting. It is easy to confuse an original written in black ink with a copy. Blue ink will copy as black, making the original and copy look different, which can reduce the possibility of error. Blue ink is also more difficult to match, making any additions to the medical record easy to spot, which can cut down on fraudulent entries. For these reasons, blue ink is the best choice for documentation.

- Use highlighting pens to call attention to specific items such as allergies. Be aware, however, that unless the office has a color copier, most colored ink will photocopy black or gray. Highlighting-pen marks may not be visible on a photocopy.
- Make sure all handwriting is legible. Take time to write names, numbers, and abbreviations clearly.
- Make any corrections to the chart by following Procedure 9-3, Correcting Medical Records.

Timeliness

Medical records should be kept up to date and should be readily available when a doctor or another health-care professional needs to see them. Follow these guidelines to ensure that a doctor can find the most recent information on a patient when it is needed.

- Record all findings from exams and tests as soon as they are available.
- If you forget to enter a finding into the record when it is received, record both the original date of receipt and the date the finding was entered into the record.
- To document telephone calls, record the date and time of the call, who initiated it, the information discussed, and any conclusions or results. You can either enter the telephone call directly into the record or make a note referring the doctor to a separate telephone log kept in the record.
- Establish a procedure for retrieving a file quickly in case of emergency. Should the patient be in a serious accident, for example, the emergency doctor will need the patient's medical history immediately.

Accuracy

The physician must be able to trust the accuracy of the information in the medical records. You must make it a priority always to check the accuracy of all data you will enter in a chart. To ensure accurate data, follow these guidelines.

- Never guess at or assume knowledge of names, procedures, medications, findings, or any other information about which there is some question. Always check all the information carefully. Make the extra effort to ask questions of the physician or senior staff member and to verify information.
- Double-check the accuracy of findings and instructions recorded in the chart. Have all numbers been copied accurately? Are instructions for taking medication clear and complete?

- Make sure the latest information has been entered into the chart so that the physician has an accurate picture of the patient's current condition.

Procedure 9-3 explains how to correct a medical chart.

Professional Attitude and Tone

Part of creating timely, accurate records is maintaining a professional tone in your writing when recording information. Record information from the patient using his own words. Also record the doctor's observations and comments as well as any laboratory or test results. Do not record your personal, subjective comments, judgments, opinions, or speculations about a patient's words, problems, or test results. You may call attention to a particular problem or observation, for example, by attaching a note to the chart. Do not, however, make such comments part of the patient's record.

Electronic Health Records

Electronic health records (EHR), also known as **electronic medical records (EMR),** are becoming increasingly essential to the quality of health care and the improvement of patient safety. However, despite some of the advantages of computerized records, adoption of this technology still remains distressingly low. Statistics show that only approximately 16 percent of primary care doctors have made the switch from paper to electronic records.

Listed are some of the advantages and disadvantages of EHRs:

Disadvantages

- costly
- retraining needed for entire staff
- may need to hire an IT staff member
- possible damage to system and to software

Advantages

- fewer lost medical records (fewer charts to pull)
- reduced transcription costs
- readability/legibility of charts
- more access to charts after hours
- easier to access patient education materials
- improved billing

Overall, the benefits outweigh the disadvantages. If your physician's office is thinking about changing to an EHR, make sure you do your homework. Make comparisons (www.physicianspractice.com/files/pdfs/theGuide_sep06.pdf) and ask questions. Here are a few questions to ask:

- Is the product licensed?
- What does each license actually provide?
- What technical support is available, and when?

- Is there a cost for technical support? How much?
- How is text imported into the system?
- Which image formats will the system support?
- What printers will the system support?
- What if you need to replace the system?
- Is everything in writing?

If your medical facility does adopt an EHR system, make sure that you continue to be sensitive to the needs of the patient; learn how to type so that you can look at the patient when inputting information into the system.

Electronic Medical Records Software Vendors

The following are several vendors and medical records software websites that produce electronic medical records.

- Medicware.com
- Allscripts (merged with Misys Computer Systems)—vendor
- Powermed.com
- Medicalcharting.com

Medical software packages range from easy-to-use to a more sophisticated approach in charting. As when considering any new technology, do your homework. Get recommendations, try demonstration models, and consider the future needs of the practice and those who will use the product. The product you choose will need to fit the practice today and be able to grow with the practice tomorrow.

 ## Additional Advantages of Computerizing Records

In a setting in which several terminals in a network are connected to a main computer, computerizing medical records presents several advantages. A physician can call up the record on her own or another computer monitor whenever the record is needed, review or update the file, and save it to the central computer again (see Figure 9-9).

Computerized records can also be used in teleconferences, where people in different locations can look at the same record on their individual computer screens at the same time. Records can also be sent by modem to the physician's home computer so that the physician will have a patient's records on hand for calls after hours. Computer access to patient records is also helpful for health-care providers with satellite offices in different cities or different parts of a city. Review the Points on Practice box for information about electronic health records.

Computers are useful for tickler files (files that need periodic attention). For example, they can alert staff members about patients who are due for yearly checkups and patients who require follow-up care. Some hospitals have begun to use electronically scanned images of patients' thumbprints to keep track of records. This system saves

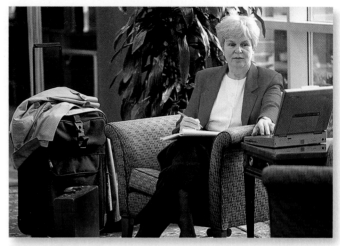

Figure 9-9. Computerized medical records, laptop computers, and the Internet provide physicians with easy access no matter where they are.

time and helps maintain the security of patient records. (Review Chapter 6 for more information on the use of computers in the medical practice.)

Security Concerns

When medical records are kept electronically, it is essential that the facility have policies in place to ensure security and confidentiality of records. In addition, electronic files must be backed up on a regular basis to avoid accidental loss of data. Whether you are documenting by hand or electronically, accuracy is always important. Careful key entry is essential to maintain accurate electronic files.

Protecting the confidentiality of patient records in computer files is the greatest concern of electronic health records. Just as paper health-care records are kept secure, so should the electronic health-care records be secure. Review Chapter 6 for more information about maintaining computer confidentiality.

Medical Transcription

Your knowledge of abbreviations, medical terminology, and medical coding will be invaluable when transcribing a doctor's notes or dictation (either recorded or direct). **Transcription** means transforming spoken notes into accurate written form. These written notes are then entered into the patient record. As is the case with information in medical charts, all dictated materials are confidential and should be regarded as potential legal documents. They are part of the patient's continuing case history. They often include findings, treatment stages, prognoses, and final outcomes. Always date and initial all transcription pages.

Strive to make transcribed material accurate and complete. Good grammar, correct spelling, and an accurate use of medical abbreviations and terminology are important in maintaining patient records. When dealing with

Points on Practice

Working with Electronic Health Records

Electronic health records (EHRs) are essentially a computer-based or a digital recording of patient information. They are also called computer records, electronic medical records (EMRs), electronic charts, and computer health records. Paper records can be lost and information is not consistent. In addition, handwriting is often illegible. EHRs provide a multitude of advantages, including the following:

- Access. Electronic records can be accessed by health-care providers at various locations, including the laboratory, pharmacy, and even the medical records department.

- Availability. Information is immediately available, so health-care providers do not have to wait for the paper document to get written and sent. The data are entered and then immediately viewed at any electronic record location.

- Security. Electronic records provide security through special passwords for each individual entering the records. Passwords can be set to open access to only the parts necessary for the type of health-care provider.

- Safety. Sophisticated programs help prevent patient identification errors by including a picture of each patient as part of the patient record.

- Extra Features. Electronic software programs can alert the health-care provider to abnormal results to tests or the need for routine tests to

be performed. More sophisticated programs can document health trends, provide voice recognition, and convert notes to complete sentences.

As a medical assistant working with electronic records, you should keep the following in mind:

- Become familiar with the software and hardware used at your facility. Make sure you are not focused on the computer when you are with the patient. Becoming comfortable with the system you are using will help you to focus on the patient. If necessary, take notes and enter them in the computer when the patient is not present until you become comfortable.

- Retrieve the patient record carefully just as you would a paper record. Make sure you have identified the patient with at least two identifiers such as the name, date of birth, and/or medical record number.

- Keep your password information secure. Change the password on a regular basis or as directed by the health-care facility.

- Secure the computer that maintains the electronic records and keep a backup of electronic files.

- Check your entries carefully before hitting the enter button. An EHR is a legal document just like a paper chart.

---

abbreviations, if there is any doubt as to the meaning or use of an abbreviation, the standard rule of thumb in health care is "when in doubt, spell it out". Use the medical dictionary and the medical computer spelling check to verify the spelling or meaning of words. Ask the physician only if you cannot find something in a reference source. Above-average typing or word processing accuracy and speed are also important. (See Chapter 5, Procedure 5-4, Using a Dictation-Transcription Machine.)

Transcribing Direct Dictation

At times the physician may wish to dictate material directly to you. He may want to get observations, comments, or treatment options into the record immediately rather than waiting until a more convenient time to dictate the material into a recorder. Follow these guidelines.

- Use a writing pad with a stiff backing or place the pad on a clipboard to make it easier to write quickly. Use a good ballpoint pen that will not smear or drag on the paper.

- Use incomplete sentences and phrases to keep up with the physician's pace. For example, say "Patient home Friday, re-check 2 wks" instead of "The patient is going home on Friday. We should see him again in 2 weeks."

- Use abbreviations for common phrases (*w/o* for "without," *s/b* for "should be," and so on); for medical terms (*q.d.* for "every day," *mg* for "milligrams," and so on); and for medications or chemicals.

- If a term, phrase, prescription, or name is unclear, ask for clarification right away (say "Excuse me, could you repeat that phrase, please?").

- If the physician speaks with a pronounced accent, ask her to speak more slowly than normal.

- Read the dictation back to the physician to verify all terms, names, figures, and other information for accuracy.

- Enter the notes into the patient record, and date and initial the notes. Procedure 9-2 details how to transcribe letters, notes, and reports from a physician.

PROCEDURE 9-2

Transcribing Letters, Reports, and Notes

Procedure Goal: To transcribe dictation from a physician.

Materials: Blank paper or stationery, transcription machine or computer with foot pedal, headphones, dictation tape or file, computer/printer, medical dictionary

Method:

1. Assemble materials. Decide what style correspondence you will choose if transcribing letters.

2. Make sure the transcription equipment has been set up properly, and you have your headphone plugged into your computer or transcription equipment.

3. Rewind the tape

Rationale
You must be sure you start transcribing at the beginning of the tape.

4. Type information while listening to dictation. Adjust tape speed as necessary to achieve a comfortable rate of transcription.

5. When you are transcribing, make sure you include the initials of both the person who is dictating and your initials as well.

Rationale
The receiver of the information needs to know who typed/transcribed the information. The format to use is TDW/smw

6. Use spell check and proofread the information carefully for grammar, punctuation, and style.

7. Make corrections as needed.

8. Finally, have the physician review for accuracy and sign if there are no corrections to be made.

Rationale
The physician is responsible for all information inserted in the medical record and all notes must be signed.

Career Opportunities

Medical Transcriptionist

To gain medical assistant credentials, you must fulfill the requirements of either the American Association of Medical Assistants (for a Certified Medical Assistant) or the American Medical Technologists (for a Registered Medical Assistant). After obtaining your medical assistant certification or registration, you may wish to acquire additional skills in specialty areas through course work or on-the-job training. Although this course work or training may not lead to an additional certification or degree, it will enable you to expand your role in the medical office and advance your career as the demand for skilled health professionals increases.

Skills and Duties

A medical transcriptionist creates written health records for patients based on the physician's dictation or notes. The records may be typewritten or input on a computer. Some transcriptionists work for a single physician; others work for a small or large group.

To create a patient record, the transcriptionist listens to an audiocassette containing information dictated by the physician. Typical information on the tape includes the physician's diagnosis and treatment of the patient. Using dictation equipment, the transcriptionist can slow down or stop and start the cassette tape as she types.

The medical transcriptionist must have excellent typing skills and a good command of medical terminology to make sure that medical terms are used accurately and spelled correctly. She will often need to edit the physician's notes to make sure that the language follows standard English grammar and usage. Sometimes she must also reorganize the physician's comments to create an understandable and easy-to- follow medical record. After she finishes transcribing the record, the medical transcriptionist checks it for correct spelling and punctuation. This last step is called proofreading.

Workplace Settings

Medical transcriptionists may work in the medical records department of a hospital or in a nursing home, clinic, laboratory, physician's practice, insurance company, or emergency or immediate health-care center. Some transcriptionists work for medical transcribing

continued ⟶

Medical Transcriptionist *(concluded)*

firms; others are self-employed and work out of their homes.

Education

Medical transcriptionists usually complete a training program at a 4-year college or university, junior or community college, vocational institute, or adult education center. They receive instruction in medical terminology, anatomy and physiology, pharmaceuticals, laboratory procedures, and medical treatments. Some transcriptionists concentrate on a particular specialty area, such as pathology, and acquire specialized training in that area. Medical transcriptionists can become certified if they meet the qualifying standards of the American Association for Medical Transcription.

For more information, visit the website of the following organization, which is available on the Online Learning Center at http://www.mhhe.com/medicalassisting4e.

American Association for Medical Transcription

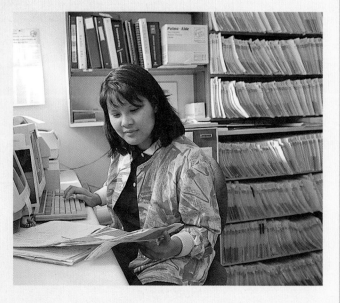

Transcription Aids

Keep a library of medical, secretarial, and transcription reference books and medical terminology texts near the transcription workstation. Abbreviations can save time, but you should use only those that are accepted as standard. Reference books will help you find the correct word quickly and easily and help you apply proper grammar, style, and usage to the copy.

Correcting and Updating Patient Records

In legal terms, medical records are regarded as having been created in "due course." All information in the record should be entered at the time of a patient's visit and not days, weeks, or months later. Information corrected or added some time after a patient's visit can be regarded as "convenient" and may damage a doctor's position in a lawsuit.

Using Care with Corrections

If changes to the medical record are not done correctly, the record can become a legal problem for the physician. A physician may be able to more easily explain poor or incomplete documentation than to explain a chart that appears to have been altered after something was originally documented. You must be extremely careful to follow the appropriate procedures for correcting patient records.

Mistakes in medical records are not uncommon. The best defense is to correct the mistake immediately or as soon as possible after the original entry was made. Procedure 9-3 shows you how to correct the patient record.

Updating Patient Records

All additions to a patient's record—test results, observations, diagnoses, procedures—should be done in a way that no one could interpret as deception on the physician's part. In a note accompanying the material, the physician should explain why the information is being added to the record. In some cases the material may simply be a physician's recollections or observations on a patient visit that occurred in the past. Each item added to a record must be dated and initialed. Sometimes a third party may be asked to witness the addition. Procedure 9-4 shows you how to maintain medical records properly.

Most hospitals and clinics have detailed guidelines for late entries to a patient's chart. You must follow these guidelines carefully to avoid potential legal problems (see Procedure 9-3).

PROCEDURE 9-3

Correcting Medical Records

Procedure Goal: To follow standard procedures for correcting a medical record

Materials: Patient file, other pertinent documents that contain the information to be used in making corrections (for example, transcribed notes, telephone notes, physician's comments, correspondence), good ballpoint pen

Method:

1. Always make the correction in a way that does not suggest any intention to deceive, cover up, alter, or add information to conceal a lack of proper medical care.

2. When deleting information, never black it out, never use correction fluid to cover it up, and never in any other way erase or obliterate the original wording. Draw a line through the original information so that it is still legible.

Rationale

All entries to a medical chart, even errors, must be legible according to law.

3. Write or type in the correct information above or below the original line or in the margin. The location on the chart for the new information should be clear. You may need to attach another sheet of paper or another document with the correction on it. Note in the record "See attached document A" or similar wording to indicate where the corrected information can be found.

4. Place a note near the correction stating why it was made (for example, "error, wrong date; error, interrupted by phone call.") Make sure you initial and date the correction. This indication can be a brief note in the margin or an attachment to the record. As a general rule of thumb, do not make any changes without noting the reason for them.

Rationale

By noting the reason as well as the correction, you clearly indicate that the correction is intentional and necessary.

5. Enter the date and time, and initial the correction.

Rationale

No correction to a medical chart is complete or acceptable without these elements.

6. If possible, have another staff member or the physician witness and initial the correction to the record when you make it.

Release of Records

All physical medical records, including x-rays, test results, and medical notes created by the physician, are considered the property of the practice. However, the information contained within the physical record belongs to the patient and is regarded as confidential. Even though the practice owns the records, no one can see them or obtain information from them without the patient's written consent. However, the law may require the physician to release them, as in the case of a patient with a contagious disease or when the records are subpoenaed by a court. Under no circumstances should you release patient information to insurance companies over the telephone. This information should be released in writing after the patient has signed a written release statement. Under HIPAA, release of information over the telephone may be problematic.

Additionally, any request to release medical records should be approved by the physician.

Procedures for Releasing Records

Physicians often receive requests from lawyers, other physicians, insurance companies, government agencies, and the patient himself for copies of a patient's records. Follow these steps for releasing medical information.

1. Obtain a signed and newly dated release from the patient authorizing the **transfer** of specific information—that is, giving information to another party outside the physician's office. *Verbal consent in person or over the telephone is not considered a valid release.* The release form should be filed in the patient's record.

2. Make photocopies of the original material. Copy and send only those portions of the record covered by the release and usually only records originating from your facility. Unless the patient specifically requests that you do so, you should not release records that were obtained from other sources, such as consultations or tests done in a hospital. Do not send original documents. (If a record will be used in a court

PROCEDURE 9-4

Maintaining Medical Records

Procedure Goal: To document continuity of care by creating a complete, accurate, timely record of the medical care provided at your facility

Materials: Patient file, other pertinent documents (test results, x-rays, telephone notes, correspondence), blue ballpoint pen, notebook, keyboard, transcribing equipment

Method:

1. Verify that you have the correct chart for the records to be filed.

   ### Rationale
   You do not want to record information in the wrong patient chart.

2. Transcribe dictated doctor's notes as soon as possible, and enter them into the patient record.

   ### Rationale
   Delays increase the chance of making errors in transcribing and recording the information. Also, for legal reasons, medical information should be entered into the record in a timely fashion.

3. Spell out the names of disorders, diseases, medications, and other terms the first time you enter them into the patient record, followed by the appropriate abbreviation (for example: "congestive heart failure [CHF]"). Thereafter, you may use the abbreviation alone.

   ### Rationale
   Using only abbreviations could cause confusion.

4. Enter only what the doctor has dictated. Do *not* add your own comments, observations, or evaluations. Use self-adhesive flags or other means to call the doctor's attention to something you have noticed that may be helpful to the patient's case. Date and initial each entry.

   ### Rationale
   Should the file be examined later in a legal proceeding, your notes and comments will be taken as part of the official record.

5. Follow office procedure to record routine or special laboratory test results. They may be posted in a particular section of the file or on a separate test summary form. If you use the summary form, make a note in the file that the results were received and recorded. Place the original laboratory report in the patient's file if required to do so by office policy. Date and initial each entry. Always note in the chart the date of the test and the results, whether or not test result printouts are filed in the record.

6. Make a note in the record of all telephone calls to and from the patient. Date and initial the entries. These entries also may include the doctor's comments, observations, changes in the patient's medication, new instructions to the patient, and so on. If calls are recorded in a separate telephone log, note in the patient's record the time and date of the call and refer to the log. It is particularly important to record such calls when the patient resists or refuses treatment, skips appointments, or has not made follow-up appointments.

   ### Rationale
   These entries can demonstrate that a doctor made every effort to provide quality care and that the patient is demonstrating noncompliant behavior.

7. Make notations in the medical record of any immunizations and vaccines that have been given to the patient. Notations should be posted in the patient's immunization record inside the medical chart. Input them into your state's public health database as well. Immunization records are kept indefinitely.

8. Read over the entries for omissions or mistakes. Ask the doctor to answer any questions you have.

   ### Rationale
   If it is not written down, from a legal perspective, it did not happen.

9. Make sure that you have dated and initialed each entry.

10. Be sure that all documents are included in the file.

11. Replace the patient's file in the filing system as soon as possible.

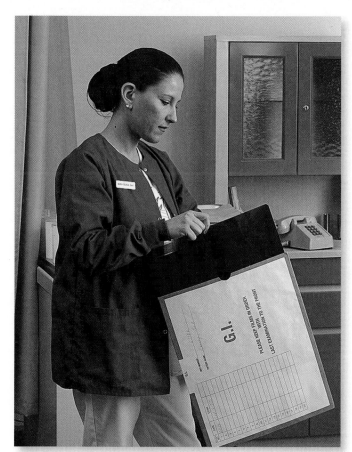

Figure 9-10. When you are preparing a patient record to be transferred, never send original material. One exception to this rule is x-rays, which should be sent with a request that the recipient return them as soon as possible.

case, however, you must submit the original unless the judge specifies that a photocopy is acceptable.) If you cannot make copies, as in the case of x-rays, send the originals, and tell the recipient that they must be returned (Figure 9-10). Follow up with the recipient until the originals have been returned and are placed in the patient's files. Often, the recipient is asked to sign a statement of responsibility for the original records until they are returned to the office. Document in the chart who has possession of the original document, the date the recipient received the originals, and the date they are returned.

3. Call the recipient to confirm that all materials were received. Avoid faxing confidential records. There is no way to tell who will see documents sent by fax.

Special Cases

It may not always be immediately clear who has the right to sign a release-of-records form. When a couple divorces, for example, both parents are still considered legal guardians of their children, and either one can sign a release form authorizing transfer of medical records. If a patient dies, the patient's next of kin or legally authorized representative, such as the executor of the estate, may see the

records or authorize their release to a third party. When you are in doubt regarding who is authorized to sign, *always* ask your supervisor before releasing confidential medical records.

Confidentiality

When children reach age 18, most states consider them adults with the right to privacy. No one, not even their parents, may see their medical records without the children's written consent. Some states extend this right to privacy to emancipated minors who are under the age of 18 and living on their own or are married, a parent, or in the armed services. This is particularly the case with minors seeking care for STDs, birth control, and drug or alcohol counseling. In these instances, the minor is considered a "mature minor" and her treatment cannot be discussed with her parents without her permission, even though the parents may still be held responsible for payment of such treatment through insurance or self-payment unless the patient pays for treatment at the time of service.

The main legal and ethical principle to keep in mind is that you must protect each patient's right to privacy at all times.

Auditing Medical Records

The auditing of medical records is a great housekeeping tool. To **audit** a record means to examine and review a group of patients' records. There are two types of audits: internal and external. The medical assistant, and generally the medical office manager, and others that handle medical records for a medical office should periodically perform an audit. Many physicians' offices are now hiring compliance specialists to do internal auditing of their charts.

Internal Audits. Internal audits can be done by the medical staff. Records are chosen randomly. Audits should be done before billing is submitted (*prospective*) and after billing is submitted (*retrospective*). The audit schedule should be determined by the medical office. Many offices prefer biannual audits, while others prefer quarterly audits. A sample chart review form created by Ronald Bradshaw MD, CPA, can be found at www.aafp.org/fpm/20000400/chartreviewform.pdf). Additionally, see Figure 9-11 for a sample of a medical record audit.

External Audits. External audits are done by government entities, managed care organizations, and private insurance carriers. Over the past few years, government audits have increased in order to recover possible overpayments. External auditors may want to investigate the medical records further by interviewing the staff, patient, and all physicians who participated in the care of the patient. If there is anything that is fraudulent in the billing that is discovered, the physician may have to refund monies or could be penalized.

Medical Record Audit

Select 10 active patient charts with at least 3–5 prior visits: the most recent visit should have taken place within the past 6-12 months. If information should be present and is not, place a 0 in the box for that chart. If information is present, rate the quality of the information with 3 = Superior, 2 = Satisfactory, and 1 = Unacceptable. Use "NA" to score items that do not apply to a given chart (e.g., patient has no allergies).

Chart number	1	2	3	4	5	6	7	8	9	10
Pages have patient ID										
Contains biographical and/or personal data										
Person providing care identified on each chart entry										
Entries are dated										
Entries are legible										
Problem list is complete										
Allergies and adverse drug reactions are prominent										
Absence of allergies and reactions prominent										
Appropriate past medical HX										
Smoking, alcohol, or substance abuse HX documented										
Pertinent HX and physical										
Lab and other tests ordered as appropriate										
Working diagnoses are consistent with findings										
Plans of action/treatment are consistent with diagnosis(es)										
Problems from previous visits addressed										
Evidence of appropriate use of consultants										
Evidence of continuity and coordination of care between primary and specialty physicians										
Consultant summaries, lab, and imaging study results reflect primary care physician review										
Completed immunization record										
Prescriptions and refills noted										
Med sheet used and appropriately located										
Chronology maintained										
Informed consent noted for all procedures and appropriate prescriptions										
Patients are adequately informed (i.e., there is documentation of patient education, follow-up instructions)										

Figure 9-11. An example of medical record audit.

Summary

9.1 Patients' records should be compiled because they serve as the chronological past, current, and future medical history of a patient's medical care and may be used in medical malpractice cases and lawsuits.

9.2 The content of a patient record consists of the patient registration form and the medical history form, the two forms that start the patient financial and medical records. The physical exam record and progress notes are added as patient care continues.

9.3 As the patient's care continues, any or all of the following may be added to the patient chart: exam results, lab and other test results, records from other physicians and hospitals, diagnosis and treatment plans, operative reports, consent forms, discharge summaries, and correspondence with or about the patient. Make sure you maintain the charts properly through documenting detailed notes about the contact with the patient, patient responses, progress, and treatment outcomes.

9.4 The most common approaches in documenting information into medical records is through conventional or source-oriented records, problem-oriented medical records (POMR), SOAP, and CHEDDAR.

9.5 Neatness, legibility, accuracy, and professional tone are musts in maintaining medical records. Remember that patients' charts are legal documents. They must be kept up-to-date and should be easy to read. Make sure you project a professional tone when recording information, and never guess at information. Always check for accuracy. Follow the 6 C's of Charting.

9.6 When performing direct transcription, make sure you use incomplete sentences or phrases to keep up with the physician's pace; use abbreviations whenever possible; if the physician speaks fast, ask him to speak slower and more clearly; read dictation back to the physician for clarity; and enter notes into the patient record. For standard dictation, follow the steps in Procedure 9-2 for accurate results.

9.7 When correcting medical records, make sure you correct as soon as possible. If there is an error, draw a single line through the error, reenter the correct information above or below the original entry, and if a separate sheet is needed for correction, note "see attached correction" and initial and date. Never use correction fluid or obliterate the original entry in any way. As a legal document, all entries, even ones that are corrected, must be legible.

9.8 Each item that is added to the patient record as an update should be dated and initialed. If the information is extremely important, get a third party to witness and initial and date as well.

9.9 Medical records can only be released with the patient's express written and signed consent. The signed consent is inserted into the medical record and copies are made of only those items listed within the consent. If records are subpoenaed by court and originals are required, make copies to keep in the chart until the originals are returned to the office. As a general rule, release only items that were ordered by the physician.

9.10 The advantages of the electronic medical record include but are not limited to, access to multiple physicians at one time, ability to have record available while seeing patient in ED or hospital setting, legibility as records are always typed, security through passwords, safety in identifying the correct chart and extra features, such as pop ups when a medication is prescribed that may interact with another medication the patient is already taking.

REVIEW

CHAPTER 9

CASE STUDY QUESTIONS

Now that you have completed this chapter, review the case study at the beginning of the chapter and answer the following questions:

1. Why is an accurate medical record important to the care of a patient?
2. Why is interviewing the patient important to the medical evaluation?
3. What are the six Cs of charting and what do they mean to you as a medical assistant?
4. What are the differences between the conventional and the POMR systems of keeping charts?
5. What are some helpful tips you might use as you perform transcription?

Multiple-Choice Questions

1. A patient's illness and reason for visit to the physician would be found in the
   a. patient's medical history.
   b. records from other health-care providers.
   c. patient registration form.
   d. informed consent form.
2. The first document(s) found in a patient medical record is the
   a. patient registration form.
   b. doctor's diagnosis and treatment plan.
   c. patient medical history.
   d. records from other physicians or hospitals.
3. The first health-care professional with whom a new patient speaks when visiting a medical office is the
   a. physician.
   b. nurse.
   c. medical assistant.
   d. laboratory technician.
4. The medical abbreviation for twice a day is
   a. BID.
   b. QI.D.
   c. BD.
   d. TID.
5. Documenting a patient's walk down a hall as "fine" violates which "C" of charting?
   a. Completeness
   b. Clarity
   c. Conciseness
   d. Chronological order

Discussion Questions

1. Select one of the six Cs of charting and discuss why it is important to maintain accurate patient records.
2. Why is confidentiality regarding medical charting so difficult to maintain? Name three areas of concern in daily chart management that could lead to a loss of confidentiality, and discuss.
3. Discuss the procedures for releasing medical records.

Critical Thinking Questions

1. A patient wants to take his medical records and x-rays to another physician's office. He insists that the records belong to him. How would you handle this situation?
2. Identify the elements of SOAP charting for the following scenario: A patient has come to see the doctor complaining of asthma. She says she has been wheezing and coughing for two days. The patient's vital signs are P–102, B/P–146/100, R–28, T–98.6. Following examination, the physician determines the patient is having an asthma attack. She gives you an order to give the patient a breathing treatment using the nebulizer and 2.5 mg of albuteral sulfate. Then you are to take her vital signs again.

Application Activities

1. After reading the following description of a patient's condition, list the patient's signs and symptoms.

   A 72-year-old man with no history of gastrointestinal problems was complaining of fatigue, back pain, appetite loss, and nausea. The patient had a hemoglobin of about 7 g, indicating marked anemia. His blood pressure was low (95/70), his heartbeat erratic—from 55 to 85 bpm—and his white blood cell count elevated.

   While in the office he experienced a headache and ringing in his right ear. A CT scan taken the next day revealed an abdominal aortic aneurysm containing a large clot. The scan also revealed a small lesion in the lining of the stomach.

2. Role-play in groups of three students. One student should play the patient, one the medical assistant, and one the observer. Role-play a scenario in which the patient requests to have her medical records released to another physician.

The medical assistant should explain to the patient the process for the release of her medical records.

The observer should not speak but should observe and take notes on the scenario as acted out by the other two students. The observer should compare the scenario to the steps provided in the text for the release of records. Note what is done well and what needs improvement.

Each student should rotate through all three roles.

3. Photocopy the blank combination medical history and physical examination form shown in Figure 9-3. Fill out the form by using the following patient information:

For medical history section: Date: 2/14/07; the patient is Heather R. MacEntee, age 35, living at 344 Westwind Lane, Apartment 28, Round Tree, IL 60012; telephone (708) 333-5555. She is a real estate broker, married, with a 6-year-old child. Her father died at age 55; her mother is 62 and has congestive heart disease. She has no siblings. The family has a history of heart disease and diabetes. The patient had chickenpox and mumps at age 7 and surgery for an ovarian cyst at 22. She has an allergy to ragweed but is not taking any medications at present.

For physical examination section: Ms. MacEntee weighs 142 lb, is 5 ft 10 in tall, and her temperature and respiration are normal. Her pulse is 74, her blood pressure is 110/75, and her chest sounds are normal. Her chief complaint is discomfort in the area of the gallbladder. She has intense pain after eating. Blood tests are normal. The doctor's initial impression is suspected gallstones, and an ultrasound scan of the gallbladder is ordered. Treatment plan depends on the scan results.

4. Working in small groups, discuss which part of a medical record you consider to be the most important and why.

5. Go on the Internet and look up the *Medical Transcriptionists Bill of Rights* for discussion in your class.

Virtual Fieldtrip

Visit the McGraw-Hill Higher Education Medical Assisting website at www.mhhe.com/medicalassisting4e to complete the following activity:

The practice manager has asked you to research and make recommendations for improvement in maintaining patient records within the office. The goal is to save time and cost.

- Describe how you would evaluate the current system and the needs of the office.
- What website might you visit to get tips for smoother management and maintenance of patient records?
- Who might you invite to your office to assist you?

Open the CD and complete this chapter's practice activities, play the games, listen to the key terms, and test yourself with the interactive review. E-mail, print, and/or save your results to document your proficiency.

CHAPTER 10

Managing the Office Medical Records

LEARNING OUTCOMES

After completing Chapter 10, you will be able to:

10.1 Identify the equipment and supplies needed for the filing of medical records.

10.2 Describe the various types of filing systems.

10.3 Explain the benefits of each type of system.

10.4 Explain the advantages of color coding files.

10.5 Model how to set up and use a tickler file.

10.6 Use each of the five steps in the filing process.

10.7 Describe the steps to take in trying to locate a misplaced file.

10.8 Differentiate between the basic file storage options and the advantages of each.

10.9 Distinguish criteria for determining whether files should be retained, stored, or discarded.

MEDICAL ASSISTING COMPETENCIES

CAAHEP COMPETENCIES

V. C (5) Identify systems for organizing medical records

V. C (6) Describe various types of content maintained in a patient's medical record

V. C (7) Discuss pros and cons of various filing methods

V. C (8) Identify both equipment and supplies needed for filing medical records

V. C (9) Describe indexing rules

V. C (10) Discuss filing procedures

V. P (3) Organize a patient's medical record

V. P (4) File medical records

V. P (8) Maintain organization by filing

V. A (1) Consider staff needs and limitations in establishment of a filing system

VII. C (7) Describe how guidelines are used in processing insurance claims

ABHES COMPETENCIES

7. **Basic Keyboarding/Computer Concepts**
   a. Perform basic keyboarding skills including:
      2) Typing medical correspondence and basic reports
   b. Identify and properly utilize office machines, computerizes systems and medical software such as:
      1) Efficiently maintain and understand different types of medical correspondence and medical reports
      2) Apply computer application skills using a variety of different electronic programs including both practice management software and EMR software

8. **Medical Office Procedures Management**
   b. Prepare and maintain medical records
   d. Apply concepts for office procedures

11. **Career Development**
    Demonstrate professionalism by:
    3) Maintaining confidentiality at all times
    4) Being cognizant of ethical boundaries
    9) Conducting work within scope of education, training, and ability

MEDICAL ASSISTING MEDIA

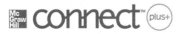 **Connect Plus+™**
connect.mcgraw-hill.com

- Electronic Health Records (E.H.R.) SpringCharts®
- eBook

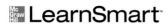 SpringCharts® Electronic Health Records

 LearnSmart™   www.mhhe.com/learnsmart   Complete Learning Module: Managing the Office Medical Records

Student CD-ROM

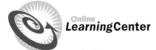 **Online Learning Center™**   www.mhhe.com/medicalassisting4e

KEY TERMS

active file	inactive file	out guide	terminal digit
alphabetic filing system	indexing	records management system	tickler file
closed file	indexing rules		unit
compactible file	lateral file	retention schedule	vertical file
cross-referenced	middle digit	sequential order	
file guide	numeric filing system	tab	

CHAPTER OUTLINE

- The Importance of Records Management
- Filing Equipment
- Filing Supplies
- Filing Systems
- The Filing Process
- Inactive and Closed File Storage

PREPARATION FOR CERTIFICATION

RMA (AMT) Exam
- Medical records management
- Protect, store, and retain medical records according to HIPAA regulations

CMA (AAMA) Exam
- Maintaining confidentiality
- Filing guidelines
- Needs, purposes, and terminology of filing systems

CMAS Exam
- Procedures

Introduction

The role of the medical assistant is both clerical and clinical in nature. The most important clerical function is the careful management of the patient chart, or record. The management of these individual files is vital to the care of each patient and to the smooth operation of the medical office.

In this chapter you will learn about various options for handling large volumes of patient records. As you work through this chapter, you will begin to have an appreciation for the very important task of records management, and you will develop an organized approach to maintaining these critical files. As you read, watch for helpful tips that teach you how to locate and access patient records quickly and efficiently.

CASE STUDY

It is the new calendar year and time to update the patient files. The office manager explains that the law in this state requires that all medical offices maintain patient records, or charts, for *seven years* from the last medical treatment or consult. The charts of current patients, of patients who have contacted the office within the last year, or of patients who have an unpaid balance are kept in the front of the office for easy access. Added to the front of each current chart will be a new sticker that indicates the new calendar year; the new sticker is placed directly on top of the previous year's sticker.

All other charts will be moved to a separate chart storage room, organized alphabetically, and grouped according to the last year in which there was contact with the patient. These older charts must remain readily available in case:

- The patient returns to the practice
- Records are subpoenaed by a court of law
- Records are requested for a medical history

The office manager reminds the staff that all original charts belong to the physician who owns the practice. Copies can be made *only* when the patient signs a release authorizing the distribution to another party. When copies are made, a notation must be added to the chart that copying occurred and the date. In this state, even with a subpoena, physicians must have patient permission to release records to the court. Originals are *never* taken out of the medical office.

At this same time, the staff will purge the chart room and shred the oldest charts. All charts that have had no activity in the last eight years will be either pulled apart and shredded in a shredding machine in the office or picked up by a local company that will shred the documents for the physician. It is essential, the office manager points out, that all documents be shredded, not just thrown away, in order to guard the confidential content of the documents.

As you read this chapter, consider the following questions:
1. What are advantages and disadvantages of different file systems?
2. What security measures might be used to protect patient files?
3. What is a tickler system and how is it set up?
4. Identify several storage options for closed charts. Which is the most secure? The easiest? The most cost-efficient?

The Importance of Records Management

The information contained in the patient medical records is the most valuable information in a medical office. For a practice to operate smoothly and efficiently, it is critical that these records be organized in a way that makes them easily retrievable. Maintaining a well-organized, easy-to-use records management system is essential to providing good patient care. The **records management system** refers to the way patient records are created, filed, and maintained.

The management of medical records is divided into two parts: (1) paper-based medical records (most of the information is on paper; however, some of the information such as payment information and billing is maintained on the computer); most medical offices still maintain paper-based records; and (2) the electronic health record (EHR), also known as the electronic medical record (EMR), where the entire record is stored on a database in the computer. When using an EHR, make sure that you discuss electronic signatures with office staff as well as the physician.

The office policies and procedures manual should include guidelines for the use of electronic signatures.

Electronic signatures are built into the software with safeguards, and accepted by HIPAA provided that the software validates identity, validates that it has not been altered in any way, and provides that the user cannot later deny the electronic signature. There are several electronic medical record software vendors . . . choose a reputable vendor.

HIPAA and the Medical Record

The primary purpose of HIPAA is to provide patients with more control over their health information. Chapter 3 provides a detailed account of the disclosure, privacy, managing, storage, and sharing of the patient's health information. For further information, visit www.hhs.gov/ocr/hipaa.

Filing Equipment

Filing equipment generally refers to the place where records, or files, are housed. Although there are various types of equipment, two of the most common options are

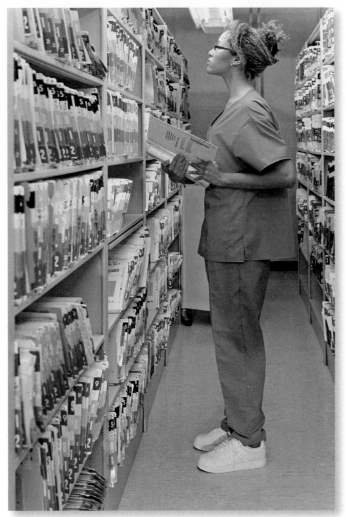

Figure 10-1. Files kept on shelves are easily accessible.

shelves and cabinets. The choice of whether to use filing shelves or filing cabinets is often made according to space considerations and personal preference.

Filing Shelves

Files can be kept on shelves, which resemble traditional shelves, as shown in Figure 10-1. Files are stacked upright on the shelves in filing containers such as boxes or large heavy-duty envelopes. Some shelf systems have doors that slide from side to side or above or below the files. These doors can be locked for security. Other shelf systems have no front covers. Some rolling file units are on wheels for ease of transporting a shelf system easily. Filing shelves are often long, sometimes extending the full length and height of an office wall or room. An advantage of keeping files on shelves is that it allows several people to retrieve and return files at the same time.

Filing Cabinets

Filing cabinets are sturdy pieces of office furniture, usually made of metal or wood. They contain a series of pullout drawers in which files are hung. Filing cabinets, unlike shelves, are best used by one person at a time because the drawer setup provides limited maneuvering room. In addition, cabinets require more floor space than filing shelves. About twice the depth of the file drawer is needed to allow it to fully open.

Although shelves are horizontal by design, filing cabinets can stand vertically or horizontally. A **vertical file** features pullout drawers that usually contain a metal frame or bar equipped to handle letter-size or legal-size documents. Hanging file folders are hung on this frame, with identifying names facing out. Vertical files may have two, three, four, or six drawers.

Horizontal filing cabinets, called **lateral files,** often feature doors that flip up and pullout drawers. Files are arranged with sides facing out. Lateral files require more wall space but do not extend as far into the room as vertical file drawers.

Compactible Files

Some offices have limited space in which to house filing cabinets or shelves. These offices may choose to use a variation of shelf filing, called compactible files. **Compactible files** are kept on rolling shelves that slide along permanent tracks in the floor.

When not in use, these files can be stored close together—even one on top of another—to conserve space. When needed, they can be rolled out into an open area so that the staff can easily use them. Compactible files can be moved manually or automatically with the touch of a button.

Rotary Circular Files

Rotary circular files are another option to consider when space is limited. These files are stored in a circular fashion, similar to a revolving door, and are accessed by rotating the files. They also can be operated either manually or electronically.

Plastic or Cardboard Tubs or Boxes

Files may be suspended in hanging files in plastic or cardboard file boxes. While this system may be adequate for a small number of files, the system is less efficient for larger numbers of files because it would require numerous boxes.

Tubs or boxes resemble open drawers. They may have a lid or be open. When not in use, all tubs or boxes must be locked in a secure storage area to protect patient confidentiality. Additionally, open tubs or boxes collect dust and are inappropriate for storage in a dirty warehouse storage area. All tubs or boxes must be stored off the floor, either on shelves or on platforms, to avoid water damage. This is a TJC requirement and is routinely checked during a survey.

Tubs or boxes are often stacked to save space, which can make it very difficult to locate files. TJC also requires that nothing be stacked within 18 inches of the ceiling. Tubs and boxes appear portable, but are usually very heavy once filled. Care should be taken to avoid injury when moving these files.

Labeling Filing Equipment

Regardless of which type of filing equipment your office uses, files should be clearly labeled on the outside of the drawer so that you do not have to open doors or drawers to know the contents. Labeling allows you to go directly to the appropriate place when retrieving a file. When labeling boxes, write on the top and on the front of the box with a permanent marker. Because labels fall off with time, writing directly on the box minimizes the chances that the labeling will be lost or unreadable. The label lists the range of files the drawer or shelf contains. For example, if the drawer includes all the files of patients whose last names begin with the letters A, B, C, and D, the drawer should be labeled "A–D."

Security Measures

All filing equipment must be secured to protect the confidentiality of medical records. *Never* place patient records in an unsecured filing system.

Most filing cabinets come with a lock and key. To protect filing shelves in a separate room, you can lock the file room. Security of the keys to that room then becomes an important issue. The number of staff members who have keys to that room should be limited—perhaps just the head doctor and the office manager. Every staff member does not need a key to the filing equipment. When the office manager comes into the office each morning, she can unlock the files. Because the files remain open during the day, it is important to make sure they are not placed in areas where unauthorized people can obtain access to them. Posting a sign on the file room door stating "Authorized Personnel Only" helps ensure that files remain secure. To ensure office security after hours, some practices install alarm systems.

Keys and locks bring a measure of security only when they are *used*. Many office staff become lazy and routinely overlook locking file rooms and cabinets. Security survey teams will always ask to see the keys to any locked door or cabinet and ask the staff to demonstrate that they work. Within a medical office, conducting regular security drills at the same time that fire drills are held will aid staff in staying sharp and aware of security risks.

Ergonomics

Ergonomics is the science of adjusting the elements of the working environment to the human body. Simply stated, it means making things around you (in your working environment) comfortable and efficient—especially for your posture. As a medical assistant, your work activities should be positioned so that you maintain healthy and safe posture. By doing this, your muscular forces will not be overexerted. By not overexerting yourself, you significantly reduce risk of injury to your body.

Common causes of workplace injury include

- Improper lifting
- Repetitiveness in body movement
- Being struck by an object
- Injuries caused by slipping and bending

Proper body mechanics can assist with preventing injuries from repetitive motion or overexertion. Here are some points that will assist you daily as a medical assistant:

- Place a footstool next to the patient's examining table so the patient can step up before sitting on the table.
- Take a brief course in proper lifting procedures.
- Make sure you have good lighting in the hallways to prevent falls.
- Wear proper shoes (do not wear slippery shoes in a medical facility).
- In selecting storage and shelving, make sure you purchase products that will assist in eliminating or minimizing muscular strain.

Equipment Safety

Safety is an important consideration for filing systems. For example, opening more than one drawer in a vertical file

---

Reflecting On . . . HIPAA

Safeguarding Protected Health Information

HIPAA law requires that every covered entity have appropriate safeguards to ensure the protection of the patient's confidential health information. Safeguards include administrative, technical, and physical measures of protection. These measures must provide a "reasonable safeguard" for protected health information from any disclosure that violates HIPAA law, whether intentional or unintentional. The use of locked, fireproof filing cabinets to store patient paper records is an important element of providing a physical safeguard for records. Computer equipment that stores electronic patient records should also be kept secure through these physical measures.

cabinet at the same time may cause it to fall forward. If the bottom drawer in a vertical file is left open, someone can easily trip over it. Shelves can be dangerous if staff members need to climb a ladder to retrieve files from the highest level.

Safety guidelines for each piece of equipment should be posted prominently in the office. Make sure that every staff member knows where the rules are posted. Then, make sure that everyone follows the rules to prevent possible injury.

Purchasing Filing Equipment

You may never be involved in the purchase of filing equipment because most medical offices already have filing systems in place. Occasionally, however, you may be responsible for setting up an office's filing system—for example, if your practice opens a new office. You may also need to buy equipment as the number of patients in the practice grows.

In either case, you will need to determine where to position the files. When purchasing filing cabinets or shelves, you need to determine how much office space is available for files. This information, along with the number of file folders to be included, will help you figure out how many cabinets or shelves to purchase. An office supply store or office supply catalog can provide you with a list of available products. Keep in mind also, that many offices now purchase filing equipment that is fireproof as additional security and protection of the personal health information contained within patient records.

Filing Supplies

Once you have chosen your filing equipment, the next step is selecting filing supplies. Figure 10-2 features an assortment of filing supplies commonly used by medical practices.

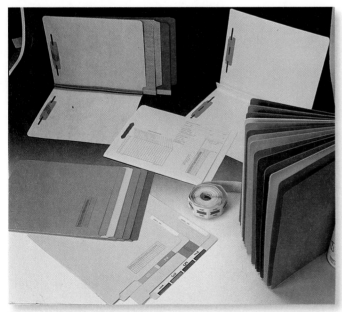

Figure 10-2. Medical offices use a wide variety of filing supplies.

File Folders

The most basic filing supply is the file folder, often referred to as a manila folder. This folder is made of heavy paper folded in half to form a pocket that can hold papers. File folders come in two sizes: letter size, which is 8½ by 11 inches, and legal size, which is 8½ by 14 inches.

Tabs. An important feature of file folders is the **tab,** the tapered rectangular or rounded extension at the top or side of the folder. Tabs may extend the full length of the folder, as with straight-cut folders, but they are usually cut to extend partway across a folder.

Using folders with a variety of tab cuts makes it easier to read the names on the tabs. One common type of folder is the third-cut folder. Tabs are one-third the width of the folder and appear at the left, center, or right side. Fourth-cut tabs are smaller. Tabs extend one-fourth the width of the folder and occupy one of four positions—left, left-center, right-center, or right.

Labels. The tabs on file folders are used to identify the contents of the individual folder. You can write directly on the tab area in pen or pencil. When creating a label manually, it is critical that each label be printed very clearly. A more desirable option is typing or printing a label and affixing it to the tab. This method is consistently easier to read and lends a more professional appearance. Printing labels can be easier from label templates that are available at any office supply store. These templates allow you to use a word processing program, such as Microsoft Word, to create several neatly printed labels at once or one at a time. Tabs should be covered with transparent tape to prevent smudging.

No matter what filing system your office uses, it is important to be consistent in preparing file labels. If all the files are labeled with the patient's last name, followed by the patient's first name and middle initial (for example, Brown, Emma L.), you should not prepare a label for a new folder giving the patient's name in a different order (for example, James P. Regan). Each member of a family must have a separate file.

File Jackets

File folders cannot be suspended inside filing cabinet drawers. File folders must be placed inside file jackets, or hanging file folders. These jackets resemble file folders, but feature metal or plastic hooks on both sides at the top, which hook onto the metal bars inside the drawers. Like file folders, jackets come in letter and legal size.

Plastic tabs, either colored or clear, and blank inserts are supplied to identify the contents of hanging file folders. The information is typed or printed on the insert and placed in the plastic tab, which is inserted into the hanging file folder. All inserts should be prepared in a consistent and legible style.

File Guides

To identify a group of file folders in a file drawer, you may use **file guides,** which are heavy cardboard or plastic inserts. For example, if a drawer contains the files for patients whose last names begin with the letters A through C, the guides might separate A from B and B from C.

Out Guides

Another filing supply is an **out guide.** An out guide is a marker made of stiff material. It is used as a placeholder when a file has been removed from the filing system. Some out guides include pockets that can hold the name of the file that belongs in that place or the name of the individual who took the file, and its due date for return. On another type of out guide, you can write the information on the out guide and cross it out when the file is returned. Out guides can be used for both shelf and cabinet filing.

Although out guides are not essential, they are extremely helpful in ensuring that files are returned to their proper places. Out guides also save the time and effort necessary to go through files to determine where a particular file belongs. Out guides work well when the entire staff, including the physicians, makes a dedicated effort to use the system.

File Sorters

File sorters are large envelope-style folders with tabs in which files can be stored temporarily. File sorters are used to hold patient records that will be returned to the files during the day or at the end of the day. The sorters help keep files in order and prevent them from being lost.

Binders

Some offices keep patient records in three-ring binders rather than in file folders. The binders are labeled on the outside spine. Documents are three-hole-punched and then placed inside the binder. Tab sheets are used to separate individual records. A binder can conveniently hold many records.

Binders are stronger than a file folder but require more storage space and so may not be functional for most medical offices. Inactive patient records can be transferred to a file folder for off-premise storage. The binder can then be used again. Binders are especially effective in the management of active patient records.

Purchasing Filing Supplies

Although you may never have to buy filing equipment, buying filing supplies may be one of your regular responsibilities as a medical assistant. (See Chapter 8 for a discussion of how to manage office supplies.)

Filing Systems

A filing system is a method by which files are organized. Any of a variety of filing systems may be used, but every system places patient records in some sort of **sequential order**—one after another in a pattern, or sequence, that can be predicted. It is important to find out which filing system your office is using and to follow it exactly. Any deviation can result in lost or misplaced records. Never make any changes in the filing system without first consulting the doctors and other staff members in the practice.

A very common filing system for maintaining patient files in sequential order is the alphabetic system. It is simple and easy to use.

Alphabetic

In the **alphabetic filing system,** files are arranged in alphabetic order (last name, first name, middle initial), as shown in Figure 10-3. Files are labeled with the patient's last name first, followed by the first, or given, name and the middle initial.

There are specific rules to follow when filing personal names alphabetically. These rules are called **indexing**

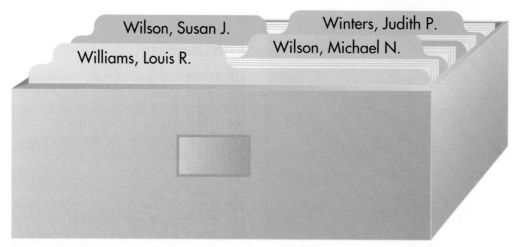

Figure 10-3. Many medical practices file patient records according to the alphabetic filing system.

TABLE 10-1 Rules for Alphabetic Filing of Personal Names

In alphabetizing, treat each part of a patient's name as a separate unit, and look at the units in this order: last name, first name, middle initial, and any subsequent names or initials. Disregard punctuation.

Name	Unit 1	Unit 2	Unit 3	Unit 4
Stephen Jacobson	JACOBSON	STEPHEN		
Stephen Brent Jacobson	JACOBSON	STEPHEN	BRENT	
B.T. Jacoby	JACOBY	B	T	
C. Bruce Hay Jacoby	JACOBY	C	BRUCE	HAY
D. Jones	JONES	D		
David Jones	JONES	DAVID		
Kwong Kow Ng	NG	KWONG	KOW	
Philip K. Ng	NG	PHILIP	K	

Treat a prefix, such as the O' in O'Hara, as part of the name, not as a separate unit. Ignore variations in spacing, punctuation, and capitalization. Treat prefixes—such as De La, Mac, Saint, and St.—exactly as they are spelled.

Name	Unit 1	Unit 2	Unit 3	Unit 4
A. Serafino Delacruz	DELACRUZ	A	SERAFINO	
Victor P. De La Cruz	DELACRUZ	VICTOR	P	
Irene J. MacKay	MACKAY	IRENE	J	
Walter G. Mac Kay	MACKAY	WALTER	G	
Kyle N. Saint Clair	SAINTCLAIR	KYLE	N	
Peter St. Clair	STCLAIR	PETER		

Treat hyphenated names as a single unit. Disregard the hyphen.

Name	Unit 1	Unit 2	Unit 3	Unit 4
Victor Puentes-Ruiz	PUENTESRUIZ	VICTOR		
Jean-Marie Vigneau	VIGNEAU	JEANMARIE		

A title, such as Dr. or Major, or a seniority term, such as Jr. or 3d, should be treated as the last filing unit, to distinguish names that are otherwise identical.

Name	Unit 1	Unit 2	Unit 3	Unit 4
Dr. George B. Diaz	DIAZ	GEORGE	B	DR
Major George B. Diaz	DIAZ	GEORGE	B	MAJOR
James R. Foster Jr.	FOSTER	JAMES	R	JR
James R. Foster Sr.	FOSTER	JAMES	R	SR
Sister Theresa	SISTER	THERESA		

Source: Adapted from William A. Sabin, *The Gregg Reference Manual*, 10th ed. (Columbus, OH: Glencoe/McGraw-Hill, 2005)

rules (Table 10-1). Indexing rules are rules used as guidelines for the sequencing of files based on current business practice. They define a consistent method for the ordering of filed materials. The Association of Records, Managers, and Administrators monitors and updates these suggested methods periodically. In this way, the best, most efficient management of paper records is continually being reevaluated for maximum outcomes. From time to time, individual medical practices may choose to deviate from some of these accepted practices. However, indexing rules are generally the norm for most medical practice filing systems.

Indexing rules define each separate part of a person's name or title as a **unit.** Indexing rules then describe the order to display and manage each unit in an alphabetized system.

Indexing rules are designed to keep alphabetizing simple. Although the alphabetic system is simple, you must know the exact spelling of a patient's name to retrieve a file. You must also know the rules of indexing.

Points on Practice

Indexing Rules

Rule 1: Individual Names

The (last name) is the first indexing unit, the (first name) is the second unit, and the (middle name) is the third unit. If an initial is used instead of a name, the single initial is viewed as the entire unit.

Name	Unit 1	Unit 2	Unit 3	Unit 4
D. Jones	Jones	D.		
David Jones	Jones	David		
David R. James Jones	Jones	David	R.	James

Rule 2: Business Names

As written (on letterhead); each word is a unit. If "The" is used as the first word, it is considered the last unit.

Name	Unit 1	Unit 2	Unit 3	Unit 4
Jones Hearing Supplies	Jones	Hearing	Supplies	
The Jones Hearing Supplies	Jones	Hearing	Supplies	The

Rule 3: Hyphenation and Abbreviations

All hyphenated names are considered to be one unit (i.e., Terry-Jones, Sheila); an abbreviated name is combined to form the unit. An abbreviated name such as Wm. for William is filed as Wm without the use of a period.

Name	Unit 1	Unit 2	Unit 3
Terry-Jones, Sheila	Terryjones	Sheila	
St. Mary, William	Stmary	William	
St. Mary, Wm.	Stmary	Wm	

Rule 4: Titles and Seniority Terms

Titles are normally disregarded unless they are used to distinguish between two patients with the same name. If there are patients with the same name and a title precedes the name, use as a fourth unit. Seniority terms such as Jr. or Sr. may be indexed as a last unit. It is important to remember that if a male child has exactly the same name as his father, he is considered Jr. until his father dies. He is a "III" if his father and his grandfather have the same name.

If II or III is used as a seniority title, the basic rule states that numbers come before letters, so David Jones, III would be filed before David Jones, Jr.

Name	Unit 1	Unit 2	Unit 3	Unit 4
David Jones Jr.	Jones	David	Jr.	
David Jones Sr.	Jones	David	Sr.	
David C. Jones	Jones	David	C.	
Rev. David C. Jones	Jones	David	C.	Rev.

Rule 5: Prefixes

If the last name has as a prefix such as Mc, Van, or de, the prefix is part of the last name. It starts the first indexing unit. The prefixes Mc and Mac are usually filed in regular order.

Name	Unit 1	Unit 2	Unit 3
Elias De Longino	Delongino	Elias	
Drew MacDreamy	MacDreamy	Drew	
Drew McDreamy	McDreamy	Drew	
Elias D. van Collins	vanCollins	Elias	D.

Rule 6: Names of Married Women

A woman may retain her maiden name as her last name instead of taking her husband's surname, or she may use both names and hyphenate them (see hyphenation). She will always keep her first and middle name as part of her original name. A married woman's name may take several forms.

Name	Unit 1	Unit 2	Unit 3
Mrs. Gisele M. Monagan-Jones	Monagan Jones	Gisele	M.
Mrs. David (Cindy M.) Jones	Jones	Cindy	M.
Mrs. Gisele Marie Jones	Jones	Gisele	Marie

Rule 7: Identical Names

If two names are identical, make sure you index them first under their names; location is next (city is the first unit, state is the second unit, street is the third unit; and street number from lowest to highest. This rule is for businesses as well as individuals.

Chronological Filing

A chronological filing system is based on dates. Chronological filing is a type of numeric arrangement that uses numeric dates as the indexing units. The most common order of units is year, month, and day, as in 12-11-06 to denote the sixth of November, 2012. It is also common practice to order the most current dates first.

In a medical practice, filing chronologically is one method used to file documents *within* a patient's chart. The most recent files (by dates) are inserted so they are on top of the documents that are dated prior to these more current dates in the file folder.

Numeric

A **numeric filing system** organizes files by numbers instead of by names. In this system each patient name is assigned a number. New patients are assigned the next unused number in sequence. Then, instead of being filed by name, the files are arranged in numeric order—1, 2, 3, 4, and so on. The resulting files are sequential by the order in which patients have come to the practice.

Only the numbers are indicated on the files. Patient names are recorded elsewhere. Such a system is often used when patient information is highly confidential—as in the case of HIV-positive patients—and patients' identities need to be protected, as well as in large offices where alphabetic filing systems become too cumbersome.

The numeric system can be expanded to indicate the location of files. For example, if the last three numbers represent the patient's number, the number 113306 may represent the file of the 306th patient, which can be found in the eleventh filing cabinet in the third drawer.

A numeric system must include a master list of patients' names and corresponding numbers. To ensure confidentiality, the office manager should keep the list in a secure place. The physician should hold a duplicate copy, which must also be kept under lock and key. Since folders are filed in numeric order, it should not be necessary for other staff members to have this list.

To find a patient's file number using a computer system, a staff member might input a password or access code, and then type in the first three letters of the patient's last name. If the patient's last name were Mulligan, for example, the staff member would type in Mul. The computer would then show all patients whose last names begin with Mul. The staff member would scroll the names, find the patient, highlight the patient name, and hit the "Enter" key. The computer would then give the number of the patient's chart.

Terminal digit filing is often used in conjunction with a general numerical system and allows for an endless number of files with minimal amount of searching to obtain the correct files. Numbers are assigned in small groups of two or three numbers, similar to a social security number, and are read from right to left. Filing is done numerically, starting with the lowest number and moving to the highest, according to the last group of numbers. For example, all files ending in 00 are filed first. They are then followed by files ending in 01, etc.

Middle digit filing is similar to terminal digit filing. Middle digit filing uses the middle group of numbers as the primary index.

Numeric, terminal digit, and middle digit filing can all be used in combination with color coding to add even more information to the filing system.

Color Coding

Color coding is used when there is a need to distinguish files within a filing system. For example, you may wish to find at a glance all the office's new patients, all patients on Medicare, or all patients whose last names begin with the letters WI. Coding by color can help you do so quickly and easily.

Patient records can be color-coded in a variety of ways. File folders are available in a range of colors, as are filing labels, plastic tabs, and stickers.

Using Classifications. To make the best use of color, you must first identify the classifications that are important to your office. For example, is it important to be able to identify all new patients easily? (A new patient is a patient who has never been seen in the practice or has not been seen at the practice in 3 years.) Once you select the classifications, choose a different color for each.

Then file the information by color, within the filing system. For example, all new patients may be kept in red folders, or you can attach a red sticker or red filing label to the folders.

An example of a typical color-coding system might be based on a combination of patient factors. The records of patients under the age of 18 might be color-coded blue. The records of patients over the age of 65 might be color-coded red. The records of patients who are insulin-dependent might be color-coded green. The records of patients who are hemophiliacs might be coded with a half-red/half-white sticker. In an emergency situation, as when a patient with diabetes passes out while in the office, the color coding could give staff quick and vital information at a glance.

After a color-coding system is finalized, the codes should be prominently posted on a chart in the file room so that all staff members are aware of them. This chart will help to ensure that records are filed correctly. Remember to update color-coded files consistently, coding new ones and revising older ones as a patient's status changes.

Using Color in an Alphabetic Filing System. One way to use color-coded filing is in conjunction with an alphabetic filing system. After files are organized alphabetically, each letter of the alphabet is assigned a color. Then the first two letters of each patient's last name are color-coded, usually with colored tabs.

The colored tabs are attached to the top of straight-edged or tabbed file folders. For example, if the letter S is coded as light blue and the letter M is coded as light green, all names starting with SM—like Smith—would have light-blue and light-green colored tabs at the top of the folders.

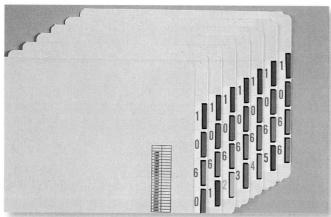

Figure 10-4. Color coding can make it easy to find a misfiled record.

The name Snyder would be filed under a different color combination, such as light blue (for S) and peach (for N). Because the colors will be the same in each segment of the file drawer, a color-coded system makes it easy to tell at a glance if files are filed correctly.

Using Color in a Numeric Filing System. Color can be used in a similar way with numeric systems. The numerals 1 to 9 may each be assigned a distinct color, as shown in Figure 10-4. Then, numerals 1, 21, 31, 41, and 51, for example, would share the same color in the ones place of their numeric designation.

As with the alphabetic system, color coding helps identify numeric files that are out of place. There are exceptions, however. For example, if a numeric system uses white stickers for the numeral 2 and red stickers for the numeral 3, the number 134 filed in place of 124 would be spotted immediately as a red sticker in a row of white, but the number 128 misfiled in the same spot could go unnoticed. To avoid this, most offices use color to identify the "key units" for each file. If the key unit is three numbers, then all three numbers of the key unit will use a colored tab to identify each file, not only two. Procedure 10-1 explains how to use your knowledge of alphabetic and numeric filing and color coding to set up a patient records system.

Tickler Files

To avoid losing track of important dates, many medical practices use tickler files. A **tickler file** is a date-ordered reminder file. Think of your home calendar; many of us write important activities on our home calendar, creating an informal tickler file for our personal activities. Any office activity that needs to be scheduled ahead of time can be noted and a reminder placed in the file. For example,

PROCEDURE 10-1

Creating a Filing System for Patient Records

Procedure Goal: To create a filing system that keeps related materials together in a logical order and enables office staff to store and retrieve files efficiently

Materials: Vertical or horizontal filing cabinets with locks, file jackets, tabbed file folders, labels, file guides, out guides, filing sorters

Method:

1. Evaluate which filing system is best for your office—alphabetic or numeric. Make sure the doctor approves the system you choose.

Rationale

The purpose of a filing system is to provide accessibility of all medical records for the entire staff.

2. Establish a style for labeling files, and make sure that all file labels are prepared in this manner. Place records for different family members in separate files.

3. Avoid writing labels by hand. Use a keyboard, a label maker, or preprinted adhesive labels.

4. Set up a color-coding system to distinguish the files (for example, use blue for the letters A–C, red for D–F, and so on). Create a chart, suitable to be hung in a professional file room, that indicates the color-coding system.

5. Use file guides to divide files into sections.

6. Use out guides as placeholders to indicate which files have been taken out of the system. Include a charge-out form to be signed and dated by the person who is taking the file.

Rationale

To quickly and easily identify a missing file and its location.

7. To keep files in order and to prevent them from being misplaced, use a file sorter to hold those patient records that will be returned to the files during the day or at the end of the day.

8. Develop a manual explaining the filing system to new staff members. Include guidelines on how to keep the system in good order.

PROCEDURE 10-2

Setting Up an Office Tickler File

Procedure Goal: To create a comprehensive office tickler file designed for year-round use

Materials: 12 manila file folders, 12 file labels, pen or typewriter, paper

Method:

1. Write or type 12 file labels, 1 for each month of the year. Abbreviations are acceptable. Do *not* include the current calendar year, just the month.

2. Affix one label to the tab of each file folder.

3. Arrange the folders so that the current month is on the top of the pile. Months should follow in chronological order.

4. Write or type a list of upcoming responsibilities and activities. Next to each activity, indicate the date by which the activity should be completed. Leave a column after this date to indicate when the activity has been completed. Use a separate sheet of paper for each month.

Rationale

Each sheet should clearly indicate when the activity has been completed and by whom. Each sheet should be filed within the appropriate month's folder.

5. File the notes by month in the appropriate folders.

Rationale

This will create a neat and orderly way to collect tickler notes for each month.

6. Place the folders, with the current month on top, in order, in a prominent place in the office, such as in a plastic box mounted on the wall near the receptionist's desk.

7. Check the tickler file at least once a week on a specific day, such as every Monday. Assign a backup person to check it in case you happen to be out of the office.

8. Complete the tickler activities on the designated days, if possible. Keep notes concerning activities in progress. Be sure to note when activities are completed and by whom.

Rationale

Keep a record of responsibilities and completed activities in case a question concerning the activity or responsibility comes up at a later date.

9. At the end of the month, place that month's file folder at the bottom of the tickler file. If there are notes remaining in that month's folder, move them to the new month's folder.

Rationale

Incomplete activities must be moved to the new month to be sure they are not overlooked.

10. Continue to add new notes to the appropriate tickler files.

Rationale

To provide for continual update to the tickler system.

---

reminders to order supplies or send patient checkup cards can be entered. When the task has been completed, the note can be crossed off the list or removed from the file and thrown away. Someone in the office should be assigned the responsibility of regularly checking the tickler files. Tickler files can be checked daily or, at a minimum, once a week. It is important to check tickler files frequently because they work only if they are used regularly.

You can organize tickler files in a variety of ways. The most common method, discussed in Procedure 10-2, is to allot one file folder to each month of the year. Tickler files can also be organized by day of the week or week of the month. This method is most useful if there are responsibilities that occur regularly on a certain day of the week or in a certain week within the month. If there are so many notes in a monthly folder that it becomes cumbersome to deal with, it may be best to organize weekly files.

Some offices keep their tickler files in three-ring binders, with tabs separating the months. Notes can be written on three-hole-punched sheets of paper, with pages added as needed. Binders offer essentially unlimited space.

Computers systems also offer tickler files in the form of a calendar. When the computer is turned on, it lists, for example, "Things to Do Today" with the tickler information posted for that date. Reminders can be set for tasks that must be done on a regular basis, such as daily, weekly, or monthly, or on a one-time basis.

Supplemental Files

Occasionally you may need to set up additional files to supplement the medical records filing system. For example, you may wish to keep some information separate from the primary file, such as older patient records or insurance information. You may also be asked to create temporary files, such as copies of patient records in the primary files. In these cases you set up supplemental files. Supplemental files allow you to keep this additional information about each patient without cluttering up the primary filing cabinets and without making it difficult to find information.

Supplemental files are usually created using the same system as the primary files, but they are kept in a different location. Depending on frequency of use, they may be stored in a less accessible, but equally secure area of the office. If you are keeping supplemental files, it is important to distinguish their content from that of the primary files. For example, you may decide that all information pertaining to certain subjects—such as patient diagnosis and treatment—will be kept in the primary files and that all other information—such as insurance company payments for each patient—will be kept in the supplemental files. This designation will help you and other office staff members know exactly where to go to retrieve specific information.

The Filing Process

Pulling and filing patient records and filing individual documents may be among your responsibilities as a medical assistant. Some practices require that records be returned to the files as soon as they are no longer in use. In other practices the timing is up to you. Still other offices schedule a specific time at the end of each day to file the current day's records and pull those for the next day.

Records waiting to be filed should be placed temporarily in a file return area, as shown in Figure 10-5. To protect patient privacy, this place should be in a secure area of the office. Clear rules should designate who may handle these files and under what conditions.

 ## How to File

Essentially, you will be filing three types of items: new patient record folders, individual documents that belong in existing patient record folders, and patient record folders that have previously been filed. There are five steps involved in filing: inspecting, indexing, coding, sorting, and storing.

Inspecting. The first step in the filing process is to make sure the item is ready to be filed. Inspect the document or patient record folder for a mark, notation, or stamp indicating that it is ready to be filed. For example, it may be initialed by the physician or stamped with the word *File* on a self-adhesive flag attached to the upper right corner. Some offices have staff members simply place folders ready for filing in a specially designated box or bin.

Remove paper clips, rubber bands, and any extraneous material that does not need to be filed. Staple loose papers to keep them together, per your specific office's protocol. Documents are less bulky when stapled than when held together by clips or rubber bands.

If the document to be filed is much smaller than standard size, it may become lost in the file or even fall

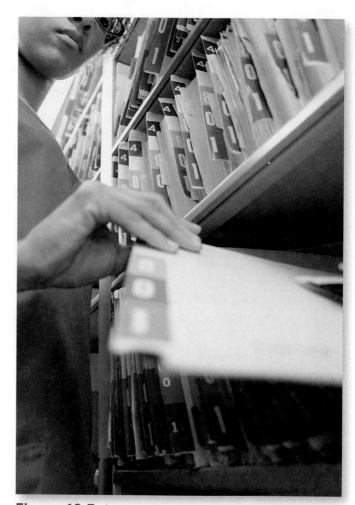

Figure 10-5. In some practices, patient records are filed once at the end of the day. Throughout the day, records are placed in a file sorter in a secure area of the office.

out. You may want to use special paper containing self-adhesive areas that allow for a smaller document to be attached to a standard size or even "shingling" the smaller document to save space and avoid its loss. If these are not available, tape or rubber cement may be used to attach it to a standard-size piece of paper before filing it within the folder. When small documents have wording on both sides of the paper, they can be placed in standard-size clear plastic envelopes and then filed.

Indexing. **Indexing** is another term for naming a file. Names should be chosen carefully because that is how the file will be known, retrieved, and replaced. Patient names are traditionally used as the file names for patient records.

If you are using a numeric system, you can assign a number instead of a name. Most offices that use a numeric system use computer software to create new patient charts and assign numbers. As part of the indexing process, color-code the file (if you use color coding in your system).

Note that some files can logically be placed in more than one location. Such files should be **cross-referenced** or filed in two or more places, with each place noted in each file. When cross-referencing a file, you may create a cross-reference form that gives the correct location to look for the file. For instance, an elderly woman might refer to herself as Mrs. John Smith. If you cannot remember her legal name, in the area where *Smith, John, Mrs.* would be located, you would place a mock folder that reads "Smith, John, Mrs., SEE Smith, Christine." You would then place the form under any heading where it is possible to look for that file. You may wish to attach it to a blank file, cutting the file folder in half so that no other documents are mistakenly filed in it.

Indexing can also be used as a step to ensure that folders are filed properly. You can take the opportunity to decide whether the name and color of the file folder are accurate or should be changed in any way.

Coding. Coding means to put an identifying mark or phrase on a document to ensure that it is placed in the correct file. To code a record, simply mark the patient's name, the number, or the subject title of the file folder. If appropriate, you can underline or highlight key words on the document itself. This step can be skipped when filing patient record folders that have previously been filed.

It is important to use a phrase or identifying code that anyone who will review the file can easily understand. Avoid medical jargon whenever possible because some terms may not be familiar to everybody. If you are unsure whether a code will be understood, attach a brief explanation to the front of the file folder for reference.

Sorting. If you have more than one folder to be filed, you must sort the files that have accumulated. Sort them in the order in which they are kept—such as alphabetically or numerically. Sorting saves you time later when you return the files to their proper places. If you will not be filing the folders immediately, store them in a temporary location, such as a file sorter. The final step in the filing process is to store the files in the appropriate filing equipment.

Storing. Documents should be stored neatly within their file folders in the proper sequence.

Careful attention to file storage will make your job easier. Make sure the folders are in good condition. Replace them whenever they appear damaged or torn to prevent file contents from spilling out during the retrieval and filing process. If a file contains too many documents, divide it into two or more folders, and label each one (for example, Glass, Ann M.—Folder 1 of 2; Glass, Ann M.—Folder 2 of 2). Also be sure when labeling records that consist of more than one chart that the content of each chart is clear (Folder 1 of 2, records prior to 2002; Folder 2 of 2, records from 2002 forward). Make sure to replace labels that are no longer legible.

Limiting Access to Files

Some offices restrict the number of people who can retrieve and return files. Limiting the number of people with access to the file room adds an extra measure of security to the practice. To obtain a file, staff members must fill out a requisition slip with their name and the name of the patient, as shown in Figure 10-6.

Springfield Medical Associates
Patient File Requisition Slip

Patient: _____
File Given to: _____
Date: _____
Time: _____
Due Back: _____

Figure 10-6. Some offices limit the personnel who have access to the file room. Staff members must fill out a requisition slip with their name and the name of the patient to obtain a patient record.

A record of who has the file is kept either in a notebook or on index cards in special boxes. The record includes the name of the file, the name of the borrower, the date the file was borrowed, and the date it is due back.

Under *no* circumstances should original patient medical records ever leave the practice. Photocopies can be made, if necessary. (Chapter 9 provides specific guidelines on releasing medical records to individuals and organizations outside your medical office.)

Filing Guidelines

There are specific rules for each filing system as well as general guidelines, or helpful hints, applicable to any system. Following these guidelines will help you file more efficiently.

- Each time you pull or file a patient record, glance at its contents. You should be familiar with the typical contents and the order of a patient record folder to help avoid filing errors.

- Keep files neat. Make sure that documents fit neatly into the file folders. Papers should not extend beyond the edge of the folder. Do not place too many papers in each file folder. Folders should be able to stay closed when laid on a flat surface.

- When inserting documents into folders already in place in the drawer, lift the folders up and out of the drawer; otherwise, this can lead to misfiling of documents. Attempting to force documents into a folder inside the drawer can damage the documents.

- Do not crowd the file drawer. Leave extra space to allow for leafing through the files and for retrieving and replacing files easily. Where possible, use a combination of uppercase and lowercase letters to label folders. This format is easier to read than labels written completely in capital letters.

- Choose file guides with a different tab position than your folders to help them stand out. Do not place guides so close together that they hide one another. A good rule of thumb is to position guides at least 5 inches apart.
- If you are unsure whether to cross-reference a file, do it. It is better to err on the side of providing too many cross-references than too few.
- File regularly so that you are not overwhelmed with too many folders to file.
- Store only files in filing cabinets or on filing shelves.
- Do not store office equipment or supplies where files belong.
- Train all staff members who will retrieve and replace files to make sure they have a thorough understanding of the system. Update them on any changes.
- Periodically evaluate your office's filing system. The Points on Practice section will help you with this task.

Locating Misplaced Files

Even in the best filing systems, there is a chance of temporarily misplacing or even losing patient medical records. No matter how good a system is, people still make errors. If a file is misplaced, here are steps you can take to try to locate it.

1. Determine the last time you or anyone else in the practice knew the file's location.
2. Go to that location, and retrace the steps of the last person who handled the file. Look for the file along the way.
3. Look in the filing cabinet where the file belongs. Check neighboring files. Possibly the file was simply put in the wrong place. Look inside other thicker files to determine if the missing file was accidentally placed inside another file.
4. Check underneath the files in the drawer or shelf to see if the file slipped out.
5. Check the pile of items to be filed or the file sorter envelope.
6. Consider possible cross-references or similar indexes (for example, similar patient names) for the file. Check those headings to see if the file was accidentally placed there.
7. Check with other staff members to determine if they have seen the file.
8. Check to make sure the missing file was not filed under the patient's *first* name instead of the last.
9. Stand back from the file cabinet and view the *top* of the folders looking at only the first three letters of the last names. A misfiled file will stand out.
10. If using a color-coded system, look for the color of the misfiled chart.
11. Even though files should always be kept in a secure area, occasionally individuals who are not part of the office staff, such as visiting physicians, may be in the area and may inadvertently pick up a file with their own materials. If you think someone could have taken the file, call the person immediately.
12. Ask another staff person to complete steps 1 through 7 to double-check your search.
13. Straighten the office, taking care to check through all piles of information where a file could be lodged.
14. Check those charts that have been pulled for next day's appointments to see if misplaced charts have been accidentally pulled.
15. Check the physician's desk.

If the misplaced file is not found within a reasonable time—24 to 48 hours—it may be considered lost. Losing a file has potentially devastating consequences. It may not be possible to duplicate the information within the file, but you can try to re-create it in a new file.

To do so, meet with the physician and office staff members to review the information needed. Record their recollections of information in the file. Note on the file document that it is a duplicate, and that the information is not official.

Then consult other office records that may include information related to the file. Contact insurance companies, laboratories, and other information providers for copies of original documents previously included in the lost file. Place copies of those records in the new file, or excerpt information. If the physician considers it appropriate, tell the patient whose file has been misplaced about its status and the steps you have taken to re-create it.

Active versus Inactive Files

At any given time, there are files that you use frequently and files that you use infrequently or not at all. Files that you use frequently are called **active files.** Files that you use infrequently are called **inactive files.** What constitutes an active, as opposed to an inactive, file? It depends on your individual practice. In a heart specialist's office, a patient who has not been seen for a year may be considered inactive, while in a dentist's office, a year may simply indicate one missed appointment.

There is a third category of files, called closed files. **Closed files** are files of patients who have died, have moved away, or for some other reason no longer consult the office. Although closed files could be moved immediately to storage, they are usually treated in the same manner as inactive files. That is, they are kept in the office for a certain length of time to make sure that there are no requests for the information in the file.

Medical records must be retained for 7 years; however, the Federal False Claims Act requires financial records be kept for 10 years. Because financial records and insurance claims must be backed up by the medical record, the American Health Information Management Association (AHIMA) and many legal experts are suggesting that medical records also be kept for 10 years instead of the legally required 7 years.

Evaluating Your Office Filing System

In a typical medical office, you retrieve and file documents daily using a filing system that may have been set up when the practice first opened. Now it is time to take a critical look at that system and determine how well it meets your needs.

The filing system you have probably does an adequate or better-than-average job of fulfilling the needs of the practice. Otherwise, retrieving and filing patient records would have become annoyingly inefficient. It is always beneficial to see where improvements can be made, however. Even a good filing system can be enhanced to increase office efficiency and save staff members valuable time.

Here are some simple guidelines for evaluating your filing system.

1. How well do you think your filing system meets your needs? Rate it on a scale of 1 to 10, with 10 representing the best. Survey staff members to determine their ratings, and calculate a composite number. *Based on this feedback, does your filing system seem to do a poor, adequate, or exceptional job?*

2. Note the type of system you use—for example, alphabetic or numeric. Then list the various reasons why files are retrieved from the system. *Would another system, a combination of systems (such as alphanumeric), or the addition of color coding save time or offer other benefits?*

3. Survey the office staff to determine whether there have been difficulties in retrieving or filing or problems with lost or misplaced files. Solicit suggestions for improvement. *If there have been problems, what steps could you take to avoid future difficulties?* (You might even ask your local office-supply representative for ideas.)

4. Consult personnel at other, similar medical practices to determine which filing system works for them. Compare and contrast their systems with yours. *How would their systems work in your office?*

Before making any major changes to your filing system, evaluate each idea in terms of the time and effort it will require and the benefits it will deliver. For example, changing from an alphabetic to a numeric system may provide a relatively small benefit to your office but require a great deal of time to prepare new files and refile current documents. In that case implementing a numeric system is probably not worthwhile.

If you do make changes to your system, make sure that all staff members are retrained on how to file documents. It is well worth the extra time required at the start to prevent having to locate misplaced files in the future.

The physician must determine when a patient file is deemed inactive or closed. You and the physician can meet regularly, perhaps once a month or once a quarter, to review these files.

Inactive and Closed File Storage

No office has unlimited space. Therefore, you may regularly need to transfer inactive and closed files from the office's filing area to a storage area.

Basic Storage Options

Before you can transfer files, you need to determine how and where they will be stored. The design and layout of file storage should make even older stored files easily accessible so that they can be periodically evaluated for retention or elimination.

There are many ways to store inactive files. For example, they can be stored in their original paper state or transferred into another format, such as onto a computer disk or tape or into microfilm or microfiche. Files can even be electronically coded with bar codes for immediate retrieval with a computer system. Regardless of the medium chosen for storing and preserving documents, keeping related material together and retrieving it should be made as easy as possible. Inactive files also must be kept secure, just as active ones are.

Paper Storage. If you choose to store files in their original form, you will be storing them as paper files. Paper files are often stored in boxes labeled with their contents. Choose boxes that are uniform in size so that they will stack well. Lift-off lids enable easy access to the contents of the box.

Paper files are bulky to store. They require roughly the same amount of space as they occupied in the office's primary files. Paper files preserve the original documents, however, and these documents can be important when providing evidence of medical treatment in legal proceedings. If paper files start to become brittle, they should be transferred to another storage medium.

Computer Storage.   If storage space is limited, there are a number of paperless options for storing files. Options include storing files on computer tapes, recordable CDs or DVDs, jump or flash drives, and external hard drives. To store records or information electronically, the office needs a computer system that can transfer documents to some type of electronic or digital format, and then read them when they are retrieved from storage. (See Chapter 6 for more information about using computers in the medical office.)

The easiest way to transfer documents directly into the computer is to use a scanner. This device copies a document onto the computer's hard drive. This process saves countless hours of rekeying (reentering) documents into the computer. Many scanners also have the capability of copying graphics and handwritten notes.

The document is then labeled and saved. When documents were originally created electronically on the computer, they can be similarly transferred to CD, DVD or tape, or external hard drive and then deleted from the computer's internal hard drive. CDs, DVDs, external hard drives, and tapes are dated and stored in file boxes or other containers.

Electronic documents are usually on the hard drive of the computer. However, the information should also be stored in a backup system in case the hard drive crashes and information is lost.

If documents are stored directly on the hard drive of the computer system, a variety of computer software programs will help in managing these records. This software checks files automatically using different criteria, such as the date the file was established or last updated. This software will help you make decisions about how long documents should be stored. When considering computer record management programs, look for user friendliness, speed and response time, and whether the features of the program meet your needs.

Microfilm, Microfiche, and Cartridges.   Other paperless storage options include microfilm, microfiche, and film cartridges. (Chapter 5 discusses these storage options.)

When considering transferring files to these formats, explore microfilm services, which index and transfer files for a fee. Using a service helps ensure that files are correctly indexed and thus easily found later on. Always have the microfilm service sign a confidentiality agreement.

Storage Facilities

You may wish to store files in a remote area of your office building, such as an unused closet or office. Check to make sure that the area is secure, accessible, and safe for storing files (for example, do not store files where hazardous materials are stored). The practice may have to pay additional rent if the space is not within the confines of its office suite.

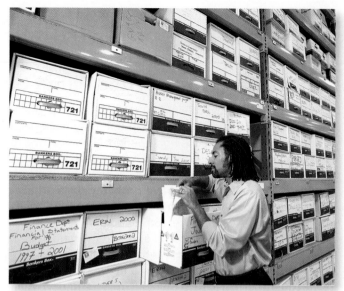

Figure 10-7. Commercial records centers manage stored documents for medical practices. Look for a center with personnel who retrieve and deliver boxes or files directly to your office.

If there is no space in the building, consider a neighboring building, perhaps one in the same office complex.

Many buildings rent space that can be used to store records. If you pursue this option, you will be responsible for managing the storage of records, including transporting them to the space, positioning them, and retrieving them as needed.

Certain storage facilities, called commercial records centers, will do some of the work for you (Figure 10-7). For a monthly fee, these centers typically house and manage stored documents. When evaluating commercial records centers, inquire about whether they will retrieve and/or deliver boxes or files and whether there is an on-site work area if someone needs to review the files at the storage location.

Beware of general storage facilities that are not specially equipped for document management. These facilities may not address safety concerns by taking precautions for fire or floods, for example.

Maintain a separate list of files stored off-site. This list can save a wasted trip to the storage site if a needed file is not housed there. The list also provides a valuable record if files are damaged or destroyed. Remember to update the list as new files are moved into storage and old files are taken out of storage and destroyed.

Storage Safety

No matter where you store files, you must consider the issue of safety as well as security. Paper, computer, and film files are easily damaged and destroyed by fire, water, and extreme temperatures. Old, brittle paper files are particularly susceptible. Therefore, it is wise to evaluate the storage site and to take some basic precautions.

- Choose a site with moderate temperatures year-round and adequate ventilation.
- Select storage containers that can withstand intense heat and are waterproof. When possible, use metal or plastic boxes that are designated as fireproof and waterproof. Cardboard boxes, although often used for storage, are not as strong or durable. If cardboard storage boxes are used, they need to be placed on shelving well off the floor to avoid water damage.
- Choose a site equipped with a smoke alarm, sprinkler system, and fire extinguishers.
- Select a site that is above ground and away from flood hazards. One way to find out if a site is susceptible to flooding is to inquire whether the facility has flood insurance, a requirement for sites at risk.
- Choose a site that is kept locked, is regularly patrolled, or has an alarm system, to prevent theft or vandalism.
- Remove old, brittle files as soon as possible, or transfer them into another format. They can then be placed in file storage again.
- Ask for references from people at other offices who have stored files at the site. Talk to these people about what they like and dislike about the storage facility and any problems they have had in storing or retrieving documents.
- If you are storing files in another form—on computer disk or microfiche—inquire about any special precautions the site owner takes to ensure safety.

Taking the time to thoroughly research storage options ultimately saves time and effort as you manage stored files.

Retaining Files in the Office

Every office will develop a length of time appropriate for the long-term storage of files. Most practices develop a records retention program.

Typically the doctor decides—based on the potential need for the information—how long to keep inactive or closed patient files in the office before sending them to storage. Working with the doctor, you should prepare a retention schedule. A **retention schedule** specifies how long to keep different types of patient records in the office after files have become inactive or closed. The schedule also details when files should be moved to a storage area and how long they should be kept in storage before being destroyed. The retention schedule should be posted in the file room to make certain that all staff members are aware of it.

Although the doctor decides how long to keep inactive or closed patient records in the office, there are legal requirements for retaining certain types of information, which determine how long these documents must be stored.

- According to the National Childhood Vaccine Injury Act of 1986, doctors must keep all immunization records on file in the office permanently. These records should not be put in storage.
- The Labor Standards Act states that doctors must keep employee health records for 3 years.
- The statute of limitations—the law stating the time period during which lawsuits may be filed—varies by state for civil suits. The most common length of time is 2 years. If a case involves a child or someone mentally incompetent, the statute of limitations extends the deadline. Regardless of the statute of limitations, it is always advisable for doctors to seek legal advice before destroying any records.
- Many legal consultants advise that doctors maintain patient records for at least 7 years to protect themselves against malpractice suits.
- The Internal Revenue Service usually requires doctors to keep financial records for up to 10 years. Doctors are required to keep medical records of minors previously under their care for 2 to 7 years after the child reaches legal age, depending on the state. Some doctors keep these records indefinitely.
- The American Medical Association, the American Hospital Association, and other groups generally suggest that doctors keep patient medical and financial records for up to 10 years after a patient's final visit or contact.

For the most updated and complete list of required record retention periods according to HIPAA law, go to the HIPAA advisory website (www.hhs.gov/ocr/hipaa). At this website you will also find a number of other federal recordkeeping laws that have specific record-keeping requirements.

This guide is updated annually. State and local retention requirements can be obtained from offices with which you regularly conduct business, such as insurance companies, state and local agencies, and medical associations. If you do business in more than one state, follow the schedule that requires the longest retention time for materials. Also, if your state's retention requirements are more stringent than HIPAA laws, follow your state's requirements.

When counting years in a retention schedule, remember not to count the year in which the document was produced but to begin counting with the following year. This way, documents produced near the end of a calendar year will be tracked more efficiently. Procedure 10-3 summarizes the steps for setting up a records retention program.

When records can finally be eliminated, they cannot simply be thrown away. Even old records hold confidential information about patients. Therefore, they must be completely destroyed by shredding. Be careful not to destroy records prematurely because they often cannot be re-created. It is vital that you retain a list of documents that have been destroyed.

Developing a Records Retention Program

Procedure Goal: To establish a records retention program for patient medical records that meets office needs as well as legal and government guidelines

Materials: Updated guide for record retention as described by federal and state law (go to the HIPAA Advisory website), file folders, index cards, index box, paper, pen or typewriter

Method:

1. List the types of information contained in a typical patient medical record in your office. For example, a file for an adult patient may include the patient's case history, records of hospital stays, and insurance information.

2. Research the state and federal requirements for keeping documents. Contact your appropriate state office (such as the office of the insurance commissioner) for specific state requirements, such as rules for keeping records of insurance payments and the statute of limitations for initiating lawsuits. If your office does business in more than one state, be sure to research all applicable regulations. Consult with the attorney who represents your practice.

3. Compile the results of your research in a chart. At the top of the chart, list the different kinds of information your office keeps in patient records. Down the left side of the chart, list the headings "Federal," "State," and "Other." Then, in each box, record the corresponding information.

4. Compare all the legal and government requirements. Indicate which one is for the longest period of time.

Rationale
Retaining all records for the longest period of time required by the laws governing your organization will assure that you are in compliance with all laws.

5. Meet with the doctor to review the information. Working together with the physician, prepare a retention schedule. Determine how long different types of patient records should be kept in the office after a patient leaves the practice and how long records should be kept in storage. Although retention periods can vary based on the type of information kept in a file, it is often easiest to choose a retention period that covers all records. For example, all records could be kept in the office for 1 year after a patient leaves the practice and then kept in storage for another 9 years, for a total of 10 years. Determine how files will be destroyed when they have exceeded the retention requirements. Usually, records are destroyed by paper shredding. Purchase the appropriate equipment, or contract with a shredding company as necessary.

Rationale
Shredding complies with HIPAA privacy rules regarding protected health information (PHI).

6. Put the retention schedule in writing, and post it prominently near the files. In addition, keep a copy of the schedule in a safe place in the office. Review it with the office staff.

7. Develop a system for identifying files easily under the retention system. For example, for each file deemed inactive or closed, prepare an index card or create a master list containing the following information:

   - Patient's name and Social Security number
   - Contents of the file
   - Date the file was deemed inactive or closed and by whom
   - Date the file should be sent to inactive or closed file storage (the actual date will be filled in later; if more than one storage location is used, indicate the exact location to which the file was sent)
   - Date the file should be destroyed (the actual date will be filled in later)

   Have the card signed by the doctor and by the person responsible for the files. Keep the card in an index box or another safe place. This is your authorization to destroy the file at the appropriate time.

8. Use color coding to help identify inactive and closed files. For example, all records that become inactive in 2008 could be placed in green file folders or have a green sticker with 08 placed on them and moved to a supplemental file. Then, in January 2010, all of these files could be pulled and sent to storage.

9. One person should be responsible for checking the index cards once a month to determine which stored files should be destroyed. Before

continued ⟶

PROCEDURE 10-3

Developing a Records Retention Program *(concluded)*

retrieving these files from storage, circulate a notice to the office staff stating which records will be destroyed. Indicate that the staff must let you know by a specific date if any of the files should be saved. You may want to keep a separate file with these notices.

10. After the deadline has passed, retrieve the files from storage. Review each file before it is destroyed. Make sure the staff members who will destroy the files are trained to use the equipment properly. Develop a sheet of instructions for destroying files. Post it prominently with the retention schedule, near the machinery used to destroy the files.

Rationale

To guard patient confidentiality and follow all HIPAA laws governing the protection of patient information.

11. Update the index card, giving the date the file was destroyed and by whom.

12. Periodically review the retention schedule. Update it with the most current legal and governmental requirements. With the staff, evaluate whether the current schedule is meeting the needs of your office or whether files are being kept too long or destroyed prematurely. With the doctor's approval, change the schedule as necessary.

Career Opportunities

Registered Health Information Technician

To gain medical assistant credentials, you must fulfill the requirements of either the American Association of Medical Assistants (for a Certified Medical Assistant) or the American Medical Technologists (for a Registered Medical Assistant). After obtaining your medical assistant certification or registration, you may wish to acquire additional skills in specialty areas through course work or on-the-job training. Although this course work or training may not lead to an additional certification or degree, it will enable you to expand your role in the medical office and advance your career as the demand for skilled health professionals increases. Should you wish to add an additional certification, the opportunity, with further training in health information technology, does exist through the American Health Information Management Association (AHIMA).

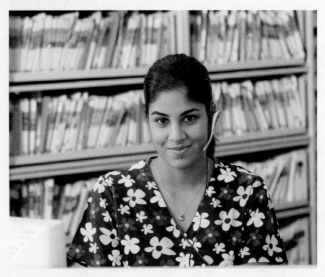

Skills and Duties

Sometimes called a medical record technician or a medical chart specialist, a Registered Health Information Technician (RHIT) maintains patient records for a physician or group of physicians. The RHIT is responsible for ensuring that all medical information is accurate and complete. In a hospital, a RHIT deals strictly with health information and has no patient contact. In a small office, however, the RHIT may have additional clerical duties such as answering the telephone.

A patient's medical record includes a medical history and statement of symptoms as well as the results of exams, laboratory tests, and x-rays. The physician's diagnoses and treatment plans are also included. The information in the patient's record may be needed for insurance purposes or to aid in further diagnosis and treatment. In addition, it may be used for research purposes.

continued ⟶

Career Opportunities

Registered Health Information Technician *(concluded)*

The Registered Health Information Technician checks all patient charts for completeness and accuracy. The RHIT makes sure that all necessary forms related to the patient's care are included, properly filled out, and signed. The RHIT checks to see that all reports and test results are attached to the chart. If necessary, the RHIT speaks with the physician to clarify information about the patient's diagnosis or treatment.

The RHIT must also code the medical record. The RHIT assigns a code to each clinical procedure and diagnosis if this coding has not already been done by another member of the health-care team. In the hospital setting, the RHIT assigns a diagnosis-related group (DRG) to the patient, using a special computer program known as a grouper. The DRG helps determine the reimbursement that the hospital will receive from Medicare or any other insurance carrier that uses a DRG system. The RHIT may also use the coded records to set up a cross-reference index, a type of file that lists the same information under several different headings.

Some medical record technicians specialize in a particular area. Coding is one example. Another is registry, which involves keeping records of all occurrences of certain diseases like bone cancer. The information the registrar collects can be used by individual physicians or as part of a research study.

Workplace Settings

The majority of RHITs work in medical record departments of hospitals. Most of the rest work in nursing homes, group practices, and health maintenance organizations (HMOs). A few RHITs work in federal or state government offices, public health departments, health and property insurance companies, or accounting and law firms. Some RHITs are self-employed and work as consultants to nursing homes or physicians' offices.

Education

Most Registered Health Information Technicians have completed a two-year associate degree program at a junior or community college. Course work includes biology, anatomy and physiology, medical terminology, data processing, coding, and statistics. The certification for RHIT is administered by the American Health Information Management Association (AHIMA).

For more information, visit the website of the following organization, which is available on the Online Learning Center at www.mhhe.com/medicalassisting4e.

American Health Information Management Association (formerly the American Medical Record Association)

Summary

10.1 Equipment needed for the filing of medical records include any one or combination of filing shelves, cabinets, rotary circular files, and plastic index boxes. Supplies necessary for efficient filing include labeling equipment, hanging file folders, folders, binders, out guides, and file guides and file labels.

10.2 There are various types of filing systems, which include alphabetic, numeric, and color coding. With the alphabetic system, files are arranged in alphabetical order. The number system organizes files by numbers instead of names, and color coding is used to distinguish files within a filing system.

10.3 The benefit of using an alphabetic system is that it is simple to use, but you have to make sure that you know the spelling of the person's name in order to retrieve the file. The numeric system keeps files confidential, as names are recorded

elsewhere and is limitless in regards to how many files may be added.

10.4 The advantage of color coding the filing system is that it distinguishes files within a system making misfiled records easier to spot. Color coding can add more information to the filing system as well. Patient records can be color-coded in a variety of ways. File folders are available in a range of colors, as are filing labels, plastic tabs, and stickers.

10.5 To set up a tickler file, write or type 12 file labels named for each month of the year and affix one label to the tab of each file folder; arrange the folders so that the current month's file is on top; write or type a list of upcoming responsibilities and activities; file the notes by month; check the tickler file at least once a week on a specific day, completing the activities on the designated date.

10.6 The five steps in the filing process are: inspect a file; index or name a file; code a file by putting an identifying mark or phrase on a document;

sort the files in order; and store documents neatly within a proper sequence.

10.7 The following are steps to assist in locating a misplaced file: Determine the last time you saw the file; go to that location and retrace steps; look in the filing cabinet where the file belongs—check neighboring files; check underneath the files in the drawer or shelf; check the pile of items to be filed; consider whether you have cross-referenced it; check with other staff members; look in the location of the patient's first name to see if it is misfiled there; stand back from the file cabinet and look down at the files (a misplaced file may "pop out"); ask other staff members to do the previous steps that you have done.

10.8 There are many ways to store inactive files. Paper storage, computer storage, and microfilm, microfiche, and cartridges are forms of basic storage options.

10.9 The criteria for retaining, storing, and discarding files vary from state to state. Medical records must be stored for 7 years, employee health records must be retained for at least three years. Immunization records should be on file permanently; they should be kept in the office and not be stored. Financial records must be kept for 10 years. It is always advisable for doctors to request legal advice before destroying records.

REVIEW

CHAPTER 10

CASE STUDY QUESTIONS

Now that you have completed this chapter, review the case study at the beginning of the chapter and answer the following questions:

1. What are advantages and disadvantages of different file systems?
2. What security measures might be used to protect patient files?
3. What is a tickler system and how is it set up?
4. Identify several storage options for closed charts. Which is the most secure? The easiest? The most cost-efficient?

Multiple-Choice Questions

1. According to the National Childhood Vaccine Injury Act of 1986, doctors must keep all immunization records on file in the office for
   a. 5 years.
   b. 7 years.
   c. permanently.
   d. 3 years.

2. Closed files are files that are of
   a. Patients who have moved.
   b. Patients who have died.
   c. Patients who are no longer seen there.
   d. All of the above

3. Which is not necessary when locating misplaced files?
   a. Determining the last time you or anyone else in the practice knew the file's location.
   b. Going to the location and retracing the steps of the last person who handled the file.
   c. Checking to make sure the missing file was not filed under the patient's first name instead of the last.
   d. Calling the patient to inform him his file is missing and to come into the office to sign a form stating he will not sue if it is not retrieved.

4. Which statement is NOT true concerning out guides?
   a. They cannot be used for both shelf and cabinet filing.
   b. The marker is made of stiff material.
   c. They can save time when going through files.
   d. They are used as a placeholder when a file has been removed from the filing system.

5. Which of the following statements is true?
   a. Terminal digit filing uses the middle group of numbers as the primary index.
   b. Indexing rules define each separate part of a person's birthdate or age as a unit.
   c. A tickler file is a date-ordered reminder file.
   d. The first step in the filing process is to make the patient make at least one payment.

Discussion Questions

1. Why is it important to use a filing system to keep medical records? What could happen if a filing system is not instituted or not followed consistently in a medical practice?

2. What is the importance of HIPAA law in the development of a medical record filing system?
3. What important behaviors should an efficient medical record technologist demonstrate?
4. What do you think is the best way to organize a filing system for a medical practice and why?

Critical Thinking Questions

1. One of the other medical assistants tells you that you really don't have to keep medical charts once the patient is no longer with the practice. What would be your response?
2. What special concerns might arise when storing records on the computer rather than in traditional (hard copy) paper files? Why do you think major clinics such as the Mayo Clinic use a completely electronic or computerized file storage system?
3. What filing system would you choose for a series of numbered insurance claim forms for patients? Why?

Application Activities

1. Arrange these 10 patient names in order as they would appear in an alphabetic filing system.
   Jordan, Larry W.
   Everett James
   Angie Jones
   John B. James
   Florence Glenn Jones
   Stafford, Samantha L.
   A. James Ingersol
   Stafford, G. E.
   Sarah Coats
   Curtis W. Weaver

2. Using your class list, develop a numeric filing system and a master list that matches each number to a specific person. Then set up an alphabetic filing system based on students' last names. Discuss with your classmates which system is most useful in an educational setting and why.
3. Set up a personal tickler file for yourself, containing personal responsibilities—such as errands, appointments, and social engagements—for the coming week. Keep your notes in a file folder or on a calendar until all activities have been completed. At the end of the week, write a brief paragraph explaining the format of your tickler system and if you found the process helpful. Give several examples to support your answer.
4. Obtain an office-supply catalog that features filing supplies. Put together a product order to set up a patient records filing system for a midsized medical office serving approximately 100 patients. Assume that the practice has already purchased the appropriate equipment, such as filing cabinets or shelves.

Virtual Fieldtrip

Visit the McGraw-Hill Higher Education Medical Assisting website at www.mhhe.com/medicalassisting4e to complete the following activity:

Research the laws in your state regarding the retention of medical records. Compare your state laws to the two states nearest your state. Determine which state has the better laws, explaining your response. What guidelines for record retention would you recommend for a medical practice in your state?

Open the CD and complete this chapter's practice activities, play the games, listen to the key terms, and test yourself with the interactive review. E-mail, print, and/ or save your results to document your proficiency.

SECTION 2

INTERACTING WITH PATIENTS

CHAPTER 11

Telephone Techniques

CHAPTER 12

Scheduling Appointments and Maintaining the Physician's Schedule

CHAPTER 13

Patient Reception

CHAPTER 14

Patient Education

CHAPTER 11

Telephone Techniques

LEARNING OUTCOMES

After completing Chapter 11, you will be able to:

11.1 Explain the importance of communication skills.

11.2 Explain how to manage incoming telephone calls.

11.3 Model how the Health Insurance Portability and Accountability Act (HIPAA) applies to telephone communications.

11.4 Describe the procedure for calling a prescription renewal into a pharmacy.

11.5 Differentiate between the types of calls the medical assistant handles and those the physician or other staff members handle.

11.6 Model how to handle various types of incoming calls from patients and from others.

11.7 Model the importance of proper telephone etiquette.

11.8 Implement the procedures for taking telephone messages.

11.9 Explain how to retrieve calls from an answering service.

11.10 Model the procedures for placing outgoing calls.

11.11 Explain the function of telephone triage in the medical office.

11.12 Explain the uses of a facsimile machine in a medical office.

MEDICAL ASSISTING COMPETENCIES

CAAHEP

Psychomotor Skills
Concepts of Effective Communication
IV. P (7) Demonstrate telephone techniques
VII. A (2) Demonstrate sensitivity in communicating with both providers and patients
VII. A (3) Communicate in language the patient can understand regarding managed care and insurance plans

ABHES

8. Medical Office Business Procedures Management
  ee. Use proper telephone techniques
  hh. Receive, organize, prioritize, and transmit information expediently

11. Career Development
Demonstrate professionalism by:
2) Exhibiting a positive attitude and a sense of responsibility
3) Maintaining confidentiality at all times
8) Being courteous and diplomatic
9) Conducting work within scope of education, training, and ability

MEDICAL ASSISTING MEDIA

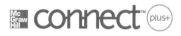 **Connect Plus+™**
connect.mcgraw-hill.com

- Electronic Health Records (E.H.R.) SpringCharts®
- eBook

SPRINGCHARTS
Electronic Health Records

 LearnSmart™ **LearnSmart™**   www.mhhe.com/learnsmart

Complete Learning Module: Telephone Techniques

 Student CD-ROM

Online Learning Center™   www.mhhe.com/medicalassisting4e

KEY TERMS

enunciation	pitch
etiquette	pronunciation
facsimile machine	telephone triage

CHAPTER OUTLINE

- Using the Telephone Effectively
- Communication Skills
- Managing Incoming Calls
- Types of Incoming Calls
- Using Proper Telephone Etiquette
- Taking Messages
- Telephone Answering Systems

- Placing Outgoing Calls
- Telephone Triage
- Telecommunications
- Telephone Slamming
- Pagers and Cell Phones
- Facsimile (Fax) Machines

PREPARATION FOR CERTIFICATION

RMA (AMT) Exam
- Professional development

CMA (AAMA) Exam
- Incoming calls management criteria
- Monitoring special calls

CMAS Exam
- Communication

Introduction

In this chapter, you will learn key terms associated with telephone techniques. You will be able to utilize a telephone professionally and effectively while handing various types of calls that are either received or initiated by a medical office. These types of calls will vary and can include calls about patient illness and injury, filling prescriptions, or requests for test results; calls from other medical offices; or calls from sales representatives. After completing this chapter, you will understand which calls may be handled by the medical assistant and which require the physician's attention.

Most medical offices have policies and procedures on handling or routing incoming calls, especially emergency calls. This chapter helps you identify which calls are considered emergencies and how to properly route these calls.

In addition, after reading this chapter, you will be able to demonstrate proper telephone etiquette by using common courtesy, proper pronunciation, tone, and enunciation while speaking. You will learn how to effectively handle difficult telephone situations or complaints and how to properly document messages taken.

A 54-year-old male patient calls in to the office and, as the medical assistant, you answer the phone. The patient obviously has shortness of breath and states rapidly, "I need to see the doctor right away."

After you establish the patient's name, you learn that the patient complains of pain in his jaw area that lasts for about 5 minutes and then goes away. He also states that he was mowing the lawn when he started sweating heavily and having difficulty breathing. Once he was inside the house, he did have some nausea and vomited once.

As you read this chapter, consider the following questions:

1. What would your first response to the patient be?
2. Explain how you would handle this situation.
3. What type of incoming call was this?
4. What type of condition did this patient's symptoms indicate?
5. What are some other symptoms of this condition?

Using the Telephone Effectively

The telephone is an important tool for promoting the positive, professional image of a medical practice. When you answer the telephone, you may be the first contact a person has with the practice. The impression you leave can be either positive or negative. Your job is to ensure that it is positive.

Good telephone management leaves callers with a positive impression of you, the physician, and the practice. Poor telephone management can result in bad feelings, misunderstandings, and an unfavorable impression. The telephone image you present should convey the message that the staff is caring, attentive, and helpful. Showing concern for a patient's welfare is a quality that patients rate highly when evaluating health-care professionals. In addition, you must sound professional and knowledgeable when handling telephone calls. Learning and using proper telephone management skills will help keep patients informed and ensure their satisfaction with the medical practice.

Communication Skills

The telephone is a communication and public relations tool that is essential to the operation of the medical office. Good communication skills are important in telephone management—they help to project a positive image and to satisfy the needs and expectations of the patient. Individuals who engage in good and effective communication employ the following communications skills:

- Using tact and sensitivity
- Showing empathy
- Giving respect
- Being genuine
- Displaying openness and friendliness
- Refraining from passing judgment or stereotyping others
- Being supportive

- Asking for clarification and feedback
- Paraphrasing to ensure an understanding of what others are saying
- Being receptive to patients' needs
- Knowing when to speak and when to listen
- Exhibiting a willingness to consider other viewpoints and concerns

As a medical assistant, you can also apply the five Cs of communication to use the telephone effectively:

- Completeness—The message must contain all necessary information
- Clarity—The message must be legible and free from ambiguity
- Conciseness—The message must be brief and direct
- Courtesy—The message must be respectful and considerate of others
- Cohesiveness—The message must be organized and logical

Managing Incoming Calls

Telephone calls must always be answered promptly, either by a telephone answering system in larger offices or by a medical assistant/receptionist answering the phone. We will address both methods of managing incoming calls in this chapter. The procedures for answering calls may vary. Guidelines are usually presented in the office policy and procedures manual. If you are in an office where the medical assistant answers the phone, general guidelines state you should greet callers with your name and the office name. Some people may feel awkward using their own name when answering the telephone. Introducing yourself to callers, however, lets them know that they are speaking to a real person, not simply an anonymous voice.

No matter how hurried you are, you should be courteous, calm, and pleasant on the telephone, devoting your full attention to the caller. If the caller does not give a name, ask for it. Many calls result in pulling the patient's file, so it is important to obtain the correct name and date of birth of the patient.

Many larger offices now utilize automated answering systems to initially answer calls, directing callers to push specific numbered buttons on their touch-tone phones to reach the person or department they are looking for. Although this frees the front office staff from every phone call, do recognize that many patients get frustrated with these automated systems and simply "push a button" to get a live person. Should that occur, you must remain pleasant, courteous, and helpful while directing the patient's call appropriately. Returning patient phone calls relating to messages they leave on these automated answering systems is covered later in this chapter.

Guidelines for Effective Telephone Communication

The following guidelines will help you use the telephone effectively and professionally:

- If answering the phone, do so promptly by the second or third ring. Hold the telephone to your ear, or use a headset to hold the ear piece securely against your ear. Do not cradle the telephone with your shoulder; doing so can cause muscle strain.
- Hold the mouthpiece about an inch away from your mouth and leave one hand free to write with.
- If answering the phone, greet the caller first with the name of the medical office and then with your name. If accepting a call routed by an automated answering system, always identify yourself by name.
- Identify the caller. Demonstrate your willingness to assist the caller by asking, "Mrs. Hernandez, how may I help you?"
- Be courteous, calm, and pleasant no matter how hurried you are.
- Identify the nature of the call and devote your full attention to the caller.
- At the end of the call, say goodbye and use the caller's name.

Following HIPAA Guidelines

As you learned in Chapter 3, the Health Insurance Portability and Accountability Act (HIPAA) was originally created in 1996 and has additions as recent as April 2006. This act is concerned with the privacy and confidentiality of patient information, including information communicated via the telephone.

In compliance with HIPAA guidelines, all medical providers have standards or written policies that require the following to be in a secure area where no one can see or overhear:

- Medical records
- Clerical forms
- Financial forms and reports
- Computer monitors
- Conversations
- Verbal reports

All employees must comply with the guidelines to safeguard patient information, including when talking on the telephone with a patient.

Health-care providers are allowed to disclose patient information for the purpose of treatment, payment, and health-care operations (known as TPO). Any use of this information outside of these reasons would require a written authorization from the patient. Exceptions include emergency situations or information that is required by governmental agencies for compliance. Follow the medical provider's policy and procedures for disclosing patient information.

Screening Calls

Part of the responsibility of answering the telephone involves screening calls before you transfer them. Even if an answering system is used you may find you have to screen calls that are directed to you. Each office has its own policy about calls that should be put through right away, those that should be returned later, and those that should be handled by other staff members. The Points on Practice section describes some guidelines for screening calls.

Routing Calls

In general, there are three types of incoming calls to a doctor's office: calls dealing mainly with administrative issues, emergency calls that require immediate action by the doctor, and calls relating to clinical issues that require the attention of the doctor, nurse, nurse practitioner, physician assistant, or clinical medical assistant.

Calls Handled by the Medical Assistant. The most common calls to a medical office involve administrative and clinical issues. As a medical assistant, you will be able to handle most of these calls yourself. They will concern the following matters:

- Appointments (scheduling, rescheduling, canceling)
- Questions concerning office policies, fees, and hours
- Billing inquiries
- Insurance questions
- Other administrative questions
- X-ray and laboratory reports
- Reports from hospitals regarding a patient's progress
- Reports from patients concerning their progress
- Requests for referrals to other doctors
- Requests for prescription renewals, where prior approval for refills is noted in the chart. If approval for the renewal is not noted in the patient's chart, prior to the renewal you should take the phone call, discuss it with the physician, chart it, and have the physician sign off on the chart. After this is completed, you

may call in the prescription renewal to the patient's pharmacy.

- Complaints from patients about administrative matters

Depending on the practice, the office manager or someone in the billing department may handle some administrative calls. The calls you handle may include scheduling appointments, receiving or requesting reports or information, insurance and billing questions, and general inquiries, such as those concerning office hours.

Calls Requiring the Doctor's Attention. Certain calls will require the doctor's personal attention. These include the following:

- Emergency calls
- Calls from other doctors
- Patient requests to discuss test results, particularly abnormal results
- Reports from patients concerning unsatisfactory progress
- Requests for prescription renewals (unless previously authorized on the patient's chart)
- Personal calls

Occasionally the patient may prefer to discuss symptoms only with the doctor. These requests should be honored. Depending on the doctor's preference and availability, you may call the doctor to the telephone to handle calls of this nature as they are received. Otherwise, the calls will be returned when the doctor has time available. As most doctors have a set time, such as a half hour in the late morning or at the end of the day, for returning nonemergency patient calls, you may tell the patient to expect a phone call from the physician at this set time. If the physician does not have a set time for returning phone calls, do not make a commitment as to the time of the return phone call.

In certain practices some of these calls may be handled by others on the staff, such as a nurse practitioner or physician assistant. For example, a nurse practitioner may be able to order a renewal of a regular prescription, provide advice for the care of a sprain, or answer well-baby questions or questions about the side effects of a drug.

The Routing List. Each medical office has a standard policy that documents how incoming telephone calls are to be routed and handled. A routing list, such as the one shown in Figure 11-1, specifies who is responsible for the various types of calls in the office and how the calls are to be handled. For example, the routing list indicates which calls should be put through to the doctor immediately and which ones can be returned later.

The routing procedure may simply identify the general title of the person responsible for handling a call. When more than one person in the office has the same

HANDLING INCOMING TELEPHONE CALLS

	Route to doctor immediately	Take message for doctor	Route to nurse or assistant
Emergencies: bleeding, drug/allergic reaction, difficulty breathing, injury, pain, poisoning, shock, unconsciousness, incoherence or hysteria	X		
Calls from other physicians	if possible		
Patient progress report		X	
Patient request for laboratory report		X (if abnormal)	Melissa (if normal)
Patient questions re medication		X	
Patient questions re billing or insurance			Jerry
Patient complaints			Melissa
Appointments			Melissa
Prescription renewals or refills		X	
Office business			Jerry
Personal business		X	
Salespeople			Jerry

Figure 11-1. A routing list identifies which office staff member is responsible for each type of incoming call.

Screening Incoming Calls

Each medical office has its own policy about how to screen incoming calls before transferring them to the appropriate person. Calls come not only from patients but also from other physicians, hospital personnel, pharmacists, insurance company personnel, sales representatives, and family members and friends of patients. Here are some general tips for screening calls.

Find out who is calling. A polite way to do this is to say, "May I ask who is calling?" Another option is, "May I tell Dr. who is calling?"

Ask what the call is in reference to. When a caller asks to speak with the physician, you should ask the purpose of the call. Depending on the answer, you may determine that you or someone else in the

office can handle the situation without disturbing the physician. The response may be as simple as solving a billing problem or clarifying instructions. Remember, however, that emergency calls should be transferred to the physician right away.

Decide whether the call should be put through. Although most calls are routed to the appropriate person, any callers who refuse to identify themselves should not be put through. In such a case suggest that the caller write a letter to the physician and mark it "Personal."

Determine what to do if the matter is personal. The physician may ask you to take a message in these instances. Inform the caller that the physician will return the call as soon as possible.

---

title, however, the name of the individual who has that particular responsibility should be specified.

Types of Incoming Calls

In dealing with incoming telephone calls, you will encounter a variety of questions and requests from numerous people. Many incoming calls are from patients. You will also receive calls from other people, including attorneys, other physicians, pharmaceutical sales representatives, and other salespeople. Procedure 11-1 reviews how to properly screen incoming telephone calls. The procedure will remain basically the same whether the calls come directly to you as you answer the phone or if they are directed to you by a telephone answering system.

Calls from Patients

Patients call the medical office for a variety of reasons, including rescheduling appointments and requesting prescription renewals. If you will be discussing clinical matters over the telephone, it is a good idea to pull the patient's chart. The information in the chart may enable you to address any problems quickly and allows you to document the conversation immediately.

Always keep in mind that the physician is legally responsible for your actions, including relaying information to patients over the telephone. The office policy manual typically specifies what you may and may not discuss with patients. If you are uncertain about giving particular information to a patient, it is best to discuss the situation with the physician or have the physician return the patient's call.

Appointment Scheduling. Follow office procedures for making or changing appointment times over the telephone. Ask the patient to provide his name, a telephone number during the day where he can be reached, and the reason for the visit. The medical assistant should repeat the information back to the patient to verify all information before ending the call. (Scheduling appointments is discussed in Chapter 12.)

Billing Inquiries. If a patient calls about a billing problem, you will need to pull the patient's billing information and possibly the medical chart as well. With this information, you can compare the charges with the actual services performed.

If a patient claims to have been overcharged, check to see if the correct fee was charged. If you find that an error was made, apologize and tell the patient the office will send a corrected statement. Ask the patient to wait for the new statement before sending payment. If in fact the proper fee was charged, it may be helpful to speak to the physician before responding to the patient. The physician may be able to tell you if there were special circumstances regarding the visit or charge in question. Allowing the patient to pay the bill in installments is usually an acceptable option. The details on arranging for payment plans is discussed in Chapter 17, Patient Billing and Collections.

Today, many offices use billing services instead of taking care of the insurance submission and monthly patient billing in the office. In that case, the patient may have called the billing service about charges and has now been referred to the office to dispute either the performance of a procedure or its cost. In this case, you may not have access to information about individual charges and need to refer the patient to the office manager. Be aware that the

PROCEDURE 11-1

Performing Telephone Screening

Procedure Goal: To properly screen incoming telephone calls

Materials: Telephone, telephone pad, pen or pencil, appointment book or computerized scheduling software (computer)

Method:

1. Make sure all of the materials are within reach of the telephone equipment.

    Rationale
    Time-saving technique.

2. Answer the telephone within two to three rings.

    Rationale
    You do not want to upset callers, nor do you want callers to feel that the office is closed or on lunch break.

3. Identify the medical office and identify yourself. Make sure you know office procedure for answering the phone in your facility even if a telephone answering system is employed to route calls to you. For example: "Genesys Medical Practice, this is Ivy Smith."

    Rationale
    Callers need to know that they have reached the correct number. Always answer with a smile. This makes callers feel welcome.

4. If the caller does not identify himself, ask him to do so and the number he is calling from, writing down this information. Get an idea what the call refers to. Listen carefully to what the caller has to say, listening for tone and feeling. Try to decide as soon as possible if this is a call that you can handle; if so, handle it. If this is a call that needs to be transferred to someone, tell the caller to whom and where you will be transferring the call.

    Rationale
    You have obtained basic information about the nature of the call to relay to the appropriate staff person, including the caller's name so that the caller does not need to repeat information needlessly. You also have the phone number to call him back if for any reason the call is unexpectedly disconnected.

5. If you need to take a message, make sure you repeat the information that is given to you, especially the name of the person and his phone number.

    Rationale
    Phone numbers can be easily transposed. The individual's name can sound a certain way, but be spelled differently.

6. If you have to transfer a caller, ask permission to place him or her on hold. Make sure you write down the caller's name and phone number in case the call is dropped. Never place a caller on hold longer than 30 seconds. Come back to the caller and let him or her know that you are still waiting for the other individual to answer. If the other staff member does not answer within a certain period or the staff member is on another line, ask the caller if he would like to call back, be transferred to the staff member's voice mail (if available), or would like to leave a message.

    Rationale
    Courtesy is the key. You must always recognize an individual as a customer and serve him to the best of your ability. Giving the caller options gives back to him some control of the situation.

7. If the caller describes a symptom that is in need of immediate care, ask questions to assess the information (ask for his or her name and telephone number). If it is indeed an emergency call and the physician or nurse is in the office, transfer the call immediately. If the doctor or nurse is not in the building, do not let the caller hang up. Have another staff member dial 911 immediately with the name and address of the patient and his symptoms, while you stay on the phone with the patient keeping him calm and aware that help is on the way.

    Rationale
    Do not put the patient at risk if this is a medical emergency. You do not want the patient to hang up and attempt to call 911, in case he is alone and loses the ability to make a call for assistance.

patient may be upset about his bill and now is being referred to yet another person. Listen patiently to the patient and take notes regarding his complaint, remaining tactful and understanding to his concerns and possible frustration that an answer does not appear to be "a simple process." No matter what your office policy is, if a patient is dissatisfied, document all appropriate comments and relay the information to the physician or office manager. If a bill has not been paid, ask if there are special circumstances affecting the patient's ability to pay. Always give this information to the physician or office manager.

Requests for Laboratory or Radiology Reports.

If a patient calls the office requesting the results of tests, pull the patient's chart to see if the report has been received. If it has not, suggest that the patient call back in a day or two. Some offices will call the laboratory or radiology office for the results.

In some offices you may be authorized to give laboratory results by telephone if they are normal, or negative, so the patient does not have to wait for results to be mailed. Make a note on the patient's chart if you provide any information about test results. If a test result is abnormal, the physician will need to speak with the patient. In such a case tell the patient that the office has received the results and that the physician will call as soon as possible. Then place the patient's chart and the telephone message on the physician's desk.

Questions About Medications.

One of the most common types of calls from patients involves questions about medication. A patient may ask about using a current prescription or may want to renew an existing prescription.

Prescription Renewals. Calls for prescription renewals occur frequently and may come from the patient's pharmacy or from the patient. A pharmacist usually calls to check before dispensing refills if more than a year has passed since the original prescription was written. If the physician has indicated on the patient's chart that renewals are approved, you may authorize the pharmacy to renew a prescription. In any other case, only the physician may authorize renewals. If the physician authorizes a renewal, you may be asked to telephone it in to the patient's pharmacy. All renewals must be documented in the patient's medical record, with the date and the initials of the person authorizing the renewal.

Old Prescriptions. Patients may call to ask if they can use a medication that was prescribed for a previous condition. In these instances, recommend that the patient come in for an appointment. Explain why the medication should not be used: it may be old and no longer effective, the current problem may not be the same as the previous one, the medication may not be helpful, and using the medication may mask the current condition's symptoms and make a diagnosis difficult.

If the patient does not want to make an appointment, relay the information to the physician. The physician will probably want to speak with the patient.

Reports on Symptoms.
Sometimes patients call the office about symptoms they wish to discuss with the physician. Here are tips for handling such calls.

- Listen attentively to the patient.
- If the patient is in real distress, try to schedule an appointment that day or as soon as possible.
- Write down all the patient's symptoms completely, accurately, and immediately. In many instances the physician may be able to suggest simple emergency relief measures that you can relay to the patient. These measures may make the patient comfortable until the time of the appointment.

Progress Reports.
Physicians often ask patients to call the office to let them know how a prescribed treatment is working. If a patient has a satisfactory progress report to make to the doctor, it is not necessary that the patient speak to the physician. It is important that the medical assistant relay the information to the doctor and log the call in the patient's medical record immediately. You may also be responsible for making routine follow-up calls to patients to verify that they are following treatment instructions.

Requests for Advice.
Although a patient may ask you for your medical opinion, do not give medical advice of any kind. Explain that you are not trained to make a diagnosis or licensed to prescribe medication. Stress that the patient must see the physician. If the patient cannot come into the office, assure her that the physician will return the call or that you will call back after discussing the problem with the physician. Occasionally a patient wants to speak only with the physician, not other staff members. You must honor this request.

In some cases the physician may feel that a patient's symptoms warrant immediate attention and will insist on seeing the patient before prescribing any treatment. If the patient refuses to come to the office, note the reason on the chart, and suggest a visit to the emergency room or to a nearby physician or urgent care center. For legal reasons, it is important to document such conversations completely in the patient's chart, including the refusal of treatment. It is always appropriate and professional to offer to take a message to have the physician return the call.

Complaints.
Even when an office provides the highest quality care, complaints still occur. When a patient calls with a complaint, such as a billing error, it is important to listen carefully, without interrupting. Take careful notes of all the details, and read them back to the caller to ensure that you have written them down correctly. Let the caller know the person to whose attention you will bring the complaint and, if possible, when to expect a response.

Always apologize to the caller for any inconvenience the problem may have caused, even if the problem occurred through no fault of the office. Make sure the proper person receives the information about the complaint.

Sometimes a patient who calls with a complaint is angry. Responding to this type of call can be difficult and

uncomfortable. Your first priority is to stay calm and try to pacify the caller. Follow these guidelines when dealing with an angry caller.

- Listen carefully, and acknowledge the patient's anger. By understanding the problem, you will be better able to work toward a solution.
- Remain calm, and speak gently and kindly. Do not act superior or talk down to the patient. Do not interrupt the patient. Do not return the anger or blame.
- Let the patient know that you will do your best to correct the problem. This message will convey that you care.
- Take careful notes, and be sure to document the call.
- Do not become defensive.
- Never make promises you cannot keep.
- Follow up promptly on the problem.
- Any time a staff member has a difficult time with a patient, it is important to inform the physician, even when the situation is resolved. Always inform the physician immediately if an angry patient threatens legal action against the office.

Emergencies. Emergency calls must be immediately routed to the physician. Emergency situations include serious or life-threatening medical conditions, such as severe bleeding, a reaction to a drug, injuries, poisoning, suicide attempts, loss of consciousness, severe burns, or whatever your medical office deems an emergency. Table 11-1 lists symptoms and conditions that require immediate help.

If someone calls the office on behalf of a patient who is experiencing any of these symptoms or conditions, you may instruct the caller to dial 911 to request an ambulance. Procedure 11-2 describes the steps for handling emergency calls. If in the office the physician should be called to the telephone immediately to offer assistance.

Other Calls

Besides calls from patients, a medical office receives many other types of calls. For example, family members and friends of patients may call the physician at the office. The use of the office telephone is never appropriate for personal calls. The physician will let you know how to handle these calls. In addition, personal cell phone use should also be limited to essential calls only as defined in your office manual which will include when and how cell phones may or may not be used in the office.

Remember that a patient's information is confidential. HIPAA requires medical providers to obtain authorization from the patient before any information can be disclosed. This is usually in the form of a written authorization, signed by the patient, and indicates what type of information may be given out and to whom. The following are guidelines for managing calls from attorneys, other physicians, and salespeople.

Attorneys. Refer to the procedures listed in your practice's office policy manual regarding how to handle calls

TABLE 11-1	Symptoms and Conditions That Require Immediate Medical Help

- Unconsciousness
- Lack of breathing or difficulty breathing
- Severe bleeding
- Pressure or pain in the abdomen that will not go away
- Severe vomiting or bloody stools
- Poisoning
- Injuries to the head, neck, or back
- Choking
- Drowning
- Electrical shock
- Snakebites
- Vehicle collisions
- Allergic reactions to foods or insect stings
- Chemicals or foreign objects in the eye
- Fires, severe burns, or injuries from explosions
- Human bites or any deep animal bites
- Heart attack. Symptoms include chest pain or pressure; pain radiating from the chest to the arm, shoulder, neck, jaw, back, or stomach; nausea or vomiting; sweating; weakness; shortness of breath; pale or gray skin color.
- Stroke. Symptoms include seizures, severe headache, slurred speech, and sudden inability or difficulty in moving a body part or one side of the body.
- Broken bones. Symptoms include being unable to move or put weight on the injured body part. The injured part is very painful or looks misshapen.
- Shock. Symptoms include paleness; feeling faint and sweaty; weak, rapid pulse; cold, moist skin; confusion or drowsiness.
- Heatstroke (sunstroke). Symptoms include confusion or loss of consciousness; flushed skin that is hot and may be moist or dry; strong, rapid pulse.
- Hypothermia (a drop in body temperature during prolonged exposure to cold). Symptoms include becoming increasingly clumsy, unreasonable, irritable, confused, and sleepy; slurred speech; slipping into a coma with slow, weak breathing and heartbeat.

from attorneys. Follow the office guidelines closely, and ask the physician how to proceed if you receive a call that does not fall within the guidelines. Remember, never release any patient information to an outside caller unless the physician has asked you to do so.

Other Physicians. Patients at your practice may be referred to surgeons, specialists, and other physicians for consultations. Consequently, you may receive calls from those physicians' offices. Route those calls to the

Handling Emergency Calls

Procedure Goal: To determine whether a telephone call involves a medical emergency and to learn the steps to take if it is an emergency call

Materials: Office guidelines for handling emergency calls; list of symptoms and conditions requiring immediate medical attention; telephone numbers of area emergency rooms, poison control centers, and ambulance transport services; telephone message forms or telephone message log

Method:

1. When someone calls the office regarding a potential emergency, remain calm.

   Rationale
   This attitude will help calm the caller and enable you to gather necessary information in the most efficient manner.

2. Obtain the following information, taking accurate notes:

   a. The caller's name

   b. The caller's telephone number and the address from which the call is being made

   Rationale
   It may be necessary for you to put the call on hold or to hang up so that you can call for medical assistance. Before you do so, however, be sure to read the information back to the caller to ensure that you have written it down correctly. If you deem the call a medical emergency, ask another medical assistant to dial 911 and give the information you have written down.

   c. The caller's relationship to the patient (if it is not the patient who is calling)

   d. The patient's name (if the patient is not the caller)

   e. The patient's age

   f. A complete description of the patient's symptoms

   g. If the call is about an accident, a description of how the accident or injury occurred and any other pertinent information

   h. A description of how the patient is reacting to the situation

   i. Treatment that has been administered

3. Read back the details of the medical problem to verify them.

Rationale
Details are necessary to determine whether or not an emergency exists and the steps you next need to take.

4. If necessary, refer to the list of symptoms and conditions that require immediate medical attention to determine if the situation is indeed a medical emergency.

If the Situation Is a Medical Emergency:

1. Put the call through to the doctor immediately, or handle the situation according to the established office procedures.

   Rationale
   Medical emergencies take precedence over all other matters.

2. If the doctor is not in the office, follow established office procedures. They may involve one or more of the following:

   a. Transferring the call to the nurse practitioner or other medical personnel, as appropriate

   b. Instructing the caller (if not the patient) to hang up and dial 911 to request an ambulance for the patient

   c. Instructing the patient to be driven to the nearest emergency room

   d. Instructing the caller to telephone the nearest poison control center for advice and supplying the caller with its telephone number

   e. Paging the doctor

If the Situation Is Not a Medical Emergency:

1. Handle the call according to established office procedures.

2. If you are in doubt about whether the situation is a medical emergency, treat it like an emergency. You must always alert the doctor immediately about an emergency call, even if the patient declines to speak with the doctor.

   Rationale
   It is better to be overly cautious than to let an emergency go untreated. The doctor should be the one to decide how to handle these situations.

physician if the caller requests that you do so. Always remember to ask if the call is about a medical emergency. Also keep in mind that you may not give out any patient information—even to another physician—unless you have a written, signed release from the patient. The exception to this rule is information requested by physicians to whom you have referred the patient for care. Because of the referral, there is a contract involved for continuity of care. You may release medical information specific to the care that the physician has been asked to provide.

Salespeople. As a medical assistant, you will probably be the contact for salespeople, unless the office policy manual states that another staff member should handle this duty. On the telephone, ask the salesperson to send you information about any new products or equipment. Pharmaceutical sales representatives may want to meet with the physician. Forward such messages to the physician with a request to let you know when to schedule the appointment. Many physicians see pharmaceutical sales representatives on certain days at certain times. Sometimes they limit the number of representatives they will see in one day. Make sure you know your office policy.

Conference Calls. Periodically, physicians may need to have a conference call with several individuals. Most newer telephone equipment can provide this type of service. The physician, the nurse, and the medical assistant may need to talk with the insurance company's representative at the same time. Telephone conferencing is an ideal setup in this case.

Additionally, there are services that provide "call-in conferencing." The host will provide a number and the time for you or your physician to call in as a participant. All of the participants are given a code and are asked to identify themselves as they call into the system. They will ask for an e-mail address to confirm the information, time, date, and pass codes that will be given to each individual. Search the Internet for more information on free conference calling.

Using Proper Telephone Etiquette

Handle all telephone calls politely and professionally. Use proper telephone **etiquette,** or good manners, so you feel confident in your role of providing quality care and assistance. Adhering to the guidelines that follow will help ensure that your telephone conversations are pleasant and constructive.

Your Telephone Voice

Customer service is critical when using the telephone. When you speak on the telephone, your voice represents the medical office. It must present your message effectively and professionally. Because you cannot rely on body language or facial expressions to help you communicate over the telephone, it is important to make the most of your telephone voice. Use the following tips to make your voice pleasant and effective.

- Speak directly into the receiver. Otherwise, your voice will be difficult to understand.
- Smile. The smile in your voice will convey your friendliness and willingness to help.
- Visualize the caller, and speak directly to that person.
- Convey a friendly and respectful interest in the caller.
- You should sound helpful and alert.
- Use language that is nontechnical and easy to understand. Never use slang.
- Speak at a natural pace, not too quickly or too slowly.
- Use a normal conversational tone.
- Try to vary your pitch while you are talking. **Pitch** is the high or low level of your speech. Varying the pitch of your voice allows you to emphasize words and makes your voice more pleasant to listen to.
- Make the caller feel important.

Pronunciation. Proper **pronunciation** (saying words correctly) is one of the most important telephone skills. Sometimes last names are difficult to pronounce. Ask patients, "How do you pronounce your name?" to make them feel welcome and important. When clarifying the spelling of a word or name, it is common practice to state the letter and then a word that begins with the letter. Examples include D as in dog, V as in Victor, M as in Mary, N as in Nancy, and B as in balloon.

Enunciation. **Enunciation** (clear and distinct speaking) is the opposite of mumbling. Good enunciation helps the person you are speaking to understand you, which is especially important when you are trying to convey medical information.

Speaking clearly over the telephone is very important because the speaker cannot be seen. Correct interpretation of the message is determined by hearing the words precisely. Activities such as chewing gum, eating, or propping the phone between the ear and shoulder hinder proper enunciation.

Tone. Because you are not face-to-face with the caller, the most important measurements of good telephone communication are voice quality and tone. Always speak with a positive and respectful tone.

Making a Good Impression

In a sense your telephone duties include public relations skills. How you handle telephone calls will have an impact on the public image of the medical practice.

Exhibiting Courtesy. Using common courtesy is a characteristic of professional office personnel. Courtesy is expressed by projecting an attitude of helpfulness. Always use the person's name during the conversation, and apologize for any errors or delays. When ending the conversation, be sure to thank the caller before hanging up. Allow the caller to hang up first. This ensures that all her questions or requests have been addressed prior to the call being ended.

Giving Undivided Attention. Do not try to answer the telephone while continuing to carry out another task. This practice may lead to errors in message taking and may give the caller the impression that you are uncaring or uninterested. Give the caller the same undivided attention you would if the person were in the office. Listen carefully to get the correct information.

Putting a Call on Hold. Although you should try not to put a caller on hold, there will be times when it is unavoidable. You may receive a call on another line, or a situation in the office may prevent you from devoting your full attention to the caller. Sometimes you may have to check a file or ask someone else in the office a question on behalf of the caller. Before putting a call on hold, however, always let the caller state the reason for the call. This step is essential so that you do not inadvertently put an emergency call on hold. Never answer the phone, "Dr. Appel's office, please hold," and immediately put the call on hold. You must ask permission to put the caller on hold and wait for the response.

The medical office may have a standard procedure for placing a call on hold. Typically, you will ask the caller the purpose of the call, state why you need to place the call on hold, explain how long you expect the wait to be, and ask the caller if this wait is acceptable. If you think the wait will be long, offer to call back rather than asking the caller to hold. Being kept on hold too long or too often makes people think the staff is inattentive to their needs. You should return to the caller on hold at no more than twominute intervals and inquire whether or not the caller wants to remain on hold.

If you know you can return to the line shortly, you can put the caller on hold, then attend to the problem. If you need to answer a second call, get the second caller's name and telephone number, and put that call on hold until you have completed the first call. You can then return to the second call.

Handling Difficult Situations. At times it will be impossible to give your undivided attention to a caller because of a pressing issue or emergency in the office. If the call itself is not an emergency one, it is best to ask if you can call back. Explain that you are currently handling an urgent matter, and offer to return the call in a few minutes. Most people will appreciate your honesty. Return the call in a reasonable amount of time, and be sure to apologize for the inconvenience.

Remembering Patients' Names. When patients are recognized by name, they are more likely to have positive feelings about the practice. Using a caller's name during a conversation makes the caller feel important. If you do not recognize a patient's name, it is better to ask, "Has it been some time since you've seen the doctor?" rather than to ask if the patient has been to the practice before.

Checking for Understanding. When communicating by telephone, you do not have visual signals to convey the caller's feelings and level of understanding of the information you are discussing. Consequently, you must ask certain questions in the right way. If a call is long or complicated, summarize what was said to be sure that both you and the caller understand the information. Ask if the caller has any questions about what you have discussed. If a situation requires a lengthy conversation, it might be best to have the patient come into the office.

Communicating Feelings. Whenever information is conveyed over the telephone, feelings are also communicated. When dealing with a caller who is nervous, upset, or angry, try to show empathy (an understanding of the other person's feelings). Communicating with empathy helps the caller feel more positive about the conversation and the medical office.

Ending the Conversation. It is not useful to let a conversation run on if you can effectively complete the call sooner. Before hanging up, however, take a few seconds to complete the call so that the caller feels properly cared for and satisfied. You can complete the call by summarizing the important points of the conversation and thanking the caller. Then let the caller hang up first. When you put the receiver down, never slam it—even if the caller has already hung up. Remember that all your actions reflect the professional image of the medical practice. Patients in the waiting room may see you when you are talking on the telephone.

Taking Messages

Always have paper and a pen or pencil near the telephone so that you are prepared to write down messages (Figure 11-2). Proper documentation protects the physician if the caller takes legal action. A record of telephone calls should also be included in a patient's file or electronic

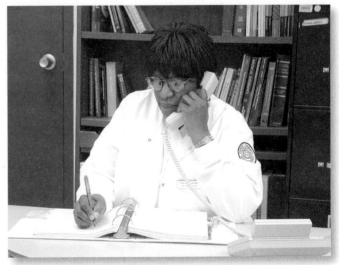

Figure 11-2. Use one hand or a telephone rest to hold the telephone so that the hand you write with is free to take messages.

TELEPHONE MESSAGE

For: _____

_____

_____

_____

_____

_____

_____

_____

Name of Caller: _____

Name of Patient (if not caller): _____

Date/Time Called: _____

Message Taken by: _____

Figure 11-3. Example of a telephone message pad that can be used for incoming calls to medical facilities.

health record as part of a complete medical history. Figure 11-3 is an example of a telephone message pad that can be used for incoming calls to medical facilities.

Documenting Calls

Documenting telephone calls is essential in a medical office. You can use telephone message pads, a manual telephone log book, or an electronic (computerized) telephone log (Figure 11-4). Again, remember that many calls (for example, those concerning clinical problems or referrals) and the actions or decisions they lead to need to be documented in patients' charts. Every entry into a patient's chart is considered a legal document; therefore, the information must be accurate and legible. Accurate documentation helps guard against lawsuits.

Telephone Message Pads. You can use telephone message pads, which often come in brightly colored paper, to record the following information:

- Date and time of the call
- Name of the person for whom you took the message
- Caller's name, or the patient's name if different from the caller
- Caller's telephone number (including area code and extension, if any)

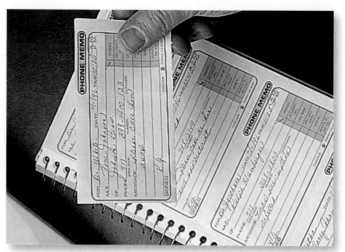

Figure 11-4. When using a telephone message pad or telephone log, be sure to fill out the form completely and accurately.

- A description or an action to be taken, including comments such as "Urgent," "Please call back," "Wants to see you," "Will call back," or "Returned your call"
- The complete message, such as "Dr. Stephenson wants to reschedule the committee meeting."
- Name or initials of the person taking the call

The Manual Telephone Log. Some medical offices use spiral-bound, perforated message books with carbonless forms to record messages. The top copy, or original, of each message is given to the appropriate person, and a copy is kept in the book for future reference.

The Electronic Telephone Log. Some medical offices use an electronic or computer-based system to record messages. The message is keyed in as it is received. A copy of the message can be stored in an electronic record, printed out, or e-mailed as needed.

Tips for Taking Messages. The following suggestions will help you provide accurate documentation for incoming messages:

- Always have a pen or pencil and paper on hand.
- Jot down notes as the information is given.
- Verify information, especially the spelling of patient or caller names and the correct spelling of medications.
- Verify the correct callback number.
- When taking a phone message for the physician, never make a commitment on behalf of the physician by saying, "I'll have the physician call you." An appropriate response would be, "I will give your message to the physician."

Ensuring Correct Information

When you are taking a message, be sure to get the proper spelling of the caller's name. Repeat the spelling to the caller to make sure it is correct. If it is necessary to pull the patient's chart, ask for the patient's date of birth, in case

PROCEDURE 11-3

Retrieving Messages from an Answering Service

Procedure Goal: To follow standard procedures for retrieving messages from an answering service

Materials: Telephone message pad, manual telephone log, or electronic telephone log

Method:

1. Set a regular schedule for calling the answering service to retrieve messages.

   Rationale

   Having a regular schedule ensures that you do not miss any messages.

2. Call at the regularly scheduled time(s) to see if there are any messages.

3. Identify yourself and state that you are calling to obtain messages for the practice.

   Rationale

   The service will only give information to approved personnel from the practice.

4. For each message, write down all pertinent information on the telephone message pad or telephone log, or key it into the electronic telephone log. Be sure to include the caller's name and telephone number, time of call, message or description of the problem, and action taken, if any.

5. Repeat the information, confirming that you have the correct spelling of all names.

   Rationale

   Many names sound alike on the phone. It is easy to make a mistake. Accurate information is important to assure that the correct medical chart is pulled and reviewed.

6. When you have retrieved all messages, route them according to the office policy.

---

there are two patient's with the same name. When you have taken down all the necessary information, repeat the key points to the caller for verification.

Maintaining Patient Confidentiality

Do not repeat information over the telephone when the information is confidential. This point is especially important if patients or others in the office may overhear the conversation. You must also maintain patient confidentiality when handling written telephone messages. If a confidential message must be brought to the doctor's attention, do not leave it on the doctor's desk where it can be seen by someone else. Instead, put the message in a file folder marked "Confidential" and place the folder on the desk. Follow the same procedure when handling confidential faxes.

Telephone Answering Systems

An office telephone system can range from a single telephone line to a complex multiline system. Most medical offices use one or more of the following pieces of equipment and services to provide efficient management of telephone calls: an automated voice mail system, an answering machine, and an answering service. Chapter 5 describes these systems. One of your telephone responsibilities may be to retrieve messages from the practice's answering service. Procedure 11-3 describes how to do so.

Placing Outgoing Calls

You will often be required to place outgoing calls on behalf of the medical office. You may need to return calls, obtain information, provide patient education, or arrange patient consultations with other physicians. Occasionally, you may be asked to assist with long-distance calls. Seek assistance as needed for these calls. It is important to determine the time zone and the time of day in the location you are calling before you place a call. Time zones can be determined by checking the front of the phone book, going online, or speaking with a telephone operator. For information on time zones, go to http://www.time.gov.

Locating Telephone Numbers

Before you can place an outgoing call, of course, you must have the correct telephone number. If you are calling a patient, the telephone number should be in the patient's chart. To find other telephone numbers, you may need to consult a telephone directory or call for directory assistance. You may also go to the Internet to find a phone directory.

The medical office should have at least one telephone directory, or telephone book, for the local calling area and perhaps additional directories for surrounding areas. Use these books to locate telephone numbers for outside calls.

The office may also have a card file, a list, or an electronic record of commonly used telephone numbers, or these numbers may be listed in the office policy manual.

If you need to find a long-distance telephone number, many offices use the directory assistance service. You can reach this service by dialing 1-[area code]-555-1212. You also can search the Internet for free "411" services. Use directory assistance only when you have exhausted other options, however, because most long-distance carriers charge a fee each time you use the service. If you are required to call out of the country, you will need to use an international dialing code. These codes, as well as area codes and long distance numbers, can be located through the Internet as well as through directory assistance.

Area Codes. There are numerous area codes for calling within the U.S. calling area. You can search the Internet to find any area code that you desire. Here are two websites that are helpful for finding information on area codes: www.nanpa.com and www.lincmad.com/areacodemap.html.

Applying Your Telephone Skills

You can apply the telephone skills you use for answering incoming calls when placing outgoing calls. Here are additional tips for handling outgoing calls.

- Plan before you call. Have all the information you need in front of you before you dial the telephone number. Plan what you will say, and decide what questions to ask so that you will not have to call back for additional information.
- Double-check the telephone number. Before placing a call, always confirm the number. If in doubt, look it up in the telephone directory. If you do dial a wrong number, be sure to apologize for the mistake.
- Allow enough time, at least a minute or about eight rings, for someone to answer the telephone. When calling patients who are elderly or physically disabled, allow additional time.
- Identify yourself. After reaching the person to whom you placed the call, give your name and state that you are calling on behalf of the doctor or practice.
- Ask if you have called at a convenient time and whether the person has time to talk with you. If it is not a good time, ask when you should call back.
- Be ready to speak as soon as the person you called answers the telephone. Do not waste the person's time while you collect your thoughts.
- If you are calling to give information, ask if the person has a pencil and piece of paper available. Do not begin with dates, times, or instructions until the person is ready to write down the information.

Arranging Conference Calls

It may be necessary for you to schedule conference calls with patients, hospitals, or other doctors to discuss tests or surgical results. When dealing with several people, suggest several time slots in case someone is not available at a particular time. Also keep in mind the various time zones in the country. Make sure that all the conference-call participants are given the proper time in their time zone to expect the call.

Telephone Triage

Some physicians delegate to other staff members some of the clinical decision making that is done over the telephone. In these instances, **telephone triage** is used as a process of deciding what necessary action to take. The word *triage* refers to the screening and sorting of emergency incidents. Performing triage correctly is an important skill. You should learn as much as possible about triage techniques.

Learning the Triage Process

Proper training of office staff is vital in providing safe, sound, and cost-effective medical care over the telephone. An increasing number of medical practices are preparing guidelines for the telephone staff to follow when patients call the office with specific medical problems or questions.

Guidelines are often written for common questions, such as how to deal with sniffles and fevers during cold and flu season or how to make a child with chickenpox more comfortable. Members of the telephone staff must realize, however, that their responsibility is to determine whether a caller needs additional medical care. They cannot diagnose or treat the patient's problem.

Office guidelines outline the specific information the telephone staff must obtain from the patient. In general, this information is the same type as that obtained during an office visit. It should include the patient's age, symptoms, when the problem began, and the patient's level of anxiety about the problem.

Automated Telephone Triage. In very busy practices, many physicians install an automated system for telephone triaging. On many occasions, medical assistants spend a great deal of time on the telephone calling patients to remind them of appointments, calling patients about no-shows, and leaving other types of messages.

Physicians feel that they can make better use of their staff's time by using automated phone systems. Many times the system pays for itself in less than a year. An automated phone system can remind patients of upcoming appointments and also allows them to leave messages for staff.

Automated phone systems offer much more than just financial benefits, however. They can conduct patient surveys and give patient test results through a privacy mechanism (patient inputs his or her password). The phone systems can assist in managing referrals from the influx of managed care. They also can assist with preventive care by giving direct access to nurses for minor problems and concerns.

Categorizing Patient Problems and Providing Patient Education

After the patient information is obtained, the guidelines help the staff categorize the problem according to severity. The telephone staff then decides if the problem can be handled safely with advice over the telephone, whether the patient needs to come into the office, or whether the problem requires immediate attention at an emergency room.

If a problem is deemed appropriate for telephone management, the guidelines may include recommendatins for nonprescription treatment that may relieve symptoms and anxiety. This information falls under the category of patient education. Advise the caller that recommendations are based on the symptoms and are not a diagnosis. Remember that only the doctor is authorized to make a diagnosis and prescribe medication. Ask the caller to repeat any instructions you give, and tell the patient to call back within a specified time if symptoms worsen. Be sure to document in the medical record the critical elements of the conversation that relate to the patient's health status.

Taking Action

Clinical triage involves determining the extent of medical emergencies and deciding on the appropriate action. If a caller is having chest pains, you would be performing a type of triage by instructing him to go to the emergency room immediately, preferably by ambulance. Telephone triage is also used in handling common minor medical problems and questions. Whatever the nature of the problem, the situation must be dealt with appropriately to protect the health and safety of the patient.

Telephone Slamming and Cramming

Telephone slamming and cramming are relatively new terms defining unauthorized charges on your phone bill. **Slamming** results when any of your telephone service providers are switched or changed without your knowledge or consent. **Cramming** occurs when unauthorized services are added to your bill either on a one time or recurring basis. To avoid paying for services or carrier changes that the office did not request, the phone bill must be carefully reviewed each month. Because both slamming and cramming are federal and state crimes, they must be reported immediately. If you believe your phone bill has incorrect or unauthorized charges, call the carrier involved immediately seeking correction and reversal of unauthorized charges. Further, if you believe any of the service providers have been changed without specific permission from the office, request a return to the providers authorized by the office. If any of these requests are not honored, legal assistance may be necessary.

Pagers and Cell Phones

A pager, sometimes called a beeper, is a simple personal telecommunications device for short messages. There are two main types of pagers. The first one is a one-way numeric pager, which can only receive a message consisting of a few digits, typically a phone number that the user is then expected to call. The second type is a two-way pager that has the ability to send and receive e-mail and numeric pages.

Another telecommunication device that is beneficial for the medical practice and the physician is the cell phone. A cell phone, also called a mobile phone, is a long-range, electronic device used for mobile voice or data communication over a network of specialized base stations known as cell sites (a term used primarily in America for a location where antennas and electronic communications equipment are placed to create a cell in a network).

When using either telecommunication device for patients or your medical facility, make sure you maintain confidentiality and privacy. Be particularly careful of any private information given over a cell phone, as it is not considered to be a secure line. It is best to have a brief, "generic" conversation by cell phone and then continue the conversation via a land-line or in person to maintain patient confidentiality.

Facsimile (Fax) Machines

Facsimile machines, more commonly referred to as fax machines, are commonly used in physicians' offices. A fax is sent over telephone lines from one fax modem to another. Fax machines may be used to send referrals, reports, insurance approvals, or medication refill approvals. Per HIPAA guidelines, a patient's confidentiality must be protected by placing the fax machine in a secure location that only authorized personnel can access. It would be helpful to keep a fax log for court-mandated documentation. These records should be kept for at least three years. Federal and state laws also must be followed in maintaining or faxing medical records. The physician's office should develop guidelines to follow when faxing information about patients. See Chapter 5 for more information regarding using a fax machine.

Summary

11.1 Communication skills are important because when communication is effective, it employs a positive image and assists with satisfying the expectations of the patient.

11.2 Incoming telephone calls must be answered promptly. You should be courteous and pleasant at all times on the telephone.

11.3 In compliance with HIPAA, information communicated via telephone should be confidential and private taking place so that others may not overhear the conversation.

Information given via a cell phone should not contain confidential information.

11.4 When calling in prescription renewals, pull the patient's chart and check if the renewal is authorized. If authorization is present, make sure you are in a private location in the office before releasing information to the pharmacy. Document the medication renewal in the patient's chart. If the renewal is not documented in the chart, refer the request to the physician per office policy.

11.5 Calls handled by the medical assistant and other staff members may vary. The medical assistant handles less complex telephone calls such as office hour inquiries, appointment requests, and previously authorized prescription renewals. Calls regarding medical advice, new prescriptions, and medical emergencies, to name a few, will be routed to the physician, nurse, or physician assistant per office policy.

11.6 The medical assistant may receive calls from patients, attorneys, and others. Always refer to your policy and procedures manual regarding how to handle incoming calls appropriately. Remember to always be courteous.

11.7 Using proper telephone techniques is a must. Customer service is critical when using the phone and provides your office with a tone of professionalism.

11.8 When taking telephone messages, always have a pen or pencil and paper near the phone. Document who the call is for, the name of the caller, the name of the patient (if different), the phone number to return a call, and a brief description of the reason for the call. Always initial the message identifying who took the call.

11.9 When retrieving messages from an answering services, always do so at set scheduled times, identify yourself, write down pertinent information, and repeat information—confirming that you understand. Route the messages per office policy.

11.10 When placing outgoing calls, check the time zone, (making sure timing of the call is appropriate), have handy all pertinent information necessary for the call, check the phone number carefully, and dial carefully. When the correct caller is reached, identify yourself, the practice, and the reason for the call.

11.11 Telephone triage is a process used to decide what actions need to be taken by the physician or other staff members regarding the caller and the reason for the call to the office. It is also used to prioritize the calls as emergent, urgent, or routine.

11.12 Fax machines may be used for various electronic transmissions such as lab reports, insurance reports, and other types of correspondence and information. Make sure that the fax machine is in a secure and private area and that a fax cover sheet with disclaimer is used for every transmission. Transmission reports should be kept near the fax machine, in a secure location for at least 3 years as legal documents.

REVIEW

CHAPTER 11

CASE STUDY QUESTIONS

Now that you have completed this chapter, review the case study at the beginning of the chapter and answer the following questions:

1. What would your first response to the patient be?
2. Explain how you would handle this situation.
3. What type of incoming call was this?
4. What type of condition did this patient's symptoms indicate?
5. What are some other symptoms of this condition?

Multiple-Choice Questions

1. Which is NOT one of the five Cs of communication to use the telephone effectively?
   - **a.** Compassion
   - **b.** Clarity
   - **c.** Conciseness
   - **d.** Cohesiveness
2. Calls from which of the following will require a doctor's immediate attention?
   - **a.** Bill collector
   - **b.** An old close friend
   - **c.** Calls from other doctors
   - **d.** A pharmaceutical salesman

3. What does HIPAA stand for?
   a. Health Issues Portability and Accountability Act
   b. Health Insurance Practice and Accountability Act
   c. Health Incompetent Practice and Accountability Act
   d. Health Insurance Portability and Accountability Act
4. Which symptom or condition does NOT require immediate medical help?
   a. Poisoning
   b. Constipation
   c. Vehicle collision
   d. Choking
5. Proper pronunciation refers to
   a. the tone of your voice.
   b. clear and distinct speaking.
   c. saying words correctly.
   d. speaking slowly.

Discussion Questions

1. What is the purpose of screening calls that come into the medical office?
2. List five communication skills that are used in effective communication.
3. Name five of the most common types of calls received in the medical office that can be handled by the medical assistant.
4. Describe the procedure for calling a prescription renewal into a pharmacy.
5. Name five symptoms or conditions that require immediate medical help.
6. List five examples of calls received by a medical office that require a doctor's attention.
7. What act does HIPAA stand for, and what is the purpose of the act?

Critical Thinking Questions

1. As a medical assistant, how would you make a positive impression over the phone?
2. Describe how you would handle a situation in which an angry patient calls to complain that he was overcharged for a recent office visit.
3. How would you handle a call from a patient who discusses symptoms he or she is experiencing?
4. A 12-year-old female patient had lab tests performed. The patient's mother calls and requests to know her daughter's lab results. What is HIPAA policy regarding this information? What should you do?

5. List the five Cs of communication and define what each means.
6. How does the way you handle telephone calls impact the public image of the medical practice?

Application Activities

1. With a partner, role-play a scenario in which a patient calls the medical office to report that he or she is experiencing chest pain. You can review Procedure 11-2 in order to demonstrate how to handle this emergency situation. If possible, ask a third student to observe and comment.
2. When speaking with patients on the telephone, how might you demonstrate the following qualities? Give several examples for each quality.
   a. concern
   b. attentiveness
   c. friendliness
   d. respect
   e. empathy
3. Your doctor's schedule is full for the day, and you have been told not to schedule any other patients. Demonstrate how you would handle the following caller: The patient states she is sick with a cough and congestion. She insists that she needs to be seen today.
4. Define telephone triage. Give examples of three different patient calls and how you would triage each call.
5. Write a paragraph about how to make a good impression in your telephone duties.

Virtual Fieldtrip

Visit the McGraw-Hill Higher Education Medical Assisting website at www.mhhe.com/medicalassisting4e to complete the following activity:

Using the Internet, research telephone etiquette and ways to handle difficult callers. Then write a brief summary of one of the most helpful articles you read, describing what you learned. Print the articles to share with the class.

Open the CD and complete this chapter's practice activities, play the games, listen to the key terms, and test yourself with the interactive review. E-mail, print, and/or save your results to document your proficiency.

CHAPTER 12

Scheduling Appointments and Maintaining the Physician's Schedule

LEARNING OUTCOMES

After completing Chapter 12, you will be able to:

12.1 Describe the importance of the appointment book in maintaining the schedule in the medical office.

12.2 Identify common scheduling abbreviations.

12.3 Describe different types of appointment scheduling systems.

12.4 Explain ways to arrange appointments for patients.

12.5 Model how to handle special scheduling situations.

12.6 Model how to properly document no-shows and late patients.

12.7 Explain how to schedule appointments that are outside the medical office.

12.8 Implement ways to keep an accurate and efficient physician schedule.

MEDICAL ASSISTING COMPETENCIES

CAAHEP

V. C (1) Discuss pros and cons of various types of appointment management systems

V. C (2) Describe scheduling guidelines

V. C (3) Recognize office policies and protocols for handling appointments

V. C (4) Identify critical information required for scheduling patient admissions and/or procedures

V. P (1) Manage appointment schedule, using established priorities

V. P (2) Schedule patient admissions and/or procedures

ABHES

8. Medical Office Business Procedures Management
  c. Schedule and manage appointments
  f. Schedule inpatient and outpatient admissions
  dd. Serve as liaison between physician and others

11. Career Development
Demonstrate professionalism by:
3) Maintaining confidentiality at all times
4) Being cognizant of ethical boundaries
8) Being courteous and diplomatic
9) Conducting work within scope of education, training, and ability

MEDICAL ASSISTING MEDIA

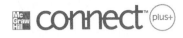 **Connect Plus+™**
connect.mcgraw-hill.com

- Electronic Health Records (E.H.R.) SpringCharts®
- eBook

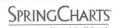

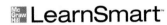 **LearnSmart™**   www.mhhe.com/learnsmart

Complete Learning Module: Scheduling Appointments and Maintaining the Physician's Schedule.

 Student CD-ROM

 Online Learning Center™   www.mhhe.com/medicalassisting4e

KEY TERMS

advance scheduling	matrix	time-specified scheduling
agenda	minutes	underbooking
cluster scheduling	modified-wave scheduling	walk-in
double-booking system	no-show	wave scheduling
itinerary	open-hours scheduling	
locum tenens	overbooking	

CHAPTER OUTLINE

- The Appointment Book
- Appointment Scheduling Systems
- Online Scheduling
- Arranging Appointments
- Special Scheduling Situations
- Scheduling Outside Appointments
- Maintaining the Physician's Schedule

PREPARATION FOR CERTIFICATION

RMA (AMT) Exam
- Appointment scheduling systems

CMA (AAMA) Exam
- Utilizing appointment schedules/types
- Appointment guidelines
- Appointment protocol

CMAS Exam
- Appointment management and scheduling
- Address cancellations and missed appointments
- Prepare information for referrals and pre-authorizations

Introduction

As a medical assistant, you need to know all aspects of how to create and utilize an appointment book. In this chapter you will learn to identify the different types of scheduling systems, how each is used, and which type of practice each system would work best in. You will also learn how to handle many types of scheduling situations within the office, including patient appointments, emergencies, pharmaceutical representatives, and the scheduling of outside appointments with other medical facilities. Legal aspects of the appointment book are discussed and proper documentation is stressed. Additional topics include appointment cards, reminder mailings, reminder calls, and recall notices for patients.

CASE STUDY

A 71-year-old female patient has a routine follow-up appointment with the physician regarding her medications. Her appointment is at 9:00 A.M. and lasts about 15 minutes. As the patient is checking out at the reception desk, she trips and falls, hitting her head on the corner of the reception desk. There is a bleeding wound on her forehead, and she complains of a headache. The physician and another medical assistant obtain a stretcher and move the patient to an exam room to assess her injuries. It is expected that this emergency will take at least 45 minutes to handle. You are managing the schedule for the day. The physician has a full schedule for this morning and has already worked in a couple of additional appointment times for patients who need to be seen this morning for acute problems.

The next scheduled appointment is for a 24-year-old male who needs an employment physical for a new job he is to start next week. He must have the physical performed prior to his first day. His appointment is scheduled for 9:15 A.M. and is expected to last 30 minutes. At 9:45 A.M., two patients are scheduled for the same 15-minute appointment. One has a sore throat and the other is scheduled for a wound check. The afternoon schedule has two appointment openings: the first at 2:00 P.M., which is for 15 minutes, and the second at 4:15 P.M., also for 15 minutes.

As you read this chapter, consider the following questions:

1. How would you adjust the schedule to allow for the emergency?
2. If it is necessary to reschedule patients, who should be rescheduled and when?
3. Would you explain anything to the patients in the waiting room about the emergency? If so, what would you say?

 ## The Appointment Book

Time is a treasured commodity for both patients and physicians. Scheduling appointments in an organized fashion shows respect for everyone's time and creates an efficient patient flow. If scheduling is changed for any reason, the medical assistant must update the physician's day slip. A well-managed appointment book, regardless of whether it is an actual book or utilizes an electronic format in a computer system, is the key to establishing this efficiency.

Scheduling is dependent upon the physician's preferences and habits, the facilities available, and the patient's need. Although most patients understand that they may have to wait in the reception area before they are seen by the physician, few patients are willing to wait more than 20 minutes. Offices that routinely have long waiting times can end up with dissatisfied patients and other problems. Some patients, in an attempt to avoid a long wait, may deliberately arrive after their scheduled appointment times. Accommodating these latecomers can throw the office schedule off track. Other patients may become resentful and decide to seek medical care with a competing practice.

Even in a well-run office, however, unexpected events can disrupt the schedule. Some patients arrive early, some arrive late, and others do not arrive at all. Some appointments take longer than expected, for example, if the physician needs to spend extra time with a patient. In addition, emergency appointments sometimes need to be squeezed into the schedule. For these reasons, making an office schedule flow smoothly can be a challenge. Through good planning and scheduling, a medical practice can run smoothly despite these obstacles.

Preparing the Appointment Book

Before you can begin scheduling appointments, you need to prepare the appointment book or electronic scheduler. The first step is to establish the **matrix,** or basic format. To create the matrix, you need to block off times within the schedule during which the doctor is not available to see patients. Time would be blocked off the schedule, for example, when the doctor is away for the following reasons:

- Hospital rounds
- Surgery
- Lunch
- Vacation days
- Holidays
- Scheduled meetings (for example, pharmaceutical, medical supply company, or in-service meetings)

The day's schedule is then built around this matrix. See Figure 12-1 for an example of a matrix for a schedule based on appointments at 15 minute increments.

Obtaining Patient Information

When the matrix has been established, you can begin scheduling appointments. You must obtain and enter certain patient information for each appointment. At some practices personnel enter the information into both traditional paper appointment books and computerized systems. Then, if the computer fails to work for some reason, the office has the book for reference. Some doctors who have been in practice for many years are used to the appointment book method and do not want to give it up for a

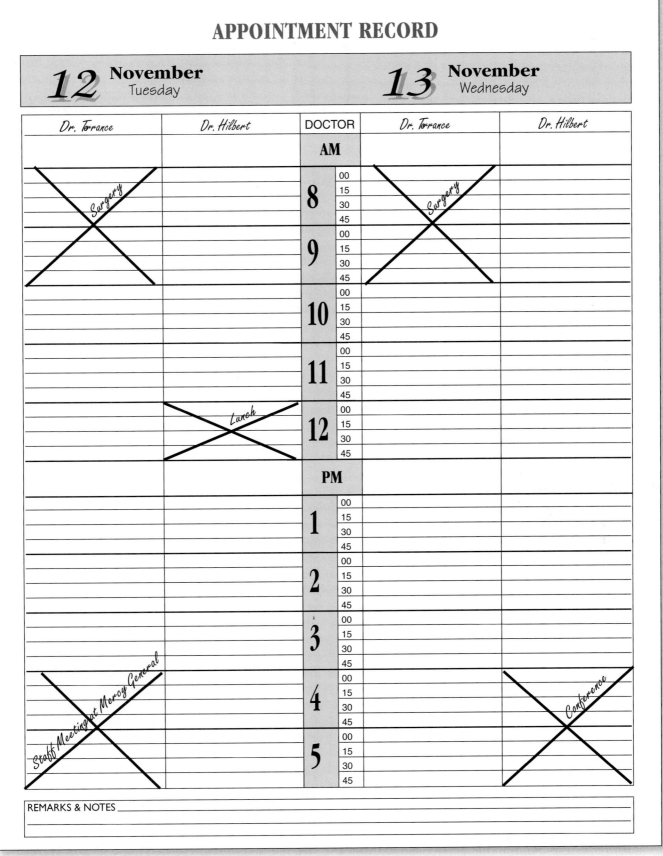

Figure 12-1. It is important to establish a matrix in the appointment book so that appointments are not scheduled for times when the doctor will be out of the office.

computer system. Other offices are completely computerized. Using either the book or computer method, obtain the necessary patient information:

- Patient's full name. Obtain the correct spelling of the patient's name.
- Home and work telephone numbers. Repeat phone numbers to ensure accuracy.
- Purpose of the visit. Use a brief description and utilize approved abbreviations when possible. Do not create your own abbreviations.

Commonly Used Abbreviations

If you are the person who maintains the appointment book, you will find that certain procedures and conditions occur frequently. To save space and time when entering information, use these abbreviations:

BP	blood pressure check
FBS/RBS	fasting blood sugar/random blood sugar
can	cancellation
c/o	complains of
cons	consultation
CP	chest pain
CPE	complete physical examination
ECG	electrocardiogram
FU or f/u	follow-up appointment
GI	gastrointestinal
I & D	incision and drainage
inj	injection
lab	laboratory studies
N & V	nausea and vomiting
NP	new patient
NS	no-show patient
P & P	Pap smear (Papanicolaou smear) and pelvic examination
Pap	Pap smear
PMS	premenstrual syndrome
pt	patient
PT	physical therapy
re	recheck
ref	referral
RS	reschedule
Rx	prescription
sig	sigmoidoscopy
SOB	shortness of breath
S/R	suture removal
STD	sexually transmitted disease
surg	surgery
URI	upper respiratory infection
US	ultrasound
UTI	urinary tract infection

Determining Standard Procedure Times

If you are to schedule appointments efficiently, you must have an estimate of how long visits will take. Working with the physician or physicians in your practice, create a list of standard procedure times. Also indicate on the list how much time to allow for tests that are commonly performed in the practice. This list, kept beside the appointment book or programmed into the electronic scheduling system, helps you identify which openings are appropriate for the procedure or test involved. This list is intended as a guide only, as each patient visit is unique. This listing will also assist you in choosing an appropriate appointment book or scheduler, as most are based on 10-, 15-, or 30-minute increments. The lengths and types of tests and procedures will depend on the practice. Following are typical lengths of common procedures:

Complete physical examination	30–60 minutes
New patient visit	30 minutes or more
Follow-up office visit	5–10 minutes
Emergency office visit	15–20 minutes
Prenatal examination	15 minutes
Pap smear and pelvic examination	15–30 minutes
Minor in-office surgery, such as a mole removal	30 minutes
Suture removal	10–20 minutes

A Legal Record

The appointment book is considered a legal record. Some experts advise holding on to old appointment books for at least 3 years. Because the appointment book could be used as evidence in legal proceedings, entries must be clear and easy to read. Management consultants suggest that because the appointment book is a legal medical document, the schedule should be written in blue ink (although many offices still prefer black ink instead of blue) and never with a pencil. Never erase a name or use correction fluid to blot the name out. Instead, draw a single line through the name and beside it write "can" for canceled or "NS" for a noshow patient. Also write the date, time, and reason (if known) why the appointment was missed or canceled, then initial the entry. This information should also be documented in the patient's chart.

Some offices permit the use of pencil to allow for changes or corrections if necessary. If pencil is used, at the end of each day you or another designated staff member should write directly over the penciled entries in ink to create a permanent document. Remember too that when a patient skips or changes her appointment, documentation should also be made in the medical record.

Appointment Scheduling Systems

There are several possible appointment scheduling systems. The method chosen usually depends on the type of practice and the physician's preferences. No matter which method your office uses, it should be regularly reviewed to see whether it is meeting its goals: a smooth flow of patients and minimal waiting time.

Open-Hours Scheduling

In the **open-hours scheduling** system, patients arrive at their own convenience with the understanding that they will be seen on a first-come, first-served basis, unless there is an extreme emergency. Depending on how many other patients are ahead of them, they may have a considerable wait. The open-hours system eliminates the problems caused by broken appointments (because there are no appointments), but it increases the possibility of inefficient downtime for the doctor. In addition, with this system the medical assistant cannot retrieve patients' charts before they arrive.

Most private practices have replaced the open-hours system with scheduled appointments. Open-hours systems are still used by rural practices and by practices specializing in urgent care, such as emergency rooms and urgent care centers. An open-hours system still requires the use of an appointment book or electronic scheduling system to record patients as they come into the office. You still also must establish a matrix so that you will know when a doctor is out of the office.

Time-Specified Scheduling

Time-specified scheduling (also called stream scheduling) assumes a steady stream of patients all day long at regular, specified intervals. Most minor medical problems, such as sore throats, earaches, or blood pressure followups, usually require only 10- to 15-minute appointment slots. More time may be required for appointments such as physical exams, which usually require 60 minutes, or new patient visits, which usually require 30 minutes (Figure 12-2). When a visit requires more time, you simply assign the patient additional back-to-back slots.

Wave Scheduling

Wave scheduling works effectively in larger medical facilities that have enough departments and personnel to provide services to several patients at the same time. This method of scheduling is based on the reality that some patients will arrive late and that others will require more or less time than expected with the physician. Wave scheduling has the flexibility to allow for appointments that require more time than anticipated or for patients who miss appointments. The goal of wave scheduling is to begin and end each hour with the overall office schedule on track. You determine the number of patients to be seen each hour by dividing the hour by the length of the average visit. If the average is 15 minutes, for example, you schedule four patients for each hour. An example of wave scheduling would be:

10:00 A.M.	Patient A	555-5683	Sore throat
10:00 A.M.	Patient B	555-7322	Low back pain
10:00 A.M.	Patient C	555-4673	FU B/P
10:00 A.M.	Patient D	555-2854	B12 inj

You ask all four to arrive at the beginning of the hour and have the physician see them in the order of their actual arrival. The main problem with wave scheduling is that patients may realize they have appointments at the same time as other patients. The result may be confusion and possibly annoyance or anger.

Modified-Wave Scheduling

The wave system can be modified in several ways. With **modified-wave scheduling,** as shown in Figure 12-3, patients might be scheduled in 15-minute increments. Another option is to schedule four patients to arrive at planned intervals during the first half hour, leaving the second half hour unscheduled. Appointments that are anticipated to require more time should be scheduled at the beginning of the hour. Appointments that are expected to be less time-consuming should be scheduled in 10- to 20-minute time slots. This method allows time for catching up before the next hour begins.

Double-Booking

With a **double-booking system,** two or more patients are scheduled for the same appointment slot. Unlike the wave or modified-wave system, however, the double-booking system assumes that both patients will actually be seen within the scheduled period. If the types of visits are usually short (5 minutes, for example), it is reasonable to book two patients for one 15-minute opening. If both patients require the entire 15 minutes, however, the office falls behind schedule.

A double-booking schedule is especially useful when one patient does not necessarily need to see the physician. This may occur when a patient can be managed by a nurse practitioner or physician assistant, such as for an immunization or blood pressure check. Double-booking systems work most effectively in practices in which more than one patient can be attended to at a time.

Double-booking can be helpful if a patient calls with a problem and needs to be seen that day but no appointments are available. You could double-book this patient with an already scheduled patient. In such cases you should explain that the caller might have to wait a bit before being seen by the doctor.

Cluster Scheduling

As the name suggests, **cluster scheduling** groups similar appointments together during the day or week. (This system is also called categorization scheduling.) For example, you might cluster all physical examinations between 9:00 A.M. and 11:00 A.M. on Tuesdays and Thursdays. Cluster scheduling is also helpful in offices where specialized equipment or services (such as physical therapy or ultrasound) are available only at certain times. Procedure 12-1 explains how to create a cluster schedule.

Advance Scheduling

In some specialties patients might be booked weeks or months in advance, as for annual gynecologic examinations.

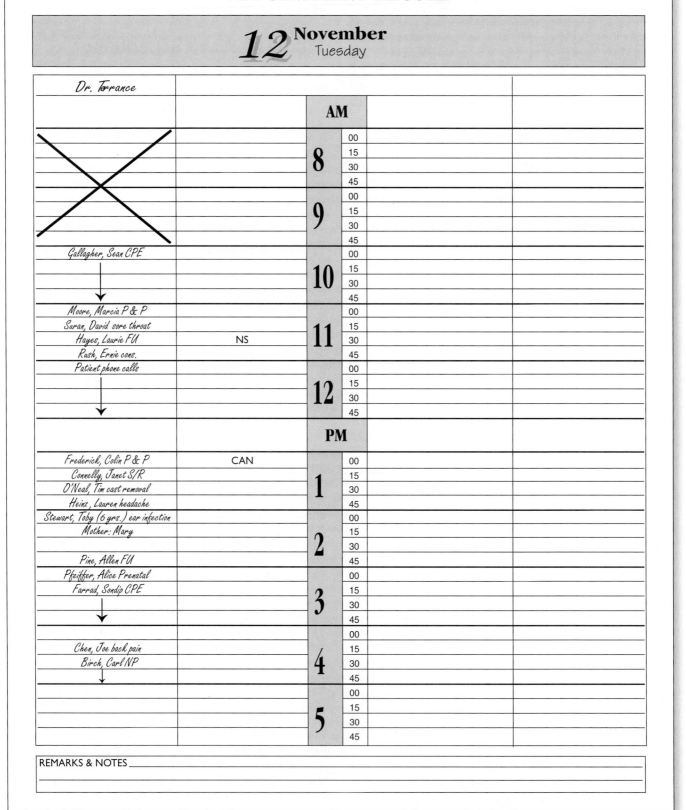

APPOINTMENT RECORD

12 November — Tuesday

Dr. Terrance

		AM			
		8	00		
			15		
			30		
			45		
		9	00		
			15		
			30		
			45		
Gallagher, Sean CPE		**10**	00		
			15		
			30		
			45		
Moore, Marcia P & P		**11**	00		
Suran, David sore throat			15		
Hayes, Laurie FU	NS		30		
Rush, Ernie cons.			45		
Patient phone calls		**12**	00		
			15		
			30		
			45		
		PM			
Frederick, Colin P & P	CAN	**1**	00		
Connelly, Janet S/R			15		
O'Neal, Tim cast removal			30		
Heinz, Lauren headache			45		
Stewart, Toby (6 yrs.) ear infection		**2**	00		
Mother: Mary			15		
			30		
Pine, Allen FU			45		
Pfeiffer, Alice Prenatal		**3**	00		
Farrad, Sondip CPE			15		
			30		
			45		
		4	00		
Chen, Joe back pain			15		
Birch, Carl NP			30		
			45		
		5	00		
			15		
			30		
			45		

REMARKS & NOTES _____

Figure 12-2. Time-specified appointment scheduling is commonly used in the medical office.

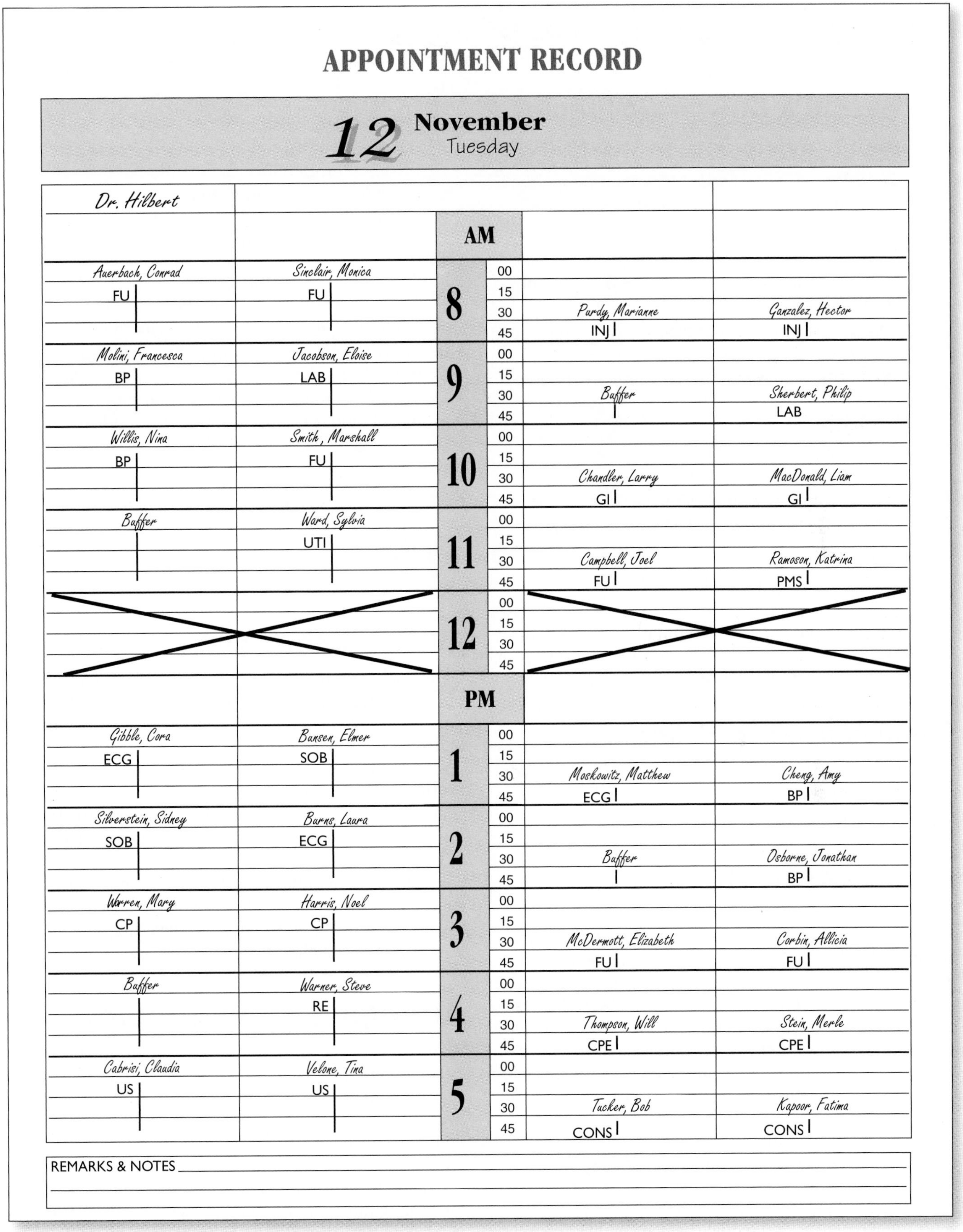

APPOINTMENT RECORD

12 November
Tuesday

Dr. Hilbert		AM			
Auerbach, Conrad **FU**	Sinclair, Monica **FU**	**8**	00 15 30 45	Purdy, Marianne **INJ**	Ganzalez, Hector **INJ**
Molini, Francesca **BP**	Jacobson, Eloise **LAB**	**9**	00 15 30 45	Buffer	Sherbert, Philip **LAB**
Willis, Nina **BP**	Smith, Marshall **FU**	**10**	00 15 30 45	Chandler, Larry **GI**	MacDonald, Liam **GI**
Buffer	Ward, Sylvia **UTI**	**11**	00 15 30 45	Campbell, Joel **FU**	Ramoson, Katrina **PMS**
✕		**12**	00 15 30 45	✕	
		PM			
Gibble, Cora **ECG**	Bunsen, Elmer **SOB**	**1**	00 15 30 45	Moskowitz, Matthew **ECG**	Cheng, Amy **BP**
Silverstein, Sidney **SOB**	Burns, Laura **ECG**	**2**	00 15 30 45	Buffer	Osborne, Jonathan **BP**
Warren, Mary **CP**	Harris, Noel **CP**	**3**	00 15 30 45	McDermott, Elizabeth **FU**	Corbin, Allicia **FU**
Buffer	Warner, Steve **RE**	**4**	00 15 30 45	Thompson, Will **CPE**	Stein, Merle **CPE**
Cabrisi, Claudia **US**	Velone, Tina **US**	**5**	00 15 30 45	Tucker, Bob **CONS**	Kapoor, Fatima **CONS**

REMARKS & NOTES _____

Figure 12-3. Modified-wave scheduling allows more flexibility than wave scheduling.

PROCEDURE 12-1 (WORK // PRODUCT)

Creating a Cluster Schedule

Procedure Goal: To set up a cluster schedule

Materials: Calendar, tickler file, appointment book, colored pencils or markers (optional)

Method:

1. Learn which categories of cases the physician would like to cluster and on what days and/or times of day.
2. Determine the length of the average visit in each category.
3. In the appointment book, cross out the hours in the week that the physician is typically not available.

Rationale

This creates the matrix of physician availability around which appointments can be booked.

4. Block out one period in midmorning and one in mid-afternoon for use as buffer, or reserve, times for unexpected needs.
5. Reserve additional slots for acutely ill patients. The number of slots depends on the type of practice.

Rationale

There needs to be room in the schedule for emergency appointments that cannot wait.

6. Mark the appointment times for clustered procedures. If desired, color-code the blocks of time. For example, make immunization clusters pink, blood pressure checks green, and so forth.

Rationale

Blocking the time or color coding it indicates that a specific type of appointment should be booked in this location.

In such practices **advance scheduling** is used. It is still advisable to leave a few slots open each day, however, for patients who call with unexpected or unusual problems.

Combination Scheduling

Some practices combine two or more scheduling methods. For example, they might use cluster scheduling for new patients and double-booking for quick follow-ups.

Computerized Scheduling

Computerized scheduling systems are becoming more common in medical offices because they have several advantages over handwritten systems (Figure 12-4). For example, they can be programmed to "lock out" selected appointment slots so that those slots will always be available for emergencies. Another advantage of using a computerized system is that the scheduling information can be accessed from all terminals located within the practice. Computerized systems can also help staff members identify patients who often are late, forget their appointments altogether, or cancel. In addition, the computer can identify patients who may require additional time with the physician because of special needs. Computerized scheduling also provides the doctor with a variety of reports about the scheduling practices of the office, which can help improve efficiency. You can use color coding when scheduling certain appointments. This can eliminate wrong entries into designated areas for other appointment types.

Online Scheduling

Online scheduling is relatively new. The patients schedule themselves via the computer and Internet. Many offices have not implemented this system because of cost and security; however, new security measures have been put in place to ensure protection of patient data online. Putting an online scheduler in your medical office takes time and requires training of the medical staff. If staffing levels are low, online scheduling may not be cost-effective.

Before you adopt an e-scheduler, assess your needs, survey patients for access to the Web, and find out about privacy issues. One of the frontrunners in e-scheduling is www.compassscheduling.com.

Arranging Appointments

Whether you are arranging appointments in person or by telephone, be polite and courteous. In scheduling an appointment, try to offer the patient a choice between two different dates, with either a morning or afternoon time slot. Once the patient decides on the date and time, always confirm the appointment by repeating it to the person before printing it in the schedule. If you are scheduling the appointment in person, write the appointment date and time on an appointment card to give to the patient. Whenever possible, try to accommodate the patient's needs while still maintaining a smoothly flowing schedule.

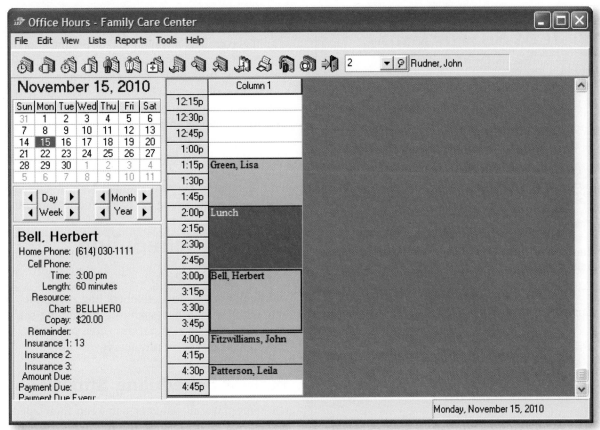

Figure 12-4. Many medical offices use computerized scheduling instead of or in addition to a traditional appointment book.

New Patients

A patient who has not been established at a medical practice is considered a new patient. Patients who have not been seen by the practice in three or more years are also considered to be new patients. Appointments for new patients are most often arranged over the telephone. Be sure to obtain all the necessary information, including the correct spelling and pronunciation of the person's name, home address, daytime telephone number, and date of birth. It is helpful to obtain insurance information at the time of new patient scheduling so that insurance verification can be made before the patient comes into the office.

When arranging the appointment, keep in mind that some physicians prefer to schedule new patients at certain times of the day, such as first thing in the morning. When scheduling an appointment for a new patient, make sure to allow enough time for filling out forms. Have the new patient arrive 15 to 30 minutes early to do this. Information about the office may be mailed out prior to the first appointment, including a patient information brochure, medical history forms, and a patient registration form if time allows. The patient should be instructed to complete the forms and bring the completed forms with him for the first appointment.

Return Appointments

It is always good practice to ask patients returning to the reception area if they need to schedule another appointment.

It may be helpful to routinely schedule return appointments at the same time and/or day that the patient has had previously. Getting them to make the appointment then will save you from having to do so by telephone later on. When patients call to arrange appointments, use the telephone techniques outlined in Chapter 11.

Appointment Reminders

Some patients may have trouble remembering their next appointment, especially if they arrange it far in advance. To help patients keep track of their appointments, you can use several types of appointment reminders.

Appointment Cards. In many offices the medical assistant fills out and hands the patient an appointment reminder card, like the one shown in Figure 12-5. To reduce the chance of error, enter the appointment in the appointment book first, then fill out the card. Otherwise, when the patient takes the appointment card, you have to rely on your memory when entering the appointment in the book.

Reminder Mailings. When making a follow-up appointment in person, you can ask the patient to address to himself a postcard on which you have written the next appointment's date and time. This postcard serves as a backup in case the patient loses the original appointment reminder card. Place the postcard in the tickler file under the day when it should be sent (usually a week or two

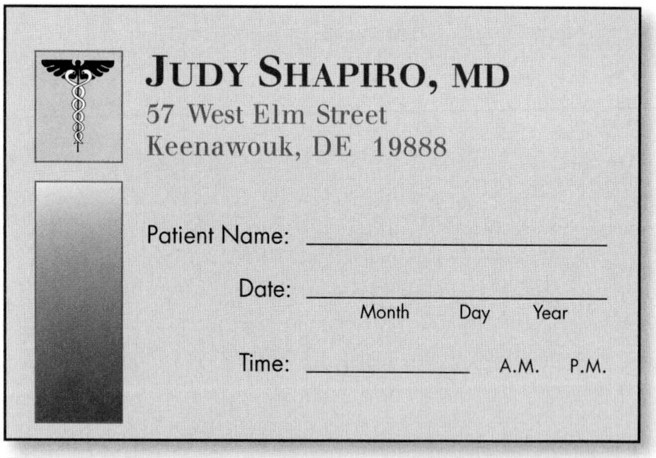
JUDY SHAPIRO, MD
57 West Elm Street
Keenawouk, DE 19888

Patient Name: ______

Date: ______
Month Day Year

Time: ______ A.M. P.M.

Figure 12-5. Before patients leave the office, be sure to give them an appointment card if they are scheduled to return to the office.

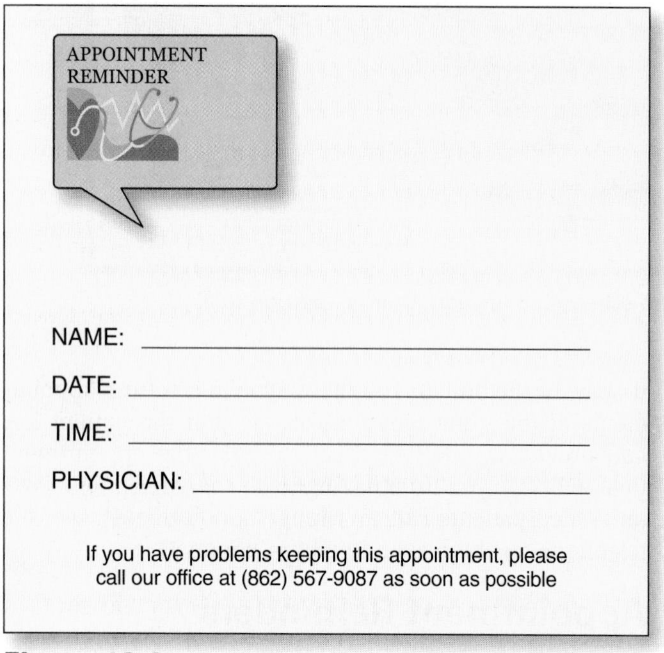
APPOINTMENT REMINDER

NAME: ______

DATE: ______

TIME: ______

PHYSICIAN: ______

If you have problems keeping this appointment, please call our office at (862) 567-9087 as soon as possible

Figure 12-6. An example of an appointment card.

before the appointment). Reminder mailings can also be sent to patients who make appointments over the telephone. In this case, of course, you must address the postcard for the tickler file yourself. Reminder mailings are useful when appointments are made many months in advance or are for geriatric patients (Figure 12-6).

Reminder Calls. Depending on office policy and available time, you might also call patients 1 or 2 days before their appointments to confirm the scheduled time. This technique can be especially helpful for patients with a history of late arrivals or for **no-shows** (patients who do not call to cancel and do not come to the appointment). Writing patients' phone numbers next to their names in the appointment book makes it convenient for you to make appointment reminder calls.

Recall Notices. Some offices book appointments no more than a few weeks in advance, or may not have the next year's schedule available when a patient is to book a return appointment. In either case, if your office has such a policy, you need a way to make sure patients do not forget to call for appointments that are 6 months—or even a year—away from their last appointments.

Suppose, for example, that the physician tells a patient she should have an annual breast examination. How can you help her remember to call to schedule one at the appropriate time? One way is to use a system of recall notices. In a tickler file enter the patient's name under the month when she should call the office. When the time arrives, send a form letter reminding her that she will soon be due for a breast examination and asking her to call for an appointment.

Special Scheduling Situations

Although a great deal of scheduling is routine, creativity and flexibility are necessary for scheduling some special cases. These special situations often involve patients, but they may also involve physicians.

Patient Scheduling Situations

On some days all patients will keep their appointments and arrive on time. On many other days, however, patients may walk in without appointments, arrive late for scheduled appointments, or miss appointments entirely. Being prepared for these possibilities allows you to handle them better and to keep the office schedule running as smoothly as possible.

Emergencies. Your training as a medical assistant will help you recognize the signs of an emergency. In some instances you will refer the caller to the nearest hospital emergency room or instruct the caller to call Emergency Medical Services (EMS) for an ambulance. In other instances you will ask the caller to come to the office right away. It is vital that doctors see emergency patients before patients who are already in the waiting area or on the schedule. It is best to explain to waiting patients that there has been an emergency (without giving details). This announcement helps them understand and accept the delay and also gives them an opportunity to reschedule their appointments. The Points on Practice section provides guidelines for scheduling emergency appointments. Procedure 11-2 in Chapter 11 details how to handle emergency calls.

Referrals. Sometimes other doctors refer patients to the practice for second opinions or special consultations. A patient seeking a second opinion before deciding on surgery, often at the request of his or her insurance carrier, should be fit into the schedule as soon as possible. Other referred patients should also be seen quickly, as a matter of professional courtesy to the referring doctor as well as good business practice.

Many office manuals contain a listing of referral physicians and facilities, including the names of facilities or

Points on Practice

Scheduling Emergency Appointments

As a multiskilled medical assistant, you will be well prepared to tell the difference between acute conditions that are emergencies and those that are not. Guidelines on types of emergencies to be seen in the office and types to be referred elsewhere will vary. If you have any doubt, interrupt the physician to ask for instructions.

Even with buffer times built into the daily schedule, emergencies are still disruptive to most practices. Your ability to stay calm, respond quickly, and remain flexible will be of great comfort to the emergency patient and to others in the waiting area. Read the following story to see how an emergency situation can be handled skillfully.

The Situation

It is 4:15 P.M. in a busy family practice. The telephone rings. The caller is the father of a 10-year-old boy. Maria, the medical assistant, can hear the panic in his voice. His son Kyle has injured his knee while playing football with friends. Kyle cannot straighten the knee, and it is quite swollen.

Maria consults the physician, who suspects torn cartilage. The physician tells Maria to have the father wrap ice in a towel, apply it to Kyle's knee, and bring him in immediately. Maria relays this advice to the father and asks him how soon he can get to the office.

"It will take about 25 minutes," he replies.

The office schedule includes a buffer time opening at 4:30, but based on the father's estimate, Kyle cannot possibly arrive until 4:40. Maria notes that Mrs. Griffin, a good-natured retiree, is scheduled to come in for her weekly blood pressure check at 4:45 P.M. Hers is the last scheduled appointment of the day.

The Solution

Mrs. Griffin lives about 5 minutes from the office. Maria calls her home and explains that there has been an emergency. She offers Mrs. Griffin three choices: she can come in at 4:30 and be seen then; she can arrive at the usual time and expect to wait; or she can be rescheduled for tomorrow.

"No problem," Mrs. Griffin says cheerfully. "I'll come right over."

Mrs. Griffin arrives at 4:35. At 4:40, Kyle hobbles in, supported by his father. Maria greets them and offers Kyle a chair on which to prop his foot.

Mrs. Griffin's blood pressure check is complete at 4:45. Kyle waits only 5 minutes before he is seen.

Thanks to Maria's quick thinking, the office stays on schedule—essentially by switching one appointment for another.

---

specialty physicians, their addresses, and their phone numbers. When arranging a referral, try to give the patient two referral names to choose from, along with the referral phone numbers and addresses. When choosing the referral names of either physicians or facilities, be sure that the facility accepts the patient's insurance. All referrals should be documented in the patient's medical record.

Fasting Patients. Some procedures and tests require patients to fast (refrain from eating or drinking anything beginning the night before). Scheduling these patients as early in the day as possible shows consideration for their needs. When scheduling appointments that require the patient to fast, be sure to inform the patient of the need to fast and when fasting should start.

Patients with Diabetes. Like fasting patients, patients with diabetes can use extra consideration when you schedule their appointments. In general, patients who take insulin must eat meals and snacks at regular times. This routine keeps their blood sugar from dropping too low—a condition that can result in confused thinking or even loss of consciousness. Therefore, you might want to avoid scheduling patients with diabetes for slots in late morning,

close to lunchtime. If the schedule is running late by the time these patients arrive, they will be waiting in your reception area at a time when they really need to eat.

If the physician sees multiple patients with diabetes, you might also ask him about keeping appropriate snacks on hand to offer these patients in emergencies. Most patients with diabetes, however, carry their own emergency snacks with them to treat low blood sugar.

Repeat Visits. Some patients need regular appointments, such as for prenatal checkups or physical therapy. If possible, schedule these appointments for the same day and time each week. Establishing a routine helps patients remember their appointments and simplifies the office schedule.

Late Arrivals. If the practice has patients who are routinely late and gentle reminders to be on time have not helped, you might try booking them toward the end of the day. Even if a patient arrives late for a late-afternoon appointment, the doctor has already seen most of the day's patients and the late patient will not disrupt the schedule. Document late arrivals or missed appointments in the patient's chart. With documentation, patients who are habitually late can be called to discuss the reasons for their lateness. The goal of the discussion should be to find a solution so that patients can make their appointments on time and the schedule will run smoothly.

Walk-Ins. From time to time, a patient (or a person who has not visited the practice before) may arrive without an appointment and still expect to see the doctor. These people are called **walk-ins.** Office policies on how to handle walk-ins vary. If the person is experiencing an emergency, handle the situation as you would handle any emergency. Otherwise, you might politely explain that the doctor is fully booked for the day and offer to schedule an appointment in the usual manner. If, by chance, the doctor is available and willing to see the walk-in, you should still ask the person to call to schedule appointments in the future. If your physician's office has a policy of no walkins, post a sign in the lobby or waiting area stating that patients are seen by appointment only.

Cancellations. When patients call to cancel appointments, thank them for calling, and try to reschedule the appointment while they are on the telephone. If patients say they will call later to reschedule, note this information in the appointment book.

You should also write "canceled" in the appointment book and draw a single line through the patient's name. To avoid confusion, cancel the first appointment *before* entering the patient's rescheduled appointment. Remember that the appointment book is a legal record. If you forget to cross out the name at the time of the first appointment, it may later seem that the doctor saw the patient twice. It is also important to note the cancellation in the patient's medical record. This notation can protect the practice from possible legal action. For example, a patient whose incision became infected could not blame the doctor if the patient canceled an appointment for a dressing change.

You may be able to fill slots created by cancellations by calling patients who have appointments scheduled for later in the day or week. Some patients may be willing to come in earlier than planned. When you make appointments, you can ask patients if they would be interested in coming in earlier if openings occur. Placing the names of interested patients in a tickler file can save time later.

Missed and Wrong-Day Appointments. It is important for legal reasons to document a no-show in the appointment book and patient record. Always inform the physician of any missed appointments in case the patient's condition requires a follow-up. The physician may want you to call the patient with a polite reminder that the patient has missed an appointment and needs to reschedule. There may have been a misunderstanding about the time, or the patient may simply have forgotten the appointment. Some offices, especially ones that use computerized scheduling systems, send out form letters when patients miss appointments. If failure to keep the appointment could endanger the patient's health, mention this possibility to the patient, or ask the physician to tell the patient over the telephone.

Periodically, physicians charge for missed appointments, especially if patients habitually miss their appointments. These missed appointment charges are for missed business opportunities and not for services rendered. If your office implements this policy, make sure that you let patients know in advance before you start charging them for missed appointments. Some offices opt for a notation on the appointment cards that states patients will be charged for appointments that are cancelled with less than 24 hours notice.

Sometimes a patient may show up on the wrong day for her appointment. If the patient lives in the local area, rescheduling makes sense. But if the patient made special transportation arrangements or traveled from a long distance, it may be best to try to work the patient into the schedule for the day. This is especially true if the patient has an appointment card verifying the appointment for that day, but she is not on the schedule. If that is the case, the office is obligated to honor the appointment if the physician is in the office. When in doubt about the best course of action, consult with the doctor or office manager.

Physician Scheduling Situations

Not all scheduling problems result from patients. Sometimes physicians disrupt the office schedule. They may be called away on an emergency, may be delayed at the hospital, or may simply arrive late. In any event, the appointment schedule may get off track.

Physicians are only human and may occasionally be late for appointments. Some physicians are frequently late, however, either when arriving in the morning or when returning from lunch or from scheduled meetings. If this situation occurs in your office, you might approach it in several ways.

At a staff meeting you could mention that the morning or afternoon schedule often seems to get off to a late start. Then you might ask if anyone has suggestions for improving this situation. The physician may recognize that she is the cause of the problem and decide to resolve it.

If the physician does not take responsibility for the problem, however, you may need to adjust the office schedule to handle the situation. Suppose, for example, that the first patient appointment slot is at 8:30 A.M., but the physician usually does not arrive until 8:35 A.M. You could simply avoid scheduling patients between 8:30 and 8:45 A.M. If a physician is often 15 minutes late returning from lunch or from meetings, you might leave open the first appointment slot after the normal arrival time. In effect, you build buffer time into the schedule.

Scheduling Outside Appointments

You may be responsible for arranging patient appointments outside the medical office. These appointments may include:

- Consultations with other physicians
- Laboratory work

- X-rays
- Other diagnostic tests
- Hospital stays
- Surgeries

Before scheduling these appointments, ask the doctor for an order that identifies the exact procedures to be performed and specifies when the results will be needed. Always verify the patient's type of insurance before choosing which facility or physician the referral will be sent to. HMOs (health maintenance organizations) often will arrange the referral themselves or at least require that only facilities and physicians who contract with the HMO see their patients. If patients are referred to noncontracted providers, the services will not be paid for by the HMO. The medical assistant or secretary requesting the referral completes the necessary forms and faxes them to the insurance company or submits the required information online via the insurance company's website. The insurance company will authorize the referral and notify the office when approved. Sometimes referrals, if not urgent, can take 30 days or longer to approve although electronic referrals usually are approved in a shorter time frame.

Once authorization has been obtained, document the authorization (referral) number in the patient's financial or insurance file. This number must appear on all forms related to this appointment for the procedure to be paid, then talk with the patient to find convenient appointment times.

This habit is not only courteous but also gives patients a sense of control over situations they may find a bit frightening. Some doctors' offices may have you call the outside laboratory or hospital with all information concerning the patient and then give the patient the number to call to set up the appointment. This approach is often easier for patients. They then have the telephone number in case they need to reschedule.

If you are calling to make the appointment for the patient, tell the medical assistant, scheduling secretary, or admissions clerk what consultation, test, or procedure is required. Then find out what your office or the patient must do to prepare for the appointment. For example, the admitting doctor may need to complete a preadmission evaluation for a patient prior to the hospitalization or the patient may need to be instructed to fast (nothing to eat or drink after midnight) the night before the procedure.

When arrangements have been made, inform the patient, and note on the chart that you have done so. You may also provide the patient with a completed referral slip or, in the case of laboratory work, a laboratory request slip. Procedure 12-2 explains how to schedule and confirm appointments for surgery. (You will find additional information on preparing patients for surgery in Chapter 14.) Figure 12-7 is an example of a surgery flow sheet that is prepared by the medical assistant for the physician. Flow sheet information varies; however, each section should be checked off before the doctor performs the surgery.

PROCEDURE 12-2

Scheduling and Confirming Surgery at a Hospital

Procedure Goal: To follow the proper procedure for scheduling and confirming surgery

Materials: Calendar, telephone, notepad, pen

Method:

1. Elective surgery is usually performed on certain days when the doctor is scheduled to be in the operating room and a room and an anesthetist are available. The patient may be given only one or two choices of days and times. (For emergency surgery the first step is to reserve the operating room.)

2. Call the operating room secretary. Give the procedure required, the name of the surgeon, the time involved, and the preferred date and hour.

3. Provide the patient's name (including birth name, if appropriate), address, telephone number, age, gender, Social Security number, and insurance information.

Rationale

This ensures that the hospital has the correct patient information for the admission.

4. Call the admissions office (or day-stay surgery office). Arrange for the patient to be admitted on the day of surgery or the day before (depending on the surgery to be performed). Ask for a copy of the admissions form for the patient record.

5. Some hospitals want patients to complete preadmission forms. In such cases, request a blank form for the patient. Depending on hospital policy, tell the patient to arrive for the appointment a few minutes early to complete the appropriate paperwork.

6. Confirm the surgery and the patient's arrival time 1 business day before surgery.

Rationale

This helps to ensure that the patient will not forget about the appointment date and time.

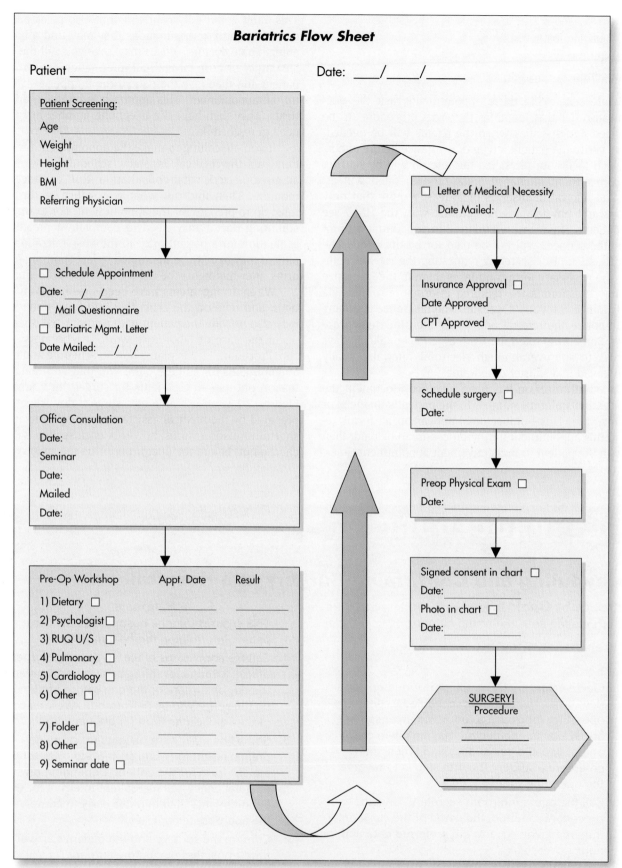

Bariatrics Flow Sheet

Patient _____   Date: ____/____/____

Patient Screening:

Age _____

Weight _____

Height _____

BMI _____

Referring Physician _____

☐ Schedule Appointment

Date: ___/___/___

☐ Mail Questionnaire

☐ Bariatric Mgmt. Letter

Date Mailed: ___/___/___

Office Consultation

Date:

Seminar

Date:

Mailed

Date:

Pre-Op Workshop	Appt. Date	Result
1) Dietary ☐	_____	_____
2) Psychologist ☐	_____	_____
3) RUQ U/S ☐	_____	_____
4) Pulmonary ☐	_____	_____
5) Cardiology ☐	_____	_____
6) Other ☐	_____	_____
7) Folder ☐	_____	_____
8) Other ☐	_____	_____
9) Seminar date ☐	_____	_____

☐ Letter of Medical Necessity

Date Mailed: ___/___/___

Insurance Approval ☐

Date Approved _____

CPT Approved _____

Schedule surgery ☐

Date: _____

Preop Physical Exam ☐

Date: _____

Signed consent in chart ☐

Date: _____

Photo in chart ☐

Date: _____

SURGERY!
Procedure

_____
_____

Figure 12-7. An example of a surgery flow sheet prepared by the medical assistant for the physician.

Maintaining the Physician's Schedule

The schedules of busy physicians are not limited to office visits with patients and hospital rounds. Physicians also need to attend professional meetings, travel to conferences, present speeches to colleagues, complete paperwork, and perform other duties. Your job is to help physicians make the most efficient use of their time.

One way is to avoid overbooking appointments with patients. **Overbooking** (scheduling more patients than can reasonably be seen in the time allowed) creates stress for the physician and the staff, and eventually causes the office schedule to fall behind.

The opposite problem, **underbooking**—leaving large, unused gaps in the schedule—does not make the best use of the physician's time. Of course, you have no control over patients who cancel or do not show for appointments. If you cannot reschedule another patient for the empty slot, the physician can use the time to catch up on telephone calls to patients or to attend to other matters.

At times you will have to cancel appointments because the physician has been delayed or called away by an emergency. Apologize to waiting patients on behalf of the physician, and offer them a choice. Explain that they can wait in the office (give an estimated waiting time), leave to run errands and return later, or reschedule their appointments for another day. Documentation should be noted in the patient's chart that because of an emergency in the office, the appointment had to be rescheduled. Be sure to write the date of the rescheduled appointment in the chart. Always make sure patients who need immediate attention are seen by another physician.

Reserving Operating Rooms

If the doctor in your office plans to perform surgery at a hospital, you will need to call the operating room secretary to reserve the facility. Give the preferred dates and times, the type of surgery, and the length of time the doctor will need the operating room. After the day and time are set, provide the secretary with all relevant patient information. Relay any requests from the doctor, such as the blood type and units of blood that may be needed. It may also be your responsibility to make arrangements for surgical assistants, an anesthetist, and a hospital bed for the patient following surgery.

The Physician's Medical Bag

Although less common than it used to be, some physicians (especially those in more rural areas) do make house calls and nursing home visits. It may be your responsibility to keep the medical bag for these visits well stocked. Some items to be included are adhesive tape/bandages, biohazard container, BP cuff and stethoscope, specimen containers, medications (such as antibiotics, epinephrine and

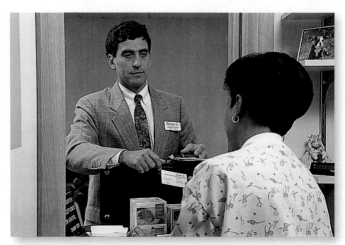

Figure 12-8. If pharmaceutical representatives come into the office without an appointment, you can ask them to leave a business card.

digitalis), ophthalmoscope and otoscope, penlight, latex gloves, face shield and gown, prescription pad and pen, scissors, dressing forceps, sterile swabs, thermometer, and sterile syringes and needles.

Scheduling Pharmaceutical Sales Representatives

Drug manufacturers often send pharmaceutical sales representatives into medical offices with printed information about new drugs as well as free samples that can be given to patients. These representatives are sometimes called detail persons. Some doctors do not want to meet with pharmaceutical representatives. Other doctors are willing to spend a few minutes if time permits and if the products are likely to be useful to the practice. Some doctors set aside a certain time 1 or 2 days a week to see detail persons. When a pharmaceutical representative who is unknown to you comes into the office, ask for a business card and check with the doctor before scheduling an appointment (Figure 12-8). (Storing drug samples is discussed in Chapter 8.)

Making Travel Arrangements

You may be responsible for arranging transportation and lodging when physicians attend meetings, speaking engagements, and other events out of town. You may contact the airline, car rental agency, hotel, or other services yourself, use an online service such as Orbitz, or you may work through a travel agent. No matter which method is used for travel arrangements, always request confirmation of travel and room reservations.

Before the day of departure, obtain an itinerary from the travel agent or online service, or create one yourself. An **itinerary** is a detailed travel plan, listing dates and times of flights and events, locations of meetings and

Dr. W. Hight's Travel Itinerary

Client Information

Traveler's Name	Dr. Will Hight
Address	560 Williamsburg Ct., Atlanta
Telephone Number	404-279-0098
Fax Number	404-279-0099
E-Mail Address	
Travel Dates	May 5 – 9, 200X

Departure Flight

Date	May 5, 200X
Airline	United International
Flight Number	567
From	Atlanta
Departure Time	6:45 am
Departure Terminal/Gate	56C
To	Los Angeles, California
Arrival Time	9:45 am pacific time
Length of Flight	5 hours
Class	First Class
Seat Number	12a
Status	confirmed

Monday – May 5, 200X

- **Morning:**

8:00 – 8:45	Physician Recruiter
9:00 – 10:00	Formal interview with Team, facilitated by Recruiter
10:00 – 11:00	Medical Director
11:00 – 12:00	Tour of UCLA including department with Area Manager

- **Afternoon:**

12:30 – 1:30	Lunch with physician(s) from another department with similar interests
2:00 – 3:00	One (1) hour with Department Chair and/or Physician Area Manager
4:00 – 6:00	One-on-one interviews with department or other physicians
	Informal time in interviewing department, as appropriate

- **Evening:**

7:00 – until	Dinner* ** (or private dinner on their own)

Figure 12-9. An example travel itinerary.

lodgings, and telephone numbers. Give several copies to the physician, and keep one for the office (Figure 12-9).

You may also be responsible for scheduling and confirming professional coverage of the practice during the physician's absence. In larger practices and more urban area, often physicians in the same or nearby practice will provide coverage while the physician is away. This coverage may be important for legal reasons, most importantly so the physician cannot be charged with "abandoning" his patients (see Chapter 3). If a local physician is not readily available, a **locum tenens,** or substitute physician, may be hired to see patients while the regular physician is away. (*Locum tenens* is Latin for "one occupying the place of another.") You may have more than one locum tenens on call, depending on the practice. In some areas special firms provide a locum tenens and other temporary medical and nursing help. Before hiring locum tenens physicians, you may want to contact some of the major insurance carriers providing health insurance coverage for your patients to find out their credentialing and claim requirements so that the services provided by the locum tenens physicians will be considered covered services.

Planning Meetings

You may help the doctor set up meetings of professional societies or committees. To do so, you will need to know how many people are expected to attend, how long the meeting will last, and the purpose of the meeting. In addition, ask the doctor if a meal is to be served.

Some groups always meet at the same location. If there is no established meeting place, you must choose and reserve one. Select a location with an adequately sized meeting room, sufficient parking, and, if needed, food services. Be sure also to arrange for necessary equipment, such as a microphone, podium, or projector. Many conference centers and hotels have an on-site catering

TABLE 12-1 Common Items on a Physician's Schedule

Payments, Dues, and Fees
- Association dues
- Health insurance premium
- Payment for laundry service
- Liability insurance premium
- Life insurance premium
- Office rent
- Property insurance premium
- Paychecks for staff
- Payment for janitorial services
- Payment for leased equipment
- Taxes
  - Quarterly federal tax payments
  - Quarterly state tax payments
  - Annual federal and state tax filing deadline

Time Commitments
- Committee meetings
- Conventions

Renewals and Accreditations
- Facility accreditation
  - State requirements
  - Certificate of necessity
  - Laboratory registration
  - Federal requirements
  - Ambulatory surgical centers
  - Physician office laboratory
- Medical license renewal
- Narcotics license renewal
- Drug Enforcement Agency registrations
- CME accreditations

manager or conference manager to assist you with these arrangements. When the facility has been booked, mail a notice to all those expected to attend the meeting. On the notice provide the topic, names of the speakers, date, time, place, and admission costs or fees associated with attending.

With direction from the physician, you may also be responsible for creating the meeting's agenda. An **agenda** is a list of topics to be discussed or presented at a meeting in order of presentation. After the meeting, you may also be asked to prepare the **minutes,** or the report of what was discussed and decided at the meeting.

Scheduling Time with the Physician

You and the physician should meet on a scheduled basis (maybe 1–2 a month) to discuss any irregularities or changes in the day-to-day workings of the office and items in the tickler file that may need his attention, as well as to keep up with any necessary paperwork. Examples of recurring deadlines include those for state medical license renewal, Drug Enforcement Agency (DEA) registrations, and documentation of the physician's continuing medical education (CME) requirements. Table 12-1 lists items that are often part of a physician's schedule.

Summary

12.1   The appointment book is important in a medical office because it creates an orderly and efficient patient flow, showing respect for both the patients' and physician's time.

12.2   Commonly used abbreviations save space and time when entering information into an appointment book. Examples of these are found in the chapter.

12.3   There are several different types of appointment scheduling systems that can be used, including both paper and electronic appointment scheduling systems. The most common types of appointment scheduling systems are open-hours, time-specified, wave and modified-wave, doubling-booking, and cluster scheduling.

12.4   When arranging appointments for patients, be courteous and polite. Offer several different dates and times; always confirm the appointment by repeating it to the patient. The goal is to accommodate the patient as much as possible while maintaining a smooth flowing schedule.

12.5   Special scheduling requires creativity and flexibility. This type of scheduling may be required not only by the physician if she is late or a patient's appointment runs longer than scheduled, but also by the patient for emergency appointments, those who need repeat visits, and those who arrive late or on the wrong date as well.

12.6   Document late arrivals and no-show patients for legal reasons within the patient's medical record. If, for example, a patient consistently misses appointments, then blames the doctor for an infected wound, the documentation of the missed appointments in the medical record shows a lack of follow up on the part of the patient for his medical care. Call patients to discuss reasons for lateness or no-show and attempt to reschedule the appointment, documenting the patient's response. If the patient's health is at stake because of missed appointments, ask the physician to speak to the patient by phone.

12.7 Before scheduling outside appointments, have the following information available: Patient name, DOB, insurance information, procedure necessary, preferred date and time. If necessary, request prior approval from the insurance carrier and document the authorization number in the patient's financial chart. Once an appointment is made, obtain any pre-appointment information needed for the patient and document the appointment in the patient's medical record.

12.8 Your job as a medical assistant is to keep the physician's schedule accurate and efficient. You can do this by not overbooking or underbooking and rearranging patient appointments as necessary to accommodate emergency appointments.

REVIEW

CHAPTER 12

CASE STUDY QUESTIONS

Now that you have completed this chapter, review the case study at the beginning of the chapter and answer the following questions:

1. How would you adjust the schedule to allow for the emergency without falling behind schedule?
2. If it is necessary to reschedule patients, who should be rescheduled and when?
3. Would you explain anything to the patients in the waiting room about the emergency? If so, what would you say?

Multiple-Choice Questions

1. The abbreviation for injection is
   a. I & J.
   c. Inj.
   b. Inj.
   d. Injc.
2. Which form of scheduling is also called stream scheduling?
   a. Time-specified scheduling
   b. Wave scheduling
   c. Open-hour scheduling
   d. Cluster scheduling
3. _____ groups similar appointments together during the day or week.
   a. Double-booking scheduling
   b. Open-hours scheduling
   c. Modified-wave scheduling
   d. Cluster scheduling
4. No-show means
   a. a patient that has passed away
   b. a person who is no longer a patient of the doctor
   c. a patient who does not call to cancel and does not come to the appointment.
   d. a patient who comes to the appointment but leaves because of other engagements.

5. What is the best approach to handling patient cancellations?
   a. Send the patient a letter pointing out that he canceled a necessary appointment.
   b. Attempt to schedule another patient in the cancellation slot.
   c. Encourage the physician to take the time off.
   d. Schedule other activities in those cancellation slots.

Discussion Questions

1. Describe situations that could cause the office to run behind schedule.
2. List the different types of appointment scheduling systems and briefly describe each.
3. Why is it important to note missed appointments and cancellations in the patient record and in the appointment book?
4. What is a matrix and why is it necessary?
5. List how long each of the following appointments should be scheduled for:
   a. earache
   b. CPE
   c. wound check
   d. Pap
   e. suture removal
   f. establish NP w/Rx prn
6. List the information that should be documented in the appointment book when scheduling.
7. Discuss how you would feel in a situation in which you had an extended wait in a physician's office. What could the medical assistant or office personnel do to ease your frustration?

Critical Thinking Questions

1. A persistent pharmaceutical representative continues to come into the office without an appointment. How would you handle this situation?
2. The physician is running about an hour and a half behind schedule and the schedule is completely filled. Describe how you would handle this problem.
3. What do you say to a patient who wishes to schedule an appointment but is reluctant to tell you the reason for the appointment? Would you make the appointment?
4. Right after lunch, a patient walks into the office and requests to see the physician. The patient does not have an appointment and is complaining of pain in her stomach that will not go away. She has vomited a few times and looks very pale. How should you handle this situation?
5. Describe the best scheduling system for the following types of physician offices:
   a. A large practice with four physicians and with x-ray and lab facilities that are available anytime
   b. A small practice with two physicians and with lab facilities that are available only between 8:00 A.M. and 10:00 A.M.

Application Activities

1. A patient arrives at 10:00 A.M. for an appointment. When you check the schedule, the patient is not listed for an appointment for today. The patient produces an appointment card that clearly states that he has an appointment on this date at 10:00 A.M. You check tomorrow's schedule and realize that the patient is scheduled for the next day at 10:00 A.M. The medical office staff member who filled out the appointment card had made a mistake. The schedule for today is completely full and is already running behind. The patient is leaving the country for two months tomorrow morning and must see the physician today. What should you do?
2. A patient is a no-show for an appointment today. List where this should be documented. Discuss why it is important to document a no-show appointment.
3. Dr. Thompson, the only physician in your office, is out of town at a medical meeting. She is due back tomorrow morning. At 4:00 P.M., Dr. Thompson calls to say that a blizzard has closed the airport and she will be forced to stay away for another day. You look at tomorrow's schedule. She has a full patient load. What should you do?

Virtual Fieldtrip

Visit the McGraw-Hill Higher Education Medical Assisting website at www.mhhe.com/medicalassisting4e to complete the following activity:

Visit The American Association of Medical Assistants website and other websites about medical practice scheduling. Prepare an oral presentation regarding topics such as electronic scheduling, different methods of medical appointment scheduling, scheduling for patients with special needs, and methods to help avoid underbooking and overbooking appointments. Present your report to the class, using all available multimedia, including PowerPoint slides or an overhead projector.

Open the CD and complete this chapter's practice activities, play the games, listen to the key terms, and test yourself with the interactive review. E-mail, print, and/or save your results to document your proficiency.

CHAPTER 13

Patient Reception

LEARNING OUTCOMES

After completing Chapter 13, you will be able to:

13.1 Identify the elements that are important in a patient reception area.

13.2 Illustrate ways to determine what furniture is necessary for a patient reception area and how it should be arranged.

13.3 Describe the housekeeping tasks and equipment needed for this area of the office.

13.4 Explain the Occupational Safety and Health Administration (OSHA) regulations that pertain to a patient reception area.

13.5 Describe the physical components associated with a comfortable and accessible patient reception area.

13.6 Describe the physical components associated with a safe and secure patient reception area.

13.7 Describe the types of reading material appropriate to a patient reception area.

13.8 Explain how modifications to a reception area can accommodate patients with special needs.

13.9 Describe special situations that can affect the arrangement of a reception area.

MEDICAL ASSISTING COMPETENCIES

CAAHEP

IV. C (14) Recognize the role of patient advocacy in the practice of medical assisting

IV. P (13) Advocate on behalf of patients

XI. C (7) Describe fundamental principles for evacuation of a health-care setting

X. P (7) Explain an evacuation plan for a physician's office

ABHES

5. Psychology of Human Relations
   b. Identify and respond appropriately when working/caring for patients with special needs
   e. Advocate on behalf of family/patients, having ability to deal and communicate with family

8. Medical Office Business Procedures Management
   e. Locate resources and information for patients and employers
   x. Maintain medical facility
   hh. Receive, organize, prioritize, and transmit information expediently

11. Career Development
Demonstrate professionalism by:
   1) Exhibiting dependability, punctuality, and a positive work ethic
   2) Exhibiting a positive attitude and a sense of responsibility
   5) Exhibiting initiative
   7) Expressing a responsible attitude
   8) Being courteous and diplomatic
   9) Conducting work within scope of education, training, and ability

MEDICAL ASSISTING MEDIA

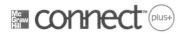 Connect Plus+™ connect.mcgraw-hill.com	• Electronic Health Records (E.H.R.) SpringCharts® • eBook	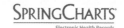
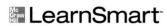 **LearnSmart™**	www.mhhe.com/learnsmart	Complete Learning Module: Patient Reception
Student CD-ROM		
Online Learning Center™	www.mhhe.com/medicalassisting4e	

KEY TERMS

access

Americans with Disabilities
 Act

color family

contagious

infectious waste

interim room

Older Americans Act
 of 1965

teletype (TTY) device

CHAPTER OUTLINE

- First Impressions
- The Importance of Cleanliness
- The Physical Components
- Keeping Patients Occupied and Informed
- Patients with Special Needs

PREPARATION FOR CERTIFICATION

RMA (AMT) Exam
- General reception of patients and visitors

CMA (AAMA) Exam
- Physical environment
- Patient advocate

CMAS Exam
- Reception
- Safety

Introduction

Going to the doctor's office can be an emotional and sometimes even a frightening event for many people. The office staff can do much to make the entry into the medical environment easier and less intimidating.

This chapter describes the patient reception area. As you look at the reception area and patient bathrooms through the eyes of patient needs, you begin to see ways to make the rooms both inviting and functional. Additionally, you will learn about the special needs of disabled patients. Well-planned and pleasant surroundings can do much to set the stage for a successful interaction between the patient and the doctor and other medical staff.

A 70-year-old patient has just arrived for his first appointment with his new primary care physician. He recently moved to Florida to be near his grown children, and today he meets his new doctor. He is apprehensive and concerned that he won't like this new doctor. He takes a deep breath and opens the door into the medical office reception room.

The first thing he notices is the cool air, which is in stark contrast to the hot humid air outside. As he enters the area, he sees a comfortable, spacious room decorated in soft color tones. The chairs and sofas are arranged in small conversational groupings. Neatly stacked on the tables is a colorful array of many different types of magazines. Playing softly in the corner of the room is a television tuned to a health channel. At the end of the room are a sliding glass window and a countertop with a sign-in clipboard. Crossing the room, he notices a family with small children playing with blocks in an adjoining room marked "Children's Reception Area." He sees a courtesy phone for patient use located in a nearby alcove. He adds his name to the list on the clipboard, noticing that all the patient names above his own have been blacked out. The glass window immediately opens and a neatly dressed medical assistant with a pleasant smile speaks to him, calling him by name. He is beginning to think this doctor might be all right after all.

As you read this chapter, consider the following questions:

1. What basic elements are *required* in every patient reception area? What other nonessential elements are nice to include as well?
2. Why is it important to think of the front patient area as the "patient reception area" and not the "waiting room"?
3. What special accommodations in the reception area are important to patients with disabilities?

First Impressions

The reception area plays a significant role in a patient's experience at the doctor's office. It is the first area patients see when entering the office. It is also a place where they have to spend time waiting for their appointments.

The appearance of the reception area creates an impression of the practice. Is the office bright and cheerful, cool and modern, or warm and cozy? The impression created by the reception area reflects on the quality of care patients can expect to receive. For example, old, tattered, or dirty furniture in the reception area will give patients the impression that the medical practice is unsuccessful and outdated. A carefully designed and well-maintained patient reception area, on the other hand, can attract and keep patients in the practice. It also ensures a pleasant and comfortable experience while they wait to receive medical care.

 ## Reception Area

The reception area includes a reception window or desk, as shown in Figure 13-1, where patients check in for their appointments. Windows are not soundproof. Care should be taken by employees to minimize noise and conversation behind the window.

The reception area also includes chairs and couches for patients to sit on while waiting. Most patient reception areas are arranged using the same basic organizational

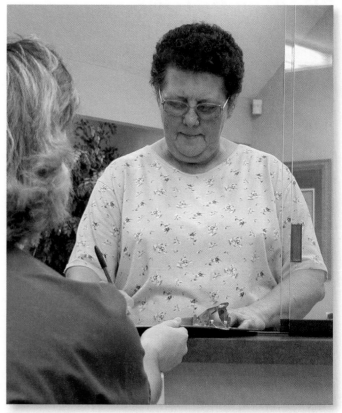

Figure 13-1. A receptionist's desk or window, where patients can check in, is part of every patient reception area.

Medical Receptionist

To gain medical assistant credentials, you must fulfill the requirements of either the American Association of Medical Assistants (for a Certified Medical Assistant) or the American Medical Technologists (for a Registered Medical Assistant). After obtaining your medical assistant certification, you may wish to acquire additional skills in specialty areas through course work or on-the-job training. Although this course work or training may not lead to an additional certification or degree, it will enable you to expand your role in the medical office and advance your career as the demand for skilled health professionals increases.

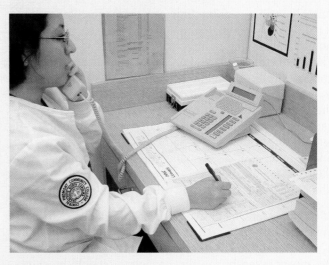

Skills and Duties

A medical receptionist, sometimes called a front office assistant or medical administrative assistant, answers telephone calls; performs triage on calls, contacting the physician or nurse with urgent needs; directs calls; assists patients with completing forms; receives patients and initiates the necessary paperwork; receives payments from patients and posts payments to patient accounts; covers all duties at the patient reception desk; schedules patient appointments; schedules surgeries; arranges referrals to other practices; calls patients as necessary; notifies patients of changes or cancellations and prioritizes appointments for rescheduling; updates patient information; maintains office bulletin boards; schedules and coordinates appointments and meetings for the physician; uses the computer to both input and retrieve data; operates the fax machine, the letter folding machine, the postage machine, and other administrative office equipment as needed; orders postage; compiles the daily mail; distributes mail to staff; maintains the patient reception area; creates patient handouts as necessary; establishes and maintains the filing system; inventories and orders office supplies as needed; and performs other administrative duties as needed.

Workplace Settings

Medical receptionists work in medical practices, including all medical specialties, as well as in outpatient clinics, hospital clinics, and all medical facilities.

Education

Medical receptionists must be a high school graduate and must complete medical receptionist training as required by state law.

For more information, visit the website of the following organization, which is available on the Online Learning Center at http://www.mhhe.com/medicalassisting4e.

The American Association of Medical Assistants

---

concepts. The impressions they create can vary widely, however, depending on the elements chosen to enhance this part of the office. Don't forget to place a waste receptacle that fits the decor. This allows patients to throw away tissues and other items.

Do not refer to the patient reception area as the "waiting room." The term has a negative connotation and implies that the patient and family members should expect a long wait. A more positive descriptive term to use is the "reception area."

Medical Office Information. As a convenience to patients, the business cards of all the physicians practicing at the location should be available. These cards are best placed at the reception window or desk, where patients can access them easily.

Other information about the practice is usually posted near the reception desk, including insurance information, workers' compensation information, and a reminder to turn off all cell phones.

Lighting. Most medical offices use fairly bright lighting in the reception area, allowing patients to see their surroundings easily. Subdued lighting, like that sometimes used in restaurants, could be hazardous because it could cause patients to trip over or bump into hard-to-see objects. In addition, bright lighting is essential for reading, which is a common activity in the patient reception area. Bright lighting also conveys an impression of cleanliness.

Lighting should not be so bright that it becomes bothersome, however. Extremely bright light can be harsh on the eyes and create an annoying glare. A specialist, such as an electrician or lighting showroom salesperson, can help determine the appropriate level of lighting for the patient reception area.

Room Temperature.
Patients will be uncomfortable if the reception area is too hot or too cold. In an uncomfortable setting, waiting time can seem much longer than it really is. Therefore, maintaining an average, comfortable temperature is important.

The thermostat should be kept at a temperature that feels comfortable to you and to the office staff. You might periodically survey patients to see if they are comfortable and adjust the setting accordingly. Many elderly people feel cold because of lowered metabolisms. You may want to increase the temperature setting for a geriatric practice or if the office sees a large number of elderly patients. The room temperature in the reception area may be a bit cooler than in the examination rooms, where patients may be required to disrobe.

Music.
Many medical offices pipe music through speakers to the reception area as well as elsewhere in the office. The music provides a soothing background sound. Because the music is meant to calm patients, it should be chosen accordingly. Classical music, light jazz, and soft rock are appropriate choices, whereas heavy metal and rap music are not. Some offices use prepared tapes or compact discs. Others tune in to an "easy listening" local (or satellite) radio station.

Decor

The patient reception area gets its distinctive look from the way it is decorated. With the appropriate elements, the decor can create whatever impression is desired—warm and friendly, modern and elegant, and so on. Some suggestions follow. It is wise to consult a professional decorator, if possible.

Colors and Fabrics.
Colors and fabrics are the primary elements that make up a room's decor. Colors can be used throughout the room—on walls, furniture, carpeting, and other items. Fabrics are used primarily on furniture and draperies.

When using several colors, it is important to decorate in color families to avoid a jarring, unprofessional look. A **color family** is a group of colors that work well together. Colors fall within two basic areas, cool and warm. Using all cool colors—like white, blue, and mauve—creates a more harmonious impression in the reception area than mixing cool colors with warm ones like red, orange, and hot pink. When choosing the color family, consider the mood you want to create. Bright colors produce a lively atmosphere, whereas softer, muted colors create a relaxing one.

Fabrics, too, add to the atmosphere in the room. Heavy fabrics like velvet or brocade are more formal, whereas lightweight or sheer fabrics create a soft, delicate appearance. Patterns on fabrics or wallpaper can immediately change the mood of the room. No matter what the design, fabrics should be easy to clean and maintain.

Many medical offices are carpeted, and carpets come in a variety of colors and patterns. Carpeting is attractive, and helps reduce noise. Carpeting also provides a comfortable cushion when people walk through the office.

Carpeting should be easy to clean and durable enough to handle a large volume of patient traffic. Wall-to-wall carpeting is preferable to scatter rugs, which can cause injuries if someone slips on or trips over them and falls.

Professional services can be contracted to deliver a clean, fresh entry carpet on a regular basis. These rubber-backed carpets lie directly on any floor surface and are commonly used at entranceways and hallways or areas of heavy traffic to catch soil from being "walked" into the rest of the office. Unlike scatter rugs, these heavyweight professional carpets lay flat and are not a hazard for tripping or falling. The service brings a fresh carpet and removes the soiled carpeting as scheduled.

Specialty Items.
Some offices include specialty items, or accessories, as part of the decor (Figure 13-2). Examples of such items include coat racks, aquariums, plants, paintings, sculptures, mobiles, and children's toys. Some items are meant to add a finishing touch, completing the desired atmosphere. Others may help to interest waiting patients by providing an activity, such as watching the fish in an aquarium.

Choosing Accessories. Although specialty items enhance the office decor, keep the number of accessories to a

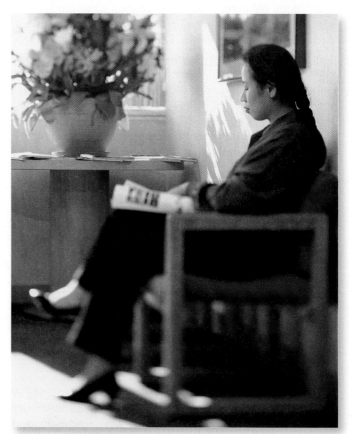

Figure 13-2. Specialty items, such as plants and paintings, enhance the patient reception area.

minimum. Too many pieces can give the room a cluttered look. Try to select specialty items that will be pleasing or helpful to patients. A clock is one example. Another useful item is a coat rack, which helps prevent clutter by providing a place for coats, umbrellas, and briefcases. Avoid accessories such as scented candles or potpourri that may be offensive to some people or cause allergic reactions.

Keeping Safety in Mind. When selecting specialty items for the medical office, be sure to consider the issue of safety. Follow these guidelines to avoid potential hazards in the patient reception area.

- Do not include any item smaller than a golf ball. Small items present a choking hazard for young children.
- Avoid objects that can be easily pulled apart and then swallowed.
- Avoid easily breakable items, such as glass vases, that might cause cuts or other injuries to patients.
- Choose furniture with rounded, not sharp, corners.
- Coffee tables or other low tables with sharp corners can be a hazard especially to the elderly and to small children.
- Secure heavy wall hangings, shelves, and coat racks to the wall so that there is no risk of their falling.
- It is preferable to display artificial plants rather than living ones. Living plants may irritate patients who have allergies or present a poisoning hazard if parts of the plants are eaten by toddlers.
- If possible, build large, heavy items (such as fish tanks) into the wall to avoid climbing children and the danger of the items falling.
- Make sure all items in the reception area get a careful daily dusting before patients arrive. Artificial flowers and plants will need to be washed upside-down in soap and water occasionally to remove any potential allergens such as dust.

Furniture

Buying furniture for a patient reception room requires thoughtful planning. Although the office in which you work will no doubt be furnished already, it is a good idea to learn the steps and decisions involved in choosing furniture. You may be included in future purchasing decisions if the office expands or moves to a new location or if the doctor wants to redecorate.

Furniture styles vary to suit the office decor. Most important, seating furniture should be firm, comfortable, safe, and easy to get in and out of. In addition, washable and fireproof fabric on the furniture minimizes care and maximizes safety. Close color coordination of the seating, floors, and walls may be difficult for an elderly person with failing eyesight. When possible, it is best to have chairs that contrast the carpet color to help prevent accidental falls.

The reception area should have enough furniture so that all patients and family members or friends who accompany them can sit, no matter how busy the office schedule. Forcing people to stand while they wait for an appointment makes the wait seem much longer. The American Medical Association (AMA) suggests that seating be sufficient to accommodate the number of patients, family members, and friends who may be in the office during a 2-hour time period. When calculating this number, be generous in allowing for family members. In some types of practices, such as pediatrics, all patients are accompanied by at least one parent or guardian and sometimes siblings as well.

Arranging Furniture. The furniture arrangement can make the office seem comfortable or uncomfortable. If furniture is too close together, patients do not have sufficient space to move around easily or to stretch their legs. They may feel cramped. To ensure that patients have adequate room, a good rule of thumb is to allow 12 square feet of space per person. By this measurement, a 120-square-foot room (10 feet by 12 feet) can accommodate ten people comfortably.

The furniture arrangement should allow maximum floor space. Patients should be able to stretch out their legs when seated and to walk around the reception area if they wish (Figure 13-3). Placing chairs against the wall usually produces the greatest amount of floor area. Additional seating in the middle of the room can be placed back-to-back to conserve space. Seats should be grouped so that families or friends can sit together. Remember to reserve room for patients in wheelchairs. This area should be carefully marked. Always allow enough space for wheelchairs with extended leg supports.

Ensuring Privacy. Some patients come to the office alone and value their privacy. Placing single chairs or

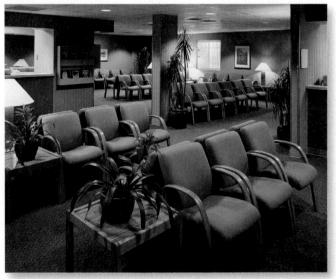

Figure 13-3. The furniture in a patient reception area can be arranged in a variety of ways.

small groups of chairs in corners of the room offers patients some measure of privacy.

Some medical offices offer more complete privacy in the form of an **interim room,** a room in which people can talk or meet without being seen or heard from the patient reception area. This interim room provides an ideal location for medical staff to confer privately with patients about appointments or bills. It also allows patients to make private telephone calls and allows people to feed or diaper babies in privacy. Not every office has the luxury of space for such a room, but it provides a valuable service to patients when it is possible.

Accommodating Children.

A pediatric reception area caters to a unique age group of patients. Reception areas for children usually have the same basic setup as those for adults, but special accommodations for children are also made.

In addition to regular chairs, for example, child-size chairs may be available. Some reception areas include playhouses or play furniture, such as small tables. The decor may also be made appealing to young children by the use of bright colors and storybook characters. It is important to make the setting feel familiar and comfortable. The reception desk may stock rolls of stickers or other inexpensive prizes to give to young patients after they have seen the doctor. Later in the chapter, you will learn how to set up a pediatric reception area.

Some pediatricians' offices have a well reception area and a sick reception area to separate children who are contagious from well children. **Contagious** means having a disease or condition that can easily be transmitted to others.

The Importance of Cleanliness

No matter how tastefully it is decorated, the reception area will be unappealing if it is not clean. Patients expect a physician's office to maintain a high standard of cleanliness. The perception is that a messy or dirty reception area or patient bathroom reflects a practice that does not meet minimum standards for cleanliness. A practice with a spotless, attractive reception area reassures patients that they have chosen a practice with high standards of cleanliness.

Housekeeping

Keeping the patient reception area clean usually falls within the duties of the medical assistant. In most cases you will be responsible for supervising the work of a professional cleaning service. In a small medical office you may be required to clean the area yourself, using appropriate antibacterial agents and a vacuum. Cleaning should occur daily, with emergency cleanups as needed.

Because professional services generally clean in the evening after business hours, you will probably not be present while the housekeeping staff is working. You may be asked to provide feedback to the cleaning company, however. It may also be your responsibility to outline the tasks you expect workers to complete, including any special requests.

One way of communicating with the cleaning staff is to create a Cleaning Communications Notebook. Arrange with the cleaning staff to leave the notebook open every evening in the same place. Date all entries. Write short, concise directions about any special requests for cleaning. Describe the nature of any stain so the service can best treat it. Sign each entry. Be sure to comment when something is done especially well. Like all of us, your cleaning staff likes to hear when they have done a particularly nice job!

Tasks.

Although housekeeping tasks vary from office to office, basic routines are applicable to areas such as the patient reception room. The Caution: Handle with Care section gives more information about maintaining a clean reception area.

Whether or not the office employs a professional cleaning service, you or another staff member will need to check for cleanliness throughout the day. As patients spend time in the office, items may become dirty or be moved out of place. Taking time between patient appointments or at midday to spot-clean small areas that have become dirty and straighten items will help keep the patient reception area in good condition.

Equipment.

If you, and not a professional service, are responsible for cleaning, the person in charge of the office budget will approve the purchase of cleaning equipment and supplies. Examples of cleaning equipment include handheld and upright vacuums, mops, and brooms. Supplies include trash bags, cleaning solutions, rags, and buckets. It is a good idea to have some basic cleaning materials on hand in case an emergency cleanup job is needed during office hours. Always wear gloves when doing cleaning of any kind and use OSHA guidelines for safety. Be sure to also obtain the MSDS for any cleaning materials stored in the office and insert the sheets in the office MSDS binder.

Cleaning Stains

If furniture, carpet, or other items in the reception area become stained, it is important to remove the stains quickly. Follow these tips for stain removal.

- Try to remove the stain right away. The longer a stain remains, the more difficult it is to remove.
- Blot as much of the stain as possible before rubbing it with a cleaning solution.
- Take special precautions in handling stains involving blood, feces, and urine. Put on latex gloves before blotting or scraping up the stain.
- Wipe the area with a cleaning solution and water.
- Blood, urine, and feces may require special cleaners with an enzyme that breaks down organic waste.

Maintaining Cleanliness Standards in the Reception Area

Cleanliness is one of the hallmarks of a medical office. Not only is cleanliness required in the examination and testing rooms, it is also expected in the patient reception area. A messy patient reception area reflects poorly on the physician and on the practice. Maintaining standards of cleanliness helps ensure that the reception area is presentable at all times.

As a medical assistant, you may be involved—along with the physician, office manager, and other staff members—in setting cleanliness standards for the office. Standards are general guidelines. In addition to setting standards, you will need to specify the tasks required to meet each standard. A checklist of the tasks required to meet all standards is a helpful document to create as well.

The following list outlines standards you may want to consider. Specific housekeeping tasks for meeting those standards are included in parentheses.

1. Keep everything in its place. (Complete a daily visual check for items that are out of place. Return all magazines to racks. Push chairs back into place.)
2. Dispose of all trash. (Empty trash cans. Pick up trash on the floor or on furniture.)
3. Prevent dust and dirt from accumulating on surfaces. (Wipe or dust furniture, lamps, and artificial plants. Polish doorknobs. Clean mirrors, wall hangings, and pictures.)
4. Spot-clean areas that become dirty. (Remove scuff marks. Clean upholstery stains.)
5. Disinfect areas of the reception area if they have been exposed to body fluids. (Immediately clean and disinfect all soiled areas.)
6. Handle items with care. (Take precautions when carrying potentially messy or breakable items. Do not carry too much at once.)

After the standards have been established, type and post them in a prominent place for the office staff to see. The checklist of cleaning activities may be posted, but the person responsible for cleaning the office should also keep a copy.

You should also produce a schedule of specific daily and weekly cleaning activities. Less frequent housekeeping duties, such as laundering drapes, shampooing the carpet, and cleaning windows and blinds, can be noted in a tickler file so that they will be performed on a regular basis.

It is always a good idea to have a second staff member responsible for periodically working with the medical assistant on housekeeping responsibilities. That person may also be responsible for handling cleaning duties when the medical assistant is away from the office.

- Use cold water instead of hot water because hot water often sets stains into the fabric.
- Keep all cleaning materials within easy reach for quick action when a stain occurs.

Removing Odors

Odors are particularly offensive in a doctor's office because people expect a high level of cleanliness and cannot readily leave to escape the odor. Some odors that may occasionally be present in a medical practice include those of urine, feces, vomit, body odors, and laboratory chemicals. A good ventilating system with charcoal filters can help minimize odors. If the system has temporary high-speed blowers, they can be activated as well. Disinfectant sprays and deodorant scents also may help. Be careful in the use of deodorant sprays because some patients may be allergic to the smell.

One odor that can be prevented is smoke. Display "Thank You for Not Smoking" signs prominently in the patient reception area. Do not provide ashtrays, and ask smokers to leave the office if they insist on smoking. Not only does smoking produce an offensive odor, it also may affect the health of other patients in the reception area. People who have asthma or other breathing disorders, or who are feeling unwell for any reason, are particularly sensitive to smoke and strong odors.

Infectious Waste

There may be times when you will need to clean up infectious waste. **Infectious waste,** also known as biohazardous waste, is waste that can be dangerous to those who handle it or to the environment. Infectious waste includes human waste, human tissue, and body fluids such as blood and urine. It also includes any potentially hazardous waste generated in the treatment of patients, such as needles, scalpels, cultures of human cells, and dressings.

Although infectious waste is not commonly generated in the patient reception area, it can be—as when a patient vomits or bleeds on the rug or on furniture. If that situation should occur, you must clean up the waste promptly.

Infectious waste must be handled in accordance with federal law. Your office may choose to purchase commercially prepared hazardous waste kits for use in cleaning up spills. After cleaning infectious waste from the patient reception area, deposit it in a biohazard container. Disinfect the site to eliminate possible contamination of other patients.

OSHA Regulations

Federal safety precautions for the workplace are mandated by the Occupational Safety and Health Administration (OSHA), a government agency. OSHA has developed general guidelines for most businesses as well as special rules for health-care practices. To determine whether the requirements are being met, OSHA periodically inspects medical offices. If the rules are not followed, medical offices may be required to pay penalties in addition to correcting the problem. All employees in a medical office must be thoroughly trained in following OSHA guidelines.

Among the OSHA requirements is regular cleaning of walls, floors, and other surfaces. OSHA requires the use of disinfectants to combat bacteria as part of a routine cleaning schedule. In addition, OSHA mandates that broken glass, which may be contaminated, be picked up using a dustpan and brush or tongs. It should not be picked up by hand, even if one wears gloves.

The Physical Components

No one arrangement of a reception area is necessarily better than another. As long as the arrangement provides clear pathways and comfortable places to sit, the reception area will be functional.

Office Access

The path patients must take to get from the parking area or street to the office and then back out again is called the office **access.** Some offices have easy access and some do not (Figure 13-4).

Parking Arrangements. Although some patients walk to the medical office or take public transportation, the majority of patients probably travel by their personal vehicles. Patients who drive to the office need a place to park.

The office can offer either on-street parking or a parking lot or parking garage. On-street parking requires patients to fend for themselves. They may have to put money into parking meters, and parking spaces may be difficult to find. Both the money required and the potential problems in finding parking spots limit the ease with which patients can gain access to the office.

A free parking lot or parking garage improves office access. Parking lots and garages should be well lit for

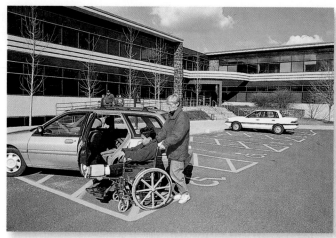

Figure 13-4. Patients should have easy, clear access from the parking lot to the medical office door.

safety. To determine the number of parking spaces the office needs, calculate the average length of time a patient spends in the office from arrival to departure and the number of appointments scheduled during that time period. Allow one parking spot per appointment if most patients drive to the office and fewer if many use public transportation. In your count be sure to include parking spaces for office staff. Periodically reevaluate the office's parking needs because they may change over time. All offices must also provide handicapped parking space for patients. Visit www.adaptiveaccess.com/handicap_parking.php for more information on handicapped parking.

Entrances. The entrance to the office should be clearly marked so that patients can find the office easily. The name of the practice and of the doctor or doctors should be on the door or beside the door. Just outside the doorway should be a doormat to help control the amount of dirt tracked into the office. If the office door opens directly to the outside, people inside will feel a sudden change in temperature each time the door is opened in hot or cold weather. A foyer or double-door arrangement helps minimize the effects of the weather and helps keep the office at a consistent, comfortable temperature.

Doorways must be wide enough to accommodate patients using wheelchairs and walkers. Hallways should be extra wide to allow patients in wheelchairs to turn around or to allow two wheelchairs to pass one another. The Americans With Disabilities Act, discussed later in this chapter, requires that doorways have a minimum width of 32 inches and that hallways have a minimum width of 5 feet. Well-lit hallways, without obstructions, are required.

Safety and Security

Safety and security are important concerns in any public building, and they are especially important in a doctor's office. To ensure safety of the patients and staff, such as protection from hazardous wiring or poorly lit hallways, there are guidelines for businesses, some of which pertain to the patient reception area. In addition, the medical office must be secure from burglary.

Building Exits. Make sure you and the office staff are familiar with all building exits. It may be necessary to leave the office quickly, as during a fire, flood, or other emergency. You and other staff members must be prepared to assist and direct patients toward the exits in such a situation. Posting evacuation plans near each exit will assist staff and patients in the event of an emergency necessitating evacuation of the building.

Ideally, the office should have at least two doorways that lead directly to the outside or to a hallway that leads to stairs. This arrangement affords patients and staff members the speediest, most direct route outside in case of an emergency. All exits must be clearly labeled with illuminated red "Exit" signs. These signs normally have a backup power system, such as a battery, so that they will remain lit even during a power outage. Posting evacuation plans and displaying the nearest exits will assist staff and patients.

Having two or more exits also allows staff members to enter and leave the office during nonemergency situations without disrupting people in the patient reception area. Deliveries can be made at the second entrance, further minimizing interruptions.

Smoke Detectors. By law, a medical office is required to install smoke detectors that sound an alarm when triggered by heat or smoke. The office staff should be trained in the proper procedure if the smoke alarm sounds—including how to evacuate patients from the building efficiently. Smoke detectors must be checked regularly to ensure that they are operating properly.

Security Systems. No matter where the medical office is located, a security alarm system is a wise investment, even if the office building is patrolled by security personnel. A security alarm system offers valuable protection for the confidential patient information housed in a medical office. After the alarm system is installed, all office staff members should thoroughly familiarize themselves with it. They should be able to arm and disarm it easily and know what to do if it is accidentally activated. Each member of the staff should have her or his own individually assigned security access number. This number is required to authorize locking or unlocking the system. Like a credit card, bank, or other security PIN (personal identification number), it should never be shared.

Keeping Patients Occupied and Informed

Many patients who come into a medical office are ill, anxious, and concerned about their health. While they wait in the reception area, they need a way to stay occupied so that the time seems to pass quickly. In addition, patients may want to be informed about a particular medical condition or about general health issues. To meet these patient needs, most medical offices provide reading materials in the patient reception area. They may also offer television or educational videotapes.

Reading Materials

The most common activity in a patient reception area is probably reading. Although some patients bring their own books or magazines, most patients expect to find reading materials at the medical office (Figure 13-5). Magazines and books are probably the most popular types of reading materials, but a variety of others may also be available.

Magazines and Books. Choosing the right mix of reading material to interest all patients is a challenge. You may know doctors' offices that have a wonderful selection of magazines and books and others that have a poor selection. Your judgment of the selection, however, is based on how those publications match your interests. The Points on Practice section gives guidelines on selecting magazines for the medical office. In addition to reading materials for adults, most offices also have children's books and magazines for younger patients and family members.

You or someone on the office staff should be sure to screen publications for medical content. You can then alert the doctors to articles that might stimulate patients' questions. Make sure magazines are current. There is nothing worse than having a patient reception area full of outdated or worn magazines.

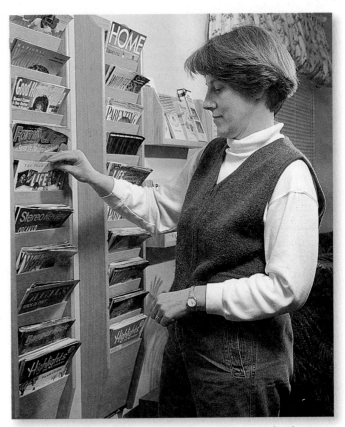

Figure 13-5. Reading materials can be organized on tables or in a wall rack.

Tailoring Office Magazines to Patient Interests

It is a common sight: Patients waiting their turn for an appointment pick up one of the many magazines in the reception area. Sometimes it is hard to choose—because every magazine is interesting or because none of them are.

As a medical assistant, you may be responsible for selecting magazines for the office's reception area. The right selection can make the difference between a pleasant wait and a tedious one. Follow these guidelines to compile a suitable mix of magazines that will be of interest to a majority of patients.

1. Patients in some practices immediately share a common ground. They fall within the category of the practice's specialty—for example, geriatrics or pediatrics. Some magazines may be a natural fit for this category. A geriatric practice, for example, may provide publications geared toward senior citizens. A pediatric practice may offer parenting and children's magazines.

2. People waiting in a doctor's office usually have an interest in their health. Therefore, health magazines geared toward the general public are good choices. Of course, the reception area is not the place for the highly technical medical journals, with graphic pictures, that the doctor may receive or for religious materials of any kind.

3. Make sure the magazines cover a variety of interests. The more topics available, the greater the chance that someone will be interested in one of them. Instead of subscribing to several magazines on one topic, try to limit subscriptions to one magazine per topic, unless the topic is of special interest to most patients.

4. Choose magazines that cover topics in a general way—travel, news, sports, fashion, or entertainment. Delving into these areas too specifically—as in a tennis magazine rather than one on a variety of sports—may not interest many patients.

5. Magazines should be discarded after three months or taken out of the patient reception area. When you discard them, replenish them with a current supply.

6. The best way to determine patients' interests is to ask for feedback. Develop a form on which patients can indicate their hobbies, interests, and favorite types of magazines. Periodically display the form in the reception area, and encourage patients to make suggestions.

Patient Information Packet. One type of reading material other than magazines is a patient information packet. This document is an easy way to inform patients about the practice. The packet can be designed in many ways, from a simple flyer to a formal folder with pockets to hold individual sheets of information. Topics covered in the packet can range from billing and insurance processing policies to biographical information on each physician in a group practice. Chapter 14 will discuss how to develop the contents of a patient information packet.

Medical Information. Another type of reading material commonly found in reception areas is medical brochures. Patients may be interested in information that pertains to their general health or to a specific condition. Brochures on a variety of topics are available to medical offices either free of charge or for a nominal fee. These brochures are usually produced by nonprofit associations that specialize in a disease or condition, such as the American Cancer Society, and by pharmaceutical companies.

Before displaying pamphlets and brochures in the reception area, be sure to read them thoroughly. Make sure they provide accurate information. You may also want to review them to prepare for questions patients may ask. The physician may also want to review them for medical accuracy.

Bulletin Board. Most patient reception areas feature a bulletin board. Bulletin boards often highlight area meetings, such as those of support groups, and offer other current information. To encourage patients to look at the bulletin board, change the format and content frequently. An interesting design with bright colors and bold headlines attracts readers. Depending on your time and inclination, you might change the bulletin board every week, month, or season.

Items on a reception area bulletin board should be tailored to patient interests. For example, an obstetrics/gynecology practice specializing in infertility might display recent birth announcements from its patients. The bulletin board might also feature support groups for parents trying to conceive, information on the latest medical studies of fertility drugs, and magazine clippings on parenting issues.

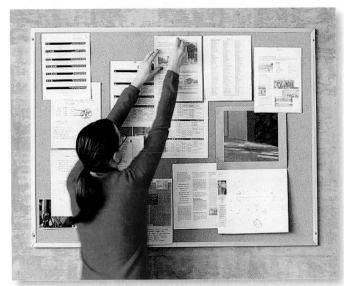

Figure 13-6. Check the office bulletin board frequently for outdated information.

Other, more general items for display on any physician's bulletin board might include the following:

- Policies and procedures for patients such as no smoking or eating in the patient reception area; information concerning late or missed appointments; and patient payment information
- Government reports on food and drugs
- Nutrition information
- Requests from the American Red Cross or the local blood bank for blood donors
- Pamphlets or flyers distributed by nonprofit health-care organizations, such as the American Heart Association
- Flyers on upcoming health fairs
- Blood pressure or other health screening notices
- Newspaper or magazine articles on interesting medical issues
- Community notices for food drives or similar charity events

The bulletin board might also feature information about staff members in the practice. Do not allow the bulletin board to become cluttered with advertising or business cards.

Finally, the bulletin board is an ideal place to display the office brochure. Put some extra copies of the brochure in an open envelope tacked to the bulletin board to encourage patients to take one home. To keep the bulletin board up to date, all time-sensitive materials, such as notices about a class or seminar, should be removed as soon as the date of the scheduled event has passed (Figure 13-6).

Television and Videotapes

Although reading remains the primary pastime in patient reception areas, watching television and videotapes is becoming a more common activity in physicians' offices across the country. Many patient reception areas now include a television, which can be tuned to regular stations or can play preselected videos. Physicians may provide informative health-care videos of general interest to their patients or videos that meet the more specific interests of the practice. Videos are helpful for patients with limited reading ability and can be helpful if customized for non-English speakers.

Items for Children

Many patient reception areas include items to occupy children while they wait. Because children—even sick ones—do not usually like to sit still for long periods, these items may include toys, games, videos, and books (Figure 13-7). If the pediatric reception area separates sick children from well children, the "well" side may include more active entertainment, such as an indoor slide or playhouse. The "sick" side may provide quieter games and activities, such as books and puzzles.

Choose toys carefully. You do not want children—even well ones—to be too active in the reception area because they might disrupt other patients and their families. Avoid balls, jump ropes, and other toys meant for outside use. Puzzles and blocks are good choices because they encourage quieter play. All toys should be easy to clean (a bleach-water solution or nonaerosol disinfectant can be used) and, for safety and health reasons, should not include stuffed animals. Stuffed animals are not appropriate because they are not easily kept clean. They can be a source of infection or the small parts on them can be a choking hazard. You might informally ask parents and children if they like the play items or if they would prefer other types of toys. Procedure 13-1 explains how to set up a pediatric playroom.

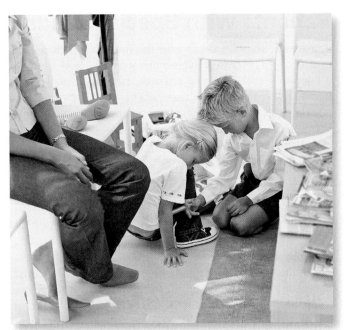

Figure 13-7. Toys and games that encourage quiet play are well suited to a reception area in a pediatric practice.

PROCEDURE 13-1

Creating a Pediatric Playroom

Procedure Goal: To create a play environment for children in the patient reception area of a pediatric practice

Materials: Children's books and magazines, games, toys, nontoxic crayons and coloring books, television and videocassette recorder (VCR) (or DVD player), children's videotapes (or DVDs), child- and adult-size chairs, child-size table, bookshelf, boxes or shelves, decorative wall hangings or educational posters (optional)

Method:

1. Place all adult-size chairs against the wall. Position some of the child-size chairs along the wall with the adult chairs.

2. Place the remainder of the child-size chairs in small groupings throughout the room. In addition, put several chairs with the child-size table.

3. Put the books, magazines, crayons, and coloring books on the bookshelf in one corner of the room near a grouping of chairs.

4. Choose toys and games carefully. Avoid toys that encourage active play, such as balls, or toys that require a large area. Make sure that all toys meet safety guidelines. Watch for loose parts or parts that are smaller than a golf ball. Toys should also be easy to clean.

Rationale
Helps ensure safety in the patient reception area.

5. Place the activities for older children near one grouping of chairs and the games and toys for younger children near another grouping. Keep the toys and games in a toy box or on shelves designated for them. Consider labeling or colorcoding boxes and shelves and the games and toys that belong there to encourage children to return the games and toys to the appropriate storage area.

6. Place the television and VCR (or DVD player) on a high shelf, if possible, or attach it to the wall near the ceiling. Keep children's videos (or DVDs) behind the reception desk, and periodically change the video in the VCR/DVD.

Rationale
Doing so helps ensure safety in the patient reception area. Videos and video equipment are easily damaged or destroyed by young patients.

7. To make the room more cheerful, decorate it with wall hangings or posters.

Patients with Special Needs

Some patients who come into the medical office will be disabled—that is, they were born with or have acquired a condition that limits or changes their abilities. A more positive way to refer to these patients who are differently abled is the use of the term special needs. For example, people who are paralyzed from the waist down have special needs; so do people who are visually impaired. This does not mean that these people cannot perform the same tasks that other people can. They may simply need special accommodations to do so.

Americans with Disabilities Act

Individuals with special needs are often singled out for their differences and are sometimes discriminated against. For example, if a company building does not have access ramps for wheelchairs, workers in wheelchairs cannot qualify for jobs there. This would violate the American with Disabilities Act, which prevents discrimination based solely on a person's physical disability.

Preventing Discrimination. In 1990 a law was enacted to prevent certain types of discrimination. The **Americans with Disabilities** Act is a federal civil rights act forbidding discrimination on the basis of physical or mental handicap. This act maintains the rights of special needs (disabled) people in many areas, including jobs, transportation, and access to public buildings. The act relates to medical practices (and reception areas) in that an office must be able to accommodate any patient who wants to see the physician.

Patients with Special Needs. With some forethought and planning, the office can accommodate patients with special needs. Ensuring wheelchair access through doors and hallways, as mentioned earlier, is just one way. Using ramps instead of steps, as shown in Figure 13-8, allows easier access not only for wheelchair users but also for others who have limited mobility. Allowing additional space in the reception area for wheelchairs, walkers, crutches, and guide dogs accommodates several types of special needs patients. Procedure 13-2 explains how to organize the patient reception area to meet the special needs of patients who are physically challenged.

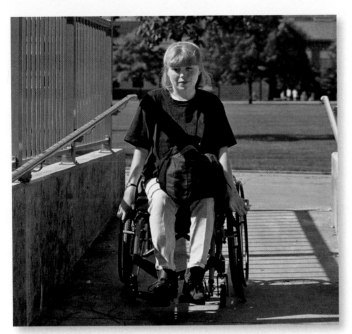

Figure 13-8. Ramps allow patients who use wheelchairs access to the medical office.

Many offices do not make special accommodations for patients with vision or hearing impairments. Post prominent signs in the reception area with information that patients need to know. A staff member should offer to assist patients with hearing or vision impairments as needed from the reception area to the examination room when it is their turn to see the doctor.

Patients who are hearing impaired may request that a certified sign language interpreter be present to assist in communicating with the medical staff. If requested, it is required by federal law that the physician provide and pay for this interpreter.

It is also helpful, but not required by law, to provide a **teletype (TTY) device,** also known as a telecommunications device for the deaf (TDD), for hearing-impaired patients. This specially designed telephone looks very much like a laptop computer with a cradle for the receiver of a traditional telephone. The receiver is placed in the cradle, and the hearing-impaired patient can then type the communication on the keyboard. The message can be received by another TTY/TDD or relayed through a specialty relay service.

Some states offer a relay service for patients with hearing impairments or those with speech disabilities. When an individual accesses this service through the TTY/TDD, the service then places the call using voice. It is important to understand that a relay service could call a medical office to make an appointment for a patient. The medical assistant needs to be careful to respond appropriately and not mistake the call as an unwanted marketing call.

Older Americans Act of 1965

A growing proportion of the American population is elderly. Like those who are disabled, many elderly people face discrimination. One reason for the discrimination

may be that with age come medical conditions and disorders that create physical limitations.

The **Older Americans Act of 1965** was passed by Congress to eliminate discrimination against the elderly. Among other benefits, the act guarantees elderly citizens the best possible health care regardless of ability to pay, an adequate retirement income, and protection against abuse, neglect, and exploitation.

What does the Older Americans Act mean for the medical office reception area? If the practice serves elderly patients, the office staff must be sensitive to their special needs. The patient reception area should be as comfortable as possible for patients with arthritis, failing eyesight, and other common ailments of the elderly. Make sure there are a few straight-backed chairs, which are easier to get into and out of than soft sofas. Arms on chairs provide support when sitting and standing for patients who are unsteady. In addition, straight-backed chairs offer greater back support than low chairs or couches with sinking cushions. These chairs should be located near the front door and near the examination rooms.

Place reading materials within easy reach of the chairs so that elderly patients do not have to get up from their chairs for them. Have large-print books and magazines available, if possible, for patients with poor eyesight. You might also offer magnifying glasses for patients who like to use them. In addition, make sure that the print on all office signs is large and easy to read. The patient reception area and restrooms should be well lit to help everyone, including elderly patients, see more clearly.

Special Situations

Patients in a medical practice are usually a diverse group of people. Their interests, needs, and medical conditions can have an impact on the design of the reception area.

Patients from Diverse Cultural Backgrounds. The United States has long been called a melting pot because of its mixture of people and cultures. Each culture lends its own special qualities, and together the cultures combine to create a unique blend of people called Americans.

You may work in a neighborhood that has a distinct culture or one in which many cultures are represented. To help patients feel comfortable, make the reception area reflect aspects of their cultural backgrounds whenever possible. This effort will help patients feel more welcome.

Suppose, for example, that the medical office where you work serves many Latino patients. Posting signs in Spanish and English acknowledges the fact that both languages are spoken in that neighborhood. Providing reading materials, such as newspapers and magazines, in a second language—for both adults and children—is another way to show respect and interest. Decorating the office for Spanish holidays in addition to American ones demonstrates that you care about what is important to

Creating a Reception Area Accessible to Patients with Special Needs

Procedure Goal: To arrange elements in the reception area to accommodate patients with special needs

Materials: Ramps (if needed), doorway floor coverings, chairs, bars or rails, adjustable-height tables, magazine rack, television/VCR or DVD player, large-type and Braille magazines

Method:

1. Arrange chairs, leaving gaps so that substantial space is available for wheelchairs along walls and near other groups of chairs. Keep the arrangement flexible so that chairs can be removed to allow room for additional wheelchairs if needed.

Rationale
To meet all the requirements of the Americans with Disabilities Act.

2. Remove any obstacles that may interfere with the space needed for a wheelchair to swivel around completely. Also remove scatter rugs or any carpeting that is not attached to the floor. Such carpeting can cause patients to trip and create difficulties for wheelchair traffic.

Rationale
Helps ensure safety in the patient reception area.

3. Position coffee tables at a height and location that is accessible to people in wheelchairs.

4. Place office reading materials, such as magazines, at a height that is accessible to people in wheelchairs (for example, on tables or in racks attached midway up the wall).

5. Locate the television and VCR/DVD within full view of patients sitting on chairs and in wheelchairs so that they do not have to strain their necks to watch.

6. For patients who have a vision impairment, include reading materials with large type and in Braille.

7. For patients who have difficulty walking, make sure bars or rails are attached securely to walls 34 to 38 inches above the floor, to accommodate requirements set forth in the Americans with Disabilities Act. Make sure the bars are sturdy enough to provide balance for patients who may need it. Bars are most important in entrances and hallways, as well as in the bathroom. Consider placing a bar near the receptionist's window for added support as patients check in.

Rationale
To meet all the requirements of the Americans with Disabilities Act.

8. Eliminate sills of metal or wood along the floor in doorways. Otherwise, create a smoother travel surface for wheelchairs and pedestrians with a thin rubber covering to provide a graduated slope. Be sure that the covering is attached properly and meets safety standards.

Rationale
Helps ensure safety in the patient reception area.

9. Make sure the office has ramp access.

Rationale
To meet all the requirements of the Americans with Disabilities Act.

10. Solicit feedback from patients with physical disabilities about the accessibility of the patient reception area. Encourage ideas for improvements. Address any additional needs.

Rationale
Doing so lets patients know that their comfort and well-being are important to you.

---

patients. Displaying artwork created by local artists and artisans is another idea.

Patients Who Are Highly Contagious. Patients may have to come into the physician's office when they are highly contagious. This fact is a concern for all patients, but it is especially critical for patients who are immunocompromised. Immunocompromised patients have an immune system—which protects against disease—that is not functioning at a normal level. Because these patients do not have the normal ability to fight off disease, they are at greater risk than the average person for becoming sick. Patients undergoing chemotherapy and patients with AIDS, for example, have compromised immune systems.

To protect patients who are immunocompromised, as well as other patients and staff members, you may need to separate a highly contagious patient from them. Instead of having contagious patients wait in the reception area, for example, you might bring them directly into an examination room to wait. By screening patients for highly contagious conditions and taking precautions, you can minimize the chances of exposing other people unnecessarily.

Summary

13.1 The elements that are important in a patient reception area include the furniture, patient information, decor, lighting, and accessibility for all patients, including those with special needs.

13.2 Furniture in a patient reception area should be firm, comfortable, safe, and easily accessible.

13.3 The housekeeping tasks include basic routine cleaning, daily dusting, and straightening of the reception area, including emptying waste containers. The medical office may provide mops, brooms, and vacuums or it may have a professional cleaning service that services the facility. Cleaning supplies for unexpected stains, spills, and odors should also be kept on hand.

13.4 OSHA requires that a medical office be cleaned regularly, and also requires the use of disinfectants to combat bacteria as a part of regular cleaning. Additionally, any broken glass must be picked up with a dustpan and tongs or brush, never by hand (even gloved ones) due to possible contamination.

13.5 As long as the arrangement to the reception area is comfortable and provides clear pathways for all patients, no arrangement is better than another. Keep in mind that office access from parking to entrances and excesses must be available for all patients.

13.6 The physical components associated with a safe and secure patient reception area are safety when exiting the office building (easy to come in and get out of), smoke detectors, and security systems within a medical facility.

13.7 The reading material that is appropriate for a patient reception area includes magazines and books, patient information packets, and medical information geared toward patients (not medical professionals). Some material should also be available in larger type for the visually impaired and in a language alternative to English if a predominant culture comes to your office.

13.8 Modifications to a patient reception area for patients with special needs includes allowing for easier access from parking areas to entrances. Be sure to allow for extra space in the reception area for wheelchairs, walkers, and the like. Be available to escort patients with visual impairments.

13.9 Special situations such as clients that are highly contagious can have an impact on the reception area. If available, bring these patients to a separate waiting area. If this is not available, every effort should be made to bring the contagious patient directly to an empty examination room.

REVIEW
CHAPTER 13

CASE STUDY QUESTIONS

Now that you have completed this chapter, review the case study at the beginning of the chapter and answer the following questions:

1. What basic elements are *required* in every patient reception area? What other nonessential elements are nice to include as well?
2. Why is it important to think of the front patient area as the "patient reception area" and not the "waiting room"?
3. What special accommodations in the reception area are important to patients with disabilities?

Multiple-Choice Questions

1. The first impression a patient gets of a medical office is the
   a. location of the practice.
   b. reception area.
   c. length of time it takes to drive there.
   d. parking facilities.
2. Which type of lighting could be hazardous and result in patients tripping or bumping into hard-to-see objects?
   a. Extremely bright
   b. Subdued
   c. Bright
   d. Dull

3. The *best* way to maintain the appropriate room temperature in the reception area is to
   a. observe the patients for signs of being too cold or hot.
   b. periodically survey patients to see if they are comfortable.
   c. allow patients to regulate the thermostat in the reception area.
   d. set the thermostat at a predetermined setting and never change it.
4. The purpose of piping music into a reception area is to
   a. keep the patients awake.
   b. provide a soothing background sound.
   c. create a conversation item for patients.
   d. eliminate the distraction to office staff of patients talking.
5. When selecting colors to decorate a medical office, it is important to
   a. choose only warm colors.
   b. mix cool and warm colors.
   c. use only cool colors.
   d. pick any colors you want.

Discussion Questions

1. What is the Americans with Disabilities Act, and what impact does it have on the patient reception area and patient bathrooms?
2. What is the Older Americans Act, and what impact does it have on the patient reception area and patient bathrooms?
3. What psychological effect does a cheerful, inviting reception room have on the patient?
4. Why do you think it is important to think of disabled patients as patients with special needs?
5. Do you think it projects a negative image to place magazines in the reception area when we do not want the patients to consider the space to be a "waiting room"? Explain your answer.

Critical Thinking Questions

1. What special difficulties might patients in wheelchairs have in a small, overcrowded reception area?
2. Who is responsible if a patient or family member or friend is hurt in the reception area or bathroom? What could be the possible consequences?
3. What would be the best design for a pediatric reception area and bathroom? Describe it.
4. What is the responsibility of the medical practice in the unlikely event of a fire?
5. Which arrangement is best for a reception area? Why?
6. Why is OSHA involved in the management of the reception area?

Application Activities

1. Design a reception area bulletin board for a family practitioner's office. List at least six items to include, and draw a rough sketch for placing these items on a rectangular bulletin board.
2. Develop a daily checklist for closing down a patient reception area at the end of the day. Be sure to include any housekeeping chores.
3. Visit a patient reception area at a clinic or a doctor's or dentist's office. Notice the decor, furniture arrangement, specialty items, and reading materials. Note what you like and dislike about the area. Then write down suggestions for improvement. Compare your results with those of your classmates.
4. Create a design for a desirable layout for a medical practice using cutouts of cardboard that represent chairs, tables, and other elements within a patient reception area. Design the entire layout to scale. In a one-page summary, explain how your plan meets safety requirements for a physician practice.
5. Develop a one-page questionnaire for patients to determine if the reception area meets their needs. Be sure to include questions that relate to the needs of special needs patients.

Virtual Fieldtrip

Visit the McGraw-Hill Higher Education Medical Assisting website at www.mhhe.com/medicalassisting4e to complete the following activity:

- Explore the occupation of a medical receptionist administrative medical assistant and compare and contrast the duties, responsibilities, education, and pay with that of a medical assistant.
- Write a one-page summary of your research, including websites accessed, for presentation to the class. You may wish to go online and visit websites in addition to the site suggested for this exercise.

Open the CD and complete this chapter's practice activities, play the games, listen to the key terms, and test yourself with the interactive review. E-mail, print, and/or save your results to document your proficiency.

CHAPTER 14

Patient Education

MEDICAL ASSISTING COMPETENCIES

CAAHEP

IV. C (7) Identify resources and adaptations that are required based on individual needs, i.e., culture and environment, developmental life stage, language, and physical threats to communication

IV. C (14) Recognize the role of patient advocacy in the practice of medical assisting

IV. P (9) Document patient education

IV. P (12) Develop and maintain a current list of community resources related to patients' health-care needs

ABHES

2. Anatomy and Physiology
 a. Comprehend and explain to the patient the importance of diet and nutrition. Effectively convey and educate patients regarding the proper diet and nutrition guidelines. Identify categories of patients that require special diets or diet modifications.

8. Medical Office Business Procedures Management
 e. Locate resources and information for patients and employers
 cc. Communicate on the recipient's level of comprehension
 dd. Serve as liaison between physician and others
 hh. Receive, organize, prioritize, and transmit information expediently
 ii. Recognize and respond to verbal and nonverbal communication
 kk. Adapt to individualized needs

9. Medical Office Clinical Procedures
 q. Instruct patients with special needs
 r. Teach patients methods of health promotion and disease prevention

11. Career Development
 Demonstrate professionalism by:
 1) Exhibiting dependability, punctuality, and a positive work ethic
 2) Exhibiting a positive attitude and a sense of responsibility
 3) Maintaining confidentiality at all times
 4) Being cognizant of ethical boundaries
 5) Exhibiting initiative
 8) Being courteous and diplomatic
 9) Conducting work within scope of education, training, and ability

LEARNING OUTCOMES

After completing Chapter 14, you will be able to:

14.1 Identify the benefits of patient education.

14.2 Explain the role of the medical assistant in patient education.

14.3 Describe factors that affect teaching and learning.

14.4 Distinguish patient education materials used in the medical office.

14.5 Distinguish how patient education can be used to promote good health habits.

14.6 Describe the types of information that should be included in the patient information packet.

14.7 Differentiate techniques for educating patients with special needs.

14.8 Describe the benefits of patient education prior to surgery, and identify types of preoperative teaching.

14.9 Select educational resources that are available outside the medical office.

MEDICAL ASSISTING MEDIA

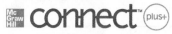 **Connect Plus+™**
connect.mcgraw-hill.com

- Electronic Health Records (E.H.R.) SpringCharts®
- eBook

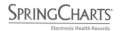

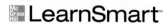 **LearnSmart™**

www.mhhe.com/learnsmart

Complete Learning Module: Patient Education

 Student CD-ROM

 LearningCenter **Online Learning Center™**

www.mhhe.com/medicalassisting4e

KEY TERMS

consumer education
dementia

modeling
philosophy

return demonstration
screening

CHAPTER OUTLINE

- The Educated Patient
- Types of Patient Education
- Promoting Health and Wellness Through Education

- The Patient Information Packet
- Educating Patients with Special Needs
- Patient Education Prior to Surgery
- Additional Educational Resources

PREPARATION FOR CERTIFICATION

RMA (AMT) Exam
- General reception of patients and visitors
- Oral and written communication

CMA (AAMA) Exam
- Adapting communication according to an individual's needs
- Patient advocate
- Patient information booklet

CMAS Exam
- Reception
- Professionalism
- Patient information and community resources

Introduction

Health education should be a lifelong pursuit for all of us. The ultimate goal of all medical professionals is to encourage and teach healthy habits and behaviors to all patients. People first have to understand what is good for them, and then they have to make a decision to follow that advice. In patient education, the medical assistant shares health information and encourages patients to make good health decisions.

In this chapter you will learn about the medical assistant's role in patient education. You will sharpen your skills in recognizing and overcoming road blocks to education. You will become more comfortable with teaching and demonstrating procedures to others. Most importantly, you will begin to recognize the incredible responsibility of the medical assistant to correctly lead others to their highest level of health.

Laura is a 26-year-old pregnant patient with hypertension (high blood pressure). She is taking blood pressure medication, but her pressure is becoming increasingly difficult to manage as she progresses with her pregnancy. The doctor has ordered a 24-hour urine collection test to help determine if Laura is in a dangerous state of preeclampsia. It is your task as a medical assistant to explain to Laura the process of urine collection that she must follow. You know that she is not going to want to carry a large jug of urine to work with her and keep it on ice all day. You know that she is not likely to accurately follow the procedures of the test. But you also know it is imperative that the doctor accurately gather this test information for the health of this woman and the infant she carries.

After first reading the 24-hour urine collection procedure yourself and ensuring that you understand it thoroughly, you sit with Laura in a quiet place and explain the test and the need for accuracy. You then listen to her and evaluate her level of understanding. You listen for any cues she gives that indicate difficulties in completing the test as ordered. Thinking creatively, you suggest that Laura conduct the test on a Sunday when she can stay at home during the day and bring the specimen directly to the doctor's office early on Monday morning. You give her all the test lab items she will need, explaining each item. Additionally, you give her written instructions that she can take with her and a phone number to call with any questions she may have over the weekend. You encourage her as she leaves. By doing everything you can to ensure this patient's compliance, you contribute to the chances that both she and her baby will be strong and healthy throughout her pregnancy and delivery.

As you read this chapter, consider the following questions:

1. What might be important to consider when creating an educational plan for a patient? How might the plan vary according to the individual?
2. What factors could block effective patient education?
3. What specific behaviors do you associate with talking down to a patient?
4. Why are good listening skills an important part of teaching?

The Educated Patient

Patient education is an essential process in the medical office. It encourages patients to take an active role in their medical care. It results in better compliance with treatment programs. When patients are suffering from illness, disease, or injury, education can often help them regain their health and independence more quickly. Simply put, patient education helps patients stay healthy. Educated patients are more likely to comply with instructions if they understand the why behind the instructions. Also, educated patients are more likely to be satisfied clients of the practice.

Patients benefit from education and the medical office benefits as well. Preoperative instruction to surgical patients, for example, lessens the chance that procedures will have to be rescheduled because surgical guidelines were not followed. Educated patients will also be less likely to call the office with questions. Thus, the office staff will have to spend less time on the telephone.

Patient education takes many forms and includes a variety of techniques. It can be as simple as answering a question that comes up during a routine visit. Patient education may involve printed materials. It can also be participatory, as with a demonstration of the procedure for changing a bandage or for giving oneself an insulin injection. No matter what type of patient education is used, the goal is the same—to help patients help themselves attain better health. Procedure 14-1 will help you create a patient education plan.

As a medical assistant, you play a vital role in the process of patient education, primarily because of your constant interaction with patients in the office. Although the initial visit is a good time to assess the need for patient education, the educational process can and should be ongoing. Continue to assess patients' needs at every visit, and be aware of situations in which you can share meaningful and helpful information.

Types of Patient Education

Patient education can take many forms. Any instructions—verbal, written, or demonstrative—that you give to patients are a type of patient education. Most formal types of patient education involve some printed information. They may also include visual materials, such as videotapes and DVDs. Patient educational materials inform patients and enable and encourage them to become involved in their own medical care.

Printed Materials

Printed educational materials come in a variety of formats. They can be as simple as a single sheet of paper, or they can be several sheets that are folded or stapled together to form a booklet.

Brochures, Booklets, and Fact Sheets. Many medical offices have materials available that explain

PROCEDURE 14-1

Developing a Patient Education Plan

Procedure Goal: To create and implement a patient teaching plan

Materials: Pen, paper, various educational aids (such as instructional pamphlets and brochures), and/or visual aids (such as posters, videotapes, or DVDs)

Method:

1. Identify the patient's educational needs. Consider the following:
   a. The patient's current knowledge
   b. Any misconceptions the patient may have
   c. Any obstacles to learning (loss of hearing or vision, limitations of mobility, language barriers, and so on)
   d. The patient's willingness and readiness to learn (motivation)
   e. How the patient will use the information

   Rationale
   All instruction must begin at the patient's point of need.

2. Develop and outline a plan using the various educational aids available. Include the following areas in the outline:
   a. What you want to accomplish (your goal)
   b. How you plan to accomplish it
   c. How you will determine if the teaching was successful

   Rationale
   Developing an educational plan ensures that all patient needs will be addressed.

3. Write the plan. Try to make the information interesting for the patient.

4. Before carrying out the plan, share it with the physician to get approval and suggestions for improvement.

5. Perform the instruction. Be sure to use more than one teaching method. For instance, if written material is being given, be sure to explain or demonstrate the material instead of simply telling the patient to read the educational materials.

6. Document the teaching in the patient's chart.

   Rationale
   All patient education must be documented in the patient's medical chart for continuity of care and as a legal record.

7. Evaluate the effectiveness of your teaching session. Ask yourself:
   a. Did you cover all the topics in your plan?
   b. Was the information well received by the patient?
   c. Did the patient appear to learn?
   d. How would you rate your performance?

8. Revise your plan as necessary to make it even more effective.

   Rationale
   Being an effective teacher means continually evaluating the methods that you use.

---

procedures performed in the medical office or give information about specific diseases and medical conditions. For example, women who have had a cesarean section delivery may be given a fact sheet describing simple exercises they can do in bed to help regain strength in the abdominal muscles. Some printed materials provide information to help patients stay healthy, such as tips for eating low-fat foods. Many educational aids are prepared by pharmaceutical companies and are provided free of charge to medical offices. Others may be written by the physician or members of the office staff. You may be asked to help prepare some of these materials.

Anytime written materials of any kind are given to a patient, it must be noted in the patient's chart. Be sure to document exactly which brochure or leaflet was distributed.

Educational Newsletters. A popular patient education tool is the medical office newsletter. Newsletters contain timely, practical health-care tips. Regular newsletters can also offer updates on office policies, information about new diagnostic tests or equipment, and news about the office staff. Newsletters are often written by the doctor or office staff. Some publishing companies and medical groups also offer newsletters that can be customized to a particular practice, using software programs such as Microsoft Publisher.

Community-Assistance Directory. Patients often require the assistance of health-related organizations within the community. For example, an elderly patient may need the services of a visiting nurse or a meals-on-wheels food program. Other patients may need the services of a day-care center, speech therapist, or weight clinic. A written community resource directory prepared by the office that is readily accessible to staff and patients is a valuable aid for referring patients to appropriate agencies.

Visual Materials

Many patients are better able to comprehend complicated medical information when it is presented in a visual format. When using visual educational materials, it is usually best to provide corresponding written materials that patients can keep for reference.

Videotapes and DVDs. Videotapes and DVDs are often used to educate patients about a variety of topics and to instruct them in self-care techniques (Figure 14-1). The use of videotapes or DVDs is especially effective when teaching about complex subjects and procedures. Examples of helpful videotapes used in patient education include videos on breast self-examination, dressing change, and infant care.

Seminars and Classes. Many physicians conduct or arrange educational seminars or classes for their patients. For example, an obstetrician might offer classes in childbirth preparation for patients and their partners.

Online Health Information. There are many wonderful online health information websites. Ask the doctor which websites to recommend to patients for general consumer health information. Be sure to recommend only sites that have been visited by a member of the office medical staff.

Promoting Health and Wellness Through Education

One of the most important goals of patient education is to promote good health. Health is not just the absence of illness. It is a complex concept that involves the body, mind, emotions, and environment. Health involves physical, mental, emotional, spiritual, and social influences working together as a whole.

Maintaining or improving your health is the best way to protect yourself against disease and illness. **Consumer education**—education that is geared, both in content and language, toward the average person—has helped Americans become more aware of the importance of good health. As a result, many people are beginning to take greater responsibility for their own health and well-being.

There are many ways to achieve good health. You can develop healthy habits, take steps to protect yourself from injury, and take preventive measures to decrease the risk of disease or illness. Patient education in the medical office should help patients achieve these goals.

Healthy Habits

When educating patients about good health, you can recommend several specific guidelines. Patient education can be used to promote good health habits by teaching patients the importance of

- Good nutrition, including limiting fat intake and eating an adequate amount of fruits, vegetables, and fiber
- Regular exercise
- Adequate rest (7 to 8 hours of sleep a night)
- The dangers of smoking and drug use
- The limiting of alcohol consumption
- Safe-sex practices
- The benefits of a balanced lifestyle of work and leisure activities (moderation)
- The benefits of safety practices

Whenever possible, these guidelines should be recommended to patients of all ages. Good health should be a top priority in life. Although it is best to incorporate healthy behavior before illness develops, remind patients that it is never too late to work toward improving their health. It is also important for medical assistants to act as models of good health practices for their patients.

Protection from Injury

Many accidents happen because people fail to see potential risks and do not develop plans of action. Following safety measures at home, at work, at play, and while

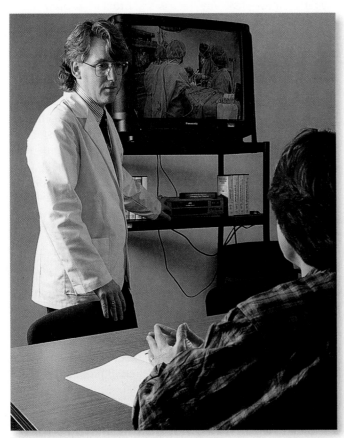

Figure 14-1. Videotapes and DVDs are an excellent educational aid for the medical office because of their visual format.

TABLE 14-1 Tips for Preventing Injury

At Home

- Install smoke detectors, carbon monoxide detectors, and fire extinguishers.
- Keep all medicines, chemicals, and household cleaning solutions out of reach of children. Purchase products in childproof containers. Lock or attach childproof latches to all cabinets, medicine chests, and drawers that contain poisonous items.
- Keep chemicals in their original containers, and store them out of children's reach.
- Install adequate lighting in rooms and hallways.
- Install railings on stairs.
- Use nonskid backing on rugs to help prevent falls, or remove rugs altogether.
- In the bathroom use nonskid mats or strips that stick to the tub floor.
- Stay with young children when they are in the bathroom.
- Don't rely on bath seats or rings as a safety device for babies and children.
- Set the water temperature on the water heater at 120°F.
- Practice good kitchen safety: Store knives and kitchen tools properly. Unplug small appliances when not in use. Wipe up spills immediately.
- Shorten long electrical cords and speaker wires, or secure them with electrical tape. Avoid plugging too many electrical appliances into the same outlet.

- Never use appliances in the bathtub or near a sink filled with water.
- Exercise caution when using electrical appliances. Use outlet covers when outlets are not in use.
- To reach high places, use proper equipment, such as stepladders, not chairs.
- Use child safety gates at the top of stairwells..
- When cooking, take care to turn all handles of pots and pans inward, toward the cooking surface, to avoid spills and burns.

At Work

- Use appropriate safety equipment and protective gear, as required.
- Lift heavy objects properly: Bend at the knees, not at the waist. As you straighten your legs, bring the object close to your body quickly. That way, strong leg muscles do the lifting, not weaker back muscles.
- Never attempt to move furniture on your own. Request that a member of the office building maintenance staff be engaged to do so.
- Use surge protectors on computer and other electronic equipment to prevent overloading outlets.
- Make sure hallways, entrance areas, work areas, offices, and parking lots are well lit.
- If your job involves desk work, practice proper posture when sitting. Do not sit for long periods of time. Get up and stretch, or walk down the hall and back.

---

traveling can help prevent injury. A discussion of ways to avoid accidents and injury should be part of the educational process. Table 14-1 lists tips for preventing injury at home and at work.

Facts from the National Safety Council data (2003) provide information on in-home deaths of people of all ages. These facts indicate that the home is not as safe as people think. According to these data, people are most likely to die in the home in the following ways:

- Falls (33%)
- Poisoning by solids (29%)
- Fires and burns (10%)
- Suffocation by ingestion (5%)
- Drowning (3%)
- Mechanical suffocation (2%)
- Poisoning by gases or vapors (1%)
- All other (15%)

Another essential aspect of educating patients about injury prevention is teaching them about the proper use of medications. A prescription includes specific instructions for taking the medication. Emphasize to the patient that these instructions must be followed exactly. In addition, the patient must not change the dosage or mix medications of any kind without first checking with the physician. Patients who do not adhere to these rules run the risk of potentially dangerous side effects. Tell patients to report to the physician any unusual reactions experienced when taking medications. Patients must also be cautioned to never share their medications with anyone else, no matter how tempting it may be to "help" a family member or friend.

When providing a patient with a new prescription, always ask the patient if he has told the doctor about all the medications he is already taking, including herbs, vitamins, and over-the-counter (OTC) medications. If the patient tells you that he has not, immediately inform the physician before the patient leaves the office. Medications taken together can change the desired drug response. The physician needs to know about all drugs as well as herbal preparations and OTC medications that the patient is taking.

Preventive Measures

Preventive health care is an area in which patient education plays a vital role. Patients need to know that they can decrease their chances of getting certain illnesses and diseases by taking preventive measures and avoiding certain behaviors. Preventive techniques can be described on three levels: *health-promoting behaviors, screening,* and *rehabilitation.*

Health-Promoting Behaviors. The first level of disease and illness prevention involves adopting the health-promoting behaviors described in the section titled Healthy Habits. This primary level of prevention also includes educating patients about the symptoms and warning signs of disease. One example is informing patients about the warning signs of cancer. The first letters of these warning signs spell the word *caution.* They are as follows:

- **C**hange in bowel or bladder habits
- **A** sore that does not heal
- **U**nusual bleeding or discharge
- **T**hickening or lump in a breast or elsewhere
- **I**ndigestion or difficulty in swallowing
- **O**bvious change in a wart or mole
- **N**agging cough or hoarseness

Screening. The second level of disease prevention is screening. **Screening** involves the diagnostic testing of a patient who is typically free of symptoms. Screening allows early diagnosis and treatment of certain diseases. Examples of screening tests include mammography and Pap smears for women and prostate examinations for men.

Annual screening is important to health maintenance. Although the requirements may differ according to the age and condition of the patient, annual screenings usually include:

- Routine blood work
- Urinalysis
- Chest x-ray
- EKG or ECG (electrocardiogram)
- Physical examination (PE)

Rehabilitation. The third level of disease prevention involves the rehabilitation and management of an existing illness. At this level the disease process remains stable, but the body will probably not heal any further. The objective is to maintain functionality and avoid further disability. Examples of this level of prevention include stroke rehabilitation programs, cardiac rehabilitation, and pain management for conditions such as arthritis.

 # The Patient Information Packet

When patients come to the medical practice, they need to learn not only about health and medical issues but also about the medical office itself. The patient information packet explains the medical practice and its policies.

Unlike most other patient education materials, the patient information packet deals mainly with administrative matters rather than with medical issues.

The patient information packet may be as simple as a one-page brochure or pamphlet. It may be a multipage brochure or a folder with multiple-page inserts.

Benefits of the Information Packet

The patient information packet is a simple, effective, and inexpensive way to improve the relationship between the office and the patients. It provides important information about the practice and the office staff. This information helps patients feel more comfortable with the qualifications of the health-care professionals involved in their care. The packet may help clarify the roles that each office staff member has in patient care.

The information packet also informs patients of office policies and procedures. Patients will learn the doctor's office hours, how to schedule appointments, the office's payment policies, and other administrative details. This information helps limit misunderstandings about these procedures.

The patient information packet also benefits the office staff. It is both an excellent marketing tool and an aid to running the office more smoothly. Providing patients with a prepared information packet saves staff time by answering a number of potential patient inquiries. The information packet is also a good way to acquaint new office staff members with office policies.

Contents of the Information Packet

Regardless of what material the information packet contains, it must be written in clear language so that patients are able to read and understand it. All materials should be written at a sixth-grade reading level to accommodate the reading level of most patients. Information should not be presented in a technical medical style. Because you may be responsible for preparing portions of the policy packet, you should be familiar with the contents of a typical packet.

Introduction to the Office. A brief introduction serves to welcome the patient to the office. It may be helpful to summarize the office's philosophy of patient care. The office's **philosophy** means the system of values and principles the office has adopted in its everyday practices.

Physician's Qualifications. The packet commonly contains information about the physician's professional qualifications and training. It includes details about education, internship, and residency. It may list credentials such as board certification or board eligibility in a certain medical specialty. It may also list the physician's membership in professional societies. The information packet for a group practice may contain a paragraph or a page for each physician.

Description of the Practice. It is helpful to include a brief description of the practice, particularly if it is a specialty practice. Explaining the types of examinations or procedures that are commonly performed in the office may be useful. It may also be helpful to list any special services the office provides, such as physical examinations for employment, workers' compensation cases, or other occupational services. Be sure to make medical terms and specialties clear by avoiding the use of initials. Spell out everything the first time the reference is made and place the appropriate initials in parentheses.

Introduction to the Office Staff. Many patients are not familiar with the qualifications and duties of the various members of the office staff. It is a good idea, therefore, to identify the staff positions according to their responsibilities and duties. Patients need to understand that some duties commonly thought to be a nurse's responsibilities may also be performed by a medical assistant. It may be helpful to include the professional credentials and licenses of key staff members.

Office Hours. This section should list the exact days and hours the office is open, including holidays. In addition, patients need to know what to do if an emergency occurs outside regular office hours. Tell the patient what number to call first (for example, the answering service, 911, or the hospital emergency room) and what to do next. Include the telephone number and address of the emergency room at the hospital with which the doctor is affiliated. Assure patients that the doctor or a physician partner can be reached at all times through the answering service. Some practices have multiple offices, and the physicians rotate from office to office on a regular schedule. List all office addresses and phone numbers along with directions to all office sites.

Appointment Scheduling. This section of the packet should explain the procedure for scheduling and canceling appointments. You might suggest that patients can benefit by scheduling routine checkups and visits as far in advance as possible. Also note if certain times of the day are reserved for sudden or unexpected office visits.

In this section encourage patients to be on time for appointments. Explain the problems that result from late or broken appointments. If the office charges a fee for breaking an appointment without advance notice, mention it here. Be careful to address these sensitive areas with a positive, nonthreatening tone. The office's written material should simply state the office policies and the problems that can result when functioning outside the policies.

Telephone Policy. Providing the office's telephone policies in the information packet can help reduce the number of unnecessary calls to the office and thus save time for the office staff. Explain which procedures can be handled over the telephone and which cannot. Explain procedures such as calling in for prescription renewals or laboratory test results. If the physician returns patients'

calls at a certain time of day, mention that policy in this section. Some practices bill patients for telephone calls in which medical advice is given but not for followup calls. For example, if a parent of a child who was vomiting uncontrollably called the physician to get immediate medical advice, the call might be billed. If the physician called to inform a patient of test results, however, the call would not be billed. It is important that patients know about these policies, particularly because many insurance plans do not cover charges for medical advice given over the phone, so the patient will be responsible for these charges.

Some offices (particularly pediatric offices) schedule a certain time of the day for patients (or parents and guardians) to call the physician for answers to their questions. This type of policy benefits both the office and the patients. The patients (or parents) have the assurance that they can speak with the physician about their concerns, and the office is spared interruptions during other times of the day.

Payment Policies. Inform patients of the office's policies regarding payment and billing. State whether payment is expected at the time of a visit or whether the patient can be billed. List accepted forms of payment (for example, cash, personal checks, and credit cards). It is not common practice to mention specific fees in an information packet.

Insurance Policies. List the major insurance carriers accepted by your office or state that *most major insurance plans are accepted.* Advise patients to bring proof of insurance coverage and a picture ID if this is their first visit to the office. A copy of this ID should be made and inserted in the patient's medical chart. State whether the office submits insurance claim forms directly to the insurance company or whether the patient has this responsibility. If the office or a billing service bills the insurance carrier, also include information regarding whether claims are submitted manually, using paper claims, or electronically. Generally, there is no charge for submission of the first insurance claim form; but if the office charges for submission of secondary insurance forms, this should be stated. Outline the practice's policy for handling Medicare coverage, including whether or not the office accepts assignment on Medicare claims. If the office does not submit insurance claims directly, explain that the staff will help patients fill out insurance forms when necessary, and providing the appropriate paperwork (usually a superbill) containing dates of service, and procedure and diagnosis codes for attachment to the claim form.

Patient Confidentiality Statement. The information packet must include a copy of the office privacy policy. Complete information regarding the privacy policy and HIPAA regulations can be found in Chapter 3 in the section titled HIPAA Privacy Rules. It is important to remember that the first step in informing patients of HIPAA compliance is the communication of patient rights. These rights are communicated through the Notice of Privacy Practices (NPP), which must adhere to the following specifications:

- Be written in plain, simple language.
- Include a header that reads "This notice describes how medical information about you may be used and disclosed and how you can get access to this information. Please review carefully."
- Describe the medical office's uses and disclosures of personal health information.
- Describe an individual's rights under the Privacy Rule.
- Describe the medical office's duties regarding patient privacy.
- Describe how patients can register complaints concerning suspected privacy violations.
- Specify a point of contact.
- Specify an effective date.
- State that the medical office reserves the right to change its privacy practices.

The information packet must also state that no information from patient files will be released without a signed authorization from the patient. Each patient who receives a copy of the privacy notice must sign a document stating that he received the privacy notice and had the opportunity to have his questions about the notice answered. This document should remain in the patient's medical file.

Other Information.   The patient information packet may include the practice's policy on referrals. It may provide information about access to available community health resources or agencies. It may also include special instructions for common office procedures (for example, whether the patient needs to fast before a procedure or to avoid certain foods).

Distributing the Information Packet

For the information packet to be effective, you must make sure that new patients receive and read it. One way is to hand the packet to new patients at the time of their first office visit and briefly review the contents with them (Figure 14-2). Explain that they can find answers to many questions in the packet. Encourage patients to take the packet home, read the information, and keep it handy for future reference.

When new patients make an appointment, many offices send them a copy of the information packet if there is enough time before the appointment to get it to them by regular mail. (It is a nice gesture to include a detailed map or written directions to the office for new patients who are not familiar with the area.) Patients can review the packet and the Consent for Treatment form before coming to the office (Figure 14-3). Additional copies of the packet should be placed in an accessible area in the office so that patients can take them home.

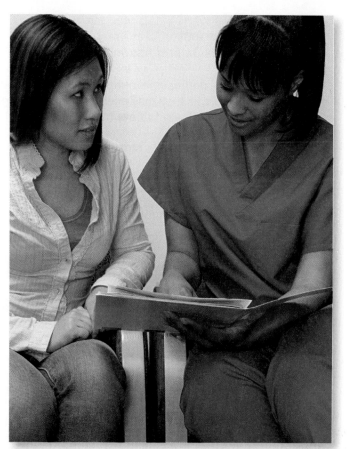

Figure 14-2.   Give patients the patient information packet on their first visit to the office, or mail it prior to their first appointment.

Special Concerns

Some practices serve patients who cannot read well or who do not speak or understand English. It may be necessary to create a second information packet that is written in very simple terms and that presents information through pictures and charts. The information packet can also be translated into one or more languages (see the section in Chapter 4 that discusses language barriers).

It is important that patients understand the office's policies and procedures. Additional one-on-one explanations may be required. Patients should still receive the printed materials to take home, however. Family members or friends may be able to read the materials for them, reinforcing what they learned in the office.

It is important to match the learning materials to the patient's needs and to her level of understanding. When possible, consider the patient's cultural background, age, medical condition, emotional state, learning style, educational background, disabilities, religious background, and readiness to learn when providing new materials. Even if a patient understands new materials, she still has the right to refuse treatment and information. If this occurs, notify the doctor and document the event in the patient's chart.

Consent for Treatment
Dr. Harry W. Jones Jr. and Associates

I voluntarily give my permission to the health-care providers of Dr. Harry W. Jones Jr. and such assistants and other health-care providers as they may deem necessary to provide medical services to me. I understand by signing this form, I am authorizing them to treat me for as long as I seek care from Dr. Harry W. Jones Jr., or until I withdraw my consent in writing.

_____

Signature of Patient or Guardian   Date

_____

Printed Name of Patient or Guardian   Relationship to Patient

Statement of Financial Responsibility/Assignment of Benefits
Dr. Harry W. Jones Jr. and Associates

I acknowledge that I am legally responsible for all charges in connection with the medical care and treatment provided by Dr. Harry W. Jones Jr. and Associates. I assign and authorize payments to Dr. Harry W. Jones Jr. I understand my insurance carrier may not approve or reimburse my medical services in full due to usual and customary rates, benefit exclusions, coverage limits, lack of authorization, or medical necessity. I understand I am responsible for fees not paid in full, co-payments, and policy deductibles and co-insurance except where my liability is limited by contract or State or Federal law.

_____

Signature of Patient or Guardian   Date

_____

Printed Name of Patient or Guardian   Relationship to Patient

A duplicate or faxed copy of this form is considered the same as the original document.

Figure 14-3. Sample patient Consent for Treatment form.

Educating Patients with Special Needs

During your career as a medical assistant, you will probably encounter many patients with special needs. Each patient's individual circumstances will affect your approach to patient education. In all cases try to see situations from the point of view of the patient. In many instances you can enlist the support of family or friends to aid in the educational process.

Elderly Patients

You will probably be called on to provide care for more and more elderly patients as the number of older people continues to grow. Patient education for elderly patients is especially valuable because it can help them prevent or manage health problems and remain independent. You may need to educate some older people about the importance of taking measures to protect their health.

You may work with elderly patients who have hearing or vision problems or physical limitations that restrict their ability to perform certain tasks. Keep the following suggestions in mind when working with elderly patients.

- Treat each patient as an individual. This point is perhaps the most important to remember when dealing with elderly patients. Some older people have trouble understanding directions. Try to communicate with them at the highest level they can understand. Never talk down to patients.

Reflecting On . . . Cultural Issues

Respecting Patients' Cultural Beliefs

Patients come from many diverse cultures and often have different beliefs about the causes and treatments of illness. These differences may affect their treatment expectations, as well as their willingness to follow medical directions. When talking with patients, it is important to understand and respect their cultural beliefs. Patients may not be willing to accept instructions or consent to treatment based on their cultural background. Consider these simple steps when giving instructions to patients of diverse cultures:

1. Speak slowly and clearly.
2. Request or provide a translator as needed.
3. Ask for and look for feedback from the patient, indicating that she understands and intends to follow the patient instructions.
4. Ask the patient if there is any reason that she will not be able to follow the instructions.
5. Address any concerns addressed by the patient, notifying the doctor if the concerns will mean that patient is not likely to follow instructions.
6. Provide educational resources in the patient's primary language, if available.

Educating the Patient

Instructing Patients with Hearing Impairments

Educating patients who have hearing impairments need not be difficult if you pay a little extra attention in the following areas.

- Try to eliminate all background noise. Talk in a quiet room, if possible.
- Make sure the room is well lit.
- Face the patient, and make sure the patient can see your mouth. Having the patient watch your mouth movements can help him understand what you are saying.
- Speak loudly and clearly, but do not shout. Use visual aids as necessary.
- Tell patients to let you know right away if they cannot hear you or do not catch something you have said. Even patients who do not have hearing impairments often appear to understand what a medical professional is saying rather than admit they are confused. It is a good idea to ask patients to repeat information to you to check their understanding. Also, periodically ask if they would like you to go over any particular part of the explanation or instructions again.

Loss of hearing can cause people to withdraw and feel isolated. Being empathic and patient greatly enhances the educational process.

Elderly Patients with Hearing Loss

Most people experience a gradual loss of hearing as they get older. In addition to the preceding suggestions, try to talk in a lower pitch whenever possible. As people get older, they often lose the ability to hear higher tones first.

Patients Who Wear Hearing Aids

When talking to a patient who wears a hearing aid, it is best to speak at a normal level. Many hearing aids make a normal voice louder but filter out loud noises. If you raise your voice, the hearing aid may filter it out. Consequently, the patient may hear only broken speech.

- Put instructions in writing. Because some elderly patients have problems with memory, detailed written instructions are an essential aspect of patient care. Patients can refer to the instructions as necessary or can ask a relative to do so.

- Adjust procedures as needed. When demonstrating a procedure to elderly patients, keep in mind any physical limitations they may have and adjust the procedure accordingly. Make sure patients understand the instructions by asking them to perform the procedure for you.

Patients with Mental Impairments

Patients with impaired mental functions include those with **dementia,** Alzheimer's disease, drug addictions, emotional problems, as well as those patients who are developmentally delayed. These patients can be challenging to deal with because communication may be difficult. Tact and empathy are important. A key to dealing with these patients is to speak at their level of understanding. Again, you must do your best to meet patients' needs without talking down to them.

Patients with Hearing Impairments

Patients with hearing impairments may have conditions ranging from mild impairment to total hearing loss. It is a common mistake to treat these patients as though they have mental impairments. Although you may have difficulty communicating with these patients, remember that their inability to hear has nothing to do with their level of intelligence. The Educating the Patient section provides techniques for educating patients who have hearing impairments.

Patients with Visual Impairments

As with hearing impairment, the level of visual impairment can vary significantly from patient to patient. Determining the severity of a patient's condition allows you to tailor your instruction to the patient's needs.

For those with mildly impaired vision, the approach may be as simple as providing instructional materials printed in large type. In addition, you can demonstrate procedures in a well-lit area and demonstrate the technique while standing or sitting close to the patient. For more severe visual impairment, adjust the level of instruction appropriately. For example, to demonstrate how to use a particular knob on a wheelchair, you might actually place the patient's hand on the knob and discuss its function.

When speaking to someone who has a visual impairment, remember to use a normal tone of voice. A patient with a visual impairment does not necessarily also have a hearing impairment. Although you should never talk down to patients, you need to verify that they understand all verbal instructions. Have the patient repeat all instructions to you.

Giving procedural instructions may be a challenge, depending on the patient's ability to perform certain tasks. Suggest that patients ask a family member or friend to help them with procedures they have trouble doing on their own.

Patient Education Prior to Surgery

One instance in which patient education is vital to a successful outcome is the instruction given before a patient undergoes a surgical procedure. Although exact instructions vary according to the procedure, their purpose is to prepare the patient for the procedure and to aid the patient during the recovery period. Instructions may include verbal, written, and demonstrative techniques (Figure 14-4).

The Role of the Medical Assistant

Patients generally receive information about the need for surgery and its nature from the physician. Educating and preparing patients for surgery will probably be your responsibility, however. You may provide support and explanations to patients. You must verify that they understand any information they may have been given by other members of the health-care team. Preoperative instruction may include discussion of postoperative care issues, such as temporary dietary restrictions.

You may also be responsible for determining whether patients have all the information they need before surgery, from both an educational and a legal standpoint. All patients who are undergoing a surgical procedure must first sign an informed consent form. As stated in Chapter 9, this legal document provides specific information about the surgical procedure, including its purpose, the possible risks, and the expected outcome. The informed consent form, along with documentation of all preoperative instruction, must be put in the patient's chart.

Benefits of Preoperative Education

Preoperative education has many benefits. It increases patients' overall satisfaction with their care. It helps reduce patient anxiety and fear, use of pain medication, complications following surgery, and recovery time. Letting the patient know what to expect during the surgery and afterward allows the patient to emotionally and educationally prepare for all aspects of the surgical procedure.

Types of Preoperative Teaching

Three types of teaching should occur during the preoperative period: factual, sensory, and participatory. The combination of these teaching methods gives the patient an overall understanding of the surgical procedure.

Factual. Factual teaching informs the patient of details about the procedure. You should tell the patient what will

Revised: 2003.06.12 Non-Hospital Medical/Surgical Facility: Schedule S-04

Patient Surgical Consent Form

Your surgeon for this procedure is: ____________________

I hereby authorize and request the surgeon, along with any assistants he/she feels are necessary, to perform upon me the following operation(s):

____

I understand that the nature and purpose of the above mentioned procedure(s) is/are to:

____

____

I also authorize the surgeon to do any therapeutic procedure or investigation that in his/her judgment may be advisable for my well-being.

The nature of the planned operation has been thoroughly explained to me by my surgeon and I have decided to proceed with this form of therapy over other alternative methods. The risks, benefits, and alternatives, including doing nothing, have been explained to me. I understand that the practice of medicine and surgery is not an exact science and I acknowledge that no guarantees have been made about the results of the operation or procedure planned. Furthermore, the risks and complications inherent in the operation have been explained to me and I accept these.

I further give permission to have such anesthetics administered to me as the surgeon or the anesthetist deems necessary or advisable.

Pictures may be taken of the treatment site for record purposes. I understand that these photographs/videos will be the property of the attending physician.

☐ I DO agree to allow these pictures to be used for publication or teaching purposes.

☐ I DO NOT agree to allow these pictures to be used for publication or teaching purposes.

If I agree, I understand that my name and identity will be kept confidential and protected.

I agree to keep the office of the surgeon informed of my post-operative progress and I agree to cooperate with instructions given for my post-operative care.

Patient or Legal Guardian (Signature) ____________________

Patient or Legal Guardian (Please Print) ____________________

Surgeon as Witness (Signature) ____________________

Surgeon as Witness (Please Print) ____________________

Date ______ Year ______ Month ______ Day

I hereby acknowledge receiving a copy of the post-operative instructions which have been reviewed with me. I understand the advice and restrictions given and agree to abide by them. I will notify my doctor immediately if any unusual bleeding, respiratory problems, or acute pain occurs after my discharge from this surgical facility.

Patient (Signature) ____________________ Witness (Signature) ____________________

Patient (Please Print) ____________________ Witness (Please Print) ____________________

Date ______ Year ______ Month ______ Day

Figure 14-4. Sample patient Surgical Consent form.

PROCEDURE 14-2

Informing the Patient of Guidelines for Surgery

Procedure Goal: To inform a preoperative patient of the necessary guidelines to follow prior to surgery

Materials: Patient chart, surgical guidelines

Method:

1. Review the patient's chart to determine the type of surgery to be performed and then ask the patient what procedure is being performed.

    Rationale

    Doing so confirms that the patient knows what surgery is being performed.

2. Tell the patient that you will be providing both verbal and written instructions that should be followed prior to surgery.

3. Inform the patient about policies regarding makeup, jewelry, contact lenses, wigs, dentures, and so on.

4. Tell the patient to leave money and valuables at home.

5. If applicable, suggest appropriate clothing for the patient to wear for postoperative ease and comfort.

6. Explain the need for someone to drive the patient home following an outpatient surgical procedure.

    Rationale

    Driving after even simple surgery can be very dangerous. Surgery can be canceled if a patient does not identify a responsible driver before surgery occurs.

7. Tell the patient the correct time to arrive at the office surgery center or the hospital for the procedure.

8. Inform the patient of dietary restrictions. Be sure to use specific, clear instructions about what may or may not be ingested and at what time the patient must abstain from eating or drinking. Also explain these points:

    a. The reasons for the dietary restrictions
    b. The possible consequences of not following the dietary restrictions.

    Rationale

    Surgery can be canceled if the patient has not followed dietary instructions.

9. Ask patients who smoke to refrain from or reduce cigarette smoking during at least the 8 hours prior to the procedure. Explain to the patient that reducing smoking improves the level of oxygen in the blood during surgery.

10. Suggest that the patient shower or bathe the morning of the procedure or the evening before.

11. Instruct the patient about medications to take or avoid before surgery.

    Rationale

    Surgery can be canceled if the patient has not followed medication instructions.

12. If necessary, clarify any information about which the patient is unclear.

13. Provide written surgical guidelines, and suggest that the patient call the office if additional questions arise.

    Rationale

    Patients may not understand or remember verbal instructions. Written instructions can be taken home and reviewed again.

14. Document the instruction in the patient's chart.

    Rationale

    All patient education must be documented in the patient's medical chart for continuity of care and as a legal record.

happen during the surgery, when it will happen, and why the procedure is necessary. Factual information also can include restrictions on diet or activity that may be necessary both before and after surgery. Procedure 14-2 describes how to inform patients of guidelines for surgery.

Sensory. Give patients a description of the physical sensations they may have during the procedure. All five senses may be involved: feeling, seeing, hearing, tasting, and smelling.

Participatory. Participatory teaching includes demonstrations of techniques that may be necessary or helpful during the postoperative period. Aspects of postoperative care include cleaning the wound, changing the dressing, and applying ice packs.

During this phase of teaching, you need to first describe the technique to the patient and then demonstrate it. The patient should repeat the demonstration for you. This practice is called **return demonstration.** If any aspects of the technique are unclear to the patient, you should

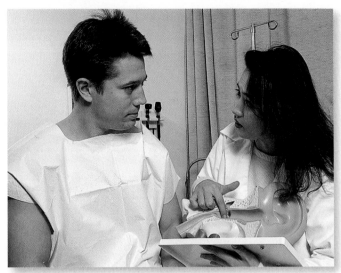

Figure 14-5. An anatomical model can help patients visualize what will happen during surgery.

demonstrate the technique again. The patient should be capable of performing the procedure properly. This process of teaching a new skill by having the patient observe and imitate is called **modeling.**

Using Anatomical Models

An anatomical model is a useful tool in preoperative education. As shown in Figure 14-5, looking at a larger-than-life model—and being able to see the actual body structures—helps patients better understand their condition. A model also allows patients to see how the surgical procedure will help correct their problem.

It may be difficult for a patient to visualize exactly what will take place in some surgical procedures. For example, think of arthroscopy of the knee. When told that the doctor will insert a viewing instrument into the knee, patients probably have no idea of the size of this scope. As a result, they may be particularly fearful of the procedure. Using a model to show exactly what will happen can ease patients' fears.

Helping Relieve Patient Anxiety

When you provide preoperative education, be aware that the fear and anxiety of patients who are about to undergo a surgical procedure can adversely affect the learning process. Consequently, allow extra time for repetition and reinforcement of material.

Always consider your choice of words carefully, stressing the positive rather than the negative whenever possible. Involving family members in the educational process is often beneficial, particularly if the patient is especially apprehensive about the surgery. Provide patients with a business card so they can contact you with further questions if necessary. Remember to present your instructions and explanations in straightforward language that they can understand. Remember to be reassuring, but to not "promise" a specific result for which the physician may be held liable if the expected result is not the actual result. Family members can often help relieve the patient's anxiety.

Verifying Patient Understanding

The key to the success of any educational process is verifying that patients have actually understood the information. A good way to check for understanding is to have patients explain in their own words what they have learned (this is a form of feedback). In addition, have them engage in return demonstrations.

Additional Educational Resources

Besides the resources available in the medical office, a vast number of outside resources are available for patient education. You can use these resources to obtain information for your own use in patient education, or you can mention them to patients who are looking for additional information. Following are several sources of patient education materials:

- Libraries and patient resource rooms. Most public libraries have an assortment of books, magazines, and electronic databases pertaining to health and medical topics. Many hospitals provide patient resource rooms, which include a variety of educational materials—such as books, brochures, and videotapes—for public use.

- Computer resources. A great deal of up-to-date medical information can be accessed through online services and CD-ROMs. The Internet is another widely used source of medical information. It will be helpful to suggest specific, reputable websites for patient research to ensure that the information obtained is valid.

- Community resources. Many local social service agencies provide specialized health information related to such topics as nursing home care, visiting nurses' care, counseling, and rehabilitation. Most of these agencies are listed in the telephone book. Area hospitals, the library, and the local chamber of commerce are other good sources for these services.

- Associations. Thousands of health organizations and associations can be contacted for information about preventive health care and virtually every known disease or disorder. The names, addresses, telephone numbers, and websites of these organizations are provided in several directories, which are available at most libraries or online. Table 14-2 provides a sample list of patient resource organizations.

TABLE 14-2 Patient Resource Organizations

Alzheimer's Disease Education and Referral Center
P.O. Box 8250
Silver Spring, MD 20907-8250
(800) 438-4380
Fax: (301) 495–3334
www.alzheimers.org

American Academy of Pediatrics
141 Northwest Point Boulevard
Elk Grove Village, IL 60007-1098
(847) 434-4000
www.aap.org

American Cancer Society
19 West 56th Street
New York, NY 10019
(212) 586-8700
www.cancer.org

American Diabetes Association
ATTN: National Call Center
1701 North Beauregard Street
Alexandria, VA 22311
(800)-DIABETES [(800) 342-2383]
www.diabetes.org

American Dietetic Association
120 South Riverside Plaza
Suite 2000
Chicago, IL 60606-6995
(800) 877-1600, ext. 4793
www.eatright.org

American Heart Association
National Center
7272 Greenville Avenue
Dallas, TX 75231
(800) 242-8721
www.americanheart.org

Arthritis Foundation
P.O. Box 7669
Atlanta, GA 30357-0669
(404) 872-7100
(404) 965-7888
(800) 568-4045
www.arthritis.org

Asthma and Allergy Foundation of America
1233 20th Street, NW
Suite 402
Washington, DC 20036
(800) 7ASTHMA [(800) 727-8462]
www.aafa.org

Centers for Disease Control and Prevention
Department of Health and Human Services
1600 Clifton Road
Atlanta, GA 30333
(404) 639-3311
www.cdc.gov

National AIDS Hotline
995 Market Street #200
San Francisco, CA 94103
(800) 342-2437
(800) 344-SIDA (Español)
(800) AIDS-TTY (hearing-impaired)
www.sfaf.org

National Cancer Institute
NCI Public Inquiries Office
6116 Executive Boulevard
Room 3036A
Bethesda, MD 20892-8322
(800) 4-CANCER
www.cancer.gov

National Clearinghouse for Alcohol and Drug
Information
P.O. Box 2345
Rockville, MD 20847-2345
(800) 729-6686
TDD: (800) 487-4889
(877) 767-8432 (Español)
www.ncadi.samhsa.gov

National Health Information Center
P.O. Box 1133
Washington, DC 20013-1133
(800) 336-4797
(The information specialists at this agency can
provide telephone numbers for associations that deal
with specific diseases or problems.)
www.health.gov/nhic

National Kidney Foundation
30 East 33rd Street
New York, NY 10016
(800) 622-9010
www.kidney.org

National Organization for Rare Disorders
55 Kenosia Avenue
P.O. Box 1968
Danbury, CT 06813-1968
(203) 744-0100
(800) 999-6673 (voicemail only)
TDD Number: (203) 797-9590
Fax: (203) 798-2291
www.rarediseases.org

President's Council on Physical Fitness and Sports
Department W, 200 Independence Avenue, SW
Room 738-H
Washington, D.C. 20201-0004
(202) 690-9000
Fax: (202) 690-5211
www.fitness.gov

Occupational Therapy Assistant

To gain medical assistant credentials, you must fulfill the requirements of either the American Association of Medical Assistants (for a Certified Medical Assistant) or the American Medical Technologists (for a Registered Medical Assistant). After obtaining your medical assistant certification or registration, you may wish to acquire additional skills in specialty areas through course work or on-the-job training. Although this course work or training may not lead to an additional certification or degree, it will enable you to expand your role in the medical office and advance your career as the demand for skilled health professionals increases.

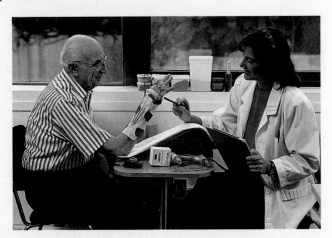

Skills and Duties

An occupational therapy assistant helps patients learn, or relearn, basic and special skills they need to function in their daily lives. Patient interaction is the focus of the occupational therapy assistant's job. An occupational therapy assistant works under the supervision of an occupational therapist.

Occupational therapists teach many different types of skills to many different types of patients. These skills include the following:

- Basic life skills, such as dressing and feeding oneself or moving about at home. For example, patients with partial paralysis or nerve damage resulting from a stroke may need this type of help.
- Vocational skills, such as typing. These skills will help patients with disabilities get jobs to support themselves.
- Designing and supervising arts and crafts activities. These activities serve as recreation and help patients develop fine motor skills in a nonthreatening, pleasant atmosphere.
- Helping accident victims who have an injured limb or a prosthetic device learn new ways to perform simple tasks. A patient with a prosthetic hand, for example, may need help learning to open jar lids.
- Working with patients who have behavioral or emotional disturbances. Occupational therapy may help these patients express their feelings in constructive ways, by building an interest in music, drama, or art.

The occupational therapy assistant also performs a number of clerical and administrative tasks. He checks inventories, orders supplies, and helps maintain the equipment in his workplace. He may also be responsible for paperwork, including writing reports on therapy sessions with patients.

Workplace Settings

Occupational therapy assistants often work in hospitals. They may also find work in clinics or long-term care facilities, such as retirement communities with assisted-care services, nursing homes, or rehabilitation centers. Some occupational therapists are employed in educational settings, including occupational workshops and schools for children with special needs.

Education

Community colleges and vocational schools offer 2-year programs for an associate degree in occupational therapy assisting. By completing a program approved by the American Occupational Therapy Association and passing a qualifying test, you can become a Certified Occupational Therapy Assistant (COTA).

For more information, visit the websites of the following organizations, which are available on the Online Learning Center at http://www.mhhe.com/medicalassisting4e.

The American Occupational Therapy Association
American Society of Hand Therapists

Summary

14.1 Patients benefit from patient education because they will be less likely to call the office with questions, and therefore the office staff can spend less time on the telephone. Educated patients take a more active role in their medical care.

14.2 Medical assistants play a vital role in patient education because of their interaction with patients; therefore, they can share vital educational information with their clients and reassess their needs at each visit.

14.3 Patients benefit from the education that is given in the office. Depending on patient need and level of understanding, teaching methods and formats are adjusted for the best possible result. Knowing your patient and his needs and abilities, as well as the goal of the instruction, will allow for the best possible education plan. Always assess your instruction at its completion and revise the plan as needed.

14.4 The types of patient education materials that are in medical offices are brochures, booklets, fact sheets, newsletters, DVDs, Internet-based sites, and community-assistance directories.

14.5 Patient education promotes good health habits by teaching patients the importance of developing healthy habits such as eating properly and exercising regularly.

14.6 The contents of the patient's information packet should include an introduction to the medical office, the physician's qualifications, a description of the practice, an introduction to the staff, office hours, appointment scheduling, telephone policies, payment and insurance policies, a confidentiality statement, and other pertinent information.

14.7 Educating patients with special needs will take flexibility on your part to accommodate the requirements of the individual patient. Explain procedures slowly and clearly; have instructions in writing and adjust demonstrations as needed for the patient's ability.

14.8 Educating patients prior to surgery is vital to a successful outcome and involves instructing them on proper procedures before surgery. The types of preoperative teaching methods are factual, sensory, and participatory.

14.9 Additional educational resources outside the medical facility can consist of libraries and patient resource rooms, computer and Internet resources, as well as community resource listings found online, in the telephone book, area hospitals, and local chambers of commerce.

REVIEW

CHAPTER 14

CASE STUDY QUESTIONS

Now that you have completed this chapter, review the case study at the beginning of the chapter and answer the following questions:

1. What might be important to consider when creating an educational plan for a patient? How might the plan vary according to the individual?
2. What factors could block effective patient education?
3. What specific behaviors do you associate with talking down to a patient?
4. Why are good listening skills an important part of teaching?

Multiple-Choice Questions

1. A benefit of the patient information packet is that it
   a. promotes better compliance with treatment programs.
   b. helps patients feel more comfortable with the qualifications of the health-care professionals who are caring for them.
   c. can answer a treatment question that may come up during an office visit.
   d. encourages patients to help themselves achieve better health.

2. The *most* important point to include when dealing with elderly patients is to
   a. put instructions in writing.
   b. treat each patient as an individual.
   c. adjust procedures as necessary.
   d. try to communicate at the highest level they can understand.
3. Which of the following should you do when educating a patient with a hearing impairment?
   a. use a higher-pitched voice.
   b. ask the patient to repeat information to check his understanding.
   c. face the patient and shout.
   d. speak at a faster rate.
4. Which of the following types of preoperative teaching gives patients a description of the physical sensations they may have during the procedure?
   a. Factual
   b. Sensory
   c. Participatory
   d. Modeling
5. When talking to a patient who wears a hearing aid, you should
   a. speak at a normal level.
   b. speak very loudly.
   c. raise the pitch of your voice.
   d. speak very slowly.

Discussion Questions

1. Why is it important to educate patients about how to take care of themselves?
2. Patients spend less time in the hospital than ever before. How does this change the role of private medical offices and the role of medical assistants in those practices?
3. What are some good ways to get patients to read printed materials?
4. How would you educate patients with diverse cultural backgrounds?

Critical Thinking Questions

1. In this chapter, you have learned that patient education is an essential process in the medical office. In your own words, describe why.

2. You are measuring the vital signs of an overweight woman. She becomes visibly upset when you ask her to step on the scale. The office has many brochures with tips on promoting good health and exercise. How might you bring up the subject of proper diet and exercise?

Application Activities

1. Practice your patient education skills by role-playing giving health-care instructions to a person who comes from a culture other than your own. Ask another student to watch and evaluate your teaching method.
2. Write the section of a patient information brochure that describes the general roles of the medical office staff. Exchange your writing sample with that of another student, and critique each other's work.
3. With a partner, role-play a medical assistant giving procedural instructions to a patient with a hearing impairment. Then switch roles, and offer suggestions for improving each other's teaching techniques.

Virtual Fieldtrip

Visit the McGraw-Hill Higher Education Medical Assisting website at www.mhhe.com/medicalassisting4e to complete the following activity:

Search the Internet for ideas on patient pamphlets that might be helpful to patients with diabetes and heart disease. What samples can you provide that you have either downloaded or created yourself?

Open the CD and complete this chapter's practice activities, play the games, listen to the key terms, and test yourself with the interactive review. E-mail, print, and/or save your results to document your proficiency.

SECTION 3

FINANCIAL RESPONSIBILITIES

CHAPTER **15**

Health Insurance Billing Procedures

CHAPTER **16**

Medical Coding

CHAPTER **17**

Patient Billing and Collections

CHAPTER **18**

Accounting for the Medical Office

Health Insurance Billing Procedures

MEDICAL ASSISTING COMPETENCIES

CAAHEP

VII. C (1) Identify types of insurance plans

VII. C (3) Discuss workers' compensation as it applies to patients

VII. C (4) Describe procedures for implementing both managed care and insurance plans

VII. C (6) Discuss referral process for patients in a managed care program

VII. C (11) Describe the concept of RBRVS

VII. C (12) Define diagnosis-related groups (DRGs)

VII. P (1) Apply both managed care policies and procedures

VII. P (3) Complete insurance claim forms

VII. P (4) Obtain precertification, including documentation

VII. P (5) Obtain preauthorization, including documentation

VII. A (1) Demonstrate assertive communication with managed care and/or insurance providers

ABHES

4. **Medical Law and Ethics**
   a. Document accurately
   f. Comply with federal, state, and local health laws and regulations

8. **Medical Office Business Procedures Management**
   s. Obtain managed care referrals and precertifications
   u. Prepare and submit insurance claims
   v. Use physician's fee schedule
   ee. Use proper telephone techniques
   hh. Receive, organize, prioritize, and transmit information expediently

11. **Career Development**
   Demonstrate professionalism by:
   5) Exhibiting initiative
   6) Adapting to change
   8) Being courteous and diplomatic

LEARNING OUTCOMES

After completing Chapter 15, you will be able to:

15.1 Describe Medicare and Medicaid.

15.2 Describe TRICARE and CHAMPVA health-care benefits programs.

15.3 Distinguish between HMOs and PPOs.

15.4 Explain how to manage a workers' compensation case.

15.5 Execute the basic steps of the health insurance claim process.

15.6 Describe your role in insurance claims processing.

15.7 Apply rules related to the coordination of benefits.

15.8 Use the health-care claim preparation process.

15.9 Explain how payers set fees.

15.10 Use a Centers for Medicare and Medicaid Service (CMS-1500) claim form.

15.11 Outline three ways to transmit electronic claims.

MEDICAL ASSISTING MEDIA

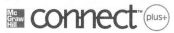 **Connect Plus+™**
connect.mcgraw-hill.com

- Electronic Health Records (E.H.R.) SpringCharts®
- eBook

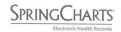

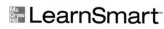 **LearnSmart™**

www.mhhe.com/learnsmart

Complete Learning Module: Health Insurance Billing Procedures

 Student CD-ROM

 Online Learning Center™

www.mhhe.com/medicalassisting4e

KEY TERMS

allowed charge
assignment of benefits
balance billing
benefits
birthday rule
capitation
Centers for Medicare and Medicaid Services (CMS)
CHAMPVA
clearinghouse
coinsurance
coordination of benefits

copayment
deductible
disability insurance
elective procedure
electronic data interchange (EDI)
exclusion
explanation of benefits (EOB)
fee-for-service
fee schedule
formulary

health maintenance organization (HMO)
liability insurance
lifetime maximum benefit
Medicaid
Medicare
Medicare Advantage plans
Medigap
Original Medicare Plan
participating physicians
preauthorization
precertification

preferred provider organization (PPO)
premium
referral
remittance advice (RA)
resource-based relative value scale (RBRVS)
third-party payer
TRICARE
X12 837 Health Care Claim

CHAPTER OUTLINE

- Basic Insurance Terminology
- Types of Health Plans
- Government Plans
- The Claims Process: An Overview
- Fee Schedules and Charges
- Preparing and Transmitting Health-Care Claims

PREPARATION FOR CERTIFICATION

RMA (AMT) Exam
- Patient billing procedures
- Medical finance terminology
- Financial applications of medical insurance
- Claim forms

CMA (AAMA) Exam
- Processing claims
- Applying managed care policies and procedures
- Fee schedules

CMAS Exam
- Insurance processing

Introduction

Health-care claims are a critical part of the reimbursement process. Accurate claims sent to payers mean that physicians receive the maximum appropriate payment for the services they provide. Patients are also concerned with their health-care plans, asking, "How much will my insurance pay?" "How much will I owe?" "Why are this doctor's fees different from my previous doctor's fees?"

You will handle questions such as these every day. Not only must you correctly prepare health-care claims, but you will also review patients' insurance coverage, explain the physician's fees, estimate what charges payers will cover, and prepare claims for patients. This chapter prepares you for these tasks by explaining the types of health-care insurance patients have, how payers calculate the amount they pay for providers' services, and how to transmit complete and accurate claims. This chapter also gives you the information you need about patients' financial responsibilities for services so that you can figure out how much patients should pay and how much will be billed to their health-care plans.

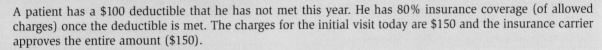

CASE STUDY

A patient has a $100 deductible that he has not met this year. He has 80% insurance coverage (of allowed charges) once the deductible is met. The charges for the initial visit today are $150 and the insurance carrier approves the entire amount ($150).

As you read this chapter, consider the following questions:
1. How much should this patient pay?
2. How much will he owe for his next visit this year, which is expected to have a charge of $200?
3. Assuming that the patient in the case study has a managed care policy, what type of policy does he probably have?
4. What term would you use to describe the part of the payment that is based on 20% of the charges?
5. If you did not know whether the deductible had been met, what procedure would you follow?

Basic Insurance Terminology

The first step in understanding insurance is to learn some basic terminology. Medical insurance, which is also known as health insurance, is a written contract in the form of a policy between a policyholder and a health plan (insurance carrier). The policyholder may also be called the insured, the member, or the subscriber.

Under the insurance policy, the policyholder pays a **premium,** which is the charge for keeping the insurance policy in effect. In exchange, the health plan provides **benefits**—payments for medical services—for a specified time period. The policy may cover dependents of the policyholder, such as a spouse or children. The contract may specify a **lifetime maximum benefit,** which is a total sum that the health plan will pay out over the patient's life.

There are actually three participants under insurance contracts. The patient (policyholder) is the *first party,* and the physician who provides medical services is the *second party.* A patient-physician contract is created when a physician agrees to treat a patient who seeks medical services. Through this unwritten contract, the patient is legally responsible for paying for services. The patient may have a policy with a health plan, the *third party,* which agrees to carry the risk of paying for those services and therefore is called a **third-party payer.**

Depending on the type of health plan, the policyholder may pay a **deductible**—a fixed dollar amount that must be paid or "met" once a year, in addition to the premium, before the third-party payer begins to cover medical expenses. The patient may also have to pay **coinsurance,** a fixed percentage of covered charges after the deductible is met. The coinsurance rate presents the health plan's percentage of the charge followed by the insured's percentage, such as 80-20, which means the insurance carrier would pay 80% of allowed charges and the patient would be responsible for the remaining 20%. If the patient belongs to a managed care health plan, such as a health maintenance organization (HMO), the patient often must pay a **copayment,** a small fixed fee that is collected at the time of the visit. The health plan then pays an agreed-upon contracted payment for the charges with any balance written off or adjusted off by the service provider.

Some expenses, such as routine eye examinations or dental care, may not be covered under the insured's contract. Uncovered expenses are **exclusions.** Many plans offer a prescription drug benefit. Such benefits usually require the use of drugs that are listed on the plan's **formulary,** a list of approved brands.

An **elective procedure** describes a medical procedure that is medically necessary but is not required to sustain life and that is requested for payment to the third-party payer by the patient or the physician. Some elective procedures are paid for by third-party payers while others are not. **Precertification** describes the process of the provider contacting the insurance plan to see if the proposed procedure is a covered service under the patient's insurance plan. **Preauthorization** or prior authorization takes this information a step further by giving the insurance carrier specific information for the particular patient's case. If the insurance plan agrees that the patient requires the procedure, in other words, it is medically necessary, they will issue a prior authorization number approving the need for the service or procedure. The prior authorization does not, however, mean they agree to pay for the service. This requires the next step of predetermination, where the insurance plan informs the physician the maximum amount they will pay for the procedure to be performed.

Two special types of insurance are liability insurance and disability insurance. **Liability insurance** covers injuries that are caused by the insured or that occurred on the insured's property. If an individual (or company) has home, business, automobile, or health liability insurance, the injured person can claim benefits under the insured's policy. To obtain details about coverage, contact the liability insurance company.

Disability insurance is a type of insurance that may be offered to (at employee expense) or provided by an employer for its employees or purchased privately by self-employed individuals. Disability insurance is activated when the insured is injured or disabled. When the insured cannot work, the insurance company pays the insured a prearranged monthly amount that covers the insured's normal expenses. Disability insurance is divided into two types; short-term policies offer coverage for shorter periods of time, usually 7 days to 6 months, and long-term disability policies that may last for a year or more, depending on policy stipulations.

 # Types of Health Plans

All insurance companies have their own rules about benefits and procedures. Many companies also have their own manuals, printed or online, that you must keep handy in the office for reference. Representatives of the insurance companies are available to work with you, however, to answer questions and help ensure that claims are correctly filed. Their business depends on it. Never hesitate to contact an insurance company. Many have toll-free numbers and websites for just this purpose.

There are many sources of health plans in the United States. The majority of individuals with insurance are covered by group policies, usually through their employers. Some people have individual plans. Many are covered under a government plan. Still others—over 40 million Americans—have no health-care insurance. The federal government through the Obama administration is again attempting a health-care plan so that all Americans have health-care coverage, but at this writing, this is not the case.

Traditionally, every insurance plan issued each of their providers an identification number, similar to the policy number given to each subscriber. Since the advent of HIPAA, individual insurers can no longer issue identifying numbers. Every physician and provider who submits a claim to any insurance carrier must now use a specific provider number, known as a National Provider Identifier (NPI), from the Centers for Medicare and Medicaid Services (CMS).

During the transition period, while providers obtained their NPIs, certain non-NPI numbers and two-character identifiers (Table 15-1) were allowed. Now that all providers have an NPI, these non-NPI numbers and their identifiers are still found on claim forms for certain payers.

Fee-for-Service and Managed Care Plans

There are two major types of health plans: fee-for-service plans and managed care plans. **Fee-for-service** plans, the oldest and most expensive type, repay policyholders for costs of health care due to illnesses and accidents. The policy lists the medical services that are covered. The amount charged for services is controlled by the physician who provides them, although the amount paid for each service is controlled by the insurance carrier. The

TABLE 15-1	National Uniform Claim Committee (NUCC) Non-NPI Qualifiers

These qualifiers are for use in CMS-1500 (and X12 837). These identifiers may be used in the following fields: 17a, 19, 24l, 32a, and 32b.

Qualifier	Description
0B	State License Number
1B	Blue Shield Provider Number
1C	Medicare Provider Number
1D	Medicaid Provider Number
1G	Provider UPIN Number
1H	CHAMPVA Identification Number
E1	Employer's Identification Number
G2	Provider Commercial Number
LU	Location Number
N5	Provider Plan Network Identification Number
SY	Social Security Number (this may not be used for Medicare)
X5	State Industrial Accident Provider Number
ZZ	Provider Taxonomy

benefit may be for all or part of the charges (as with the 80/20 plans discussed previously).

Managed care plans, in contrast, control both the financing and the delivery of health care to policyholders. They enroll policyholders, and they also enroll physicians and other providers, controlling the delivery of health care. The managed care organizations (MCOs) that set up managed care health plans reach agreements with physicians and other health-care providers that control fees. Many people who are insured through their employers are covered by some form of a managed care plan.

Physicians who enroll with managed care plans are called **participating physicians.** They have contracts with the MCOs that stipulate physician fees, the credentials they must have, and their responsibilities and that also explain the MCO's duties. For example, the MCO usually publishes the participating physicians' names in booklets and on a website so that policyholders can choose a provider from the list.

Managed care plans pay their participating physicians in one of two ways—either by contracted fees or a fixed prepayment called **capitation.** In a capitated managed care plan, providers (usually the primary care physicians or PCPs) are paid a fixed amount per month to provide necessary, contracted services to patients who are plan members. The rate the provider is paid is based on several factors, including the number of plan members in the insured pool and their ages. The capitated rate per enrollee is paid to the provider

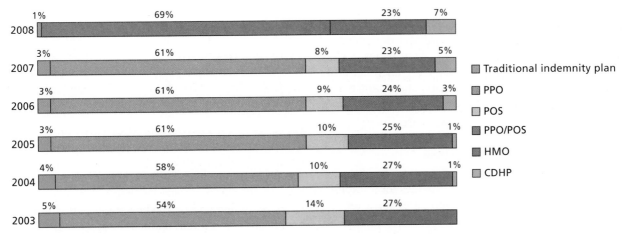

Figure 15-1. Types of health plans.

Source: Mercer's National Survey of Employer Sponsored Health Plans, 2007. Copyright 2007, The Managed Care Information Center.

even if the provider does not provide any medical services to the patient during the time period covered by the payment. Similarly, the provider receives the same capitated rate if a patient is treated more than once during the time period. In other plans, negotiated per-service fees are paid. These fees are less than the regular rate for a service that the provider normally charges. Most specialists who participate in MCOs are reimbursed for their services in this manner.

As shown in Figure 15-1, more than half of all health plans are **preferred provider organizations (PPOs).** A PPO is a managed care plan that establishes a network of providers to perform services for plan members. In exchange for the PPO sending them patients, the physicians agree to charge discounted fees. In most PPOs, plan members may also choose to receive care from doctors or providers outside the network, but if they do so, they are responsible for paying a higher percentage of the charges for these visits and may also be subject to a deductible that they would not be responsible for if they saw in-network providers.

Another common type of managed care system is a **health maintenance organization (HMO).** Physicians with HMO contracts are often paid a capitated rate, or they may be employees of the organization who are paid salaries. Patients who enroll in an HMO pay premiums and usually also pay a copayment, often $10 to $20, at the time of the office visit. No other fees are required for any covered service that a member needs. In HMOs, patients must usually choose from a specific group of health-care providers for care. If they seek services from a provider who is not in the health plan, the HMO does not pay for the care. Patients also pay for excluded services.

Government Plans

Government plans are generally designed to offer health care to retirees, low-income and disadvantaged individuals, and active or retired military personnel and their families. Some of these plans still maintain many of the features of managed care plans.

Medicare

Several federal programs provide health care. The largest is **Medicare,** which provides health insurance for citizens aged 65 and older. Certain patients under the age of 65 may also be entitled to Medicare. Such patients include those who are blind or widowed or who have serious long-term disabilities, such as chronic joint pain or kidney failure. The Medicare program is managed by the **Centers for Medicare and Medicaid Services (CMS),** www.medicare.gov (for patient and beneficiary information) and www.cms.gov (includes provider and claims information for both Medicare and Medicaid).

Part A. Medicare has two main parts. Part A is hospital benefit, which is billed by hospitals (or other health-care facilities). It pays most of the benefits for the following individuals:

- A patient who has been hospitalized (as an inpatient) up to 90 days for each benefit period. A benefit period begins the day a patient goes into the hospital and ends when that patient has not been hospitalized or placed in a skilled nursing facility for a period of 60 continuous days after discharge.

  The 90-day benefit period is divided into two parts. The Medicare benefit period is 60 days where after the patient pays a deductible, hospital coverage is at 100%. After the first 60 days the patient enters into a 30-day period called coinsurance days. During this 30-day period, the patient must pay an additional per-day payment or co-insurance. If the hospital stay extends beyond the 30 coinsurance days, the patient may use up to 60 lifetime reserve days, which also include a per-day charge.

- A patient who has been an inpatient in a skilled nursing facility (SNF) for no more than 100 days in each benefit period. A benefit period is usually 1 calendar year.

- A patient who is receiving medical care at home.
- A patient who has been diagnosed as terminally ill and needs hospice care. Medicare defines *terminally ill* as having a prognosis (prediction of the probable course of a disease in an individual and the chances of recovery) of 6 months or less to live. A hospice is a medical organization that provides pain relief and other end-of-life care to terminally ill patients and emotional support for these patients and their families.
- A patient who requires psychiatric treatment. Currently Medicare covers only 190 days of psychiatric hospitalization in a patient's lifetime.
- A patient who requires respite care. In certain, clearly defined circumstances, Medicare provides for a respite, or short break, for the person who cares for a terminally ill patient at home. The terminally ill patient is moved to a care facility for the respite.

Anyone who receives Social Security benefits is automatically enrolled in Part A and does not have to pay a premium. Individuals aged 65 or older who are not eligible for Social Security benefits may enroll in Part A, but they must pay premiums for the coverage.

Part B. Part B helps pay for a wide range of outpatient procedures and supplies. For example, it covers physician services, outpatient hospital services, diagnostic tests, clinical laboratory services, and outpatient physical and speech therapy as long as these services are considered medically necessary. Individuals entitled to Part A benefits automatically qualify for Part B benefits. In addition, U.S. citizens and permanent residents over the age of 65 are also eligible. Part B is a voluntary program; eligible persons may or may not take part in it. However, those desiring Part B must enroll because coverage is not automatic. The Medicare beneficiary has a 6 month time frame to apply, beginning 3 months prior to his 65th birthday until 3 months after it. If the deadline is missed, the beneficiary must wait until open enrollment, which is from January 1–March 31 of each year. Unlike Part A, Part B coverage is not premium-free. Starting in 2007, the Medicare Part B premium is based on the beneficiary's income. The cost ranges between $0 and $211.90 per month, and the premium usually increases annually.

Each Medicare enrollee receives a health insurance card. This card lists the beneficiary's name, sex, effective dates for Part A and Part B coverage, and Medicare number. The Medicare number is assigned by CMS and usually consists of the Social Security number followed by an alpha or alphanumeric suffix.

Medicare Part C and Part D. Medicare Part C was introduced in 1997 and provides several choices for individuals in the types of plans they utilize. They are called Medicare Advantage plans and include PPOs, HMOs, private fee-for-service (PFFS) plans, special needs plans, and Medicare medical savings plans (MSA). The MSA plan started in 2007.

Medicare Part D was passed in 2003 and coverage began January 1, 2006. It is the prescription drug plan. All persons with Medicare can join a plan that is provided through the Medicare Prescription Drug plan, Medicare Advantage and other Medicare plans, and employers and unions. Figure 15-2 is the Medicare Part D Coverage Determination Request Form.

Types of Medicare Plans. Medicare beneficiaries can choose from among a number of insurance plans, including traditional fee-for-service and Medicare Advantage, which consists of a group of different managed care plans.

Fee-for-Service: The Original Medicare Plan. The Medicare fee-for-service plan, referred to by Medicare as the **Original Medicare Plan,** allows the beneficiary to choose any licensed physician certified by Medicare. Each time the beneficiary receives services, a fee is billable. Part of this fee is generally paid by Medicare and part is due from the beneficiary. An annual deductible of $135 is the patient's responsibility. If the patient sees a participating provider, Medicare pays 80% of approved charges directly to the provider and the patient is responsible for the remaining 20% as well as any disallowed charges. Providers who accept the Medicare allowed charge as payment in full are known as those who "accept assignment." These providers cannot charge the patient more than the Medicare-allowed charge, no matter what the original fee may have been. A Medicare beneficiary may choose a provider who does not participate in the Medicare program and who does not accept assignment. In that case, the provider does not have to accept the Medicare allowable as payment in full and may charge the patient up to the "limiting charge" as described by Medicare. The limiting charge is usually defined as 115% of the nonparticipating allowable fee. This arrangement usually results in an increased out-of-pocket expense for the patient.

To help with payment of the 20% coinsurance, individuals enrolled in Medicare Part B Original Medicare Plan often buy additional insurance called a **Medigap** plan. These plans frequently reimburse the patient's Part B deductible and pick up the 20% of the Medicare allowed charge. If Medicare does not pay a claim, Medigap is not required to pay the claim either. Although private insurance carriers offer Medigap plans, coverage and standards are regulated by federal and state law. In exchange for Medigap coverage, the policyholder pays a monthly premium. A number of different options are available. These choices are labeled A through J. Monthly premiums vary widely across the different plan levels as well as within a single plan level, depending on the insurance company selected. While coverage varies from policy to policy, a set of core benefits is common to all Medigap plans, including the Part B coinsurance amount (usually 20% of approved charges) after the deductible ($135). A fiscal intermediary (an insurance company that contracts with the federal government to review and pay Medicare claims) handles and processes Medicare claims for each state. Payments for services are standardized nationally.

Medicare Advantage Plans. Medicare also offers a group of plans called the **Medicare Advantage plans.**

Plan Name _____

Phone # _____

Fax # _____

Medicare Part D Coverage Determination Request Form

This form cannot be used to request:
- Medicare non-covered drugs, including barbiturates, benzodiazepines, fertility drugs, drugs prescribed for weight loss, weight gain or hair growth, over-the-counter drugs, or prescription vitamins (except prenatal vitamins and fluoride preparations).
- **Biotech or other specialty drugs for which drug-specific forms are required. [See <Part D plan website.>] OR [See links to plan websites at http://www.cms.hhs.gov/PrescriptionDrugCovGenIn/04_Formulary.asp]**

Patient Information	**Prescriber Information**
Patient Name:	Prescriber Name:
Member ID#:	NPI# (if available):
Address:	Address:
City: State:	City: State:
Home Phone: Zip:	Office Phone #: Office Fax #: Zip:
Sex (circle): M F DOB:	Contact Person:

Diagnosis and Medical Information		
Medication:	Strength and Route of Administration:	Frequency:
☐ New Prescription OR Date Therapy Initiated:	Expected Length of Therapy:	Qty:
Height/Weight: Drug Allergies:	Diagnosis:	
Prescriber's Signature:		Date:

Rationale for Exception Request or Prior Authorization
FORM CANNOT BE PROCESSED WITHOUT REQUIRED EXPLANATION

☐ Alternate drug(s) contraindicated or previously tried, but with adverse outcome (eg, toxicity, allergy, or therapeutic failure)

→ Specify below: (1) Drug(s) contraindicated or tried; (2) adverse outcome for each; (3) if therapeutic failure, length of therapy on each drug(s);

☐ Complex patient with one or more chronic conditions (including, for example, psychiatric condition, diabetes) is stable on current drug(s); high risk of significant adverse clinical outcome with medication change

→ Specify below: Anticipated significant adverse clinical outcome

☐ Medical need for different dosage form and/or higher dosage

→ Specify below: (1) Dosage form(s) and/or dosage(s) tried; (2) explain medical reason

☐ Request for formulary tier exception

→ Specify below: (1) Formulary or preferred drugs contraindicated or tried and failed, or tried and not as effective as requested drug; (2) if therapeutic failure, length of therapy on each drug and adverse outcome; (3) if not as effective, length of therapy on each drug and outcome

☐ Other:_____   → Explain below

REQUIRED EXPLANATION:_____

_____

_____

Request for Expedited Review

☐ REQUEST FOR EXPEDITED REVIEW [24 HOURS]

→ BY CHECKING THIS BOX AND SIGNING ABOVE, I CERTIFY THAT APPLYING THE 72 HOUR STANDARD REVIEW TIME FRAME MAY SERIOUSLY JEOPARDIZE THE LIFE OR HEALTH OF THE MEMBER OR THE MEMBER'S ABILITY TO REGAIN MAXIMUM FUNCTION

Information on this form is protected health information and subject to all privacy and security regulations under HIPAA.

Figure 15-2. Medicare Part D Coverage Determination Request Form.

Beneficiaries can choose to enroll in one of three major types of plans instead of the Original Medicare Plan:

1. Medicare Managed Care Plans
2. Medicare Preferred Provider Organization Plans (PPO)
3. Medicare Private Fee-for-Service Plans

Medicare Managed Care Plans charge a monthly premium and a small copayment for each office visit, but not a deductible. Like private payer managed care plans, Medicare managed care plans often require patients to use a specific network of physicians, hospitals, and facilities. Some plans offer the option of receiving services from providers outside the network for a higher fee. However, they offer coverage for services not reimbursed in the Original Medicare Plan, such as physical examinations and inoculations. Participants are generally required to select a primary care provider (PCP) from within the network. The PCP provides treatment and manages the patient's medical care through **referrals.**

In the *Medicare Preferred Provider Organization Plan (PPO),* patients pay less when they use doctors within a network, but they may choose to go outside the network for additional costs, such as a higher copayment or higher coinsurance. Patients do not need a PCP, and referrals are not required.

Under a *Medicare Private Fee-for-Service Plan,* patients receive services from the provider they choose, as long as Medicare has approved the provider or facility. The plan is operated by a private insurance company that contracts with Medicare to provide services to beneficiaries. The plan sets its own rates for services, and physicians are allowed to bill patients the amount of the charge not covered by the plan. A copayment may or may not be required.

Recovery Audit Contractor (RAC) Program.

In 2008, CMS announced aggressive new steps to find and prevent waste, fraud, and abuse in Medicare. CMS is working closely with beneficiaries and providers, consolidating its fraud detection efforts, strengthening its oversight of medical equipment suppliers and home health agencies, and launching the national recovery audit contractor (RAC) program.

CMS took the next steps in the agency's comprehensive efforts to identify improper Medicare payments and fight fraud, waste, and abuse in the Medicare program by awarding contracts to four permanent RACs, each of which will audit one-fourth of the country, designed to guard the Medicare Trust Fund.

The goal of the recovery audit program is to identify improper payments made on claims of health-care services provided to Medicare beneficiaries. Improper payments may be overpayments or underpayments. Overpayments can occur when health-care providers submit claims that do not meet Medicare's coding or medical necessity policies. Underpayments can occur when health-care providers submit claims for a simple procedure, but the medical record reveals that a more complicated procedure was actually performed. Health-care providers that might be reviewed include hospitals, physician practices, nursing homes, home health agencies, durable medical equipment suppliers, and any other provider or supplier that bills Medicare Parts A and B. For further information, go to www.cms.hhs.gov/RAC/.

Medicaid

Medicaid, also run by CMS, is a health-benefit program designed for low-income, blind, or disabled patients; needy families; foster children; and children born with birth defects. Medicaid is a health cost assistance program, not an insurance program. The federal government provides funds to all 50 states to administer Medicaid (covering specified mandated services), and states add their own funds (for optional services in addition to the federally funded services). Every state has a program to assist with medical expenses for citizens who meet its qualifications. Such programs may have different names and slightly different rules, but they provide basically the same assistance. This assistance includes:

- Physician services
- Emergency services
- Laboratory services and x-rays
- Skilled nursing facility (SNF) care
- Early diagnostic screening and treatment for minors (those aged 21 and younger)
- Vaccines for children

Accepting Assignment. A physician who agrees to treat Medicaid patients also agrees to accept the established Medicaid payment for covered services. This agreement is called accepting assignment. It means that the physician will accept the amount of money that Medicaid will pay as payment in full for the Medicaid-covered service. If the physician's fee is higher than the Medicaid payment, the patient cannot be billed for the difference. The physician can bill the patient for services that Medicaid does not cover, however. It is important to note that, as a federally funded assistance program, Medicaid is known as the *payer of last resort.* This means that if a patient is covered by both a private insurance plan and Medicaid, the private plan must be billed before Medicaid. It is considered fraud to knowingly bill Medicaid if another insurance company provides medical coverage for a patient.

Medi/Medi. Older or disabled patients who have Medicare and who cannot pay the difference between the bill and the Medicare payment may qualify for Medicare and Medicaid. This type of coverage is known as Medi/Medi. In such cases, Medicare is the primary payer, and Medicaid is the secondary payer. The patient with Medi/Medi is never billed for a balance unless the service provided is a non-covered service, or Medicare/Medicaid states that the patient may be billed.

State Guidelines. Medicaid benefits can vary greatly from state to state. Eligibility for Medicaid is based on how much income the patient reported for the previous month. It is important to understand the Medicaid guidelines in your state so that your office's Medicaid reimbursement is prompt and trouble-free. Here are some suggestions:

- Do not submit a claim to Medicaid without verification of Medicaid membership and benefit eligibility. Doing so may constitute fraud. You should always contact Medicaid to verify eligibility.
- Ensure that the physician signs all claims, unless claims are submitted electronically, in which case the physician's signature is kept on file. Then send them to the state's Medicaid-approved contractor (which pays on behalf of the state) or to the state department that administers Medicaid (for example, the state department of social services or public health). Check the regulations with the state Medicaid office if you are unsure where to send the claim.

- Unless the patient has a medical emergency, Medicaid often requires authorization before services are performed. Authorization must be obtained from the state Medicaid office in advance.
- Check the time limit on claim submissions. It can be as short as 2 months or as long as 1 year. Verify deadlines with your local Medicaid office.
- Meet the deadlines. If a Medicaid claim is submitted after the time limit, the claim may be rejected. If a claim deadline is missed, it is considered provider error and the patient cannot be billed for the services.
- Treat Medicaid patients with the same professionalism and courtesy that you extend to other patients. Simply because a patient qualifies for Medicaid assistance does not mean that the patient is in any way inferior to those with private insurance.

TRICARE and CHAMPVA

The U.S. government provides health-care benefits to families of current military personnel, retired military personnel, and veterans through the TRICARE and CHAMPVA programs. Unless you work in a military-related facility, you will probably see TRICARE and CHAMPVA patients only for emergency services or for nonemergency care that a military base cannot provide.

TRICARE. Run by the Defense Department, **TRICARE** (formerly known as CHAMPUS or Civilian Health and Medical Program for Uniformed Sevices) is not a health insurance plan. Rather, it is a health-care benefit for families of uniformed personnel and retirees from the uniformed services, including the Army, Navy, Marines, Air Force, Coast Guard, Public Health Service, and National Oceanic and Atmospheric Administration (Figure 15-3). TRICARE offers families three choices of health-care benefits:

1. TRICARE Prime, a health maintenance organization
2. TRICARE Extra, a managed care network of health-care providers that families can use on a case-by-case basis without a required enrollment
3. TRICARE Standard, a fee-for-service plan

Another program, TRICARE for Life, is aimed at Medicare-eligible military retirees and Medicare-eligible family members. TRICARE for Life offers the opportunity to receive health care at a military treatment facility to individuals aged 65 and older who are eligible for both Medicare and TRICARE.

In the past, individuals became ineligible for TRICARE once they reached age 65, and they were required to enroll in Medicare to obtain any health-care coverage. Beneficiaries could still seek treatment at military treatment facilities, but only if space was available. Under TRICARE for Life, enrollees in TRICARE who are aged 65 and older can continue to obtain medical services at military hospitals and clinics as they did before they turned 65. TRICARE for Life acts as a secondary payer to Medicare; Medicare pays first, and the remaining out-of-pocket expenses are paid by TRICARE.

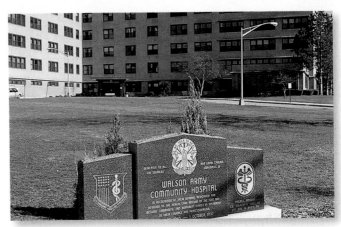

Figure 15-3. TRICARE covers health-care services for family members of military personnel and military retirees at facilities such as the military base hospital pictured here.

CHAMPVA. **CHAMPVA** (Civilian Health and Medical Program of the Veterans Administration) covers the expenses of the families (dependent spouses and children) of veterans with total, permanent, service-connected disabilities. It also covers surviving spouses and dependent children of veterans who died in the line of duty or as a result of service-connected disabilities.

TRICARE and CHAMPVA Eligibility. You must verify TRICARE eligibility. All TRICARE patients should have a valid identification card. To receive TRICARE benefits, eligible individuals must be enrolled in the Defense Enrollment Eligibility Reporting System (DEERS), a computer database.

Eligibility for CHAMPVA is determined by the nearest Veterans Affairs medical center. Contact this center if any questions arise. Patients can choose the doctor they wish after CHAMPVA eligibility is confirmed.

Under TRICARE and CHAMPVA, participating doctors have the option of deciding whether to accept patients on a case-by-case basis. Make sure you know the policy of the doctor or doctors in your office on this issue.

Blue Cross and Blue Shield

Many people think that Blue Cross and Blue Shield (BCBS) is one large corporation. Rather, it is a nationwide federation of nonprofit and for-profit service organizations that provide prepaid health-care services to BCBS subscribers. Each local organization operates under its own state laws, and specific plans for BCBS can vary greatly.

State Children's Health Plan

In 2009, the State Children's Health Plan (SCHIP) was reauthorized. The plan was originally enacted in 1997. The plan allows states to provide health coverage to uninsured children in families whose incomes are too high to qualify for Medicaid but too low to afford private insurance. States have raised eligibility levels to provide coverage to more families. Check your state's requirements for this plan through its website.

Workers' Compensation

Workers' compensation insurance covers employment-related accidents or diseases. Federal law requires employers to purchase and maintain a certain minimum amount of workers' compensation insurance for their employees. Workers' compensation laws vary from state to state. In most states, workers' compensation includes these benefits:

- Basic medical treatment.
- A weekly amount paid to the patient for a temporary disability. This amount compensates workers for loss of job income until they can return to work.
- A weekly or monthly sum paid to the patient for a permanent disability.
- Death benefits.
- Rehabilitation costs to restore an employee's ability to work again.

Not all medical practices accept workers' compensation cases. Every procedure or treatment that is deemed necessary must be approved in order for payment to be made. Make sure you know your office's policy. Records management of workers' compensation varies by state. If you see a patient privately and then she comes to you for a work-related illness or injury, be sure to keep the medical and financial records of the private care and the care related to the workers' compensation case separate. Because the employer and the insurer have contracted with the physician to provide care, they have the right to see any and all treatment and applicable financial records related to the workers' compensation claim without patient consent. It is up to the office to maintain the patient's confidentiality related to any care provided to her that is not related to the workers' compensation claim and keeping separate files makes it easier to do so.

Procedure 15-1 outlines the steps for verifying a patient's workers' compensation coverage.

PROCEDURE 15-1 — WORK // PRODUCT

Verifying Workers' Compensation Coverage

Procedure Goal: To verify workers' compensation coverage before accepting a patient

Materials: Telephone, paper, pencil

Method:

1. Call the patient's employer and verify that the accident or illness occurred on the employer's premises or at an employment-related work site.

2. Obtain the employer's approval to provide treatment. Be sure to write down the name and title of the person giving approval, as well as his phone number.

   Rationale
   Without approval, treatment costs may not be covered.

3. Ask the employer for the name of its workers' compensation insurance company. (Employers are required by law to carry such insurance. It is a good policy to notify your state labor department about any employer you encounter that does not have workers' compensation insurance, although you are not required to do so.)

   You may wish to remind the employer to report any workplace accidents or injuries that result in a workers' compensation claim to the state labor department within 24 hours of the incident.

   Rationale
   Without this form on file, the claims may not be approved.

4. Contact the insurance company and verify that the employer does indeed have a policy with the company and that the policy is in good standing.

   Rationale
   The insurance company will not pay for services without a valid policy.

5. Obtain a claim number for the case from the insurance company. This claim number is used on all bills and paperwork.

   Rationale
   All invoices must include the claim number in order for the practice to receive payment.

6. At the time the patient starts treatment, create a patient record. If the patient is already one of the practice's regular patients, create separate medical and financial records for the workers' compensation case.

   Rationale
   This is the legal procedure to protect the patient confidentiality with regard to private medical care. Confidentiality does not exist with regard to care related workers' compensation cases.

The Claims Process: An Overview

From the time the patient enters a doctor's office until the time the insurer pays the practice for that office visit and associated services, several steps are carried out. In brief, the doctor's office performs the following services:

- Obtains patient information
- Delivers services to the patient and determines the diagnosis and fee (Table 15-2)
- Records charges and codes, records payment from the patient, and prepares health-care claims
- Reviews the insurer's processing of the claim, remittance advice, and payment

Most medical assistants use a medical billing program to support administrative tasks such as:

- Gathering and recording patient information
- Verifying patients' insurance coverage
- Recording procedures and services performed
- Records applicable diagnosis and codes for each procedure performed
- Filing insurance claims and billing patients
- Reviewing and recording payments

Billing programs streamline the important process of creating and following up on health-care claims sent to payers and bills sent to patients. For example, a large medical practice with a group of providers and thousands of patients may receive a phone call from a patient who wants to know the amount owed on an account. With a billing program, the medical assistant can key the first few letters of the patient's last name and the patient's account data will appear on the screen. The outstanding balance can then be communicated to the patient.

TABLE 15-2 Common Abbreviations Used in Claims Form Processing

Abbreviations Related to Diagnosis		Abbreviations Related to Procedures	
AHF	Acute heart failure	AKA	Above-knee amputation
Ca	Cancer	BKA	Below-knee amputation
CC	Chief complaint	Bx	Biopsy
CHF	Congestive heart failure	CABG	Coronary artery bypass graft
CO	Complains of	CT	Computed tomography
COPD	Chronic obstructive pulmonary disease	CXR	Chest x-ray
CVA	Cerebrovascular accident	D & C	Dilation and curettage
DJD	Degenerative joint disease	ERCP	Endoscopic retrograde cholangiopancretography
DVT	Deep vein thrombosis	I & D	Incision and drainage
Dx	Diagnosis	IF	Internal fixation
ESRD	End-stage renal disease	IVP	Intravenous pyelogram
ESRF	End-stage renal failure	MRI	Magnetic resonance imaging
FAS	Fetal alcohol syndrome	PE	Physical examination
FBD	Fibrocystic breast disease	PET	Positron emission tomography
FUO	Fever of unknown origin	PFT	Pulmonary function test
Fx	Fracture	PTCA	Percutaneous transluminal coronary angioplasty
GI	Gastrointestinal	T & A	Tonsillectomy and adenoidectomy
HA	Headache		
HPV	Human papillomavirus	TKA	Total knee arthroplasty
Hx	History	Tx	Treatment
RO	Rule out		
SOM	Serous otitis media		

Billing programs are also used to exchange health information about the practice's patients with health plans. Using **electronic data interchange (EDI),** similar to the technology behind ATMs, information is sent quickly and securely.

 ## Obtaining Patient Information

You will need certain information to be able to complete insurance claims and bill correctly for the patients of the medical practice where you work. This information is usually completed on a patient registration form, as shown in Chapter 9.

Basic Facts. When the patient first arrives, obtain or verify the following personal information:

- Name of patient (be sure to get the correct spelling of the patient's legal name)
- Current home address
- Current home telephone number
- Date of birth (month, day, and the four digits of the year)
- Social Security number
- Next of kin or person to contact in case of an emergency

Obtain the following insurance information:

- Current employer (may be more than one)
- Employer address and telephone number
- Insurance carrier and effective date of coverage
- Insurance group plan number
- Insurance identification number
- Name of subscriber or insured

Depending on state law, obtain the following release signatures:

- Patient's signature on a form authorizing release of information to the insurance carrier
- Patient's signature on a form for assignment of benefits

Eligibility for Services. After you obtain personal and insurance information and release signatures from the patient, scan or copy the patient's insurance card, front and back, to include in the patient's financial record. Also verify the effective date of insurance coverage because services performed before this date may be excluded from claims. To reduce possible payment problems, remind the patient before a service is performed if it might not be covered. Many offices now have a patient sign a waiver of liability form, giving the reason it is believed that a procedure will not be covered. By signing the form, the patient agrees to accept responsibility for payment should the insurer not pay for the service.

Coordination of Benefits. Coordination of benefits clauses are legal clauses in insurance policies that prevent duplication of payment. These clauses restrict payment by insurance companies to no more than 100% of the cost of covered benefits. In many families, husband and wife are both wage earners. They and their children are frequently eligible for health insurance benefits through both employers' plans. In such cases the two insurance companies coordinate their payments to pay up to 100% of a procedure's cost. A payment of 100% includes the policyholder's deductible and copayment. The *primary*, or main, plan is the policy that pays benefits first. Then the *secondary*, or supplemental, plan pays the deductible and copayment. A policyholder's primary plan is always his employer group health plan. If both a husband and wife have insurance through their employers, the husband's plan is his primary plan and the wife's insurance plan is her primary plan. To determine which plan is the primary for dependents, in many states, the **birthday rule** is followed. It states that the insurance policy of the policyholder whose birthday comes first in the calendar year is the primary payer for all dependents.

For example, if a husband's birthday is July 14 and his wife's birthday is June 11, following the birthday rule, the wife's insurance plan is the primary payer for their children and the husband's is the secondary payer. If a husband and wife were born on the same day, the policy that has been in effect the longest is the primary payer.

The birthday rule is applied in most states in which dependents are covered by two or more medical plans. Not all states are covered by the birthday rule, so be sure to check with your state's insurance commission whenever you are in doubt. Table 15-3 describes widely used coverage guidelines.

Delivering Services to the Patient

To ensure accuracy in claims processing, any services delivered to the patient in the office by the physician or other members of the health-care team must be entered into the patient record. Referrals to outside physicians or specialists must be entered into the record.

Physician's Services. The physician who examines the patient notes the patient's symptoms in the medical record. The physician also notes a diagnosis and treatment plan (including prescribed medications) and specifies if and when the patient should return for a follow-up visit. After completing the visit with the patient, the physician writes the diagnosis, treatment, and sometimes the fee on a charge slip and instructs the patient to give you the charge slip before leaving.

Medical Coding. The next step is to translate the medical terminology on the charge slip from precise descriptions of medical services into procedural and diagnostic codes on the health-care claim. Today, most offices use charge slips (encounter forms) with the appropriate charge and procedure codes printed next to the descriptions. It is, however, critical to verify that the procedure checked off on the form was actually completed by comparing the charge slip to the medical record. This necessary step ensures that the patient is not inadvertently charged for a procedure that did not take place. This topic is covered in depth in Chapter 16.

TABLE 15-3 Guidelines for Determining Primary Coverage

- If the patient has only one policy, it is primary.

- If the patient has coverage under two plans, the plan covering the employee for the longest period of time is primary. However, if an active employee has a plan with the present employer and is still covered by a former employer's plan as a retiree or a laid-off employee, the current employer's plan is primary.

- If the patient is also covered as a dependent under another insurance policy, the patient's plan is primary.

- If an employed patient has coverage under the employer's plan and additional coverage under a government-sponsored plan, the employer's plan is primary. An example of this is a patient enrolled in a PPO through employment who is also on Medicare.

- If a retired patient is covered by the plan of the spouse's employer and the spouse is still employed, the spouse's plan is primary, even if the retired person has Medicare.

- If the patient is a dependent child covered by both parents' plans and the parents are not separated or divorced (or have joint custody of the child), the primary plan is determined by which parent has the first birth date in the calendar year (the birthday rule).

- If two or more plans cover the dependent children of separated or divorced parents who do not have joint custody of their children, the children's primary plan is determined in this order:

  1. The plan of the custodial parent
  2. The plan of the spouse of the custodial parent (if the parent has remarried)
  3. The plan of the parent without custody

Referrals to Other Services. You may be asked to secure authorization from the insurance company for additional procedures. If so, contact the insurance company to explain the procedures and obtain approval and an authorization number. Enter this referral number in the billing program for inclusion in claims related to this procedure.

Frequently you will be asked to arrange an appointment for the referred services, particularly if the physician believes they are urgently needed. For example, a physician may send a patient for a specialist's evaluation or x-ray on the same day the patient visits your office.

Preparing the Health-Care Claim

Everyone who receives services from a doctor in the practice where you work is responsible for paying the practice for those services. When the patient brings you the charge slip from the doctor, you may perform one or more of the following procedures, depending on the policy of your practice:

- Prepare and transmit a health-care claim on behalf of the patient directly to the insurance company.

- Accept payment from the patient for the full amount. The patient will submit a claim to the insurance carrier for reimbursement.

- Accept an insurance copayment.

Filing the Insurance Claim. If you are going to transmit the claim directly to the payer, you will prepare an insurance claim, often electronically. After the physician reviews the claim, you will transmit the claim to the insurance carrier for payment. The billing program will create a log of transmitted claims, or a register such as the one shown in Figure 15-4 may be maintained.

Patient's Name	Insurance Company	Claim Filed		Payment Received		Difference (owed by patient)
		Date	Amount	Date	Amount	

Figure 15-4. After submitting a claim to an insurer, track each claim in an insurance claim register, such as the one pictured here.

Time Limits. Claims must be filed in a timely manner. Time limits for filing claims vary from company to company. For example, some insurers will not pay a claim unless it is filed within 8 weeks of the date of service, others will allow up to a year for claim submission.

Medicare states that for services rendered from January 1 to September 30, claims must be filed by December 31 of the following year; for services rendered from October 1 through December 31, claims must be filed no later than December 31 of the second year following the service. For example, if a patient was seen on September 15, 2010, you would have until December 31, 2011, to file the claim. If the patient was seen on November 8, 2010, you would have until December 31, 2012, to submit that claim.

Medicaid states that claims must be filed no later than 1 year from the date of service. The time frame for refiling rejected claims varies by state. In Indiana (which allows one year from the date of rejection for resubmission of claims), for example, if you filed a claim for a service performed on January 2, 2009, and the claim was rejected on May 31, 2009, you would have until May 31, 2010, to refile the claim. Other states may allow only 60–90 days for re-filing a claim, so it is important to know your individual state rules and regulations.

Although Medicare and Medicaid allow quite a long time for claims to be filed, it is poor business practice to wait so long. In the typical medical practice, claims are transmitted within a few business days after the date of service. Many large practices file claims every day or twice a week.

Insurer's Processing and Payment

Your transmitted claim for payment will undergo a number of reviews by the insurer. Currently, much of the review process occurs electronically.

Review for Medical Necessity. The insurance carrier reviews each claim to determine whether the diagnosis and accompanying treatment are compatible and whether the treatment is medically necessary, as explained in Chapter 16.

Review for Allowable Benefits. The claims department also compares the fees the doctor charges with the benefits provided by the patient's health insurance policy. This review determines the amount of deductible or coinsurance the patient owes. This amount—that is, what the patient owes—is called subscriber liability.

Payment and Remittance Advice. After reviewing the claim, the insurer pays a benefit, either to the subscriber (patient) or to the practice, depending on what recipient the claim requested. With the payment, the insurer sends a **remittance advice (RA),** formerly called an **explanation of benefits (EOB).** A patient who receives the payment receives an RA containing only his information and the practice receives a practice RA that typically contains information for multiple patients at one time. The RA or the EOB explains the medical claim. For each

service submitted to an insurer, the RA or EOB form gives the following information:

- Name of the insured and identification number
- Name of the beneficiary
- Claim number
- Date, place, and type of service (coded)
- Amount billed by the practice
- Amount allowed (according to the subscriber's policy)
- Amount of subscriber liability (coinsurance, copayment, deductible, or noncovered services)
- Amount paid and included in the current payment
- A notation of any services not covered and an explanation of why they were not covered (for example, many insurance plans do not cover a woman's annual gynecologic examination and only a certain dollar amount of well-baby visits for infants)

Reviewing the Insurer's RA and Payment

Verify all information on the RA, line by line, using your records for each patient represented on the RA. In a large practice, you will frequently receive payment and an RA for multiple patients at one time. An example of a Medicare RA, which is called a Medicare Remittance Notice, is shown in Figure 15-5.

If all numbers on the RA agree with your records, you can make the appropriate entries in the insurance follow-up log for claims paid. In a small practice, the insurance follow-up log is used to track filed claims, using such information as patient name, date the claim was filed, services the claim reflects, notations about the results of the claim, and any balance due from the patient. Larger practices tend to track claims in the computer billing program in a file called, for example, "Unpaid Claims." If all the numbers do not agree, you will need to trace the claim with the insurance company.

When a claim is rejected, the RA states the reason. You will need to review the claim, examining all procedural and diagnosis codes for accuracy and comparing the claim with the patient's insurance information. You will probably need to contact the insurance company by telephone to find out how to resolve the claim problem.

Fee Schedules and Charges

Physicians establish a list of their usual fees for the procedures and services they frequently perform. The usual fees are those that they charge to most of their patients most of the time under typical conditions. These fees are listed on the office's **fee schedule.**

Medicare Payment System: RBRVS

Third-party payers also set the fees they are willing to pay providers, and often these fees are less than the physician's fee schedule. Most payers base their fees on the amounts

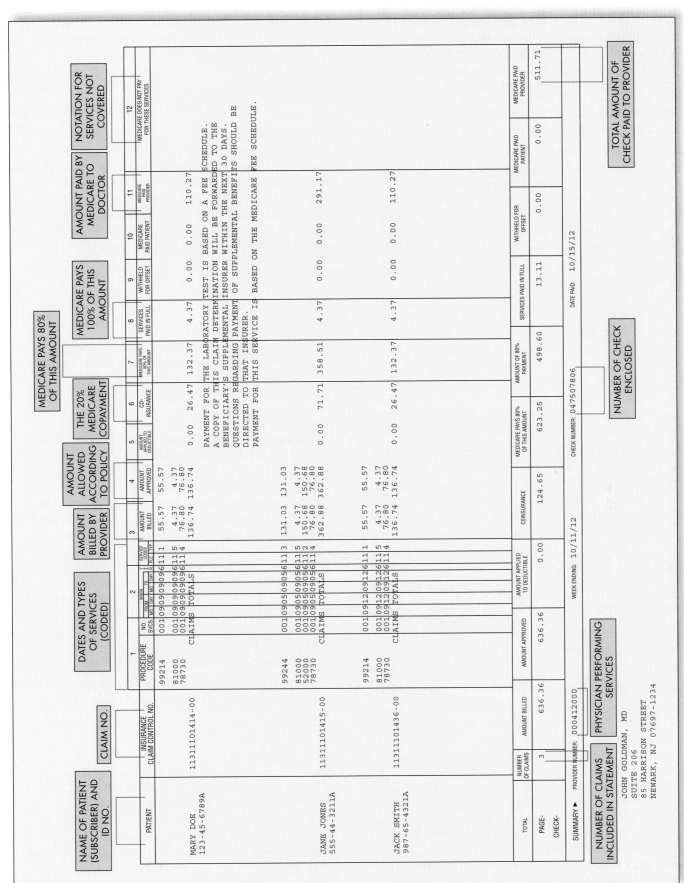

Figure 15-5. The insurer sends the remittance advice form to the medical practice.

that Medicare allows because the Medicare method of fee setting takes into account important factors other than only the usual fees.

The payment system used by Medicare is called the **resource-based relative value scale (RBRVS).** The RBRVS establishes the relative value units for services, replacing providers' consensus on fees (the "usual" or historical charges) with amounts based on resources (what each service really costs to provide).

There are three parts to an RBRVS fee, of which the formula is RVU $\times$ GAF $\times$ CF. Listed below is an explanation for each part of this formula:

1. The nationally uniform relative value unit (RVU). The relative value of a procedure is based on three cost elements: the physician's work, the practice cost (overhead), and the cost of malpractice insurance. For example, the relative value unit for a simple office visit, such as to administer a flu shot, is much lower than the relative value for a complicated encounter such as planning the treatment of uncontrolled diabetes in a patient.

2. A geographic adjustment factor (GAF). A geographic adjustment factor is used to adjust each relative value to reflect a geographical area's relative costs, such as office rents.

3. A nationally uniform conversion factor (CF). A uniform conversion factor is a dollar amount used to multiply the relative values to produce a payment amount. It is used by Medicare to make adjustments according to changes in the cost-of-living index.

When RBRVS fees are used, providers receive considerably lower payments than when usual fees are used. Each part of the RBRVS—the relative values, the geographic adjustment, and the conversion factor—is updated each year by CMS. The year's Medicare fee schedule (MFS) is published by CMS in the *Federal Register*.

Payment Methods

Most third-party payers use one of three methods for reimbursing physicians:

1. Allowed charges
2. Contracted fee schedule
3. Capitation

Allowed Charges. Many payers set an **allowed charge** for each procedure or service. This amount is the most the payer will pay any provider for that work. The term *allowed charge* has many equivalent terms, including *maximum allowable fee, maximum charge, allowed amount, allowed fee,* or *allowable charge.*

The physician's usual charge is often greater than a plan's allowed charge. If the physician participates in the plan, only the allowed charge will be the basis for the payment by the payer. The plan's rules govern whether the provider is permitted to bill a patient for the part of a usual charge that the payer does not cover. Billing a patient for the difference between a higher usual fee and a lower allowed charge is called **balance billing.** Under most contracts, participating providers may not bill the patient for the difference. Instead, the provider must write off the difference, meaning that the amount of the difference is subtracted from the patient's bill and never collected. The common term for this write-off is *adjustment.*

For example, Medicare-participating providers may not receive an amount greater than the Medicare-allowed charge that is based on the Medicare fee schedule. The Original Medicare Plan is responsible for paying 80% of this allowed charge (after patients have met their annual deductible). Patients are responsible for the other 20%.

Here is an example of a Medicare billing. A Medicare-participating provider reports a usual charge of $200 for a service, and the Medicare-allowed charge is $84. The provider must write off the difference between the two charges. The patient is responsible for 20% of the allowed charge, not of the provider's usual charge:

Provider's usual fee:	$200.00
Medicare-allowed charge:	$84.00
Medicare pays 80%	$67.20
Patient pays 20%	$16.80

The total that the provider can collect is $84. The provider must write off the difference between the usual fee and the allowed charge, or $116.00 in this example. It is important to remember that in this example, it is assumed that the patient has paid her deductible for the year.

Contracted Fee Schedule. Some payers, particularly PPOs, establish fixed fee schedules with their participating physicians. The terms of the plan determine what percentage of the charges, if any, the patient owes and what percentage the payer covers. Participating providers can typically bill patients their usual charges for procedures and services that are not covered by the plan.

Capitation. The fixed prepayment for each plan member in capitation contracts is determined by the managed care plan that initiates contracts with providers. The plan's contract with the provider lists the services and procedures that are covered by the cap rate. For example, a typical contract with a primary care provider might include the following services:

- Preventive care, including well-child care, adult physical exams, gynecological exams, eye exams, and hearing exams
- Counseling and telephone calls
- Office visits
- Medical care, including medical care services such as therapeutic injections and immunizations, allergy immunotherapy, electrocardiograms, and pulmonary function tests
- The local treatment of first-degree burns, the application of dressings, suture removal, the excision of small skin lesions, the removal of foreign bodies or cerumen from the external ear

These services are covered in the per-member charge for each plan member who selects the PCP. Noncovered services can be billed to patients using the physician's usual rate. Plans often require the provider to notify the patient in advance that a service is not covered and to state the fee for which the patient will be responsible.

Calculating Patient Charges

The patients of medical practices have a variety of health plans, so they have different financial responsibilities. In addition to premiums, patients may be obligated to pay deductibles, copayments, coinsurance, excluded and over-limit services, and balance billing (only if allowed by the insurance contract between the provider and the insurance plan).

All payers require patients to pay for excluded (non-covered) services. Physicians generally can charge their usual fees for these services. Likewise, in managed care plans that set limits on the annual usage (or other period) of covered services, patients are responsible for usage beyond the allowed number. For example, if one preventive physical examination is permitted annually, additional preventive examinations are paid for by the patient.

Communications with Patients About Charges

When patients have office visits with a physician who participates in the plan under which they have coverage, such as a Medicare-participating (PAR) provider, they generally sign an **assignment of benefits** statement. When this occurs, the provider agrees to prepare health-care claims for patients, to receive payments directly from the payers, and to accept a payer's allowed charge. Patients are billed for charges that payers deny or do not pay. When patients have encounters with nonparticipating (nonPAR) providers, the procedure is usually different. To avoid the difficulty of collecting payments at a later date from a patient, practices may require that the patient either (1) assigns benefits or (2) pays in full at the time of services.

Many times patients want to know what their bills will be. For example, suppose a patient receives a bill for $100 from your practice. She calls to say that she has paid her deductible for the year, so her insurance company should have paid 80% of the bill. You call the patient's insurance company and learn that she still has to pay $100 to meet her deductible. If she pays the $100 bill in full, her deductible will then be met. You would have to explain these facts to the patient.

To estimate patients' bills, you should check with the payer to find out:

- The patient's deductible amount and whether it has been paid in full, the covered benefits, and coinsurance or other patient financial obligations
- The payer's allowed charges for the services that the provider anticipates providing

If the patient's request comes after the appointment, the encounter form can be used to tell the payer what procedures are going to be reported on the patient's claim to determine the likely payer reimbursement.

Patients should always be reminded of their financial obligations under their plans, including claim denials, according to practice procedures. The practice's financial policy regarding payment for services is usually either displayed on the wall of the reception area or included in a new patient information packet. The policy should explain what is required of the patient and when payment is due. For example, the policy may state the following:

- For unassigned claims: Payment for the physician's services is expected at the end of your appointment, unless you have made other arrangements with our practice manager.
- For assigned claims: After your insurance claim is processed by your insurance company, you will be billed for any amount you owe. You are responsible for any part of the charges that are denied or not paid by the carrier. All patient accounts are due within 30 days of the date of the invoice you receive.
- For managed care members: Copayments must be paid before patients leave the office.

It is also a good practice to notify patients in advance of the probable cost of procedures that are not going to be covered by their plan. For example, many private plans as well as Medicare do not pay for most preventive services, such as annual physical examinations. Many patients, however, consider preventive services a good idea and are willing to pay for them. Patients should be asked to agree in writing to pay for any noncovered services. A letter of agreement, also known as a waiver of liability, should also specify why the service will not be covered and the cost of the procedure.

The Advance Beneficiary Notice of Noncoverage (ABN) is a notice given to beneficiaries in the Original Medicare Plan to convey that Medicare is not likely to provide coverage in a specific case. "Notifiers" include physicians, providers (including institutional providers like outpatient hospitals), practitioners, and suppliers paid under Part B (including independent laboratories), as well as hospice providers and religious nonmedical health care institutions (RNHCIs) paid exclusively under Part A. As of March 1, 2009, the ABN-G (general) and ABN-L(laboratory) were invalid; and notifiers began using the revised Advance Beneficiary Notice of Noncoverage (CMS-R-131). See Figure 15-6.

The ABN must be verbally reviewed with the beneficiary or his or her representative, and any questions raised during that review must be answered before it is signed. The ABN must be delivered far enough in advance that the beneficiary or representative has time to consider the options and make an informed choice. Employees or subcontractors of the notifier may deliver the ABN. ABNs are never required in emergency or urgent care situations. Once all blanks are completed and the form is signed, a copy is given to the beneficiary or representative. In all cases, the notifier must retain the original notice on file.

(A) Notifier(s):

(B) Patient Name: _____ *(C)* Identification Number: _____

ADVANCE BENEFICIARY NOTICE OF NONCOVERAGE (ABN)

<u>NOTE</u>: If Medicare doesn't pay for *(D)*_____ below, you may have to pay.

Medicare does not pay for everything, even some care that you or your health care provider have good reason to think you need. We expect Medicare may not pay for the *(D)*_____ below.

*(D)*_____	*(E)* Reason Medicare May Not Pay:	*(F)* Estimated Cost:

WHAT YOU NEED TO DO NOW:

- Read this notice, so you can make an informed decision about your care.
- Ask us any questions that you may have after you finish reading.
- Choose an option below about whether to receive the *(D)*_____ listed above.
    - **Note:** If you choose Option 1 or 2, we may help you to use any other insurance that you might have, but Medicare cannot require us to do this.

(G) OPTIONS: **Check only one box. We cannot choose a box for you.**
❑ **OPTION 1.** I want the *(D)*_____ listed above. You may ask to be paid now, but I also want Medicare billed for an official decision on payment, which is sent to me on a Medicare Summary Notice (MSN). I understand that if Medicare doesn't pay, I am responsible for payment, but **I can appeal to Medicare** by following the directions on the MSN. If Medicare does pay, you will refund any payments I made to you, less co-pays or deductibles.
❑ **OPTION 2.** I want the *(D)*_____ listed above, but do not bill Medicare. You may ask to be paid now as I am responsible for payment. **I cannot appeal if Medicare is not billed**.
❑ **OPTION 3.** I don't want the *(D)*_____ listed above. I understand with this choice I am **not** responsible for payment, and **I cannot appeal to see if Medicare would pay.**

(H) **Additional Information:**

This notice gives our opinion, not an official Medicare decision. If you have other questions on this notice or Medicare billing, call **1-800-MEDICARE** (1-800-633-4227/**TTY**: 1-877-486-2048).

Signing below means that you have received and understand this notice. You also receive a copy.

(I) **Signature:**	*(J)* **Date:**

According to the Paperwork Reduction Act of 1995, no persons are required to respond to a collection of information unless it displays a valid OMB control number. The valid OMB control number for this information collection is 0938-0566. The time required to complete this information collection is estimated to average 7 minutes per response, including the time to review instructions, search existing data resources, gather the data needed, and complete and review the information collection. If you have comments concerning the accuracy of the time estimate or suggestions for improving this form, please write to: CMS, 7500 Security Boulevard, Attn: PRA Reports Clearance Officer, Baltimore, Maryland 21244-1850.

Form CMS-R-131 (03/08)   Form Approved OMB No. 0938-0566

Figure 15-6. Advance Beneficiary Notice of Noncoverage.
Source: Centers for Medicare and Medicaid Services.

Preparing and Transmitting Health-Care Claims

Health-care claims are a critical communication between medical offices and payers on behalf of patients. Processing claims is a major task in most offices, and the numbers can be huge. For example, a 40-physician group practice with 55,000 patients served annually typically processes 1000 claims daily!

HIPAA Claims and Paper Claims

Two types of claims are in use: (1) the predominant HIPAA electronic claim transaction and (2) the older CMS-1500 paper form. The electronic claim transaction is the HIPAA Health-Care Claim or Equivalent Encounter Information; it is commonly referred to as the "HIPAA claim." Its official name is **X12 837 Health Care Claim.** The paper format is the "universal claim" known as the CMS-1500 claim form (formerly, the HCFA-1500).

As of October 2003, Medicare mandated the X12 837 transaction for all Medicare claims except those from very small practices. Third-party payers may continue to accept paper transactions. But practices that elect to use paper claims must have two versions of their medical billing software: one to capture the necessary data elements for HIPAA-compliant electronic Medicare claims and another version to generate CMS-1500 claims. Also, under HIPAA regulations, only medical offices that do not handle any other HIPAA-related transactions can still use paper claims. It is anticipated that eventually, for cost reasons, all payers will require electronic submissions and add this provision to their contracts with providers.

Preparing HIPAA Claims. The information entered on claims is called data elements. Many elements, such as the patient's personal and insurance information, are entered in the billing program before patients' appointments, based on forms patients fill out and on communications with payers. After patients' office visits, their claims are completed when the medical assistant enters the billing transactions—the services, charges, and payments—as detailed on the superbill (encounter form). The medical assistant then instructs the software to prepare claims for editing and transmission.

Follow these tips when entering data in medical billing programs:

- Enter data in all capital letters
- Do not use prefixes for people's names, such as Mr., Ms., or Dr.
- Unless required by a particular insurance carrier, do not use special characters such as hyphens, commas, or apostrophes
- Use only valid data in all fields; avoid words such as "same"

The X12 837 transaction requires many data elements, and all must be correct. Most billing programs or claim transmission programs automatically reformat data such as dates into the correct formats. These data elements are reported in five major sections:

1. Provider
2. Subscriber (the insured or policyholder)
3. Patient (who may be the subscriber or another person) and payer
4. Claim details
5. Services

Not all data elements are required. Some are considered situational and are required only when a certain condition applies. When it does apply, then that data element also becomes required. For example, if a claim involves pregnancy, the date of the last menstrual period is required. If the claim does not involve pregnancy, that date should not be reported.

Before the HIPAA mandate for standard transactions, some payers required additional records, such as their own information sheet, when providers billed them. Some payers also used their own coding systems. The HIPAA Electronic Health Care Transactions and Code Sets (TCS) mandate means that health plans are required to accept the standard claim submitted electronically.

Other standard transactions also support the claim process, such as advising the office of claim status, payment, and other key information. These transactions standards apply to the treatment, payment, and operations information that is exchanged between medical offices and health plans. Each electronic transaction has both a title and a number. Each number begins with X12, which is the number of the EDI format, followed by a unique number that stands for the transaction. Here are some examples of titles and numbers that medical assistants may encounter while processing X12 837 health-care claims:

Number	Title
X12 276/277	Claim status inquiry and response
X12 270/271	Eligibility inquiry and response
X12 278	Referral authorization inquiry and response
X12 835	Payment and remittance advice
X12 820	Health plan premium payments
X12 834	Enrollment in and withdrawal from a health plan

Preparing Paper Claims. The process for preparing paper claims is similar to the X12 837 claim. Usually, the medical billing program is updated with information about the patient's office visit. Then the program is instructed to print the data on a CMS-1500 paper form, shown in Figure 15-7. This claim may be mailed or faxed to a third-party payer.

Because of the HIPAA mandate, the paper claim is not as widely used as previously; however, the information it contains is essentially very similar to the X12 837. For this reason, you should study Procedure 15-2, Completing the CMS-1500 Claim Form. This exercise will give

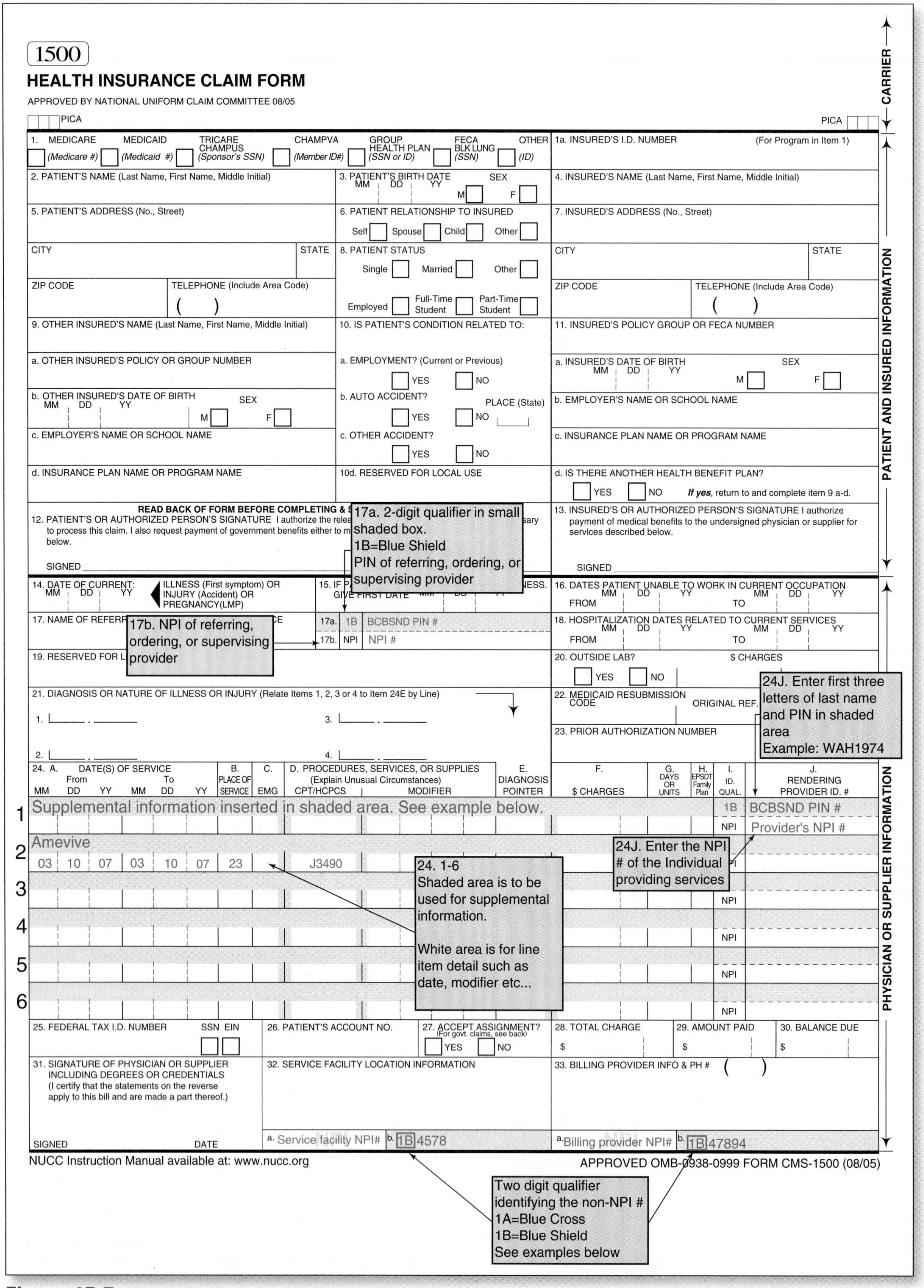

1500

HEALTH INSURANCE CLAIM FORM

APPROVED BY NATIONAL UNIFORM CLAIM COMMITTEE 08/05

PICA | PICA

CARRIER

1. MEDICARE (Medicare #) | MEDICAID (Medicaid #) | TRICARE CHAMPUS (Sponsor's SSN) | CHAMPVA (Member ID#) | GROUP HEALTH PLAN (SSN or ID) | FECA BLK LUNG (SSN) | OTHER (ID)

1a. INSURED'S I.D. NUMBER (For Program in Item 1)

2. PATIENT'S NAME (Last Name, First Name, Middle Initial)

3. PATIENT'S BIRTH DATE MM DD YY SEX M F

4. INSURED'S NAME (Last Name, First Name, Middle Initial)

5. PATIENT'S ADDRESS (No., Street)

6. PATIENT RELATIONSHIP TO INSURED Self Spouse Child Other

7. INSURED'S ADDRESS (No., Street)

CITY STATE

8. PATIENT STATUS Single Married Other

CITY STATE

ZIP CODE TELEPHONE (Include Area Code) ( )

Employed Full-Time Student Part-Time Student

ZIP CODE TELEPHONE (Include Area Code) ( )

9. OTHER INSURED'S NAME (Last Name, First Name, Middle Initial)

10. IS PATIENT'S CONDITION RELATED TO:

11. INSURED'S POLICY GROUP OR FECA NUMBER

a. OTHER INSURED'S POLICY OR GROUP NUMBER

a. EMPLOYMENT? (Current or Previous) YES NO

a. INSURED'S DATE OF BIRTH MM DD YY SEX M F

b. OTHER INSURED'S DATE OF BIRTH MM DD YY SEX M F

b. AUTO ACCIDENT? YES NO PLACE (State)

b. EMPLOYER'S NAME OR SCHOOL NAME

c. EMPLOYER'S NAME OR SCHOOL NAME

c. OTHER ACCIDENT? YES NO

c. INSURANCE PLAN NAME OR PROGRAM NAME

d. INSURANCE PLAN NAME OR PROGRAM NAME

10d. RESERVED FOR LOCAL USE

d. IS THERE ANOTHER HEALTH BENEFIT PLAN? YES NO *If yes*, return to and complete item 9 a-d.

READ BACK OF FORM BEFORE COMPLETING & S...

12. PATIENT'S OR AUTHORIZED PERSON'S SIGNATURE I authorize the relea... to process this claim. I also request payment of government benefits either to m... below.

SIGNED

13. INSURED'S OR AUTHORIZED PERSON'S SIGNATURE I authorize payment of medical benefits to the undersigned physician or supplier for services described below.

SIGNED

PATIENT AND INSURED INFORMATION

17a. 2-digit qualifier in small shaded box.
1B=Blue Shield
PIN of referring, ordering, or supervising provider

14. DATE OF CURRENT: MM DD YY ILLNESS (First symptom) OR INJURY (Accident) OR PREGNANCY(LMP)

15. IF P... GIVE FIRST DATE ...NESS.

16. DATES PATIENT UNABLE TO WORK IN CURRENT OCCUPATION FROM MM DD YY TO MM DD YY

17. NAME OF REFERR...

17b. NPI of referring, ordering, or supervising provider

17a. 1B BCBSND PIN #

17b. NPI NPI #

18. HOSPITALIZATION DATES RELATED TO CURRENT SERVICES FROM MM DD YY TO MM DD YY

19. RESERVED FOR L...

20. OUTSIDE LAB? YES NO $ CHARGES

24J. Enter first three letters of last name and PIN in shaded area
Example: WAH1974

21. DIAGNOSIS OR NATURE OF ILLNESS OR INJURY (Relate Items 1, 2, 3 or 4 to Item 24E by Line)

1. ___ . ___ 3. ___ . ___

2. ___ . ___ 4. ___ . ___

22. MEDICAID RESUBMISSION CODE ORIGINAL REF. NO.

23. PRIOR AUTHORIZATION NUMBER

	24. A. DATE(S) OF SERVICE From MM DD YY	To MM DD YY	B. PLACE OF SERVICE	C. EMG	D. PROCEDURES, SERVICES, OR SUPPLIES (Explain Unusual Circumstances) CPT/HCPCS MODIFIER	E. DIAGNOSIS POINTER	F. $ CHARGES	G. DAYS OR UNITS	H. EPSDT Family Plan	I. ID. QUAL.	J. RENDERING PROVIDER ID. #
1	Supplemental information inserted in shaded area. See example below.									1B	BCBSND PIN #
										NPI	Provider's NPI #
2	Amevive										
	03 10 07	03 10 07	23		J3490					NPI	
3										NPI	
4										NPI	
5										NPI	
6										NPI	

24J. Enter the NPI # of the Individual providing services

24. 1-6
Shaded area is to be used for supplemental information.

White area is for line item detail such as date, modifier etc...

PHYSICIAN OR SUPPLIER INFORMATION

25. FEDERAL TAX I.D. NUMBER SSN EIN

26. PATIENT'S ACCOUNT NO.

27. ACCEPT ASSIGNMENT? (For govt. claims, see back) YES NO

28. TOTAL CHARGE $

29. AMOUNT PAID $

30. BALANCE DUE $

31. SIGNATURE OF PHYSICIAN OR SUPPLIER INCLUDING DEGREES OR CREDENTIALS (I certify that the statements on the reverse apply to this bill and are made a part thereof.)

SIGNED DATE

32. SERVICE FACILITY LOCATION INFORMATION

a. Service facility NPI# b. 1B 4578

33. BILLING PROVIDER INFO & PH # ( )

a. Billing provider NPI# b. 1B 47894

NUCC Instruction Manual available at: www.nucc.org

APPROVED OMB-0938-0999 FORM CMS-1500 (08/05)

Two digit qualifier identifying the non-NPI #
1A=Blue Cross
1B=Blue Shield
See examples below

Figure 15-7. The CMS-1500 is a paper health insurance claim form.

Completing the CMS-1500 Claim Form

Procedure Goal: To complete the CMS-1500 claim form correctly

Materials: Patient record, CMS-1500 form, typewriter or computer, patient ledger card or charge slip

Method:

Note: The numbers below correspond to the numbered fields on the CMS-1500.

Patient Information Section

1. Place an *X* in the appropriate insurance box.

   ### Rationale
   Check marks are not recognized by computer programs.

1a. Enter the insured's insurance identification number as it appears on the insurance card.

   ### Rationale
   If the insurance identification number is incorrect, payment will be denied.

2. Enter the patient's name in this order: last name, first name, middle initial (if any).

3. Enter the patient's birth date using two digits each for the month and day. For example, for a patient born on February 9, 1954, enter 02-09-1954. Indicate the sex of the patient: male or female.

4. If the insured and the patient are the same person, enter SAME. If not, enter the policyholder's name. For TRICARE claims, enter the sponsor's (service person's) full name. For Medicare, leave blank.

5. Enter the patient's mailing address, city, state, and zip code.

6. Enter the patient's relationship to the insured. If they are the same, mark SELF. For TRICARE, enter the patient's relationship to the sponsor. For Medicare, leave blank.

7. Enter the insured's mailing address, city, state, zip code, and telephone number. If this address is the same as the patient's, enter SAME. For Medicare, leave blank.

8. Indicate the patient's marital, employment, and student status by placing an *X* in the boxes.

9. Enter the last name, first name, and middle initial of any other insured person whose policy might cover the patient. If the claim is for Medicare and the patient has a Medigap policy, enter the patient's name again. Keep in mind that block 9 is for secondary insurance coverage; block 11 is for the patient's primary insurance plan.

9a. Enter the policy or group number for the other insured person. If this is a Medigap policy, enter MEDIGAP before the policy number. If Medicare, leave blank.

9b. Enter the date of birth and sex of the other insured person (field 9).

9c. Enter the other insured's employer or school name. (Note: If this is a Medicare claim, enter the claims-processing address for the Medigap insurer from field 9. If this is a Medicaid claim and other insurance is available, note it in field 1a and in field 2, and enter the requested policy information.

9d. Enter the other insured's insurance plan or program name. If the plan is Medigap and CMS has assigned it a nine-digit number called PAYERID, enter that number here. On an attached sheet, give the complete mailing address for all other insurance information, and enter the word ATTACHMENT in 10d.

10. Place *X*s in the appropriate YES or NO boxes in a, b, and c to indicate whether the patient's place of employment, an auto accident, or other type of accident precipitated the patient's condition. If an auto accident is responsible, for PLACE, enter the two-letter state postal abbreviation for the location of the accident.

    For Medicaid claims, enter MCD and the Medicaid number at line 10d. For all other claims, enter ATTACHMENT here if there is other insurance information. Be sure the full names and addresses of the other insurers appear on the attached sheet. Also, code the insurer as follows: MSP Medicare Secondary Payer, MG Medigap, SP Supplemental Employer, MCD Medicaid.

   ### Rationale
   If any of these questions are answered *yes*, a workers' compensation plan, automobile insurer, or other liability insurer may be responsible for charges.

11. Enter the insured's policy or group number. For Medicare claims, fill out this section only if there is other insurance primary to Medicare; otherwise, enter NONE and leave fields 11a–d blank.

continued ⟶

Completing the CMS-1500 Claim Form (continued)

Rationale
The word NONE lets Medicare know that there is no payer primary to Medicare. Without this notation, Medicare will assume another payer is primary.

11a. Enter the insured's date of birth and sex as in field 3, if the insured is not the patient.

11b. Enter the employer's name or school name here. This information will determine if Medicare is the primary payer.

11c. Enter the insurance plan or program name.

11d. Place an *X* to indicate YES or NO related to another health benefit plan. If YES, you must complete 9a through 9d. Failure to do so will cause the claim to be denied.

> *Note:* It is important to remember that section 11 is for the primary insurer and section 9 is for any secondary insurance coverage.

12. Have the patient or an authorized representative sign and date the form here. If a representative signs, have the representative indicate the relationship to the patient.

Rationale
The signature indicates that the patient has given permission to release medical information to the insurance company and is required for payment. If a signature is kept on file in the office, indicate by inserting "Signature on file."

13. Have the insured (the patient or another individual) sign here.

Rationale
Required for payment to be sent directly to the provider. Otherwise, payment will be sent to the patient.

Physician Information Section

14. Enter the date of the current illness, injury, or pregnancy, using eight digits.

15. Enter date patient was first seen for illness or injury. Leave it blank for Medicare.

16. Enter the dates the patient is or was unable to work. This information could signal a workers' compensation claim.

17. Enter the name of the referring physician, clinical laboratory, or other referring source.

17a. Depending on insurance carrier instructions, enter an approved 2-digit qualifier (refer to Table 15-1) in the small space and the appropriate provider identifier next to it. If the carrier requires only the NPI, leave this box blank.

17b. Enter the provider NPI number.

Rationale
This number identifies the referring physician. NPI numbers generally replace all other provider identifiers.

18. Enter the dates the patient was hospitalized, if at all, with the current condition.

19. Use your payer's current instructions for this field. Some payers require you to enter the date the patient was last seen by the referring physician or other medical professional. Other payers ask for certain identifiers. If a non-NPI is used, be sure to use the appropriate non-NPI qualifier to identify the identifier used.

20. Place an *X* in the YES box if a laboratory test was performed outside the physician's office, and enter the test price if you are billing for these tests. Ensure that field 32 carries the laboratory's exact name and address and the insurance carrier's nine-digit provider identification number (PIN). Place an *X* in the NO box if the test was done in the office of the physician who is billing the insurance company.

21. Enter the multidigit *International Classification of Diseases, 9th edition, Clinical Modification* (ICD-9-CM) code number diagnosis or nature of injury (see Chapter 16). Enter up to four codes in order of importance. *Note:* Some insurers are allowing up 6 or 8 diagnoses, particularly on electronic claims. Be sure to check with each carrier for its regulations.

Rationale
The first code should relate to the primary reason the patient was seen.

22. Enter the Medicaid resubmission code and original reference number if applicable.

23. Enter the prior authorization number if required by the payer.

Rationale
If prior authorization was required and not obtained, the claim will be denied.

24. The six service lines in block 24 are divided horizontally to accommodate NPI and other

continued ⟶

Completing the CMS-1500 Claim Form *(concluded)*

proprietary identifiers. The upper shaded area may also be used to provide supplemental information regarding services provided, but you must verify requirements for the use of this area with each payer prior to use. Otherwise, use the nonshaded areas.

24A. Enter the date of each service, procedure, or supply provided. Add the number of days for each, and enter them, in chronological order, in field 24G.

24B. Enter the two-digit place-of-service code (see Table 15-4). For example, 11 is for office, 12 is for home, and 25 is for birthing center. Your office should have a list for reference.

24C. EMG stands for *emergency care*. Check with provider to see if this information is needed. If it is required and emergency care was provided, enter *Y;* if it is not required or care was not on an emergency basis, leave this field blank. For Medicare, leave blank.

24D. Enter the CPT/HCPCS codes with modifiers for the procedures, services, or supplies provided (see Chapter 16).

24E. Enter the diagnosis code (or its reference number—1, 2, 3, or 4—depending on carrier regulations) that applies to that procedure, as listed in field 21.

Rationale
Identifies the medical necessity for each procedure or service performed

24F. Enter the dollar amount of fee charged.

24G. Enter the days or units on which the service was performed. If a service took 3 days or was performed 3 times, as listed in 24A, enter 3.

24H. This field is Medicaid-specific for early periodic screening diagnosis and treatment programs.

24I. If required by the insurance carrier, enter the appropriate non-NPI indentifier here. If not required, leave this area blank.

24J. If a non-NPI number is required by the carrier, enter the PIN identified in 24I in the shaded area. Use the nonshaded area below this to enter the provider's NPI in 24I.

25. Enter the physician's or care provider's federal tax identification number or Social Security number.

26. Enter the patient's account number assigned by your office, if applicable.

27. Place an *X* in the YES box to indicate that the physician will accept Medicare or TRICARE assignment of benefits. The check will be sent directly to the physician.

28. Enter the total charge for the service.

29. Enter the amount already paid by any primary insurance company or the patient, if it pertains to his deductible. Do not enter payments by the patient if it pertains to the coinsurance amount. For primary Medicare claims, leave blank.

Rationale
Bill the insurance carrier for the full charge owed to the office. The physician's allowed amounts are based on this and must be consistent each time a claim is filed. If the coinsurance is deducted prior to billing the insurer, it may be assumed that the provider has decreased his charges and the payment from the insurer will be decreased.

30. Enter the balance due your office (subtract field 29 from field 28 to obtain this figure). For primary Medicare claims, leave blank.

31. Have the physician or service supplier sign and date the form here.

Rationale
The provider is verifying that the services were provided, which is required for payment.

32. Enter the name and address of the organization or individual who performed the services. If performed in the patient's home, leave this field blank.

   a. In field 32a, enter the NPI for the service facility.

   b. Use field 32b if required by the insurance carrier. In this case, enter the appropriate two-digit qualifier immediately followed by the identification number being used. Do not place any spaces or punctuation between the qualifier and the identification number.

33. List the billing physician's or supplier's name, address, zip code, and phone number.

   a. In field 33a, enter the NPI of the billing provider.

   b. If required by the insurance carrier, enter the non-NPI qualifier in field 33b, immediately followed by the identification number being used. Do not place any spaces or punctuation between the qualifier and the identification number.

TABLE 15-4	Place of Service Codes for CMS 1500 Form
Code	**Place of Service**
11	Office
12	Home
21	Inpatient hospitalization
22	Outpatient hospitalization
23	Emergency room—hospital
23	Ambulatory surgical center
25	Birthing center
36	Military hospital or clinic
31	Skilled nursing facility
32	Nursing facility
33	Custodial care facility

you a good understanding of the data elements needed on all claims.

The CMS-1500 contains 33 form locators, which are numbered items. Form locators 1–13 refer to the patient and the patient's insurance coverage. Form locators 14–33 contain information about the provider and the transaction information, including the patient's diagnoses, procedures, and charges.

Transmission of Electronic Claims

Practices handle the transmission of electronic claims—which may be called electronic media claims, or EMC—in a variety of ways. Some practices transmit claims themselves; others hire outside vendors to handle this task for them.

Claims are prepared for transmission after all required data elements have been posted to the medical billing software program. The data elements that are transmitted are not seen physically, as they would be on a paper form. Instead, these elements are in a computer file.

Three major methods are used to transmit claims electronically: direct transmission to the payer, clearinghouse use, and direct data entry.

Transmitting Claims Directly. In the direct transmission approach, medical offices and payers exchange transactions directly. To do this, providers and payers need the necessary information systems, including a translator and communications technology, to conduct electronic data interchange (EDI).

Using a Clearinghouse. Many offices whose medical billing software vendors do not have translation software must use a **clearinghouse** in order to send and receive data in the correct EDI format. Clearinghouses can take in nonstandard formats and translate them into the standard format. To ensure that the standard format is compliant, the clearinghouse must receive all the required

data elements from the physician. Clearinghouses are prohibited from creating or modifying data content.

Medical offices may use a clearinghouse to transmit all their claims, or they may use a combination of direct transmission and a clearinghouse. For example, they may send claims directly to Medicare, Medicaid, and a few other major commercial payers, and use a clearinghouse to send claims to other payers.

Using Direct Data Entry. Online direct data entry (DDE) is offered by some payers. It uses an Internet-based service into which employees key the standard data elements. Although the data elements must meet the HIPAA standards requirements regarding content, they do not have to be formatted for EDI. Instead, they are loaded directly in the health plans' computer.

Generating Clean Claims

Although health-care claims require many data elements and are complex, often simple errors prevent you from generating "clean" claims—that is, those accepted for processing by the payer. Claims should be carefully checked before transmission or printing. Be alert for common errors (see Table 15-5).

Many offices use a specialized software program called a "claim scrubber" to check claims before they are released and to allow errors to be fixed. Clearinghouses also apply software checks to claims they receive and transmit back reports of errors or missing information to the sender.

Claims Security

Electronic data about patients are stored on a computer system. Most medical offices use computer networks in which personal computers are connected to a local area network (LAN), so users can exchange and share information and hardware. The LAN is linked to remote networks such as the Internet by a router that determines the

TABLE 15-5	Common Errors When Filing Claims
• Missing or incomplete service facility name, address, and identification for services rendered outside the office or home; this includes invalid ZIP codes or state abbreviations.
• Missing Medicare assignment indicator or benefits assignment indicator.
• Missing part of the name or the identifier of the referring provider
• Missing or invalid subscriber's birth date
• Missing information about secondary insurance plans, such as the spouse's payer
• Missing payer name and/or payer identifier, required for both primary and secondary payers

Points on Practice

Data Elements for HIPAA Electronic Claims

The X12 837 health-care claim requires many of the same data elements as a paper claim, but some elements require understanding new terms. Here are tips for locating these types of information.

Reporting Provider Information

The *billing provider* is the entity that is transmitting the claim to the payer. Medical offices often use a billing service or a clearinghouse to serve as the billing provider and transmit their claims. When this is done, the outside organization is the billing provider, and the practice is the *pay-to provider* that receives the payment from the insurance carrier. If an office sends claims directly to the payer, it is the billing provider and there is no additional pay-to provider to report.

Another term associated with claim preparation is *rendering provider.* A rendering provider is the physician who, as a member of the practice, treats the patient.

Reporting Taxonomy Information

A *taxonomy code* is a 10-digit number representing a physician's medical specialty. Physicians select the taxonomy code that most closely matches their education, license, or certification. The code is reported on claims because payment for some services is impacted by the particular specialty of the doctor performing them and by payers' contracts. For example, nuclear medicine is usually a higher paid specialty than internal medicine. An internist who also has a specialty in nuclear medicine would report the nuclear medicine taxonomy code when billing for that service and use the internal medicine taxonomy code when reporting internal medicine claims.

Reporting HIPAA National Identifiers

HIPAA *national identifiers* are established for:

- Employers
- Health-care providers
- Health plans
- Patients

Identifiers are numbers of predetermined length and structure, such as a person's Social Security number. As the HIPAA rules establishing these identifiers are passed, the correct data elements must be reported on the claim. For example, the employer identifier has been adopted; it is the Employer Identification Number (EIN) issued by the Internal Revenue Service.

Until the identifiers for the three other entities are adopted, these rules are in effect:

- For health care providers, report the tax identification number or Social Security number
- For health plans, report the appropriate code; here are some common codes

Code	Definition
09	Self-pay
12	Preferred provider organization (PPO)
15	Indemnity insurance
BL	Blue Cross/Blue Shield
CH	TRICARE
CI	Commercial insurance company
HM	Health maintenance organization
MB	Medicare Part B
MC	Medicaid
WC	Workers' compensation health claim

- For patients, report the policyholder's health plan identification number

---

best route for data to travel across the network. Packets of data traveling between the LAN and the Internet—such as electronic claims—must usually pass through a firewall, a security device that examines information (for example, e-mails) that enter and leave a network, determining whether to forward them to their destination.

The HIPAA rules set standards for protecting individually identifiable health information when it is maintained or transmitted electronically. Medical offices must protect the confidentiality, integrity, and availability of this information. A number of security measures are used:

- Access control, passwords, and log files to keep intruders out
- Backups (saved copies of files) to replace items after damage to the computer
- Security policies to handle violations that do occur

Medical assistants participate in the protection of patients' health information. One way is to select a good password for your computer. Never give out your password, nor allow anyone to use a computer terminal where you are logged in. Before you walk away from a computer, be sure you log out. Doing so will require that anyone else needing to use the computer logs in, using her or his own password. Here are tips for selecting a good password:

- Always use a combination of letters and numbers that are not real words and also not an obvious number string such as 123456 or a birth date.
- Do not use a user ID (log-on or sign-on) as a password. Even if it has both numbers and letters, it is not secret.
- Select a mixture of both uppercase and lowercase letters if the system can distinguish between them, and, if possible, include special characters such as @, $, or &.
- Use a minimum of six or seven alphanumeric characters. The optimal minimum number varies by system, but most security experts recommend a length of at least six or seven characters.
- Change passwords periodically, but not too often.

Forcing frequent changes can actually make security worse because users are more likely to keep passwords written down.

Summary

15.1 Medicare provides health care for citizens aged 65 and over; certain patients under 65 that have long-term disabilities and some other illnesses also may qualify for Medicare. Medicaid is a health benefits program for low-income, blind, or disabled patients; needy families; foster children; and children born with birth defects.

15.2 TRICARE is a health benefit program for families of uniformed personnel and retirees from the uniformed services. CHAMPVA covers the expenses of families of veterans with total, permanent, service-connected disabilities, as well as the surviving spouses and children of veterans in this same category.

15.3 HMOs are programs where members must generally seek services from a specific group of providers within their plan in order to receive benefits. PPOs establish a network of providers to perform services for their plan members at discounted rates, but members may seek care from out-of-network providers and still have coverage, but the member's share of the cost will likely be higher.

15.4 Prior to providing any service, contact the employer and verify the injury or illness is work-related and will be covered by the W/C insurance plan. Obtain the name and number of the person verifying this information. Next contact the insurance carrier for the WC plan and verify coverage is in effect. Obtain a case number which must be placed on every document pertaining to this case. Keep medical and financial records of workers' compensation cases separate from other employee records and maintain confidentiality.

15.5 The claims process consists of obtaining patient information; determining procedures, codes, and fees; recording charge codes and fees; preparing and submitting the claim; reviewing the processing of the claim and remittance advice; and recording any payments and adjustments to the correct patient account.

15.6 Medical assistants gather and record patient information; verify coverage; record procedures and services performed and the applicable diagnoses and codes; file claims; bill patients; and review and record payments.

15.7 The rules that determine the coordination of benefits are guidelines for payments from insurance companies so that no more than 100% of charges are ever paid by the insurance carriers. Table 15-3 states each rule as applicable to patients.

15.8 Preparing the health-care claim consists of filing the claim; meeting the time limits for filing claims; reviewing the claim for medical necessity; and reviewing for allowable benefits, reviewing payment, and remittance advice to verify that the claim was paid correctly and that payments and adjustments will be posted correctly. Also note any noncovered services for possible resubmission or patient billing.

15.9 Payers set fees generally base their payment amounts on the amounts that Medicare allows. Medicare bases its fee schedule on a payment system known as RBRVS. The formula for this is RVU (consisting of physician work, practice overhead, and malpractice insurance) $\times$ GAF (geographic adjustment factor) $\times$ CF (conversion factor).

15.10 The CMS-1500 form contains numbered items that refer to the patient and the patient's insurance coverage. Follow the steps in Procedure 15-2 for completing the CMS-1500 claim form.

15.11 Three ways to transmit electronic claims are to transmit claims directly to the insurance carrier; use a clearinghouse to prepare and send claims; and use direct data entry utilizing an Internet-based service known as DDE.

CASE STUDY QUESTIONS

Now that you have completed this chapter, review the case study at the beginning of the chapter and answer the following questions:

1. How much should this patient pay?
2. How much will he owe for his next visit this year, which is expected to have a charge of $200?
3. Assuming that the patient in the case study has a managed care policy, what type of policy does he probably have?
4. What term would you use to describe the part of the payment that is based on 20% of the charges?
5. If you did not know whether the deductible had been met, what procedure would you follow?

Multiple-Choice Questions

1. The first national health insurance for Americans age 65 and older is
   a. Medicaid.
   c. Disability insurance.
   b. Medicare.
   d. Liability insurance.
2. The authorization for an insurance carrier to pay the physician or practice directly is the
   a. copayment.
   b. provider of medical services.
   c. assignment of benefits.
   d. health insurance provider.
3. A fixed dollar amount the subscriber must pay or "meet" each year before the insurer begins to cover expenses is the
   a. copayment.
   c. premium.
   b. deductible.
   d. coinsurance.
4. The goal of Blue Cross/Blue Shield was to
   a. cover only the frequent disasters of the era.
   b. cover lost income because of a disability.
   c. make health insurance accessible to as many people as possible.
   d. negotiate for fringe benefits of employment.
5. TRICARE and CHAMPVA cover
   a. active military families.
   b. veterans who served in active combat.
   c. nonmilitary government employees.
   d. families of all military personnel.

Discussion Questions

1. How do HMOs and PPOs compare?
2. How would you explain the purpose of the assignment of benefits form to a patient?

3. Why do insurers coordinate benefits?
4. How would you explain to a patient what an allowable charge is?

Critical Thinking Questions

1. How is the increasing cost of medical procedures affecting the insurance industry?
2. Why is it important to remind patients of their financial obligations?
3. What are the advantages of electronic claims?

Application Activities

1. Apply the birthday rule in this situation: Both parents of the patient have health-care coverage through their employers. The father's birthday is December 5 and the mother's is June 4. Which plan is primary for the child?
2. A patient's insurance policy states: Annual deductible: $300; Coinsurance: 70-30. This year, the patient has made payments totaling $533 to all providers. Today, the patient has an office visit (fee: $80). The patient presents a credit card for payment of today's bill. What is the amount that the patient should pay?
3. A patient is a member of an HMO with a capitation plan and a $10 copayment. The usual charges for the day's services would be $480. What does the patient pay?
4. You need to calculate how much a patient needs to pay. He is a member of a preferred provider organization (PPO) that has a contract that allows all members a 25% discount. The patient's total bill for services rendered today is $300.00. The patient has a copayment of 20%. The patient states that he can only pay $50.00 today. Does the patient have enough to cover the amount due today?

Virtual Fieldtrip

Visit the McGraw-Hill Higher Education Medical Assisting website at www.mhhe.com/medicalassisting4e to complete the following activity:

Visit a Medicaid website and determine the requirements to qualify for Medicaid services in your state. Write a one-page summary for submission to your instructor.

 Open the CD and complete this chapter's practice activities, play the games, listen to the key terms, and test yourself with the interactive review. E-mail, print, and/or save your results to document your proficiency.

CHAPTER 16

Medical Coding

LEARNING OUTCOMES

After completing Chapter 16, you will be able to:

16.1 Describe the purpose and format of the ICD-9-CM volumes that are used by medical offices.

16.2 Model how to analyze diagnoses and locate correct codes using the ICD-9-CM.

16.3 Describe the purpose and format of the CPT.

16.4 Distinguish three key factors that determine the level of Evaluation and Management codes that are selected.

16.5 Differentiate between the two types of codes in the Health Care Common Procedure Coding System (HCPCS).

16.6 Carry out the process used to locate correct procedure codes using CPT.

16.7 Explain how medical coding affects the payment process.

16.8 Distinguish fraud and provide examples of fraudulent billing and coding.

MEDICAL ASSISTING COMPETENCIES

CAAHEP

VIII.C (1) Describe how to use the most current procedural coding system

VIII.C (3) Describe how to use the most current diagnostic coding classification system

VIII.C (4) Describe how to use the most current HCPCS coding

VIII.P (1) Perform procedural coding

VIII.P (2) Perform diagnostic coding

VIII.A (1) Work with the physician to achieve the maximum reimbursement

ABHES

3. **Medical Terminology**
   d. Recognize and identify acceptable medical abbreviations

4. **Medical Law & Ethics**
   a. Document accurately
   f. Comply with federal, state, and local health laws and regulations

8. **Medical Office Business Procedures Management**
   t. Perform diagnostic and procedural coding
   hh. Receive, organize, prioritize, and transmit information expediently

11. **Career Development**
   Demonstrate professionalism by:
   1) Exhibiting dependability, punctuality, and a positive work ethic
   4) Being cognizant of ethical boundaries
   9) Conducting work within scope of education, training, and ability

MEDICAL ASSISTING MEDIA

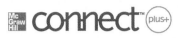 **Connect Plus+™**
connect.mcgraw-hill.com

- Electronic Health Records (E.H.R.) SpringCharts®
- eBook

SPRINGCHARTS
Electronic Health Records

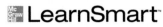 **LearnSmart™**

www.mhhe.com/learnsmart

Complete Learning Module: Medical Coding

 Student CD-ROM

 Online Learning Center™

www.mhhe.com/medicalassisting4e

KEY TERMS

add-on code

Alphabetic Index

code linkage

compliance plan

conventions

cross-reference

Current Procedural Terminology (CPT)

diagnosis (Dx)

diagnosis code

E code

E/M code

established patient

global period

HCPCS Level II codes

Health Care Common Procedure Coding System (HCPCS)

International Classification of Diseases, Ninth Revision, Clinical Modification (ICD-9-CM)

modifier

new patient

panel

procedure code

Tabular List

V code

CHAPTER OUTLINE

- Diagnosis Codes: The ICD-9-CM
- Procedure Codes: The CPT
- HCPCS
- Avoiding Fraud: Coding Compliance

PREPARATION FOR CERTIFICATION

RMA (AMT) Exam

- ICD-9/CPT coding applications
- HIPAA-mandated coding systems
- Medical insurance terminology

CMA (AAMA) Exam

- Processing claims
- Fee schedules
- Applying managed care policies and procedures
- Relationship between procedure and diagnosis codes

CMAS Exam

- Coding
- Insurance processing
- Insurance billing and finances

Introduction

Welcome to the world of coding! In this introduction, you will learn that in order to correctly report on health-care claims the conditions that patients have and the services they receive during office visits, medical assistants need to understand the basics of medical coding. Medical coding is the translation of medical terms for diagnoses and procedures into code numbers selected from standardized code sets. Codes on health-care claims explain to payers that the services patients received were medically necessary and complied with the payer's rules. Finding the correct codes can require detective work! The reward is accurate claims that bring the maximum appropriate reimbursement to the physicians in your medical office.

A patient who has asthma has an office visit for her chest pain and shortness of breath. The physician performs a cardiovascular stress test using submaximal treadmill (with continuous electrocardiographic monitoring, physician supervision, and interpretation/report) to assess the patient's heart function. While the patient is in the office, the physician also evaluates her asthma and increases her prescription for asthma medication.

As you read this chapter, consider the following question:

1. How would you select the ICD-9 and CPT codes for a health-care claim for this visit?
2. What diagnosis and procedure codes will result in the correct payment for these services?
3. How should the claim show the medical necessity of the procedures?
4. Locate the ICD-9 code for the patient's asthma. How many digits are required? What code did you assign?
5. Locate the CPT code for the cardiovascular stress test. What information did you use to select it from the list of related codes?

Diagnosis Codes: The ICD-9-CM

Patients present physicians with a description of their medical problems, called their chief complaints (CC) in the documentation of their visits. To diagnose a patient's condition, the physician follows a complex process of decision making based on the patient's statements, an examination, and the physician's evaluation of this information. The physician establishes a **diagnosis (Dx)** that describes the primary condition for which a patient is receiving care. Additional conditions or symptoms that affect the patient's management are called coexisting conditions. These conditions may be related or totally unrelated to the primary condition, but if they currently affect the patient's condition or treatment, they must also be noted in the chart, coded, and reported to the insurance carrier. The diagnoses listed on a health-care claim form should prove medical necessity for the treatment provided.

The diagnosis is communicated to the third-party payer through a **diagnosis code** on the health-care claim. The diagnosis codes used in the United States are found in the *International Classification of Diseases, Ninth Revision, Clinical Modification,* commonly referred to as the **ICD-9-CM** or simply ICD-9. Also available on CD-ROM, this code set is based on a system maintained by the World Health Organization (WHO) of the United Nations.

The use of the ICD-9 codes in the health-care industry is mandated by the Health Insurance Portability and Accountability Act (HIPAA) for reporting patients' diseases, conditions, or their signs and symptoms if no actual diagnosis has been assigned. The codes are updated every year and new ICD-9 manuals are available prior to October 1, which is when the new diagnosis codes are to be used on claims. Medical offices should have the current year's reference book and should update office forms and computer programs that contain diagnosis codes; using outdated codes can result in denied claims. The edition of diagnosis code being used is based on the date of service, not on the date the claim is submitted. For instance when completing claims on October 1, 2011, you would use 2011 ICD-9 codes on a claim for services provided on September 30, 2011. However, for a claim reporting services provided on October 1, 2011, the new 2012 ICD-9 codes would be used.

Using the ICD-9

To find the correct diagnosis codes, you follow a five-step process, working with the diagnostic information provided by the physician and the ICD-9 manual. Coding becomes easier with practice, but do not be tempted to take shortcuts. Every case is different, and additional terms or digits may be necessary to make a diagnosis code as specific as possible. If a step is skipped, important information may be missed. If more than one diagnosis is described in a patient's chart, work on only one diagnosis at a time to avoid coding errors, which may result in decreased or denied payment of a patient's claim.

The ICD-9-CM used in medical offices has two parts, the Tabular List, known as Volume 1, and the Alphabetic Index, known as Volume 2, which is actually found at the beginning of the manual.

Diseases and Injuries: Tabular List, Volume 1. The **Tabular List** has 17 chapters of disease descriptions and codes, with two additional types of codes and five appendixes.

Diseases and Injuries: Alphabetic Index, Volume 2. The **Alphabetic Index** provides the following:

- An index of the disease descriptions in the Tabular List
- An index in table format of drugs and chemicals that cause poisoning
- An index of external causes of injury, such as accidents and poisonings

Diagnoses are listed two ways in the ICD-9, as illustrated in Figure 16-1. In the Alphabetic Index, diagnoses appear in

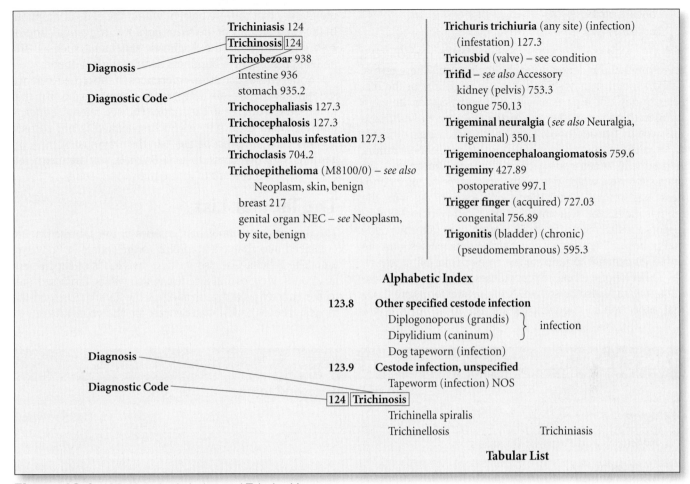

Figure 16-1. ICD Alphabetic Index and Tabular List.

Source: International Classification of Diseases, Ninth Revision, Clinical Modification, 2009, Volumes 1 and 2.

alphabetic order with at least the main portion of their corresponding diagnosis codes. In the Tabular List, the diagnosis codes are listed in numerical order with additional instructions that are necessary to choose the final diagnosis code. Both the Alphabetic Index and the Tabular List are used to find the right code. The Alphabetic Index is *never* used alone because it does not contain all the necessary information. After you locate a code in the index, look it up in the Tabular List. Notes in this list may suggest or require the use of additional codes, or indicate that conditions should be coded differently because of exclusion from a category.

Although the official order of the volumes puts the Tabular List before the Alphabetic Index, the correct use is to examine the Alphabetic Index when you are researching a term and then to verify your selection in the Tabular List. For this reason, commercial printers usually reverse the order, printing the Alphabetic Index at the front and the Tabular List behind it.

The Alphabetic Index

The Alphabetic Index contains all the medical terms in the Tabular List. For some conditions, it also has common terms that are not found in the Tabular List. The index is organized by the condition, not by the body part in which the condition occurs. To use the Alphabetic Index, think

about what is wrong (the problem) and not where the problem occurred. For example, you would find the term *wrist fracture* by looking under *fracture* (the condition) and then, below it, *wrist* (the location), rather than by looking under *wrist* to find *fracture*. In fact, if you look up the word *wrist*, you will be told "See also condition," telling you to look up the problem with the wrist.

The assignment of the correct code begins with looking up the medical term that describes the patient's condition in the Alphabetic Index. The following example illustrates the index's format. Each main term is printed in boldface type and is followed by its code number. For example, if the diagnostic statement is "the patient presents with blindness," the main term *blindness* is located in the Alphabetic Index.

Blindness (acquired) (congenital) (both eyes) 369.00
   blast 921.3
      with nerve injury—see Injury, nerve, optic
   Bright's—see Uremia
   color (congenital) 368.59
      acquired 368.55
      blue 368.53
      green 368.52
      red 368.51
      total 368.54

concussion 950.9
cortical 377.75

Any other terms that are needed to select correct codes are printed and indented after the main term. These terms, called *subterms,* may show the cause or source of the disease, or describe a particular type or body site for the main term. In this shortened example, the main term *blindness* is followed by five additional terms, each indicating a different type—such as color blindness—for this medical condition. Additionally, when coding color blindness, note that each of its subterms, which denote the actual type of color blindness, has its own code. When cross-referencing with the tabular index, you will note that the main code of 368 represents a visual disturbance. The fourth digit (after the decimal point) of 5 represents color vision deficiencies, and the fifth digit changes to indicate the type of color blindness.

Other helpful terms, in parentheses, known as *nonessential terms,* may also be shown. Nonessential terms are those that assist you in choosing the correct code, but it is not mandatory that they be present within the code description. In the example, any of the terms *acquired, congenital,* and/or *both eyes* may be in the diagnostic statement, such as "the patient presents with blindness acquired in childhood."

Some entries use **cross-references.** If the cross-reference *see* appears after a main term, you *must* look up the term that follows the word *see* in the index. The **see** reference means that the main term where you first looked is not correct; another category must be used. In the previous example regarding color blindness, to code *Bright's,* you are instructed to *See* the term *Uremia* to locate the correct code.

The Tabular List

The diseases, conditions, and injuries in the Tabular List are organized into chapters according to the source or body system. The Tabular List also includes two kinds of supplementary codes, V codes and E codes, which will be discussed later in the chapter. The organization of the Tabular List and the ranges of codes each chapter covers are shown in Table 16-1.

TABLE 16-1 Tabular List Organization

Classification of Diseases and Injuries

Chapter	Categories
1 Infectious and Parasitic Diseases	001–139
2 Neoplasms	140–239
3 Endocrine, Nutritional, and Metabolic Diseases, and Immunity Disorders	240–279
4 Diseases of the Blood and Blood-Forming Organs	280–289
5 Mental Disorders	290–319
6 Diseases of the Central Nervous System and Sense Organs	320–389
7 Diseases of the Circulatory System	390–459
8 Diseases of the Respiratory System	460–519
9 Diseases of the Digestive System	520–579
10 Diseases of the Genitourinary System	580–629
11 Complications of Pregnancy, Childbirth, and the Puerperium	630–679
12 Diseases of the Skin and Subcutaneous Tissue	680–709
13 Diseases of the Musculoskeletal System and Connective Tissue	710–739
14 Congenital Anomalies	740–759
15 Certain Conditions Originating in the Perinatal Period	760–779
16 Symptoms, Signs, and Ill-Defined Conditions	780–799
17 Injury and Poisoning	800–999
Supplementary Classifications	
V Codes—Supplementary Classification of Factors Influencing Health Status and Contact with Health Services	V01–V83
E Codes—Supplementary Classification of External Causes of Injury and Poisoning	E800–E999

Code Structure. ICD-9-CM diagnosis codes are made up of three, four, or five digits. The system uses three-digit categories for diseases, injuries, and symptoms. Many of these categories are divided into four-digit codes. Some codes are further subdivided into five-digit codes. For example:

415 Acute pulmonary heart disease *[three digits]*

   415.1 Pulmonary embolism and infarction *[four digits; more specific]*

      415.11 Iatrogenic pulmonary embolism and infarction *[five digits; most specific]*

When listed in the ICD-9, four- and five-digit diagnosis codes should be reported on claims because they represent the most specific diagnosis documented in the patient medical record. When they are available, the use of fourth and fifth digits is not optional; payers require them. For example, the Centers for Medicare and Medicaid Services (CMS) rules state that a Medicare claim will be rejected when the most specific code available is not used. In the above example, it would be incorrect to use code 415 or 415.1 because code 415.11 is available and so, as the most specific code, it must be used. Always keep in mind that the minimum code contains 3 digits, but if a 4th digit is available, it must be used, and if a 5th digit is available, it also must be used. The fourth and fifth digits are preceded by a decimal point.

V Codes and E Codes. Two additional types of codes follow the chapters of the Tabular List:

1. **V codes** identify encounters for reasons other than illness or injury, such as annual checkups, immunizations, and normal childbirth. The descriptions for V codes are found throughout the main portion of the Alphabetic Index. V codes can be used either as primary codes for an encounter or as additional codes. You should be aware that some insurance carriers, such as Medicare, do not cover V codes, so the charges associated with them may become the patient's responsibility.

2. **E codes** identify the external causes of injuries and poisoning. E (for external) codes are used for injuries resulting from various environmental events, such as transportation accidents, accidental poisoning by drugs or other substances, falls, and fires. Some beginning coders find it easy to remember that if a diagnosis makes you question "How did that happen?" at least one E code will be required to answer the question. An E code is never used alone as a diagnosis code. It always supplements the code that identifies the injury or condition itself. You might find it helpful to also think that in addition to "external," that the E also stands for "extra," so you will not be tempted to let an E code stand by itself. E codes are often used in collecting public health information. The alphabetic descriptions for E codes are found at the end of the Alphabetic Index in two sections. Section 2 is the alphabetic Table of Drugs and Chemicals, which is used to identify drugs and chemicals responsible for poisonings. Immediately following this, in Section 3, is the alphabetic index for all E codes.

Both V and E codes are alphanumeric; they contain letters followed by numbers. For example, the code for a complete physical examination of an adult is V70.0. The code for a fall from a ladder is E881.0. The same rule for specificity applies to E and V codes regarding 4th and 5th digits; that is, if a 4th or 5th digit is available, it must be utilized or the code will be rejected by the insurance carrier.

ICD-9-CM Conventions

A list of abbreviations, punctuation, symbols, typefaces, and instructional notes appears at the beginning of the ICD-9. These items, called **conventions,** provide guidelines for using the code set. Here are some important conventions:

- NOS. This abbreviation means "not otherwise specified," or "unspecified." It is used when a condition cannot be described more specifically. In general, codes with *NOS* should be avoided unless no other option is available. The physician should be asked for more specific information to help select a more specific code, if possible. Most of the NOS codes end with the number 9.

- NEC. This abbreviation means "not elsewhere classified." It is used when the ICD-9 does not provide a code specific enough for the patient's condition. Only use these codes when you are sure a more specific code does not exist. In general, the NEC codes end with the number 8.

- [ ] Brackets. These are used around synonyms, alternative wordings, or explanations.

- ( ) Parentheses. These are used around descriptions that do not affect the code, that is, nonessential or supplementary terms.

- : Colon. This is used in the Tabular List after an incomplete term that needs one of the terms that follows the colon to make it assignable to a given category.

- } Brace. This encloses a series of terms, each of which is modified by the statement that appears to the right of the brace.

- § Section mark symbol. This symbol, preceding a code, denotes the placement of a footnote at the bottom of the page that is applicable to all subdivisions in that code. Not all editions of ICD-9 utilize the section mark symbol.

- *Includes.* This note indicates that the entries following it further define the content of a preceding entry. For example, after the three-digit diagnosis code for acute sinusitis, the word *includes* is followed by the types of sinusitis that the code covers.

- *Excludes.* These notes, which are boxed and italicized, indicate that an entry is not classified as part of the preceding code. The note may also give the correct location of the excluded condition to assist you in locating the correct code.

- *Use additional code.* This note indicates that an additional code should be used, if available. The additional code is always listed after the primary code. For instance, when looking up a urinary tract infection NOS (599.0), you are asked to also code the causative organism (if given), such as *E. coli* (041.4). The complete coding sequence would be 599.0, 041.4.
- *Code first underlying disease.* This instruction appears when the category is not to be used as the primary diagnosis. These codes may not be used as the first code; they must always be preceded by another code for the primary diagnosis. An example of this would be any diabetic complication, such as diabetic retinopathy for a noninsulin-dependent diabetic. Under diabetic retinopathy (362.01), you are instructed to *Code first diabetes* (250.5). The correct coding order would be 250.50, 362.01. The fifth digit with the diabetes code indicates *noninsulin-dependent diabetes not stated as uncontrolled.* You will note when coding diabetes that the instructions state that all diabetes codes require fifth digits.

Locating the Diagnosis in the Patient Chart. If the physician uses a SOAP note format (Chapter 9), you can locate the diagnosis in the assessment area. If a more "free-hand" approach is used, a little detective work may be needed.

Example #1, from a Patient Medical Record:

CC: *Chest and epigastric pain; feels like a burning inside. Occasional reflux.*

Exam: *Abdomen soft, flat without tenderness. No bowel masses or organomegaly.*

Dx: *Peptic ulcer.*

The diagnosis is peptic ulcer.

Now, decide what the main term is for the condition or the diagnosis. For the diagnosis in the above scenario, the main term is *ulcer.* The word *peptic* (meaning stomach) describes the type of ulcer and is considered a subterm. Because there is an exact diagnosis, the pain and reflux will not be coded in outpatient facilities such as physician offices. Inpatient facilities such as hospitals have different rules and the symptoms would be coded.

Example #2:

The diagnosis is sebaceous cyst. Look under *cyst,* the condition, and not *sebaceous,* the descriptive subterm. Many entries in the Alphabetic Index are crossreferenced, so if you look up a descriptive word, the ICD-9 will lead you to alternate words to assist you in finding the correct description. For example, *sebaceous* is followed by instructions in parentheses that say "(*see also* Cyst, sebaceous)." Be sure to follow all cross-reference instructions.

Once you find the description, locate the code given for that description; it is usually to the right of the description or just below it. Now go to Volume 1, the Tabular Index, to verify the code. Be sure to read all instructions in this section because there are often more specific instructions

in the Tabular Index that will help you find the right code or affirm that you have the correct code.

Examples:

1. For the first diagnosis of peptic ulcer, the main 3-digit code for peptic ulcer is 533. The 4th digit, 9, indicates that the ulcer is not specified as acute or chronic and there is no mention of hemorrhage or perforation. The 5th digit, 0, is chosen as there is no mention of obstruction. The final code for the peptic ulcer is 533.90.

2. In the second scenario, the sebaceous cyst, the main code is 706, which denotes diseases of the sebaceous glands. The 4th digit, 2, indicates that the "disease" is a sebaceous cyst. In this example, there is no 5th digit, so the final code for a sebaceous cyst is 706.2.

In both of these cases, the level of specificity of each diagnosis was greatly increased by the addition of the 4th and 5th digits, underlining the importance of these "optional" additions to the main codes; they truly are not optional at all.

Lastly, don't forget to look for instructions for additional codes that may be needed to completely code the diagnosis. These instructions may include *Code also* and *Code first underlying condition,* as well as *includes* and *excludes* notes that assist you in deciding on the correct code or codes.

Procedure 16-1 outlines the steps for locating an ICD-9-CM code.

A New Revision: The ICD-10-CM and ICD-10-PCS

When the United States modified ICD-9 to create ICD-9--CM more than 30 years ago, a third volume was added to capture (primarily hospital) procedure codes; what we know today as ICD-9 Volume 3. However, instead of appending a short volume of procedure codes to ICD-10-CM, a complete classification, ICD-10-PCS (procedural coding system), was developed. This procedural coding system is much more detailed and specific than the short number of procedure codes included in ICD-9-CM volume 3.

PCS is used only in the hospital inpatient setting by those reporting ICD-9-CM procedure codes. All other entities will continue to report CPT and HCPCS codes.

The ICD-10-CM system consists of more than 68,000 diagnosis codes, compared to approximately 13,000 ICD-9-CM diagnosis codes. ICD-10-PCS consists of 87,000 procedure codes.

Transitioning to ICD-10-CM/ICD-10-PCS is more complex than implementation of new code sets in the past because the uses of coded data are more complex than those for which ICD-9-CM was designed. The ICD-10-C/ICD-10-PCS include several features:

- *Combination codes* are available including those for external causes and poisonings (E codes), with information combined into one code (including the drug involved) making those difficult sequencing rules obsolete. For poisoning codes, alpha extensions are added to identify the

PROCEDURE 16-1

Locating an ICD-9-CM Code

Procedure Goal: To analyze diagnoses and locate the correct ICD code.

Materials: Patient record, charge slip or superbill, ICD-9-CM manual

Method:

1. Locate the patient's diagnosis.

   a. This information may be located on the superbill (encounter form) or elsewhere in the patient's chart. If it is on the superbill, verify documentation in the medical chart.

   Rationale

   All diagnosis codes must be referenced in the patient's medical record for legal purposes.

2. Find the diagnosis in the ICD's Alphabetic Index. Look for the condition first, then locate the indented subterms that make the condition more specific. Read all cross-references to check all the possibilities for a term, including its synonyms and any eponyms.

   Rationale

   The goal is to attain the highest level of specificity possible to avoid denial of the claim.

3. Locate the code from the Alphabetic Index in the ICD's Tabular List.

   Rationale

   Never code directly from the Alphabetic Index. Important coding instructions are found only in the Tabular Index.

4. Read all information to find the code that corresponds to the patient's specific disease or condition.

   a. Study the list of codes and descriptions. Be sure to pick the most specific code available. Check for the symbol that shows that a four-or five-digit code is required.

   Rationale

   When available, 4th and 5th digits are mandatory for accurate coding. Claims will be denied if these "optional" digits are available and not used when submitting a claim.

5. Carefully record the diagnosis code(s) on the insurance claim and proofread the numbers.

   a. Be sure that all necessary codes are given to completely describe each diagnosis. Check for instructions stating an additional code is needed. If more than one code is needed, be sure instructions are followed and the codes are listed in the correct order.

   Rationale

   Coding order is important for claims to be considered "clean" and paid in a timely fashion.

---

type of encounter; a is an *initial encounter* d for a *subsequent encounter* and q for *sequela*. Examples include,

- I25.110 – Atherosclerotic heart disease of native coronary artery with unstable angina pectoris
- T36.0x1 – Poisoning by penicillins, accidental (unintentional)

- ICD-10-CM includes *Codes for Laterality* (unclassified in ICD-9-CM) at the 5th or 6th character level. An example of these types of codes includes
  - C50.511, Malignant neoplasm of the lower-outer quadrant of the right female breast
- *Expanded codes capture more detail.* Expanded codes are available in many sections of ICD-10-CM, particularly in the injury, diabetes, alcohol and substance abuse, and postoperative complication sections. An example of the new expanded codes includes,

- E11.610 – Type 2 diabetes mellitus with diabetic neuropathic arthopathy
- *Flexibility and expandability of the ICD-10-CM coding system.* Because of the flexibility and expandability of the ICD-10-CM coding system, it is possible to provide more specificity in the coding of many conditions. An example of more specific codes includes
  - S72.324A, Nondisplaced transverse fracture of the shaft of the right femur; initial encounter for closed fracture

Because the ICD-10-CM codes are much more specific, providers will have to give detailed diagnosis information so that the most accurate code can be assigned, but it is generally acknowledged that experienced ICD-9 coders will require only brief training to work effectively and efficiently with ICD-10-CM.

Surgery

General

10021   Fine needle aspiration; without imaging guidance
CPT Assistant Aug 02:10, Mar 05:11; *CPT Changes: An Insider's View* 2002

10022   with imaging guidance
CPT Assistant Nov 02:1, Jun 07:10; *CPT Changes: An Insider's View* 2002
Clinical Examples in Radiology Summer 05.1, 6

(For radiological supervision and interpretation, see 76942, 77002, 77012, 77021)

▷(For percutaneous needle biopsy other than fine needle aspiration, see 20206 for muscle, 32400 for pleura, 32405 for lung or mediastinum, 42400 for salivary gland, 47000, 47001 for liver, 48102 for pancreas, 49180 for abdominal or retroperitoneal mass, 60100 for thyroid, 62267 for nucleus pulposus, intervertebral disc, or paravertebral tissue, 62269 for spinal cord)◁

(For evaluation of fine needle aspirate, see 88172, 88173)

Integumentary System

Skin, Subcutaneous and Accessory Structures

Incision and Drainage

(For excision, see 11400, et seq)

10040   Acne surgery (eg, marsupialization, opening or removal of multiple milia, comedones, cysts, pustules)
CPT Assistant Fall 92:10, Feb 08:8

10060   Incision and drainage of abscess (eg, carbuncle, suppurative hidradenitis, cutaneous or subcutaneous abscess, cyst, furuncle, or paronychia); simple or single

10061   complicated or multiple

10080   Incision and drainage of pilonidal cyst; simple
CPT Assistant Fall 92:13, Dec 06:15, May 07:5

10081   complicated
CPT Assistant Fall 92:13, Dec 06:15, May 07:5

(For excision of pilonidal cyst, see 11770-11772)

10120   Incision and removal of foreign body, subcutaneous tissues; simple

10121   complicated
CPT Assistant Spring 91:7, Dec 06:15

(To report wound exploration due to penetrating trauma without laparotomy or thoracotomy, see 20100-20103, as appropriate)

(To report debridement associated with open fracture(s) and/or dislocation(s), use 11010-11012, as appropriate)

10140   Incision and drainage of hematoma, seroma or fluid collection
CPT Changes: An Insider's View 2002

(If imaging guidance is performed, see 76942, 77012, 77021)

10160   Puncture aspiration of abscess, hematoma, bulla, or cyst
CPT Changes: An Insider's View 2002

(If imaging guidance is performed, see 76942, 77012, 77021)

10180   Incision and drainage, complex, postoperative wound infection

(For secondary closure of surgical wound, see 12020, 12021, 13160)

Excision—Debridement

(For dermabrasions, see 15780-15783)

(For nail debridement, see 11720-11721)

(For burn(s), see 16000-16035)

11000   Debridement of extensive eczematous or infected skin; up to 10% of body surface
CPT Assistant May 99:10

(For abdominal wall or genitalia debridement for necrotizing soft tissue infection, see 11004-11006)

+△ 11001   each additional 10% of the body surface, or part thereof (List separately in addition to code for primary procedure)
CPT Assistant May 99:10; *CPT Changes: An Insider's View* 2009

(Use 11001 in conjunction with 11000)

11004   Debridement of skin, subcutaneous tissue, muscle and fascia for necrotizing soft tissue infection; external genitalia and perineum
CPT Changes: An Insider's View 2005

△ = Revised code   ◎ = New code   ▷ ◁ = Contains new or revised text   ⊘ = Modifier 51 exempt

Figure 16-2. Examples of CPT codes, surgical section.
Source: American Medical Association, *Current Procedural Terminlolgy,* copyright 2009.

Procedure Codes: The CPT

After an office visit, each procedure and service performed for a patient is reported on health-care claims using a **procedure code.** These codes represent medical procedures, such as surgery and diagnostic tests, and medical services, such as physical examinations to evaluate a patient's condition. Medical assistants often choose procedure codes based on the information given to them by the physician on the charge slip and use them to report physicians' services.

The most commonly used system of procedure codes is found in the *Current Procedural Terminology,* a book published by the American Medical Association (AMA) that is commonly known as **CPT.** CPT is the HIPAA required code set that translates descriptions for physicians' procedures into 5-digit codes.

Like ICD-9-CM, the CPT manual is updated yearly with the new codes being used beginning January 1 of each new year. In each new edition, newly developed procedures are added and old ones are revised or, if they have become obsolete, are deleted. These changes are also available in a computer file because some medical offices use a computer-based version of the CPT. As with ICD-9, the choice of which set of codes to use is based on the date of service not the date of the claim. If claims are being submitted January 2, 2012, and the date of service was December 23, 2011, CPT codes from 2011 would be used; for services provided on January 2, 2012, the 2012 edition of the CPT codes would be used.

Medical offices should have the current year's CPT available for reference and keep forms up to date. Like ICD-9 codes, if current codes are not used, medical claims are often denied. Previous years' books should also be kept in case there is a question about health-care claims that were previously submitted.

Organization of the CPT Manual

CPT codes are organized into six main sections:

Section	Range of Codes
Evaluation and Management	99201–99499
Anesthesiology	00100–01999, 99100–99140
Surgery	10021–69990
Radiology	70010–79999
Pathology and Laboratory	80048–89356
Medicine (except for anesthesia)	90281–99199, 99500–99602

Except for the first section, the CPT reference book is arranged in numerical order. Codes for evaluation and management, which describe care given by the physician, are listed first, out of numerical order, because they are used most often.

Each section opens with important guidelines that apply to its procedures. This material should be checked carefully before a procedure code is chosen. The sections of the CPT are divided into categories. These in turn are further divided into headings according to the type of test, service, or body system. Code number ranges included on a particular page are found in the upper-right corner. This helps to locate a code quickly after using the index. An example is shown in Figure 16-2.

Locate correct procedure codes by first looking up the term in the CPT's index, which is found in the back of the manual. Boldfaced main terms may be followed by descriptions and groups of indented subterms. The correct code is selected by reviewing each description and indented term under the main term.

Although it may seem tempting to record the procedure code directly from the index, resist the shortcut. Explanations and notes in the guidelines and main sections more accurately lead to finding main numbers and modifiers that reflect the services performed. That is the <u>only</u> way to ensure reimbursement at the highest allowed level.

Add-On Codes. A plus sign (+) is used for **add-on codes,** indicating procedures that are usually carried out in addition to another procedure. For example, code 90471 covers one immunization administration and code 90472 covers administering an additional shot. Add-on codes are never reported alone. They are used together with the primary code. Figure 16-3 includes symbols that appear in the 2009 *Current Procedural Terminology* code manual.

Modifiers. One or more two-digit **modifiers** (up to three per procedure) may be assigned to the five-digit main number. Modifiers are written in a separate column on the CMS-1500 Claim Form (Centers for Medicare and Medicaid Services Claim Form; see Figure 15-7). The use of a modifier shows that one or more special circumstance applies to the service or procedure the physician performed. For example, in the surgery section, the modifier-62 indicates that two surgeons worked together, each performing part of a surgical procedure during an operation. Each physician will be paid part of the amount normally reimbursed for that procedure code. Appendix A of the CPT explains the proper use of each modifier. Some section guidelines also discuss the use of modifiers with the section's codes (see Table 16-2).

;	= SEPARATES COMMON AND UNIQUE PORTIONS OF CODES
•	= NEW PROCEDURE
▲	= REVISED CODE DESCRIPTION
▶◀	= OTHER REVISED TEXT
⊘	= MODIFIER 51 EXEMPT (FORBIDDEN/PROHIBITORY SYMBOL)
+	= ADD-ON CODE; CAN'T BE ASSIGNED ALONE, DO NOT USE -51 WITH THIS SYMBOL
⚡	= CODES FOR PRODUCTS PENDING FDA APPROVAL
○	= CODE INCLUDES MODERATE SEDATION

Figure 16-3. Symbols that appear in the 2009 *Current Procedural Terminology* code manual.

Source: American Medical Association, *CPT 2009 Professional Edition,* copyright 2009.

TABLE 16-2 CPT Selected Modifiers That Are Used in the Medical Office

Modifier	Description
-21	Prolonged evaluation and management services
-22	Increased procedural services (not used for E/M services)
-26	Professional component
-32	Mandated service
-47	Anesthesia by surgeon (not including local anesthesia)
-50	Bilateral procedure—this code is added to the second (bilateral) procedure performed at the same operation
-51	Multiple procedures (performed at the same session)
-52	Reduced services
-54	Surgical care only—this code is used when another physician provides preoperative and postoperative care
-55	Postoperative management only
-56	Preoperative management only
-57	Decision for surgery (added to an E/M code when the physician makes the decision for surgery during an E/M visit)
-58	Staged or related procedure by the same physician during postoperative session
-59	Distinct procedural service
-90	Reference (outside) laboratory
-91	Repeat clinical diagnostic laboratory test
-92	Alternative laboratory platform testing
-99	Multiple modifiers

Note: You can see a complete listing of all the modifiers in the *Current Procedural Terminology* manual, Appendix A.

Source: American Medical Association, *Current Procedural Terminology,* 2009 Professional Edition, copyright 2009.

Category II Codes, Category III Codes, and Unlisted Procedure Codes. Category II codes are optional, supplemental tracking codes used to track healthcare performance measures, such as programs and counseling to avoid tobacco use. Category III codes are temporary CPT codes for emerging technology, services, and procedures. If available, these codes should be used instead of the *unlisted codes* found throughout the CPT manual.

When no code is available to completely describe a procedure, a code for an unlisted procedure is selected. Unlisted procedure codes are used for new services or procedures that have not yet been assigned codes in CPT. When these codes are used, which is rare, a procedure or service description (usually from the medical record) is sent with the submission of the claim.

Evaluation and Management Services

To diagnose conditions and plan treatments, physicians use a wide range of time, effort, and skill for different patients and circumstances. Evaluation and management codes (**E/M codes**) are often considered the most important of all CPT codes because they can be used by all physicians in any medical specialty.

The E/M section guidelines explain how to code different levels of these services. Three key factors documented in the patient's medical record help determine the level of service:

1. The extent of the patient history taken
2. The extent of the examination conducted
3. The complexity of the medical decision making

Payers also want to know whether the physician treated a **new patient** or an **established patient.** Physicians often spend more time during new patients' visits than during visits from established patients, so the E/M codes for the two types of patients are separate for some of the E/M codes. For reporting purposes, the CPT considers a patient "new" if that person has not received professional services from the physician within the past three years. An established patient is one who has seen the physician within the past three years. Most insurers also consider a patient to be an established patient if, within the past three years, she had seen a different physician in the same practice with the same specialty as the "new" physician she is seeing. Emergency patients are not classified as either new or established patients.

The CPT has a range of five codes each for new patient or established patient encounters. The lowest-level code is often called a Level I code; the highest-level code is a Level V code. For example, code 99213 is the Level III code for an established patient's office visit. The higher the level, the more labor-intensive the service, the higher the reimbursement.

The location of the service is also important because different E/M codes apply to services performed in a physician's office or other outpatient location, a hospital inpatient room, a hospital emergency department, a nursing facility, an extended-care facility, or a patient's home.

Surgical Procedures

Figure 16-2 illustrated a series of codes from the integumentary part of the surgical section. Codes listed in the surgery section represent all the procedures that are normally a part of that operation, including preoperative testing, local anesthesia, the surgery itself, and routine follow-up care. This combination of services is called a *surgical package.* Payers assign a fee to each of these packaged codes that pays for all the services provided in this package. If other than local anesthesia is used, an anesthesia code would be used by the anesthesiologist billing for his services.

The period of time that is covered for follow-up care is called the **global period.** For example, the global period for repairing a tendon might be set at 15 days. A global period for major surgery such as an appendectomy might be set at 100 days. During the global period, any care provided related to the surgical procedure is included in the surgical fee and cannot be billed separately; any attempt to do so is called *unbundling* and is considered fraud. If a patient is seen for an unrelated problem, the procedure may be billed separately using a modifier (24 for E/M services, 79 for a surgical procedure), identifying the procedure as being unrelated. After the global period ends, additional services related to the initial surgery can be reported separately for payment.

To make the coding process more efficient, medical offices often list frequently used procedures and their applicable CPT codes on superbills. After seeing the patient, the physician checks off the appropriate procedures or services. An example of a dermatology practice's superbill is shown in Figure 16-4. This sample superbill lists the E/M codes for

VALLEY ASSOCIATES, P.C.
David Rosenberg, M.D. - Dermatology
555-321-0987
FED I.D. #06-2345678

PATIENT NAME				APPT. DATE/TIME			
Scott Yeager				10/14/12		11:00am	

PATIENT NO.				DX			
YEAGESCO				1. 919.7 superficial foreign body without 2. major open wound. Infected 3. 4.			

DESCRIPTION	✓	CPT	FEE	DESCRIPTION	✓	CPT	FEE
EXAMINATION				PROCEDURES			
New Patient				Acne Surgery		10040	
Problem Focused		99201		I&D Cyst/Abscess		10060	
Expanded Problem Focused	✓	99202	50	I&D Multiple		10061	
Detailed		99203		I&D Remove Foreign Body	✓	10120	60
Comprehensive		99204		Debridement		11000	
Comprehensive/Complex		99205		Paring/Curett. (Benign)		11055	
Established Patient				Paring/Curett. (2-4)		11056	
Minimum		99211		Paring/Curett. (Over 4)		11057	
Problem Focused		99212		Excision Skin Tags (1-15)		11200	
Expanded Problem Focused		99213		Cyrosurgery		17340	
Detailed		99214		Skin Biopsy		11100	
Comprehensive/Complex		99215		Skin Biopsy (EA additional)		+11101	

Figure 16-4. Superbill with procedure codes.

new and established patient office visits as well as common procedures for the office. If superbills are used in the office, it is important to remember to update both the ICD-9 and CPT codes on the superbills and in any computer programs when the new codes are available each year (October for ICD-9 codes and January for CPT codes).

Laboratory Procedures

Organ or disease-oriented **panels** listed in the pathology and laboratory section of the CPT include tests frequently ordered together. An electrolyte panel, for example, includes tests for carbon dioxide, chloride, potassium, and sodium. Each element of the panel has its own procedure code. However, when the tests are performed together, the code for the panel must be used rather than the separate procedure codes. To code a panel correctly, the physician must order each test listed within the panel and there must be a need for each of them. If a panel is appropriate but one or two laboratory tests are also ordered that are not included in the panel, code the panel and then the additional tests separately.

If each test in a panel or procedure in a surgical package is listed separately, it will cause unbundling of the panel or package. The review performed by the insurance carrier's claims department will rebundle the services under the appropriate code, which could delay payment. Remember that when unbundling is done intentionally or repeatedly to receive more payment than is correct, you and the practice can come under investigation for fraud.

Immunizations

Injections and infusions of immune globulins, vaccines, toxoids, and other substances require two codes, one for giving the injection and one for the particular vaccine or toxoid that is given. An E/M code is not used along with the codes for immunization unless a significant evaluation and management service is also performed and documented appropriately by the doctor. Modifier 59 would be appended to the E/M code in this case indicating the need for both procedures.

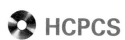 **HCPCS**

The **Health Care Common Procedure Coding System,** commonly referred to as **HCPCS,** was developed by the Centers for Medicare and Medicaid Services (CMS) for use in coding services for Medicare patients. The HCPCS (pronounced "hic-picks") coding system has two levels:

1. HCPCS Level I codes are more commonly known as CPT codes.
2. **HCPCS Level II codes,** issued by CMS, are called national codes and cover many supplies, such as sterile trays, drugs, injections, and DME (durable medical equipment). If both CPT and HCPCS have an appropriate code, the HCPCS Level II code should be used, especially for Medicare claims, because they are

generally more specific then the CPT codes. Level II codes also cover services and procedures not included in the CPT.

The HCPCS codes for Level II have five characters, either numbers, letters, or a combination of both. At times there are also two-character modifiers, either two letters or a letter with a number. These modifiers are different from the CPT modifiers, but may be used with CPT codes as well as with Level II codes. For example, HCPCS modifiers may indicate social worker services or equipment rentals.

Examples of Level II codes are:

Code Number	Description
A0225-QN	Ambulance service, neonatal transport, base rate, emergency transport, one way, furnished directly by the provider of services
E0781	Ambulatory infusion pump
G0001	Routine venipuncture
G0104	Colorectal cancer screening; flexible sigmoidoscopy
Q0091	Screening Papanicolaou (Pap) smear; obtaining, preparing, and conveyance of cervical or vaginal smear to laboratory
V5299	Hearing service, miscellaneous

In medical offices where the HCPCS system is used, regulations issued by CMS are reviewed to determine the correct code and modifier for use on a particular payers' claims. Procedure 16-2 outlines the steps for locating a HCPCS code.

Using the CPT

Before you can use the CPT manual, you must first become familiar with the format and guidelines regarding the use of CPT. To begin with, read the introduction and main section guidelines and notes for each section. For example, look at the guidelines for the evaluation and management section. They include definitions of key terms, such as *new* and *established patient, chief complaint, concurrent care,* and *counseling.* They also explain the method for selecting E/M codes. You may find it helpful to actually highlight important information within the guidelines and section notes.

The next step is to find the procedures and services provided by the office. As with diagnosis codes, these may be found on the superbill, but remember to check the patient's chart to verify that documentation on the procedures and services exists within the medical chart (if it is not written down, it did not happen). When coding E/M codes, remember that you must keep in mind *where* the service took place, as well as whether the patient is a new client or an established one. You may find it easiest to go directly to the E/M section in the front of the CPT manual to choose the correct code. For all other procedures, you will need to use the alphabetic listing of procedures found in the back of the CPT manual.

The number or number range in the index to the right of the description represents the coding possibilities

PROCEDURE 16-2

Locating a HCPCS Code

Procedure Goal: To locate the proper HCPCS code for a service or piece of equipment

Materials: HCPCS manual, patient record, charge slip or superbill

Method:

1. Locate the service, supplies, and equipment requiring a HCPCS code from the charge slip or from the patient's record.

Rationale

The charge slip or superbill usually identifies the procedure performed. However, having the patient's record nearby makes it convenient to identify more details about the services, and so on.

2. Use the index at the back of the manual to locate the section in which the category of codes is found.

3. Find the code or code range by seeking first the initial letter and then the four-digit number. They are arranged alphabetically and numerically. Make sure you read the description thoroughly and determine the correct code. Do not code from the index.

Rationale

You cannot be sure that you have identified the correct code without reading the description of the code. You also may find additional information in the section to help you code properly.

4. Make sure the code is valid for the type of insurance the patient carries.

Rationale

Some HCPCS codes are valid for some insurers, but invalid for others, particularly Medicare and Medicaid.

5. Enter the correct code(s) on the superbill or charge slip, encounter form (if necessary), and, if the office uses a computerized billing program, in the patient's computerized record so that it can be used for billing purposes. Otherwise, the codes will be stored on the encounter form to be inserted appropriately on the insurance claim form.

Rationale

Reimbursement is made by insurance companies on the basis of the codes that are submitted. They *must* be accurate and reflect the service or procedure that is performed.

---

for the description. If a hyphen is between 2 codes, this indicates a code range and each code in the range will need to be checked in the numeric index to choose the correct code. Code numbers with commas between them indicate that there is more than one location possibility. Again, all codes will have to be checked. In some cases, the patient's medical record may show an abbreviation, an *eponym* (a person or place for which a procedure is named), or a synonym. For example, the record might state "treated for bone infection." In CPT's index, the entry for "Infection, Bone," is followed by the instruction "See Osteomyelitis." The greater your knowledge of anatomy and physiology and terminology, the easier it will be for you to code.

Example 1: To find the code for "dressing change," first look alphabetically in the index for that procedure. Then find the procedure code in the body of the CPT to be sure the code accurately reflects the service performed. The procedure code 15852 explains the dressing change is for "other than burns" and "under anesthesia (other than local)." (A dressing change without anesthesia would be included in an E/M code.) Per the notes in CPT, a dressing for a burn is found in procedure codes 16010–16030.

Example 2: To code the excision of a vaginal cyst, you would first look under "Excision" (the main term). There is a listing for the subterm "Cyst" beneath "Excision," followed by a list of organs, regions, or structures involved. Note that each subterm is indented under the main term. Additionally, the subterms relating to cyst locations are indented even further under that subterm. This is a common occurrence in the CPT manual. Look for "Vagina" to find the code (57135). Another way to find the code is to look under "Vagina" as the main term and then find the listing for "Cyst Excision" as a subterm beneath it.

Once you decide on the appropriate CPT code(s), the next step is to check for any applicable modifiers. The use of modifiers can greatly enhance your reimbursement and can cut down on claim inquiries from the insurance carrier, but the ability to use modifiers correctly and proficiently will require practice. Appendix A contains all CPT modifiers and many times the section guidelines also contain information regarding the use of modifiers within that section. This is not an optional step. Modifier use is required if there is one that is available for the situation.

Example: A bilateral breast reconstruction requires the modifier -50. Find the code for "breast reconstruction

PROCEDURE 16-3

Locating a CPT Code

Procedure Goal: To locate correct CPT codes

Materials: Patient record, superbill or charge slip, CPT manual

Method:

1. Find the services listed on the superbill (if used) and in the patient's record.

   a. Check the patient's record to see which services were documented. For E/M procedures, look for clues as to the location of the service, extent of history, examination, and medical decision making that were involved.

   Rationale
   Every billed procedure or service must be backed up by the medical record.

2. Look up the procedure code(s) in the alphabetic index of the CPT manual.

   a. Verify the code number in the numeric index, reading all notes and guidelines for that section.

   b. If a code range is noted, look up the range and choose the correct code from the range given. If the correct description is not found, start the process again. Use the same process if multiple codes are given.

   Rationale
   CPT codes must accurately reflect the services or procedures provided to the patient. Payment is based on the codes chosen and must be backed up by the medical record.

3. Determine appropriate modifiers.

   a. Check section guidelines and Appendix A to choose a modifier if needed to explain a situation involving the procedure being coded, such as bilateral procedure, surgical team, or a discontinued procedure.

   Rationale
   The goal of coding is specificity. Modifiers, when available for the circumstance, provide specificity to CPT codes.

4. Carefully record the procedure code(s) on the health-care claim. Usually the primary procedure, the one that is the primary reason for the encounter or visit, is listed first.

   Rationale
   Checking for transposed figures is important as the code they produce could represent procedures other than those performed, affecting claim status and reimbursement.

5. Match each procedure with its corresponding diagnosis. The primary procedure is often (but not always) matched with the primary diagnosis.

   Rationale
   Matching each procedure to the correct diagnosis gives the insurance carrier the reason the procedure was done, which verifies medical necessity.

with free flap": 19364. To show the insurance carrier that the procedure was performed on both breasts, attach the -50: 19364-50. (Some insurers will require that you list the code once and then a second time with the modifier: 19364, 19364-50.) The insurance company will often pay the full charge for the first procedure and then pay the second procedure at 50%.

Once all procedures and services have been assigned a CPT code and modifier as needed, carefully enter the 5-digit code(s) and modifiers in the appropriate area of the CMS-1500 form. After the procedure code is verified, it is posted to the health-care claim. The primary procedure, often the one that is most labor intensive or is the principal reason for the patient's encounter, is listed first and is often matched with the primary diagnosis.

Be sure to match up each procedure with its applicable diagnosis. This step verifies medical necessity for the insurance carrier.

Procedure 16-3 outlines the correct steps for locating a CPT code.

Avoiding Fraud: Coding Compliance

Physicians have the ultimate responsibility for proper documentation and correct coding as well as for compliance with regulations, and many expect their medical assistants to have working knowledge of this as well. Medical assistants help ensure maximum appropriate reimbursement for reported services by submitting correct health-care claims. These claims, as well as the process used to create them, must comply with the rules imposed by federal and state law and with payer requirements.

Code Linkage

On correct claims, each reported service is connected to a diagnosis that supports the procedure as necessary to investigate or treat the patient's condition. Insurance company representatives analyze this connection between the diagnostic and the procedural information, called **code linkage,** to evaluate the medical necessity of the reported charges. Correct claims also comply with many other regulations from government agencies.

The possible consequences of inaccurate coding and incorrect billing include:

- Denied claims
- Delays in processing claims and receiving payments
- Reduced payments
- Fines and other sanctions
- Loss of hospital privileges
- Exclusion from payers' programs
- Prison sentences
- Loss of the physician's license to practice medicin

To avoid errors, the codes on health-care claims are checked against the medical documentation. A code review, also known as a coding audit, checks these key points:

- Are the codes appropriate to the patient's profile (age, gender, condition; new or established), and is each coded service billable?
- Is there a clear and correct link between each diagnosis and procedure?
- Have the payer's rules about the diagnosis and the procedure been followed?
- Does the documentation in the patient's medical record support the reported services?
- Do the reported services comply with all regulations?

Insurance Fraud

The majority involved in the delivery of health care are trustworthy persons devoted to patients' welfare. However, some people are not. For example, according to the Department of Health and Human Services (DHHS), in 1 year alone, the federal government recovered more than $1.3 billion in judgments, settlements, and other fees in health-care fraud cases. Fraud is an act of deception used to take advantage of another person or entity. For example, it is fraudulent for people to misrepresent their credentials or to forge another person's signature on a check.

Claims fraud occurs when physicians or others falsely represent their services or charges to payers. For example, a provider may bill for services that were not performed (phantom billing), overcharge for services, or fail to provide complete services under a contract. A patient may exaggerate an injury to get a settlement from an insurance company or ask a medical assistant to change a date on a chart so that a service is covered by a health plan.

A number of coding and billing practices are fraudulent. Investigators reviewing physicians' billings look for patterns like these:

- Reporting services that were not performed.

  Example: A lab bills Medicare for a general health panel (CPT 80050), but fails to perform one of the tests in the panel.

- Reporting services at a higher level than was carried out.

  Example: After a visit for a flu shot, the provider bills the encounter as an evaluation and management service plus an injection

- Performing and billing for procedures that are not related to the patient's condition and therefore not medically necessary.

  Example: After reading an article about Lyme disease, a patient is worried about having worked in her garden over the summer and requests a Lyme disease diagnostic test. Although no symptoms or signs have been reported, the physician orders and bills for the Lyme disease test.

- Billing separately for services that are bundled in a single procedure code.

  Example: When a physician orders a comprehensive metabolic panel (CPT 80053), the provider bills for the panel as well as for a quantitative glucose test, which is in the panel.

- Reporting the same service twice.

Note that HIPAA calls for penalties for giving remuneration to anyone eligible for benefits under federal health-care programs. The forgiveness or waiver of copayments may violate the policies of some payers; others may permit forgiveness or waiver if they are aware of the reasons for the forgiveness or waiver, such as the patient's inability to pay (be sure to have documentation of such inability to avoid charges of discrimination). Routine forgiveness or waiver of copayments or deductibles constitutes fraud when billing federal programs such as Medicare or TRICARE. The physician practice should ensure that its policies on copayments are consistent with applicable law and with the requirements of their agreements with payers.

Compliance Plans

To avoid the risk of fraud, medical offices have a **compliance plan** to uncover compliance problems and correct them. A compliance plan is a process for finding, correcting, and preventing illegal medical office practices. Its goals are to:

- Prevent fraud and abuse through a formal process to identify, investigate, fix, and prevent repeat violations relating to reimbursement for health-care services provided
- Ensure compliance with applicable federal, state, and local laws, including employment laws and environmental laws as well as antifraud laws

Medical Coder, Physician Practice

Medical coding specialists work in a number of health-care settings, including medical practices, hospitals, government agencies, and insurance companies. Coders who work in physician practices review patients' medical records and assign diagnosis and procedure codes. They are knowledgeable about the coding rules and procedures for physicians' work, which are different than those for coding hospital services. The position of medical coding specialist is growing in importance in physician practices. Accurate coding is a critical part of ensuring that claims follow the legal and ethical requirements of Medicare and other third-party payers as well as HIPAA regulations. Accurate coding also ensures optimum reimbursement for submitted claims.

Medical office employees may gain required health-care work experience and then attain coding positions through coding education from seminars or college classes. Certification as a professional coder offers an excellent route to success as a medical coder in the medical practice setting. Some employers require certification for employment; others state that certification must be earned after a certain amount of time in the position, such as 6 months. Coding classes followed by examinations are used to obtain certification. Three physician-office coding certifications are available. All require a high school diploma or equivalent.

- The American Health Information Management Association offers the Certified Coding Associate (CCA) credential and the Certified Coding Specialist—Physician-based (CCS-P) credential. The CCA is an entry-level title; completion of either a training program or 6 months' job experience is recommended. The CCS-P requires at least 3 years of coding experience.

- The American Academy of Professional Coders offers the Certified Professional Coder (CPC) credential, also requiring coursework and on-the- job experience. AAPC also offers an entry-level certification, the CPC-A (apprentice). Once documentation of two years of work experience as a coder is received and if the CPC-A maintains the required number of CEUs (continuing education units), the credential will be converted to a CPC.

Medical assistants who hold these credentials and have coding experience may advance to coding management and coding compliance auditor positions. Becoming expert in a specialty such as surgical coding also offers advancement opportunities.

- Help defend physicians if they are investigated or prosecuted for fraud by showing the desire to behave compliantly and thus reduce any fines or criminal prosecution

When a compliance plan is in place, it demonstrates to payers such as Medicare that honest, ongoing attempts have been made to find and fix weak areas of compliance with regulations. The development of this written plan is led by a compliance officer and committee with the intention to (1) audit and monitor compliance with government regulations, especially in the area of coding and billing; (2) develop written policies and procedures that are consistent; (3) provide for ongoing staff training and communication; and (4) respond to and correct errors.

Although coding and billing compliance are the plan's major focus, it covers all areas of government regulation of medical practices, such as equal employment opportunity (EEO) regulations (for example, hiring and promotion policies) and OSHA regulations (for example, fire safety and handling of hazardous materials such as bloodborne pathogens). For further information, go to www.oig.hhs.gov/fraud/docs/complianceguidance/thirdparty.pdf.

Summary

16.1 The purpose of the ICD-9-CM manual is to find diagnosis codes for patients' medical conditions. It is formatted with the Alphabetic Index (Volume 2) and the Tabular List (Volume 1).

16.2 To analyze diagnoses think about the condition first and then think about the affected body part or location. This will assist you in finding the correct codes much more easily. Locate the diagnosis description in the alphabetic index and then verify the code in the tabular index.

16.3 The CPT-4 is used for locating medical procedure codes. It is organized from Evaluation/Management (E/M) sections to Medicine sections. The alphabetic index is found in the back of the book and the numeric index is in the front.

16.4 The three levels that determine E/M service are the extent of patient history taken; the extent of the exam conducted; and the complexity of the medical decision making.

16.5 The two types of HCPCS codes are Level I codes (also called CPT codes) and Level II codes, which are national codes describing services, procedures, equipment, and supplies either not listed in CPT or containing more detail than CPT.

16.6 In locating a procedure code, you first become familiar with the format and guidelines. First look up the procedure description in the alphabetic listing in the back of the CPT manual. Then verify the correct code, codes, or code range in the numeric index. For detailed information in completing this process, see Procedure 16-3.

16.7 Medical codes must be correctly linked (one diagnosis for each procedure) when reporting them for reimbursement because payers analyze this connection to determine the medical necessity for the charge.

16.8 Insurance fraud is an act of deception used to take advantage of another entity. An example of billing and coding fraud is when a physician reports services that were not performed.

REVIEW

CHAPTER 16

CASE STUDY QUESTIONS

Now that you have completed this chapter, review the case study at the beginning of the chapter and answer the following questions:

1. How would you select the ICD-9 and CPT codes for a health-care claim for this visit?
2. What diagnosis and procedure codes will result in the correct payment for these services?
3. How should the claim show the medical necessity of the procedures?
4. Locate the ICD-9 code for the patient's asthma. How many digits are required? What code did you assign?
5. Locate the CPT code for the cardiovascular stress test. What information did you use to select it from the list of related codes?

Multiple-Choice Questions

1. The Alphabetic Index for ICD-9-CM is organized by
   a. the part of the body involved.
   b. symptoms the patient displays.
   c. codes found in the Tabular List.
   d. the condition.
2. The Tabular List of ICD-9-CM is organized by
   a. the condition of the patient.
   b. the codes found in the Alphabetic Index.
   c. the symptoms of the patient.
   d. the part of the body involved.
3. The _____ codes are considered to be the most important of the CPT codes.
   a. modifier   c. add-on
   b. E/M   d. unlisted procedure

4. For reporting purposes, CPT considers a patient "new" if he or she has not received professional services within the past _____ year(s).
   a. one   c. three
   b. two   d. five
5. The Health Care Common Procedure Coding System (HCPCS) was developed for use in coding services for
   a. Blue Cross.
   b. HMOs.
   c. Medicare patients.
   d. Managed care organizations.

Discussion Questions

1. What are the differences among the three code sets discussed in the chapter?
2. Are see cross-references in the Alphabetic Index of the ICD-9 followed by codes? Why?
3. Would you expect to locate codes for the following services or procedures in CPT? What range or series of codes would you investigate?
   a. Routine obstetric care including antepartum care, cesarean delivery, and postpartum care
   b. Echocardiography (cardiac)
   c. Radiologic examination, nasal bones, complete
   d. Home visit for evaluation and management of an established patient
   e. Drug test for amphetamines
   f. Anesthesia for cardiac catheterization
4. Why are both the ICD-9 and CPT codes updated each year?
5. What three main changes in coding are included in the ICD-10-CM revision?
6. What is the value of modifiers in coding?

1. What is the proper order in which to select a diagnosis code?
2. What are some of the possible consequences of inaccurate coding and incorrect billing?
3. Why is accurate coding important to the financial management of a medical practice?
4. How can improving physicians' documentation of diagnoses and procedures help ensure compliance?
5. A patient asked a medical assistant to help her out of a tough financial spot. Her medical insurance authorized her to receive four radiation treatments for her condition, one every 35 days. Because she was out of town, she did not schedule her appointment for the last treatment until today, which is 1 week beyond the approved period. The health plan will not reimburse her for this procedure. The patient asks the MA to change the date on the record to last Wednesday so that it will be covered, explaining that no one will be hurt by this change, and anyway, she pays the insurance company plenty.

    What type of action is the patient asking the MA to do? How should the request be handled?
6. What does the existence of a compliance plan in the workplace indicate about the medical practice?

1. A. A female patient is taking a medication that is known to affect the lining of the endometrium. She received an endometrial biopsy and pelvic ultrasound to monitor changes. What type of ICD-9 code is used to describe the medical need for these services?

    B. A patient fell off a ladder while on the job, spraining his left ankle and fracturing the right femur. In addition to the main code, what type of ICD-9 code is used to report his diagnosis?
2. Review Figure 16-2. What is the correct code for nail debridement?
3. Underline the main term in each of the following diagnoses and then determine the correct ICD-9 codes.
    a. Cerebral atherosclerosis
    b. Spasmodic asthma with status asthmaticus
    c. Congenital night blindness
    d. Recurrent inguinal hernia with obstruction
    e. Incomplete bundle branch heart block
4. Find the following codes in the index of CPT. Underline the key term you used to find the code.
    a. Intracapsular lens extraction
    b. Coombs test
    c. X-ray of duodenum
    d. Unlisted procedure, maxillofacial prosthetics
    e. DTAP immunization
5. Review Table 16-1, Tabular List Organization. What is the category number range for congenital abnormalities?
6. According to Figure 16-1, the ICD Alphabetic Index and Tabular List, what is the diagnosis code for Trichocephalus infestation?
7. According to Figure 16-4, the superbill with procedure codes, what is the correct code for a detailed evaluation of a new patient?

Visit the McGraw-Hill Higher Education Medical Assisting website at www.mhhe.com/medicalassisting4e to complete the following activity:

Use the American Association of Medical Assistants and other websites related to medical practice coding. Prepare an oral presentation about one of the following topics:

- Code structuring
- The Alphabetic Index and its use
- The Tabular List and its use
- Special codes such as V codes and E codes
- A career in medical billing

Ask your instructor how many references and citations you should minimally include in your research. Present your report to the class, using all available multimedia including PowerPoint slides or an overhead projector if possible.

Open the CD and complete this chapter's practice activities, play the games, listen to the key terms, and test yourself with the interactive review. E-mail, print, and/or save your results to document your proficiency.

Patient Billing and Collections

MEDICAL ASSISTING COMPETENCIES

CAAHEP

VI. C (9) Explain both billing and payment options

VI. C (13) Discuss types of adjustments that may be made to a patient's account

VII. C (8) Compare processes for filing insurance claims both manually and electronically

VII. C (9) Describe guidelines for third-party claims

VII. P (2) Apply third-party guidelines

VII. A (1) Demonstrate assertive communication with managed care and/or insurance providers

VII. A (2) Demonstrate sensitivity in communicating with both providers and patients

IX. C (6) Describe liability, professional, personal injury, and third-party insurance

ABHES

8. Medical Office Business Procedures Management
  i. Perform billing and collections procedures
  r. Apply third-party guidelines
 ee. Use proper telephone techniques
 hh. Receive, organize, prioritize, and transmit information expediently

11. Career Development
Demonstrate professionalism by:
1) Exhibiting dependability, punctuality, and a positive work ethic
3) Maintaining confidentiality at all times
5) Exhibiting initiative
7) Expressing a responsible attitude

LEARNING OUTCOMES

After completing Chapter 17, you will be able to:

17.1 Explain the importance of accounts receivable to a medical practice.

17.2 Model how to accept and account for payment from patients.

17.3 Execute a patient statement.

17.4 Execute a billing cycle efficiently.

17.5 Use standard collection techniques.

17.6 Explain how to perform a credit check.

17.7 Identify credit arrangements.

17.8 Describe common collection problems.

MEDICAL ASSISTING MEDIA

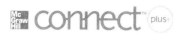 **Connect Plus+™**
connect.mcgraw-hill.com

- Electronic Health Records (E.H.R.) SpringCharts®
- eBook

SPRINGCHARTS

LearnSmart **LearnSmart™**   www.mhhe.com/learnsmart   Complete Learning Module: Patient Billing and Collections

 Student CD-ROM

Online
LearningCenter **Online Learning Center™**   www.mhhe.com/medicalassisting4e

KEY TERMS

accounts payable (A/P)	credit bureau	overpayment
accounts receivable (A/R)	cycle billing	punitive damages
age analysis	damages	single-entry account
charge slip	disclosure statement	statement
class action lawsuit	encounter form	statute of limitations
credit	legal custody	superbill
credit balance	open-book account	written-contract account

CHAPTER OUTLINE

- Basic Accounting
- Standard Payment Procedures
- Standard Billing Procedures
- Standard Collection Procedures
- Credit Arrangements
- Common Collection Problems

PREPARATION FOR CERTIFICATION

RMA (AMT) Exam
- Collection procedures
- Patient billing procedures
- Medical insurance terminology

CMA (AAMA) Exam
- Applying managed care policies and procedures
- Accounts receivable (billing procedures, aging/collection procedures)
- Processing claims (tracing claims)

CMAS Exam
- Insurance billing and finances
- Patient accounts

Introduction

Medical assisting is a multifaceted career. As such, a person in that career may be required to take on many duties in the medical office that are administrative in nature. The medical office has customers who have various payment arrangements, such as third-party payers (usually insurance carriers) and payment plans, and who may also have large outstanding balances. A proper understanding and administration of billing—for both third-party payers and patients—as well as payment collection methods is therefore required.

Basic Accounting

In any business, basic accounting involves managing accounts receivable and accounts payable. **Accounts receivable (A/R)** is the term for income, or money, owed to the business. **Accounts payable (A/P)** is the term for money owed by the business. In a medical practice, accounts receivable represents the money patients owe in return for medical services. Accounts payable describes the money the medical practice must pay out to run the practice.

Billing and collections are vitally important tasks because they convert the practice's accounts receivable into income, or cash flow, from which the accounts payable can be paid. Unless billing and collections are carried out effectively, a practice might have plenty of money due in accounts receivable without having enough cash flow for accounts payable.

There are methods of improving billing and collection procedures to increase income for the practice. You will need to know about standard payment, billing, and collection procedures as well as about credit arrangements and common problems in collecting payment.

Standard Payment Procedures

Most physicians prefer to collect payment from patients at each office visit particularly if the money owed to the practice is in the form of co-payment, which is a small sum owed by the patient for each visit as their part of the insurance contract for most HMOs and PPOs. Immediate payment not only brings income into the practice faster, but it saves the cost of preparing and mailing bills and collecting on past-due accounts. For these reasons, many physicians' offices post a small sign at the reception desk that states, for example, "Payment is requested when services are rendered unless other arrangements are made in advance."

As a medical assistant, you are responsible for collecting these payments. If the patient cannot pay at the time of the visit, it may be your responsibility to bill for the physician's services. A bill, the paperwork sent to patients to inform them of payment or balance due, is referred to as a statement.

Determining Appropriate Fees

A fee schedule is a price list for the medical practice. Figure 17-1 shows an example. The fee schedule lists the services the doctor offers and the corresponding charges for those services. Fees are not randomly assigned. They reflect the cost of services, the doctor's experience, charges of other doctors in the area, and other factors. Sometimes the fee allowed by insurance policies is a determining factor. The practice may use a particular system to determine how much to charge for each service. Following are descriptions of these systems.

Usual and Customary Fees. A usual fee is the fee a doctor normally charges for a service or procedure. A customary fee is either the average fee charged for a service or procedure by all comparable doctors in the same region or the 90th percentile of all fees charged by comparable doctors in the same region for the same procedure. There is a growing tendency, however, to determine fees by national rather than regional trends.

Relative Value Unit. Section 121 of the Social Security Act Amendments of 1994 required CMS to develop a methodology for a resource-based system. This system was created to determine practice expense relative value units (RVUs) for all Medicare physician fee schedule services. Effective January 1, 1999, Phase 1 of resource-based practice expense was put into effect.

For each medical service, an RVU is assigned that reflects the following factors:

- The doctor's skill and time required
- The professional liability expenses related to that service, such as malpractice insurance
- The overhead costs associated with that service

The RVUs are converted to dollar amounts. These dollar amounts form the basis of the RVU fee schedule. This schedule creates uniform payments that are adjusted for geographic differences.

This methodology has reduced the growth rate of spending for doctors' professional services, related services and supplies, and other Medicare Part B services.

John Q. Davis, MD

Adult and Pediatric Urology-Infertility

SERVICE RENDERED	CPT	FEE
Initial OV	99204	$100.00
Follow-up Visit	99214	$65.00
Fertility Consultation	99243	$140.00
Office Consultation	99244	$140.00
Hospital Admission	99223	$150.00
Hospital Consultation	99254	$150.00
ER Visit	99284	$75.00–$150.00
Hospital Visit	99232	$55.00
Urinalysis w/ Micro	81000	$14.00
Culture	87086	$45.00
Stone Analysis	32360	$60.00
Venipuncture	36415	$10.00

SERVICE RENDERED	CPT	FEE
Condyloma Treatment	54050	$40.00
Cystoscopy	52000	$300.00
Catheterization	93975	$45.00
Vasectomy	55250	$775.00
Ultrasonic Guide Needle Biopsy	76942	$395.00
Prostate Biopsy	55700	$325.00
Biopsy Gun	A9270	$45.00
Uroflowmeter	51741	$80.00
Renal Ultrasound	76775	$295.00
Scrotal Ultrasound	76870	$295.00
Acidic Acid	99070	$20.00
Foley Catheter Starter Set	A4329	$35.00

Figure 17-1. The fee schedule shows the charges for services provided by the practice.

DATE	DESCRIPTION-CODE	CHARGE	PAYMENT	CURRENT BALANCE

(918) 555-9680   Tax ID No. 11-0004004

Patricia Belden, MD
111 Roosevelt Boulevard
Lawrence, OK 77527

99205	Office Visit, New Patient	36425	Venipuncture	59025	NST
99215	Office Visit, Established Patient	57454	Colposcopy with Biopsy	54150	Circumcision
99213	Office Visit, Established, Brief	57511	Cryosurgery	58300	IUD Insertion
88155	Pap	58100	Endometrial Biopsy	57170	Diaphragm Fitting
84703	Urine Pregnancy Test	56600	Vulva Biopsy		

NAME _____ DX _____   No. 0005807

Figure 17-2. A charge slip shows the services performed for a patient and the charges for those services.

You may refer back to Chapter 15 for more detailed information on RVUs and the RBRVS system that calculates the final allowable charge for Medicare, and increasingly for other payers as well.

Processing Charge Slips

Fees must be determined in order to create a **charge slip**, the original record of the doctor's services and the charges for those services. Figure 17-2 shows an example of a charge slip. Charge slips are also called fee slips, encounter forms, or transaction slips. They are usually numbered consecutively. Charge slips that are preprinted with common services, CPT, and ICD-9 codes, and charges for the practice are known as "superbills" because they contain all of the information needed to submit a claim form to the insurance carrier. Superbills will be discussed in more detail later in the chapter. Charge slips are used in several ways.

Some doctors keep a pad of charge slips on their desk. After seeing a patient, they fill in the services and charges on the charge slip. They give the charge slip to the patient and ask the patient to give it to you on the way out of the office.

In other offices, you may write the patient's name on the charge slip and give the slip to the doctor along with the patient's medical record. In practices with computerized billing systems, the superbills are often included in the program. When a patient arrives in the office, with a few clicks of the mouse or a few key strokes a superbill is produced with the patient's name and insurance information printed on it. The doctor then fills in the services performed and asks you to fill in the charges according to the fee schedule. If questions arise about the fee for a particular service, you can refer to the fee schedule and tell the patient how much that service will cost.

Accepting Payment

When the patient comes to you with the charge slip, you complete the charge slip and ask for payment. There are several effective yet diplomatic ways to request payment. Two examples are, "For today's visit, the total charge is $50. How would you like to pay?" and "The charge for your laboratory work today is $80. Would you like to pay for that now?" The first example is the preferred method because in the second example, asking the patient if he would like to pay for the service now leaves him open to say, "No, bill me," which will slow your cash flow and cost the practice the expense of sending an invoice. Most practices accept several forms of payment, including cash, check, debit card, credit card, and insurance. Insurance payment is discussed in detail in Chapter 15.

Cash. If the patient chooses to pay in cash, count the money carefully to be sure you have received the proper amount. Next, record the payment on the patient's ledger card or, with a computerized system, credit the patient's account as per system instructions and give the patient a receipt. (Patient ledger cards are explained in Chapter 18.)

Once the money is posted to the account, a computerized billing program will give you the option of printing a receipt which you can give to the patient. A superbill, a carbonless form consisting of 2–3 copies, automatically creates a receipt, as one of the copies is given to the patient. If your office does not use either of these methods, prepare a cash receipt manually, as shown in Figure 17-3. Be sure that whatever method is used, the office also retains a copy of the receipt. Then place the money in the cash drawer or cash box.

No. ______ Date ______________, 20______

Received of ______________________________

____

________________________________ Dollars

For Professional Services Amount Account $______

This Payment $______

Balance $______

Thank You!

Lauren Harris, MD

Medical Arts Bldg. 117 City Line Road Newtown, NJ 08944 (201) 555-0000

Figure 17-3. After writing a receipt for cash, record the payment on the patient's ledger card.

Check. If the patient pays by check, be sure the check is written properly, including the current date. The amount of the check should match the total amount listed on the charge slip, unless the patient has made prior arrangements to pay only part of the amount. The name of the doctor or practice should appear in the "Pay to the Order of" section and should be properly spelled. The check should be signed by the person whose name is printed on the check. After accepting the check, endorse it immediately, and deposit it in the practice bank account. If a check is returned for insufficient funds, notify the patient immediately, asking for payment in full by another payment method. It is acceptable to also charge the patient an additional fee for the inconvenience and expense of processing the bad check. Most offices then see that patient on a *cash-only* basis unless the patient can provide a current credit card.

Debit Card. Some patients may pay through the use of a debit card. A debit card looks like a credit card but is used differently. When the patient presents a debit card for payment, he is allowing the immediate removal of funds from his checking or savings account to the account of the practice. If there are insufficient funds in the patient's account to cover the payment, it is known immediately and other arrangements can be made with the patient. A debit card is processed much like a credit card. It is read by swiping it through an electronic reader that transmits the information to the patient's bank or credit union. The patient must input his PIN (personal identification number), which is a four-digit number, to release the funds for transfer.

Credit Card. Many doctors' offices accept credit cards, such as Visa or MasterCard. This payment method offers advantages for both the practice and the patient. For the practice, it provides prompt payment from the credit card company, thus increasing cash flow. It also reduces the amount of time and money spent on preparing and mailing invoices, thus decreasing expenses. For the patient, it is convenient and allows a large bill to be paid in several smaller amounts, usually once a month.

Credit cards have one major disadvantage for the practice—cost. The credit card company deducts a percentage of each transaction for its collection service, usually between 1% and 5%. If a patient charges $100 in services on a credit card, for example, the practice receives only $95 to $99. The credit card company keeps the difference. A disadvantage for patients is the accrued interest charges on unpaid balances.

If the practice accepts credit card payments, the American Medical Association (AMA) suggests several guidelines.

- Do not set higher fees for patients who pay by credit card.

- Do not encourage patients to use credit cards for payment.

- Do not advertise outside the office that the practice accepts credit cards.

If a patient chooses to pay by credit card, process the transaction carefully to ensure that the credit card company charges the patient correctly. To begin, inform the patient of the amount due and ask for the credit card.

Check the expiration date on the front of the credit card. If the card has expired, it cannot be used for payment. If the card has not expired, it may be swiped through an electronic reader or recorded through the use of a credit card machine that mechanically records the information on the card. To operate a credit card machine, place the credit card in the machine and place a credit card voucher on top of it. Slide the imprint arm firmly to the right and back across the machine. Remove the voucher from the machine. Write in the date and circle the type of credit card, such as Visa or MasterCard, after it is removed from the machine. Return the credit card to the patient.

Next, obtain the authorization code from the credit card company. Some offices have devices that read the magnetic strip on the credit card and automatically transmit the information to the credit card company by telephone line (Figure 17-4). If your office has such a device,

type in the amount to be charged on its keypad. Then, the credit card company issues an authorization code, which appears on the device's screen.

If your office does not have such a device, call the credit card company for the authorization code. Give the operator the patient's credit card number and the amount of the payment. The operator then gives you the authorization code.

Write the authorization code in the box marked "Authorization" on the credit card voucher. Initial the voucher in the appropriate box. Then, fill in the services provided and the amount of the charges. Enter the total charges in the box marked "Total."

Give the receipt to the patient to sign. Compare the patient's signature on the receipt with the signature on the back of the credit card (they should, of course, be identical). Keep one copy of the receipt for the office. Give the other copy and the credit card to the patient.

Using the Pegboard System for Posting Payments

While not often used, some physicians' offices still use the pegboard system to post payments and generate receipts for patients. If your office uses the pegboard system, you may use the pegboard to record the payment on the ledger card and receipt simultaneously. You handle this task in basically the same way, whether the patient pays immediately or later, in response to a bill. (See Chapter 18 for more information about pegboard systems.)

Determining Payment Responsibility

Generally the patient is responsible for payments for medical services. To help promote timely payments, however, you need to know exactly who is responsible for them.

Third-Party Liability. Third-party liability refers to the responsibility of the patient's insurance company to pay for certain medical expenses, which may include doctors' services. Each practice decides how to handle its patients' health insurance claims.

Some practices do not accept any insurance, although these practices are rare. The patient must pay the doctor directly and file an insurance claim for reimbursement. If you work in such a practice, you must give the patient the necessary medical information to fill out the insurance claim. A completed superbill or encounter form (discussed later in this chapter) provides the information.

Practices increasingly handle all their patients' insurance paperwork to ensure accuracy, timely submission, and prompt payment. Rarely practices charge a fee for handling patients' insurance claims, although for some insurance plans such as Medicare, participating providers are required to submit claim forms except under very specific circumstances. Some practices handle paperwork only for patients who find it particularly difficult, such as those who are frail or disabled.

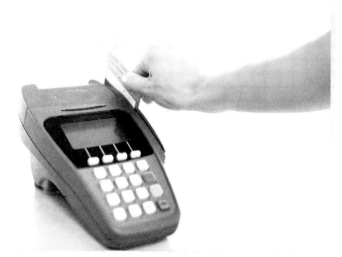

Figure 17-4. Using a device like this one, you can swipe the patient's card through the machine and obtain instant authorization from the credit card company.

If you work in an office that handles insurance paperwork, you can submit insurance claims manually or electronically. Regardless of which method you use, be sure to use the proper forms, complete them correctly, and submit them within the time limits set by insurers to ensure timely and accurate reimbursement. (Procedures for completing insurance forms and filing claims are discussed in Chapter 15.)

TRICARE, which provides health insurance for dependents of active-duty and retired military personnel, operates differently from other insurers. TRICARE pays the doctor through a local fiscal agent. TRICARE gives the service-person's dependents the choice of three plans. The plans are TRICARE Standard, TRICARE Prime, and TRICARE Extra. The Standard package is an indemnity package where TRICARE pays a percentage of allowed charges and the patient is responsible for the balance of the allowed fee. TRICARE Prime is an optional HMO-type plan, and TRICARE Extra is the PPO-like option that allows individuals to seek care from out-of-network providers on a visit-by-visit basis. As with all PPOs, this "opt-out" option allows for more freedom to choose a provider but cost is less if the patient stays in-network.

Responsibility for Minors. When a child's parents are married, either parent may consent (agree) to treatment for the minor child (child younger than age 18). Both parents are responsible for payment for the minor's treatment. If you must send them a bill, you should address it to both parents to ensure payment. There is one exception to this process. Anyone younger than the age of 18 who is no longer living at home and is self-supporting is considered an emancipated minor and is responsible for payment. For example, a 16-year-old girl who is pregnant and leaves her parents' home to set up a household with her boyfriend is considered an emancipated minor. In addition to this example, emancipation may also occur if a minor is in the military, is married, or obtains a court order.

Divorce or separation can create confusion about which parent can consent to the child's treatment and which of the two is responsible for payment. The parent who has **legal custody,** or the court-decreed right to make decisions about a child's upbringing, is the parent who has consent ability and payment responsibility. A divorced couple's legal and financial arrangements are considered private information, however. Therefore, you should assume that the parent who brings the child for treatment has consent ability and payment responsibility. The physician should inform the responsible parent of this assumption before providing treatment. Occasionally, a custodial parent brings in a minor for care and states that the other parent is responsible for medical bills. Any time someone states that someone else is responsible for his or her bill, it is important to have documentation to support the claim. Otherwise, if the office policy is that payment is due at the time of service; whoever brings the child in for treatment should expect to pay for the service at the time of the visit. Some practices have a policy of asking for a copy of the divorce agreement so that proof of responsibility for

payment can be filed in the patient record. It is important to know the policy of your medical practice.

Responsibility for Elderly Patients and Patients with Disabilities. Sometimes elderly patients or patients with disabilities are brought in for medical care. The medical assistant may be asked to send the bill to another party. In general, it is considered good practice to request proof of legal guardianship before sending the bill to another person. Always check your medical practice's policies to learn how to handle these situations correctly and confidentially.

Refunding and Overpayment. Periodically, the insurance payments and patient payments exceed the allowed charges. This is called an **overpayment.** Sometimes this happens when patients who feel they have not met their annual deductible pay their balance and then the insurance carrier also makes a payment. After posting the payments, the account balance will be a negative number, which is called a **credit balance.** When this happens, the medical office owes the patient. In some medical offices, if this amount is small they leave it in place so that the next scheduled visit's new charges will be applied against this amount. Procedure 17-1 outlines the steps for processing a credit balance.

Most times, however, the medical assistant will refund these monies to the patient. This refunded amount is notated in the patient's account, bringing the balance to zero. When this happens, the medical assistant generates a letter explaining how the overpayment occurred with the check for the refund amount. Procedure 17-2 outlines the steps for processing refunds to patients.

Professional Courtesy. Although much less common then in years past, a doctor may treat some patients free of charge or for just the amount covered by the patient's insurance. This practice is known as professional courtesy. These patients often include other doctors and their families, the practice's staff members (including medical assistants) and their families, other health-care professionals (including pharmacists and dentists), clergy members, and hospital employees. If the patient is part of a managed care organization or has Medicare, the provider must collect any copayment or deductible as part of the contracted agreement with the insurance carrier. It is considered fraud to consistently not collect copayments or deductibles if the collection of such payments is stipulated in the provider-insurer contract.

Be sure you know the doctor's policy so that you do not bill these patients in error. If, for example, the doctor agrees to accept only the amount paid by the patient's insurance, note this professional courtesy on the patient's account or ledger card and do not request payment from the patient.

Standard Billing Procedures

If the physician extends credit to patients, you need to know how to prepare invoices. You also have to manage related billing responsibilities, such as establishing and maintaining billing cycles.

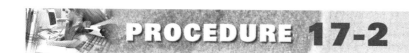

PROCEDURE 17-1

Processing a Credit Balance

Procedure Goal: To process a credit balance

Materials: Daily log sheet (also known as a day sheet), checks, ledger card, computer, calculator, RA (Remittance Advice) also known as an Explanation of Benefits (EOB)

Method:

1. Locate the patient's account in the computer or pull the patient's ledger card for paper-based systems.

    Rationale

    All financial transactions must be entered in the correct patient account.

2. Review the policy manual to make sure you are following the guidelines for posting credit balances.

    Rationale

    Medical assistants should follow proper policies and procedures of the medical facility.

3. Review the EOB and check to be sure that the payment is being credited to the correct patient account.

4. Post the payment to the patient's account.

5. Check calculations carefully if it appears that an overpayment has been made.

6. Review the account thoroughly in case more insurance payments are expected on the patient's account.

    Rationale

    If more activity is expected on the account, do not proceed with a refund until all expected payments are received on the account.

7. Adjust the credit balance of the patient's account by issuing a refund.

    Rationale

    To give the patient a refund, if one is due.

PROCEDURE 17-2

Processing Refunds to Patients

Procedure Goal: To process refunds to patients

Materials: Payment (check), ledger card, computer, calculator, Remittance Advice (RA) also known as an Explanation of Benefits (EOB)

Method:

1. Calculate the amount to be refunded.

    Rationale

    To make sure that the correct amount is refunded to the patient.

2. Write a check to the patient for the amount to be refunded.

3. Ask the physician or business manager to sign the check so that it can be given or mailed to the patient.

Rationale

Checks are not negotiable without a legal signature.

4. Post the refund as a negative payment (credit) to the patient's ledger card or to the patient's account if a computerized system is being used.

5. Make a copy of the check, retaining a copy in the patient's financial record. Give or mail the check to the patient (verify the correct address of the patient). Mail the check certified return receipt.

Rationale

To make sure the check was properly received by the patient, and to obtain a signature for verification.

Preparing Invoices

As a medical assistant, part of your job may be to prepare an invoice to mail to the patient who does not pay when services are rendered or who makes only a partial payment. Figure 17-5 shows an invoice with an itemized list of services.

You can obtain most of the information for the invoice from the patient ledger card or from the patient's computerized account. The invoice should include the following information:

- Physician's name, address, and telephone number (usually preprinted on the invoice, or prepared by the computer program)

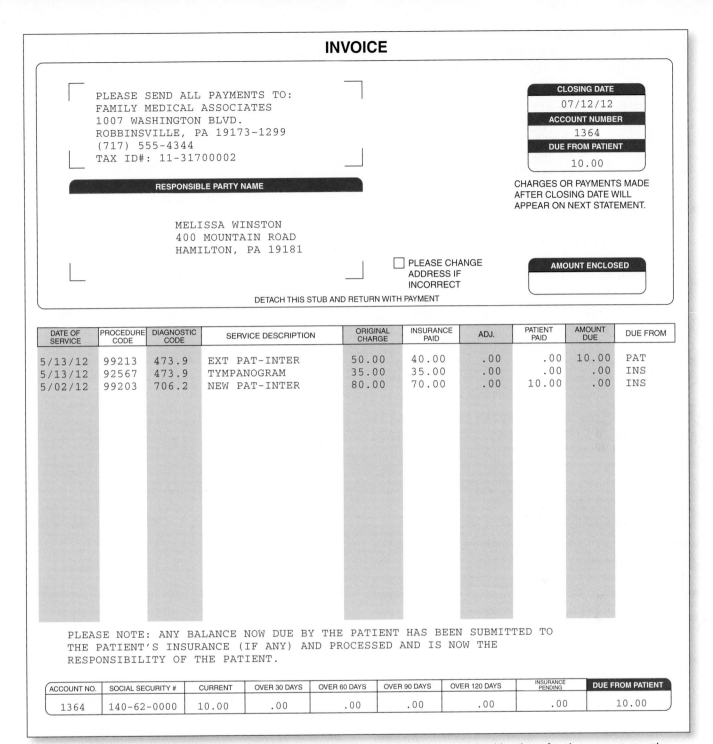

INVOICE

PLEASE SEND ALL PAYMENTS TO:
FAMILY MEDICAL ASSOCIATES
1007 WASHINGTON BLVD.
ROBBINSVILLE, PA 19173-1299
(717) 555-4344
TAX ID#: 11-31700002

CLOSING DATE
07/12/12
ACCOUNT NUMBER
1364
DUE FROM PATIENT
10.00

CHARGES OR PAYMENTS MADE
AFTER CLOSING DATE WILL
APPEAR ON NEXT STATEMENT.

RESPONSIBLE PARTY NAME

MELISSA WINSTON
400 MOUNTAIN ROAD
HAMILTON, PA 19181

☐ PLEASE CHANGE
ADDRESS IF
INCORRECT

AMOUNT ENCLOSED

DETACH THIS STUB AND RETURN WITH PAYMENT

DATE OF SERVICE	PROCEDURE CODE	DIAGNOSTIC CODE	SERVICE DESCRIPTION	ORIGINAL CHARGE	INSURANCE PAID	ADJ.	PATIENT PAID	AMOUNT DUE	DUE FROM
5/13/12	99213	473.9	EXT PAT-INTER	50.00	40.00	.00	.00	10.00	PAT
5/13/12	92567	473.9	TYMPANOGRAM	35.00	35.00	.00	.00	.00	INS
5/02/12	99203	706.2	NEW PAT-INTER	80.00	70.00	.00	10.00	.00	INS

PLEASE NOTE: ANY BALANCE NOW DUE BY THE PATIENT HAS BEEN SUBMITTED TO
THE PATIENT'S INSURANCE (IF ANY) AND PROCESSED AND IS NOW THE
RESPONSIBILITY OF THE PATIENT.

ACCOUNT NO.	SOCIAL SECURITY #	CURRENT	OVER 30 DAYS	OVER 60 DAYS	OVER 90 DAYS	OVER 120 DAYS	INSURANCE PENDING	DUE FROM PATIENT
1364	140-62-0000	10.00	.00	.00	.00	.00	.00	10.00

Figure 17-5. The invoice shows an itemized list of services and charges, organized by date, for the current month.

- Patient's name and address.
- Guarantor's name (if different from the patient)
- Balance (if any) from the previous month(s)
- Itemized list of services and charges, by date, for the current month
- Payments from the patient or insurer during the month
- Total balance due

Whatever invoicing procedure you use, enclose a self addressed envelope with the invoice to encourage prompt payment. Some offices have found that using a lightly colored return envelope, such as pale yellow, actually encourages faster payment because the color stands out against the usual white envelopes, jogging the patient's memory to "pay that one."

Using Codes on the Invoice. Write the name of each procedure on the itemized list, or use abbreviations for common procedures, such as OV for office visit. If you use abbreviations, be sure that an explanation of the abbreviations appears with the invoice. (Many practices use invoices with a key to the abbreviations printed at the bottom.) Using an itemized list on invoices is standard procedure in most physicians' offices and is required by all health insurance plans. After completing the invoice, fold it in thirds, and mail it in a typewritten or window business envelope.

Using the Patient's Ledger Card as an Invoice. A common alternative to writing or typing the invoice, is to photocopy the patient's ledger card and fold the photocopy so that the patient's address shows through the window in a window envelope. If you prepare invoices this way, be sure there are no stray marks or comments written on the card. Also, be sure the photocopy is clean and easy to read.

Generating the Invoice by Computer. In computerized offices, you may print out an invoice for each patient account that has a balance due. Follow the instructions in the software manufacturer's manual. You can then fold the printouts and mail them in window envelopes.

Using an Independent Billing Service. Large practices may have invoices handled by an independent billing service. The billing service may rapidly copy ledger cards or produce computer-generated invoices from the office computer for patients with balances due. Then it mails the invoices to patients, usually with an envelope for sending payment directly to the physician's office.

Sending Claims Electronically to Insurance Companies. Claims to insurance companies may be prepared by hand using paper claims or physicians' offices that have a computer and modem may bill insurance companies electronically, as discussed in Chapter 15.

Using the Superbill

Some doctors' offices use a **superbill,** which includes the charges and procedure codes (CPT) for services rendered on that day, including appropriate diagnoses and codes (ICD-9), an invoice for payment or insurance copayment, and all the information for submitting an insurance claim. In many facilities, the superbill is also known an **encounter form.** Figure 17-6 shows an example of a superbill. Having all this information on one form saves time and paperwork. These forms are often printed on NCR (no-carbon-required) paper with copies for the practice, patient, and insurance company. Encounter forms can also be generated and transmitted electronically as part of electronic health records.

Complete as much of the superbill as possible at the beginning of the patient's visit. (See Procedure 17-3 for specific instructions.) Some practices use a computerized version of the superbill, printing it out instead of completing the initial information by hand. Attach the superbill to the patient's medical record, and give them both to the doctor before he sees the patient. The doctor circles or checks the appropriate procedures and diagnoses after seeing the patient and it is returned to the front desk to begin the billing cycle.

Managing Billing Cycles

Many practices send out their bills just after the end of each month. You can send out bills at any regular time, however,

such as once a week or twice a month. You may also send bills at a particular time of the month at the patient's request.

Cycle billing is a common billing system that bills each patient only once a month but spreads the work of billing over the month. Using this system, you send invoices to groups of patients every few days.

For example, you may bill on the fifth of the month for patients whose last names begin with A through D. Then, on the tenth of the month, you may bill patients whose names begin with E through H, and so on. In a larger office with more patients, you may prefer to bill more frequently but to smaller groups of patients.

Standard Collection Procedures

Although most patients pay invoices within the standard 30-day period, some do not. When a patient does not pay an invoice during the standard period, you need to take steps to collect the payment. For example, you may need to call or write the patient to determine the reason for non-payment or to set up a payment arrangement.

Whether you use telephone calls, notes, or letters, there are laws, such as statutes of limitations, and professional standards to guide your efforts to collect overdue payments from patients.

State Statute of Limitations

A **statute of limitations** is a state law that sets a time limit on when a collection suit on a past-due account can legally be filed. The time limit varies with the type of account and the state in which the debt was incurred.

Open-Book Account. An **open-book account** is one that is open to charges made occasionally as needed. Most of a physician's long-standing patients have this type of account. An open-book account uses the last date of payment or charge for each illness as the starting date for determining the time limit on that specific debt.

Written-Contract Account. A **written-contract account** is one in which the physician and patient sign an agreement stating that the patient will pay the bill in more than four installments. Some states allow longer time limits for these accounts than for open-book accounts. Written-contract accounts are regulated by the Truth in Lending Act, discussed later in this chapter.

Single-Entry Account. A **single-entry account** is an account with only one charge, usually for a small amount. For example, someone vacationing in your area might come in for treatment of a cold. This person's account would list only one office visit. If the vacationer did not become a regular patient, the account would be considered a single-entry account. Some states impose shorter time limits on single-entry accounts than on open-book accounts.

Lakeridge Medical Group
262 East Pine Street, Suite 100
Santa Cruz, CA 95062

☐ PRIVATE ☐ BLUECROSS ☐ IND. ☐ MEDICARE ☐ MEDI-CAL ☐ HMO ☐ PPO

PATIENT'S LAST NAME	FIRST	ACCOUNT #	BIRTHDATE / /	SEX ☐ MALE ☐ FEMALE	TODAY'S DATE / /

INSURANCE COMPANY	SUBSCRIBER	PLAN #	SUB. #	GROUP

ASSIGNMENT: I hereby assign my insurance benefits to be paid directly to the undersigned physician. I am financially responsible for non-covered services.
SIGNED: (Patient, or Parent, if Minor)　　　　DATE: / /

RELEASE: I hereby authorize the physician to release to my insurance carrers any information required to process this claim.
SIGNED: (Patient, or Parent, if Minor)　　　　DATE: / /

✔	DESCRIPTION	M/Care	CPT/Mod	DxRe	FEE	✔	DESCRIPTION	M/Care	CPT/Mod	DxRe	FEE	✔	DESCRIPTION	M/Care	CPT/Mod	DxRe	FEE
	OFFICE CARE						PROCEDURES						INJECTIONS/IMMUNIZATIONS				
	NEW PATIENT						Tread Mill (In Office)		93015				Tetanus		90718		
	Brief		99201				24 Hour Holter		93224				Hypertet	J1670	90782		
	Limited		99202				If Medicare (Set up Fee)		93225				Pneumococcal		90732		
	Intermediate		99203				Physician Interpret		93227				Influenza		90724		
	Extended		99204				EKG w/Interpretation		93000				TB Skin Test (PPD)		86585		
	Comprehensive		99205				EKG (Medicare)		93005				Antigen Injection-Single		95115		
							Sigmoidoscopy		45300				Multiple		95117		
	ESTABLISHED PATIENT						Sigmoidoscopy, Flexible		45330				B12 Injection	J3420	90782		
	Minimal		99211				Sigmoidos., Flex. w/Bx.		45331				Injection, IM		90782		
	Brief		99212				Spirometry, FEV/FVC		94010				Compazine	J0780	90782		
	Limited		99213				Spirometry, Post-Dilator		94060				Demerol	J2175	90782		
	Intermediate		99214										Vistaril	J3410	90782		
	Extended		99215										Susphrine	J0170	90782		
	Comprehensive		99215				LABORATORY						Decadron	J0890	90782		
							Blood Draw Fee		36415				Estradiol	J1000	90782		
	CONSULTATION-OFFICE						Urinalysis, Chemical		81005				Testosterone	J1080	90782		
	Focused		99241				Throat Culture		87081				Lidocaine	J2000	90782		
	Expanded		99242				Occult Blood		82270				Solumedrol	J2920	90782		
	Detailed		99243				Pap Handling Charge		99000				Solucortef	J1720	90782		
	Comprehensive 1		99244				Pap Life Guard		88150-90				Hydeltra	J1690	90782		
	Comprehensive 2		99245				Gram Stain		87205				Pen Procaine	J2510	90788		
	Dr.						Hanging Drop		87210								
	Case Management		98900				Urine Drug Screen		99000				INJECTIONS - JOINT/BURSA				
													Small Joints		20600		
	Post-op Exam		99024										Intermediate		20605		
							SUPPLIES						Large Joints		20610		
													Trigger Point		20550		
													MISCELLANEOUS				

DIAGNOSIS:	ICD-9									
__ Abdominal Pain	789.0	__ Gout	274.0	__ C.V.A. - Acute	436.	__ Electrolyte Dis.	276.9	__ Herpes Simplex	054.9
__ Abscess (Site)	682.9	__ Asthma	493.90	__ Cere. Vas. Accid. (Old)	438	__ Fatigue	780.7	__ Herpes Zoster	053.9
__ Adverse Drug Rx	995.2	__ Asthmatic Bronchitis	493.90	__ Cerumen	380.4	__ Fibrocys. Br. Dis	610.1	__ Hydrocele	603.9
__ Alcohol Detox	291.8	__ Atrial Fib.	427.31	__ Chestwall Pain	786.59	__ Fracture (Site)	829.0	__ Hyperlipidemia	272.4
__ Alcoholism	303.90	__ Atrial Tachi.	427.0	__ Cholecystitis	575.0	__ Open/Close		__ Hypertension	401.9
__ Allergic Rhinitis	477	__ Bowel Obstruct.	560.9	__ Cholelithiasis	574.00	__ Fungal Infect. (Site)	110.8	__ Hyperthyroidism	242.9
__ Allergy	995.3	__ Breast Mass	611.72	__ COPD	492.8	__ Gastric Ulcer	531.90	__ Hypothyroidism	244.9
__ Alzheimer's Dis.	290.1	__ Bronchitis	490	__ Cirrhosis	571.5	__ Gastritis	535.0	__ Labyrinthitis	386.30
__ Anemia	285.9	__ Bursitis	727.3	__ Cong. Heart Fail.	428.9	__ Gastroenteritis	558.9	__ Lipoma (Site)	214.9
__ Anemia - Pernicious	281.0	__ Cancer, Breast (Site)	174.9	__ Conjunctivitis	372.30	__ G.I. Bleeding	578.9	__ Lymphoma	202.8
__ Angina	413.9	__ Metastatic (Site)	199.1	__ Contusion (Site)	924.9	__ Glomerulonephritis	583.9	__ Mit. Valve Prolapse	424.0
__ Anxiety Synd.	300.00	__ Colon	153.9	__ Costochondritis	733.99	__ Headache	784.0	__ Myocard. Infarction (Area)	410.9
__ Appendicitis	541	__ Cancer, Rectal	154.1	__ Depression	311.	__ Headache, Tension	307.81	__ M.I., Old	412
__ Arterioscl. H.D.	414.0	__ Lung (Site)	162.9	__ Dermatitis	692.9	__ Migraine (Type)	346.9	__ Myositis	729.1
__ Arthritis, Osteo.	715.90	__ Skin (Site)	173.9	__ Diabetes Mellitus	250.00	__ Hemorrhoids	455.6	__ Nausea/Vomiting	787.0
__ Rheumatoid	714.0	__ Card. Arrhythmia (Type)	427.9	__ Diabetic Ketosis	250.1	__ Hernia, Hiatal	553.3	__ Neuralgia	729.2
__ Lupus	710.0	__ Cardiomyopathy	425.4	__ Diverticulitis	562.11	__ Inguinal	550.9	__ Nevus (Site)	216.9
		__ Cellulitis (Site)	682.9	__ Diverticulosis	562.10	__ Hepatitis	573.3	__ Obesity	278.0

DIAGNOSIS: (IF NOT CHECKED ABOVE)

SERVICES PERFORMED AT: ☐ Office ☐ E.R. ☐ CLAIM CONTAINS NO ORDERED REFERRING SERVICE ☐ ☐

REFERRING PHYSICIAN & I.D. NUMBER

RETURN APPOINTMENT INFORMATION: 5 - 10 - 15 - 20 - 30 - 40 - 60 [DAYS] [WKS.] [MOS.] [PRN]	NEXT APPOINTMENT M - T - W - TH - F - S DATE / / TIME:	AM PM	ACCEPT ASSIGNMENT? ☐ YES ☐ NO	DOCTOR'S SIGNATURE

INSTRUCTIONS TO PATIENT FOR FILING INSURANCE CLAIMS:	☐ CASH	TOTAL TODAY'S FEE
1. Complete upper portion of this form, sign and date. 2. Attach this form to your own insurance company's form for direct reimbursement. **MEDICARE PATIENTS - DO NOT SEND THIS TO MEDICARE. WE WILL SUBMIT THE CLAIM FOR YOU.**	☐ CHECK #_____ ☐ VISA ☐ MC ☐ CO-PAY	OLD BALANCE TOTAL DUE AMOUNT REC'D. TODAY

INSUR-A-BILL ® BIBBERO SYSTEMS, INC. • PETALUMA, CA • UP. SUPER. © 6/94 (BIBB/STOCK)

Figure 17-6. A superbill is a form that can also be used as a charge slip and invoice, and can be submitted with insurance claims.

How to Bill with the Superbill

Procedure Goal: To complete a superbill accurately (make sure the doctor's name and address appear on the form)

Materials: Superbill, patient ledger card, patient information sheet, fee schedule, insurance code list, pen

Method:

1. From the patient ledger card and information sheet, fill in the patient data, such as name, sex, date of birth, and insurance information.

2. Fill in the place and date of service.

3. Attach the superbill to the patient's medical record, and give them both to the doctor.

Rationale

The doctor must have the superbill to add the charges for the day.

4. Accept the completed superbill from the patient after the patient sees the doctor. Make sure that the doctor has indicated the diagnosis and the procedures performed. Also make sure that an appropriate diagnosis is listed for each procedure.

Rationale

Ensures medical necessity for payment by the insurance carrier.

5. If the doctor has not already recorded the charges, refer to the fee schedule for procedures that are marked. Then fill in the charges next to those procedures.

Rationale

Each procedure must have a charge to ensure accurate billing.

6. In the appropriate blanks, list the total charges for the visit and the previous balance (if any).

7. Calculate the subtotal.

8. Fill in the amount and type of payment (cash, check, money order, or credit card) made by the patient during this visit.

Rationale

This helps to ensure accurate posting to the patient's account.

9. Calculate and enter the new balance.

10. Have the patient sign the authorization-and-release section of the superbill.

Rationale

Without this signature (or one on file), there is no permission to release information to the insurance carrier, nor is there agreement for the carrier to pay the provider directly.

11. Keep a copy of the superbill for the practice records. Give the original to the patient along with one copy to file with the insurer.

Using Collection Techniques

Individual practices have their own ways of approaching the task of collection. Most begin the process with telephone calls, letters, or statements.

Initial Telephone Calls or Letters. When calling a patient (or sending a letter) about collections, be friendly and sympathetic. (Do not call a patient at work and leave a message. That type of phone call is an invasion of privacy. Call the patient at home unless you have permission to call the patient at work and you have been unable to reach the patient at home.) The first phone call to the patient should occur if payment has not been received after 30–45 days (remember the patient received his first bill at the time of the visit, so the invoice received in the mail is essentially a second notice of payment due). Assume that the patient forgot to pay or was temporarily unable to pay. You should ask the patient for the full amount due. If the patient states that he cannot afford full payment, ask him what amount he feels could be sent (you should have a minimum amount in mind), and obtain a date you can expect to receive the payment. If you do not receive the payment within 24 hours of the stated date, an initial collection letter may be sent. This letter may need to be more urgent in tone because the patient did not respond to your phone call and the tone of any subsequent letters will be still more urgent. Standard collection letters, such as the one shown in Figure 17-7, are available for you to fill in the details, or you can create a letter to reflect the style of the practice.

Preparing Statements. You might send the patient a statement for an account that is 30 days past due. A **statement** is similar to an invoice except that it contains a courteous reminder that payment is due. This reminder can be a typewritten note on the statement, a brightly colored sticker, or prepared message produced by the computer billing program.

If an account is 60 days past due, you could send a collection letter that says, for example, "If you are unable to pay your account in full this month, please telephone our office at (number) to make payment arrangements."

If an account is 90 days past due, your collection letter can contain stronger wording. For example, it might say,

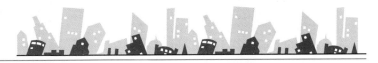

City Medical Group

1234 Wayne Street
Smithtown, OR 93689
(503) 555-1217

Internal Medicine
Marianne Harris, MD
Karen Payne-Johnson, MD

May 5, 2012

Mr. J. J. Andrews
1414 First Avenue
Smithtown, OR 93668

Dear Mr. Andrews:

It has been brought to my attention that your account in the amount of <u>$240.00</u> is past due.

Normally at this time the account would be placed with a collection agency. However, we would prefer to hear from you regarding your preference in this matter.

(   )   Payment in full is enclosed.

(   )   Payment will be made in _____ days.

(   )   I would like to make regular weekly/monthly payments of $ _____ until this account is paid in full. My first payment is enclosed.

(   )   I would prefer that you assign this account to a collection agency for enforcement of collection. (Failure to return this letter within 30 days will result in this action.)

(   )   I don't believe I owe this amount for the following reason(s):

Signed: _____

Please indicate your preference and return this letter within 30 days. Please do not hesitate to call if you have any questions regarding this matter.

Sincerely,

Diana Sanchez
Office Manager

Figure 17-7. Standard collection letters are available for you to fill in the details.

"Please let us know when you plan to pay the $250 past-due balance. We have sent you three monthly reminders. If you cannot pay in full now, please contact us at (number) to make payment arrangements. We want to be understanding but need your cooperation."

If an account is 120 days or more past due, you can send a final letter. It might state, "Every courtesy has been extended to you in arranging for payment of your long overdue account. Unless we hear from you by (date), the account will be given to (name of collection agency) for collection." Be sure to note the cutoff date on the patient's ledger card. By law, you cannot threaten to send an account to a collection agency unless it will actually be sent on that cutoff date. Therefore, you must be sure you are ready to do so before you send such a letter. This collection letter should be mailed by certified mail with return receipt so you have proof that the letter was sent and that the intended recipient received the letter.

If you still cannot collect payment, the physician may indeed choose to hire an outside collection agency. Once an agency has taken over the account, there should not be any more correspondence on this matter between the physician's office and the patient. If the patient contacts you or sends a payment after the account has been sent to collection, you are to refer the patient to the collection agency.

 ## Preparing an Age Analysis

Age analysis is the process of classifying and reviewing past-due accounts by age from the first date of billing. A monthly age analysis, such as that shown in Figure 17-8, helps you keep on top of past-due accounts and determine which ones need follow-up.

You can do an age analysis by computer (most computer programs generate one automatically) or by hand. An age analysis should list all patient account balances, when the charges originated, the most recent payment date, and any special notes concerning the account. Procedure 17–4 outlines the steps for preparing an age analysis.

In a single doctor's office or a small group practice, information for the age analysis may come from the patient ledger cards. You may place color-coded tags on the patient ledger cards to indicate the number of days past due. For example, a yellow tag might be placed on the ledger card of an accoun t that is 60 days past due. An orange tag might be used for an account that is 90 days past due. A red tag might be used for an account that is 120 days or more past due. The use of patient ledger cards is being phased out as more practices have become computerized.

Following Laws That Govern Debt Collection

Federal and state laws govern debt collection. Table 17-1 outlines the penalties for violating laws that regulate credit and debt.

ACCOUNTS RECEIVABLE–AGE ANALYSIS

Date: October 1, 2012

Patient	Balance	Date of Charges	Most Recent Payment	30 days	60 days	90 days	120 days	Remarks
Black, K.	120.00	5/24	5/24			75.00	45.00	3rd Notice
Brown, R.	65.00	8/30	8/30	65.00				
Green, C.	340.00	8/25						Medicare filed
Jones, T.	500.00	6/1	6/30		125.00	125.00	250.00	3rd Notice
Perry, S.	150.00	7/28	7/28	75.00	75.00			1st Notice
Smith, J.	375.00	6/15	7/1			375.00		2nd Notice
White, L.	200.00	6/24	7/5	20.00	30.00	150.00		2nd Notice

Figure 17-8. An age analysis organizes past-due accounts by age.

PROCEDURE 17-4 [WORK//PRODUCT]

Preparing an Age Analysis

Procedure Goal: To create and examine an age analysis

Materials: Computer, patient accounts, ledger cards (if being done by hand), accounts receivable aging record analysis form (optional), policy and procedure manual, pen

Method:

1. Using the reporting section of your billing computer program, create an age analysis report for patients and insurance companies. This also can be done manually by pulling patient ledger cards, noting balances due and dates of last payments. Use Figure 17-8 as a guide to create a spreadsheet for your findings.

   Rationale
   The computerized report can generate the report of all overdue accounts and can do it faster.

2. Review the accounting report. Check the report—highlight for proposed actions for each account according to your office policy.

   Rationale
   Efforts to collect on outstanding accounts will get increasingly more active as the account ages.

3. Mark the accounts that are under 31 days as NO ACTION TO BE TAKEN AT THIS TIME.

   Rationale
   Accounts that are less than 31 days are considered current.

4. Bills that are unpaid at more than 31 days should be marked as "Contact or follow up with insurance company."

   Rationale
   Patients generally do not make payments until their insurance company has paid or they find out what their portion of the charges will be. If the insurance payment is overdue, you must follow up with the insurance company as soon as possible.

5. Accounts that are 31–60 days old should be marked according to your office policy. An initial phone call may be made inquiring as to payment arrangements.

6. Accounts that are 61–90 days old should be marked according to your office policy. Make notations such as "Account Past Due." A follow-up phone call and/or more insistent letter for payment may be in order.

7. Accounts that are 91–120 days old should be marked according to your office policy. A last phone call to attempt discussing the account and more insistent collection statement/letter should be sent.

8. For accounts older than 120 days, make sure you review previous collection attempts. At this point, after discussion with the physician, a letter stating the account will be turned over to the collection agency will take place with a specific date listed in the letter. This letter should be mailed by certified, return receipt mail.

   Rationale
   After 120 days without any activity, it is unlikely that the patient will pay this amount without a more aggressive means of action.

9. Record all actions that have been taken beside each account.

   Rationale
   This notation provides a written record of all actions that have been taken in an attempt to collect this debt.

10. Finally, write follow-up letters to patients and document any agreements that you and the patient have discussed via telephone. Be sure to keep a copy of any correspondence mailed to the patient in the financial record.

    Rationale
    This will provide documentation if any legal actions have to be taken.

Fair Debt Collection Practices Act of 1977. This act (also called Public Law 95-109) governs the methods that can be used to collect unpaid debts. It prevents you from threatening to take an action either that is illegal or that you do not actually intend to take. The aim of this law is to eliminate abusive, deceptive, or unfair debt collection practices. For example, the law requires that after you have said you are going to give an account to a collection agency if it is not paid within 1 month, you must actually do so. Not doing what you threaten to do can be construed as harassment, and your practice can be liable for a harassment charge. Following are guidelines for sending letters and making calls requesting payment from patients. For

TABLE 17-1 Laws That Govern Credit and Collections

Law	Requirements	Penalties for Breaking Law
Equal Credit Opportunity Act (ECOA) www.ftc.gov/bcp/edu/pubs/consumer/credit/cre15.shtm	• Creditors may not discriminate against applicants on the basis of sex, marital status, race, national origin, religion, or age. • Creditors may not discriminate because an applicant receives public assistance income or has exercised rights under the Consumer Credit Protection Act.	• If an applicant sues the practice for violating the ECOA, the practice may have to pay **damages** (money paid as compensation), penalties, lawyers' fees, and court costs. • If an applicant joins a class action lawsuit against the practice, the practice may have to pay damages of up to $500,000 or 1% of the practice's net worth, whichever is less. (A **class action lawsuit** is a lawsuit in which one or more people sue a company that wronged all of them the same way.) • If the Federal Trade Commission (FTC) receives many complaints from applicants stating that the practice violated the ECOA, the FTC may investigate and take action against the practice.
Fair Credit Reporting Act (FCRA) www.ftc.gov/os/statutes/fcra.htm	• This act requires credit bureaus to supply correct and complete information to businesses to use in evaluating a person's application for credit, insurance, or a job.	• If one applicant sues the practice in federal court for violating the FCRA, the practice may have to pay damages, **punitive damages** (money paid as punishment for intentionally breaking the law), court costs, and lawyers' fees. • If the FTC receives many complaints from applicants stating that the practice violated the FCRA, the FTC may investigate and take action against the practice.
Fair Debt Collection Practices Act (FDCPA) www.ftc.gov/bcp/edu/pubs/consumer/credit/cre27.pdf	• This act requires debt collectors to treat debtors fairly. It also prohibits certain collection tactics, such as harassment, false statements, threats, and unfair practices.	• If one debtor sues the practice in a state or federal court for violation of the FDCPA, the practice may have to pay damages, court costs, and lawyers' fees. • If the debtor joins a class action suit against the practice, the practice may have to pay damages of up to $500,000 or 1% of the practice's net worth, whichever is less. • If the FTC receives many complaints from debtors stating that the practice violated the FDCPA, the FTC may investigate and take action against the practice.
Truth in Lending Act (TLA) www.occ.treas.gov/handbook/til.pdf	• This act requires creditors to provide applicants with accurate and complete credit costs and terms, clearly and obviously.	• If one applicant sues the practice in a federal court for violation of the TLA, the practice may have to pay damages, court costs, and lawyers' fees. • If the FTC receives many complaints from applicants stating that the practice violated the TLA, the FTC may investigate and take action against the practice.

further information, visit www.ftc.gov/bcp/edu/pubs/consumer/credit/cre27.pdf.

- Do not call the patient before 8 A.M. or after 9 P.M. Calling outside those hours can be considered harassment.

- Do not make threats or use profane language. For example, do not state that an account will be given to a collection agency in 7 days if it will not be.

- Do not discuss the patient's debt with anyone except the person responsible for payment. If the patient is represented by a lawyer, discuss the problem only with the lawyer, unless the lawyer gives you permission to talk to the patient.

- Do not use any form of deception or violence to collect a debt. For example, do not pose as a government employee or other authority figure to try to force a debtor to pay.

Telephone Consumer Protection Act (TCPA) of 1991. This act protects telephone subscribers from unwanted telephone solicitations, commonly known as telemarketing. The act prohibits autodialed calls to emergency service providers, cellular and paging numbers, and patients' hospital rooms. It prohibits prerecorded calls to homes without prior permission of the resident, and it prohibits unsolicited advertising via fax machine.

Choosing a Collection Agency

If a patient does not respond to your final collection letter or has twice broken a promise to pay, the doctor may choose to seek the help of a collection agency. This step should be taken carefully, however. Some collection agencies use illegal and unethical tactics to obtain payment. For example, some collectors have made repeated, profane phone calls to frighten debtors. Others have threatened debtors with prison for nonpayment. A good collection agency reflects the humanitarian and ethical standards of the medical profession.

To help select an effective—and ethical—collection agency, ask for a referral from the doctor's colleagues, fellow specialists, or hospital associates. You may also contact the following organizations:

American Collectors Association International
ACA International
P.O. Box 390106
Minneapolis, MN 55439
(952) 926–6547
www.acainternational.org

After obtaining a referral, contact the agency and request samples of its letters, reminder notices, and other print material for debtors. Be sure this material is courteous and reflects the way you would handle the collection. Also, be sure the agency uses a persuasive approach rather than simply suing debtors. Ask if the agency reports cases that deserve special consideration to the doctor's office.

Determine what methods the agency uses for out-of-town accounts. For example, it may use out-of-town services to help with those collections. Ask the agency about its collection percentage and fees for large, small, and out-of-town accounts. Be sure the percentages and fees are appropriate for the collection amounts.

After selecting a collection agency, supply all pertinent data to the agency, such as the patient's name, address, and full amount of the debt. Mark the patient's ledger card so that you do not call or write to the patient about the debt. If the patient contacts the office about the account, refer the patient to the collection agency.

If you receive any payments from the debtor, alert the collection agency immediately. (The agency takes a portion of any payments it collects.) Also, contact the agency if you learn anything new about the patient's address or employer.

These regulations do not apply to people who have an established business relationship with the telemarketing firm or people who have previously given the telemarketing firm permission to call. The law also does not apply to telemarketing calls placed by tax-exempt nonprofit organizations, such as charities.

Although most provisions of this federal law do not apply to medical practices, you should be aware of the law. One way to avoid an unknowing violation of this law is to limit your calls to patients to the hours between 8 A.M. and 9 P.M. (some states, however, have exceptions for the TCPA provisions). Also, place your calls yourself. Do not use an automated dialing device for calls to patients.

Observing Professional Guidelines for Finance Charges and Late Charges

According to the AMA, it is appropriate to assess finance charges or late charges on past-due accounts if the patient is notified in advance. Advance notice may be given by posting a sign at the reception desk, giving the patient a pamphlet describing the practice's billing practices, or including a note on the invoice.

The physician must adhere to federal and state guidelines that govern these charges. The physician should also use compassion and discretion when assigning charges, especially in hardship cases.

Using Outside Collection Agencies

If your collection efforts do not result in payment, the doctor may wish to select a collection agency to manage the account. Because collection agencies keep a percentage of any funds they collect for their clients (usually between 40% and 60% of the collected amount), the office staff should use all reasonable methods to collect unpaid balances prior to sending an account to collection. Because doctors adhere to the humanitarian and ethical standards of the medical profession, they must be careful to avoid collection agencies that use harsh or harassing collection practices. The Points on Practice section gives information about selecting an outside collection agency.

When giving a patient's account to an agency, supply the following information about the patient:

- Full name and last known address
- Occupation and business address
- Name of spouse, if any
- Total debt
- Date of last payment or charge on the account

- Description of actions you took to collect the debt
- Responses to collection attempts

Color-coded tabs on the patient ledger cards make this information easy to gather. Note on the patient ledger card that the account has been given to a collection agency. When the agency reports progress toward a settlement, record that information on the card too.

After the account is given to the agency, do not send bills to or contact the patient in any way. If the patient wants to discuss payment, refer the patient to the agency. If the patient sends a payment, forward it to the agency; or, if the agency and the practice agree, keep the payment for the practice and forward the collection fee to the agency.

The arrangement with the agency should give the doctor the final word on the uncollected account. In other words, the doctor should decide whether to write off the debt or take the matter to court.

Insuring Accounts Receivable

To protect the practice from lost income because of non-payment, the practice may buy accounts receivable insurance. One type of accounts receivable policy pays when a large number of patients do not pay and the physician must absorb the lost income. It protects the practice's cash flow and helps ensure that the practice will have sufficient income to cover expected expenses.

Credit Arrangements

Sometimes a doctor agrees to extend credit to a patient who is unable to pay immediately. This situation is not uncommon when a patient's medical bills are high. By extending **credit,** the doctor gives the patient time to pay for services, which are provided on trust. If the doctor knows the patient well, she may offer credit without checking the patient's credit history. However, to avoid charges of discrimination under the Equal Credit Opportunity Act (ECOA), you will normally perform a credit check prior to extending credit. The ECOA is discussed in further detail later in the chapter.

Performing a Credit Check

To perform a credit check, be sure you have the most current information. You will need the patient's address, telephone number, and Social Security number and the patient's employer's name, address, and telephone number. With this information you can verify employment and generate a credit bureau report.

Employment Verification. Explain to the patient that you will be calling his employer to verify employment. Many employers have someone designated to handle such calls. The patient may be able to give you that name before you call the place of employment.

After calling, record the updated information on the patient's registration card, along with any credit references you obtain from the patient.

Credit Bureau Report. A **credit bureau** is a company that provides information about the creditworthiness of a person seeking credit. If a patient's credit history is in question, you may request a report from a credit bureau. A sample credit report is shown in Figure 17-9. A credit bureau collects information about an individual's payment history on credit cards, student loans, and similar accounts. Three leading national credit bureaus are TRW Inc., Equifax Inc., and Trans Union Credit Information Company.

The physician may decide not to extend credit, based on the credit report. If so, the Fair Credit Reporting Act states that you must inform the patient in writing that credit was denied based on the credit report. You must also provide the name and address of the credit bureau; however, you do not need to discuss the information obtained from the report. The patient may contest the credit report and may correct any incorrect information the credit bureau may have. Once the information has been corrected, the provider may then decide to extend the patient credit.

Following Laws Governing Extension of Credit

When you help the doctor decide whether to grant credit to a patient, you must comply with certain laws governing extension of credit.

Equal Credit Opportunity Act. This act states that credit arrangements may not be denied based on a patient's sex, race, religion, national origin, marital status, or age. Also, credit cannot be denied because the patient receives public assistance or has exercised rights under the Consumer Credit Protection Act, such as disputing a credit card bill or a credit bureau report.

Under the Equal Credit Opportunity Act, the patient has a right to know the specific reason that credit was denied. Some reasons might include having too little income or not being employed for a certain period of time. Vague reasons about not meeting minimum standards or not receiving enough points on a credit-scoring system are not acceptable.

Truth in Lending Act. This act is Regulation Z of the Consumer Credit Protection Act. The Truth in Lending Act covers credit agreements that involve more than four payments. It requires the physician and patient to discuss, sign, and retain copies of a **disclosure statement** (frequently called a federal Truth in Lending statement), which is a written description of the agreed terms of payment (Figure 17-10).

According to the Truth in Lending Act, a disclosure statement must meet the following two requirements.

1. The agreement must be discussed with the patient when the terms are first determined. The physician and the patient must agree on the payment terms.

2. Both the physician and the patient must sign the document to indicate mutual agreement on the written terms.

File No.

Date
1/8/12

Amount Received
$15.00

Payment Type

Credit Card No.

Exp. Date

In File Since 10/94

Consumer Name and Address

SSN

Date Rptd.

Spouse Name SSN

Tel.

Date Rptd.

Former Address

Present Employer and Address

Position Income

Empl. Date

Date Verif.

Former Employer and Address

Spouse's Employer and Address

Subscriber Name	Subscriber Code	Date Opened	High Credit	Date Verif.	Present Status		Payment Pattern	Type Account & MOP
					Balance Owed	Amount Past Due	1–12 Months 13–24 Months	
Account Number		Terms	Credit Limit	Dated Closed	Maximum Delinquency		Historical Status	
Collateral					Remarks	Type Loan	No. of Months | 25–39 | 40–59 | 60+	
MIDLANTIC	B382D021	4/92 MIN10	$850	11/98A	$325	$0	111111111111 X11111111111 12 0 0 0	R01
LINCOLN SAV B	B814M006	6/88 360M34	$30.5K	10/94A	$16K	$0	1111X11X1111 111X11111X1X 29 0 0 0	M01
BANK AMER	B196P017	11/89 10M	$5000	10/96A	$1136	$0	111111111111 11111111111X 48 0 0 0	R01
MACY D	D787D008	1/84 MIN20	$475 $1000	11/97A	$0	$0*	111XXXXXXXXX 1111111111XX 48 0 0 0	R01
			*CREDIT LINE CLOSED BY CUSTOMER					
UJ BK MC	33DB0002	7/91 MIN20	$3000	3/96A	$310	$0	111111111111 111X111111XX 47 0 0 0	R01

Figure 17-9. Credit reports are generated by credit bureaus.

Further, a disclosure statement must include the following six pieces of information:

1. The amount of total debt (the amount for which the patient is receiving credit).
2. The amount of the down payment (which is sometimes greater than the weekly or monthly payments that follow).
3. The amount of each payment (which may be weekly or monthly or for another period) and the date it is due. (Frequently the total number of payments to be made after the down payment is also included.)
4. The due date for the final payment.
5. The interest rate, if interest is to be paid, expressed as an annual percentage.
6. The total finance charges, if any. (If interest is charged, the total amount of interest accrued during the course of the debt will be entered here.)

The practice and the patient should each keep a copy of the signed disclosure agreement.

Under the Truth in Lending Act, you must send the patient a statement of account at the end of each billing cycle. This statement must include the previous balance, any payments or charges, the periodic and annual interest rates, finance charges (if any) for the billing cycle, the new balance, and a description of how the new balance was obtained.

Extending Credit

If the doctor decides to extend credit, several possible arrangements can be made. Two common arrangements are the unilateral decision and the mutual agreement.

Unilateral Decision. The doctor may decide that the patient will be billed every month for the full amount owed and should make whatever payment is possible each month. This type of arrangement is considered a unilateral decision of the doctor and is not regulated by the Truth in Lending Act.

Mutual Agreement. Another option is a mutual, or bilateral, agreement between physician and patient.

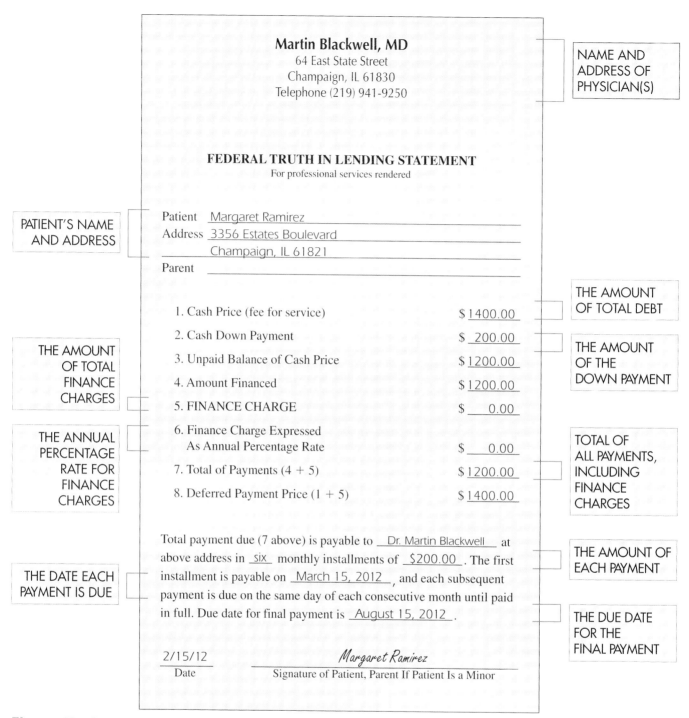

Figure 17-10. The federal Truth in Lending Act mandates that a written disclosure statement be completed and signed by the physician and patient.

They might agree that the patient will be billed for the full amount owed each month and will pay a minimum amount each month. If the physician does not assess finance charges, and if the total number of payments is four or fewer, this type of agreement is also not covered by the Truth in Lending Act. If the physician and patient make a bilateral agreement that includes more than four payments, or if the physician assesses finance charges, the agreement is subject to the requirements of the Truth in Lending Act.

Common Collection Problems

There are two common collection problems that medical practices encounter. The first is patients who cannot pay—also called hardship cases—and the second is patients who have moved and have not received an invoice.

Hardship Cases

A physician may decide to treat some patients without charge—or at a deep discount—simply because they

Coding, Billing, and Insurance Specialist

To gain medical assistant credentials, you must fulfill the requirements of either the American Association of Medical Assistants (for a Certified Medical Assistant) or the American Medical Technologists (for a Registered Medical Assistant). After obtaining your medical assistant certification or registration, you may wish to acquire additional skills in specialty areas through course work or on-the-job training. Although this course work or training may not lead to an additional certification or degree, it will enable you to expand your role in the medical office and advance your career as the demand for skilled health professionals increases.

Skills and Duties

A coding, billing, and insurance specialist analyzes the data in patients' charts to provide accurate information for insurance claims. She is also responsible for processing insurance forms and obtaining fees for procedures performed, either from patients or from their insurance companies.

For the purpose of processing insurance claims, there is a code for every recognized disease, condition, problem, and diagnosis. The codes used in medical records come from the International Classification of Disease (ICD) system, issued by the World Health Organization (WHO). There is also a separate system of codes for medical procedures, known as the *Physicians' Current Procedural Terminology, released* annually by the AMA. Coders are encouraged to take courses each year to stay informed about coding changes and updates.

After coding the medical record, the specialist bills the responsible party for the charges incurred by the patient's diagnosis and treatment. She may bill the patient, Medicare or Medicaid, and/or an insurance company. If the insurance company has questions about a bill, it may request the patient's medical records to verify that a particular procedure was medically necessary.

The coding, billing, and insurance specialist may also assist patients with the claims process. She can explain what information the patient must provide to streamline the process. When patients are responsible for submitting claims to their insurance companies, the coding, billing, and insurance specialist may tell the patient what forms to use and assist the patient with the forms completion.

The coding, billing, and insurance specialist also processes responses from the insurance companies, including the explanation of benefits (EOB) form. She checks the EOB against the claim form to make sure that the insurance company addressed all procedures that were performed. Sometimes a balance remains because the insurance company did not pay the total amount due on all procedures. In those cases the coding, billing, and insurance specialist sends a bill to the patient or responsible party, or adjusts balances as required by contracted agreement. She may discover an error in the EOB. In such instances she looks for the source of the error and then contacts the insurance company to correct it.

Workplace Settings

Coding, billing, and insurance specialists work in many health-care settings, including hospitals, nursing homes, and physicians' practices. Some are employed by insurance companies.

Education

Billing and Coding specialists may receive their training through accredited programs, continuing education courses, workshops, and seminars, as well as through on-the- job training. A high school diploma or its equivalent is required to be eligible for this training. After completing the training, a coding specialist may take certification examinations through the American Health Information Management Association (AHIMA) or the American Academy of Professional Coders (AAPC). Billing Specialists may receive certification through the American Medical Billing Association (AMBA).

For more information, visit the websites of the following organizations, which are available on the Online Learning Center at www.mhhe.com/medicalassisting4e.

American Health Information Management Association (AHIMA)

American Academy of Professional Coders (AAPC)

American Medical Billing Association (AMBA)

cannot pay. These patients may be poor, uninsured, underinsured, or elderly and on a limited income. They may be patients who have suffered a severe financial loss or family tragedy. Medical ethics require physicians to provide care to individuals who need it, regardless of their ability to pay. Nevertheless, free treatment for hardship cases is at the physician's discretion.

Keep in mind that under the Equal Credit Opportunity Act (ECOA), if a patient is given free or reduced-fee treatment based on her inability to pay and another patient under similar circumstances is treated, she must also be extended the same financial consideration or a charge of discrimination may be levied against the physician. Some providers treat such patients for urgent problems and then refer the patients to federally funded clinics that are allowed to provide free or reduced-fee services related to their government funding.

Patient Relocation and Address Change

Sometimes an invoice remains unpaid because the patient has moved without leaving a forwarding address and has not received the invoice. Obviously, you will have a problem if you are trying to call such a patient about an invoice.

Remember not to discuss a debt with anyone except the person responsible for the charges. When you make a telephone call for collection, however, you may ask a third party for the patient's new address. If the third party claims not to know the new address, do not call again unless there is reason to believe that the third party has learned of the person's address since the first inquiry. You may ask the post office for a forwarding address, but if the patient cannot be located, the patient may be labeled a "skip." It is acceptable to refer the patient to the office collection agency. Be sure to keep the returned invoice stamped by the post office as "addressee unknown" or "no forwarding address" to prove a reasonable attempt to collect the debt.

Summary

17.1 Accounts receivable is an important component of any business including a medical practice because it represents the money that is owed to the practice for services provided to patients. An understanding of accounts receivable within the accounting process ensures that money is collected, managed, and documented properly.

17.2 Payments from patients can be accepted by check, debit card, cash, and credit cards. Make sure you give a receipt to the patient and place a copy of the receipt in the financial record. Record all payments on the ledger card or in the patient's electronic financial record if a computer program is used, to track accounts receivable.

17.3 Preparing a patient statement is essential in the medical office in order to bill a patient for his portion of the cost of medical care. Statements can be computer generated, typewritten or created by photocopying a clean copy of the patient ledger card.

17.4 To manage a billing cycle efficiently, maintain consistency in sending out bills (e.g., send monthly on the 15th for patients with last names starting with A–L; send monthly on the 30th for patients with last names M–Z).

17.5 Standard collection techniques include payment at the time of service and, for those charges not paid at that time, calling or writing patients to determine the reason for nonpayment or to set up a payment arrangement.

17.6 To perform a credit check, you must have current information such as the date of birth, the social security number, and the address of the patient. Make sure you get the patient's consent to perform a credit check. You may then call her employer to verify employment and contact one of three credit bureaus to obtain credit information.

17.7 Credit arrangements for patients include extending credit based on trust, or setting up a bilateral agreement of more than four payments based on the Truth and Lending Act.

17.8 Two of the most common collection problems are (1) patients who are financially unable to make payments and (2) patients relocating without leaving forwarding information, commonly known as a "skip."

REVIEW

CHAPTER 17

CASE STUDY QUESTIONS

Now that you have completed this chapter, review the case study at the beginning of the chapter and answer the following questions:

1. What is the total owed for this patient's visits?
2. How much of the total is not covered by insurance and should be billed to the patient?

Multiple-Choice Questions

1. Which of the following is a diplomatic way to ask a patient for payment?
   a. "I need $50 for today's visit."
   b. "For today's visit, the total charge is $50. How would you like to pay?"
   c. "That will be $50. What is your check number?"
   d. "Your charge for today's visit is $50. We take cash, check, credit, and debit cards."

2. A medical practice that handles patients' insurance claims
   a. devotes a lot of time to processing these claims.
   b. ensures an accurate and timely submission of the claims and prompt payment.
   c. always charges a fee for handling a patient's insurance claims.
   d. has extra expenses related to the processing of the claims.
3. CHAMPUS/TRICARE provides insurance to
   a. people over the age of 65 years.
   b. dependents of active-duty and retired military personnel.
   c. low-income, blind, or disabled parents; families receiving aid to dependent children; foster children; and children born with birth defects.
   d. families of veterans with total, permanent, service-connected disabilities. ·
4. Who is responsible for payment and for giving consent for the treatment of a 5-year-old child of divorced parents?
   a. The mother
   b. The father
   c. The parent who has legal custody
   d. The grandparents
5. Which of the following information should be included on a patient statement?
   a. The patient's income
   d. The balance from the previous month and an itemized list of charges
   c. The patient's credit card information
   d. The patient's occupation and place of employment

Discussion Questions

1. Discuss the procedure for handling a parent who brings in a child for care and asks you to bill the other parent.
2. What information is required to prepare invoices?
3. What are some of the techniques used in the task of collections?
4. Discuss the difference between a unilateral and a bilateral or mutual agreement.

Critical Thinking Questions

1. What are the most common collection problems? Give examples of how you would handle these problem cases. Who has the final decision on who receives discounted rates for services?
2. How is the use of a debit card a more reliable payment method than accepting a check from a patient?

Application Activities

1. With a partner, role-play a scenario in which you, as a medical assistant, are making an initial request for payment over the phone to a patient who is late in paying a bill but has not yet been sent any collection letters. Your partner should act as the patient, offering any information or explanation she wants.
2. Explain to another student the difference between accounts receivable and accounts payable. Use an example of each in your explanation.
3. Using the guidelines described in this chapter, write a collection letter to a fictional patient. The patient owes the doctor $125, and the account is 60 days past due. Share your letter with a classmate to analyze how well you complied with federal collection guidelines.

Virtual Fieldtrip

Visit the McGraw-Hill Higher Education Medical Assisting website at www.mhhe.com/medicalassisting4e to complete the following activity:

Go online and visit a website that offers "free" credit reports. Some examples are:

- Free Credit Report Instantly
- Free3BureauCreditReport
- Credit Smart

Write one to two paragraphs answering these questions. Is the credit report really "free"? Do you have to join first? Specifically state the disclaimer. What do the warnings on the website say?

Open the CD and complete this chapter's practice activities, play the games, listen to the key terms, and test yourself with the interactive review. E-mail, print, and/or save your results to document your proficiency.

CHAPTER 18

Accounting for the Medical Office

LEARNING OUTCOMES

After completing Chapter 18, you will be able to:

18.1 Describe traditional bookkeeping systems.

18.2 Explain the benefits of performing bookkeeping tasks on the computer.

18.3 Describe banking tasks in a medical office.

18.4 Explain the logistics of accepting, endorsing, and depositing checks from patients and insurance companies.

18.5 Model how to reconcile the office's bank statements.

18.6 Carry out several examples of disbursements.

18.7 Classify and record disbursements in a disbursement journal.

18.8 Describe how to set up and maintain a petty cash fund.

18.9 Use an employee payroll information sheets.

18.10 Explain an employee's gross earnings, total deductions, and net earnings.

18.11 Execute an employee earnings record and payroll register.

18.12 Implement the practice's tax liability accounts.

18.13 Use federal, state, and local tax forms.

18.14 Carry out employment taxes to government agencies.

MEDICAL ASSISTING COMPETENCIES

CAAHEP

VI. C (3) Describe banking procedures

VI. C (6) Differentiate between accounts payable and accounts receivable

VI. C (10) Identify procedure for preparing patient accounts

VI. C (13) Discuss types of adjustments that may be made to a patient's account

VI. P (1) Prepare a bank deposit

VI. P (2) Perform accounts receivable procedures, including
   a. Post entries on a daysheet
   e. Process a credit balance
   g. Post nonsufficient funds (NSF) checks

VI. A (1) Demonstrate sensitivity and professionalism in handling accounts receivable activities with clients

ABHES

4. **Medical Law and Ethics**
   f. Comply with federal, state, and local health laws and regulations

8. **Medical Office Business Procedures Management**
   g. Prepare and reconcile a bank statement and deposit record
   h. Post entries on a day sheet
   j. Perform accounts payable procedures
   k. Perform accounts receivable procedures
   l. Establish and maintain a petty cash fund
   m. Post adjustments
   n. Process credit balance
   o. Process refunds
   p. Post non-sufficient funds (NSF)
   q. Post collection agency payments
   r. Apply third-party guidelines
   w. Use manual or computerized bookkeeping systems
   hh. Receive, organize, prioritize, and transmit information expediently

11. **Career Development**
   Demonstrate professionalism by:
   1) Exhibiting dependability, punctuality, and a positive work ethic
   2) Exhibiting a positive attitude and a sense of responsibility
   3) Maintaining confidentiality at all times
   4) Being cognizant of ethical boundaries
   7) Expressing a responsible attitude
   9) Conducting work within scope of education, training, and ability

MEDICAL ASSISTING MEDIA

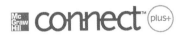 **Connect Plus+™**
connect.mcgraw-hill.com

- Electronic Health Records (E.H.R.) SpringCharts®
- eBook

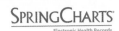

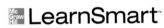 **LearnSmart™**

www.mhhe.com/learnsmart

Complete Learning Module: Accounting for the Medical Office

 Student CD-ROM

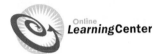 **Online Learning Center™**

www.mhhe.com/medicalassisting4e

KEY TERMS

ABA number
bookkeeping
cash flow statement
cashier's check
certified check
check
counter check
dependent
endorse

Federal Unemployment Tax Act (FUTA)
gross earnings
journalizing
limited check
money order
negotiable
net earnings
patient ledger card

pay schedule
payee
payer
pegboard system
petty cash fund
power of attorney
quarterly return
reconciliation

State Unemployment Tax Act (SUTA)
tax liability
third-party check
tracking
traveler's check
voucher check

CHAPTER OUTLINE

- The Business Side of a Medical Practice
- Patient Accounting Methods
- Banking for the Medical Office
- Managing Accounts Payable
- Managing Disbursements
- Handling Payroll
- Calculating and Filing Taxes

PREPARATION FOR CERTIFICATION

RMA (AMT) Exam
- Financial calculations and accounting procedures
- Employee payroll
- Office banking procedures
- Fundamental medical office accounting procedures

CMA (AAMA) Exam
- Banking procedures (processing accounts receivable, preparing bank deposit)
- Accounts payable
- Bookkeeping principles

CMAS Exam
- Fundamental financial management
- Patient accounts
- Payroll

Introduction

Accounting is another of the administrative competencies for the medical assisting career. A person in this career may be required to take on many duties in the medical office that would typically be done by an office manager. This chapter describes the key areas of accounting and bookkeeping that may be encountered.

CASE STUDY

Ben is a medical assistant at a family practice clinic. A patient gave him a check for $85 for payment on her account.

As you read this chapter, consider the following question:

1. What should Ben do to properly record the payment?

The Business Side of a Medical Practice

A medical practice is a business. If it is to prosper, its income must exceed its expenses. In other words, it must produce a profit. To determine whether the business is making a profit, you may be asked to do **bookkeeping,** or systematic recording of business transactions. Your records will later be analyzed by an accountant or by a more experienced medical assistant.

Bookkeeping and banking are two key responsibilities of medical assistants. To fulfill these responsibilities, you need an understanding of basic accounting systems and certain financial management skills.

Importance of Accuracy

Whenever you do bookkeeping or banking, strive for 100% accuracy. Because bookkeeping records form a chain of information, an undetected error at the first link will be carried through all other links in the chain. Undetected errors can result in billing a patient twice for the same visit, omitting bank deposits, or making improper payments to suppliers. These actions can result in lost money—and patients—for the practice.

Establishing Procedures

A consistent procedure not only helps you remember important aspects of bookkeeping and banking but also helps ensure that your books are accurate. Here are some general suggestions for maintaining accuracy in bookkeeping and banking procedures for a medical practice.

- Maintain the practice's bookkeeping and banking procedures in a logical and organized way.
- Be consistent. Always handle the same kinds of transactions in exactly the same way. For example, endorse all checks with the same information, regardless of who wrote them or when you will be depositing them.
- Use check marks as you work to avoid losing your place if you are interrupted. For example, place a red check mark on each check stub as you reconcile the bank statement.
- Write clearly, and always use the same type of pen. If more than one person performs bookkeeping and banking tasks, each person should initial her part of the procedure to identify her work. It is recommended that as

few people as possible perform these tasks, however. You may use pencil for trial balances and worksheets, but you should use pen for bookkeeping entries.

- Double-check your work frequently to detect—and correct—any errors. To correct errors, draw a straight line through the incorrect figure, and write the correct figure above it. Do not erase errors or delete them with correction fluid or tape. As with medical records, the office financial records are legal documents and every entry, even corrected ones, need to be readable at all times.
- Keep all columns of figures straight, so that decimal points align correctly.

Using set procedures will help you organize your work, help ensure accuracy, and make you a more valuable member of the practice staff.

Patient Accounting Methods

Patient accounting methods within a medical practice may be computerized or manual. Computerized patient accounting is the most commonly used type of system. Three types of manual accounting systems may be used by medical practices that are not computerized: single-entry, double-entry, and pegboard (also known as the write-it-once system). All accounting systems record income, charges (money owed to the practice), disbursements (money paid out by the practice), and other financial information. The choice of system is based on the size and complexity of the practice.

Bookkeeping on the Computer

Physicians or office managers who choose to set up the practice's bookkeeping system on the computer enjoy several important benefits over traditional bookkeeping methods. Computerized bookkeeping saves time; many repetitive tasks are done by the computer. The computer also performs mathematic calculations. Most bookkeeping software programs include built-in tax tables, which can calculate tax liabilities and so on.

As discussed in Chapter 6, many bookkeeping software programs or practice management software programs are available on the market. Any bookkeeping software package performs the same tasks as manual bookkeeping methods, so knowing these tasks is essential to performing computerized bookkeeping. Understanding these tasks is an essential part of managing books on a computer. The practice in which you work may already have a computerized bookkeeping program in place, which you should learn. It is also

Dr. _____			Date _____	
Hour	Patient	Service Provided	Charge	Paid
	1			
	2			
	3			
	4			
	5			
	6			
	7			
	8			
	9			
	10			
	11			
	12			
	13			
	14			
	15			
	16			
		Totals		

Figure 18-1. A daily log is used to record charges and payments.

a good idea to stay current by reading computer software magazines. You may learn about a new software program you might recommend to the physician or office manager, or you may read about a new or more efficient way to use the practice's current software program.

Single-Entry System

As the name implies, the single-entry system requires only one entry for each transaction. Therefore, it is the easiest system to learn and use. Unlike the double-entry system, however, the single-entry system is not self-balancing. In addition, it does not detect errors as readily and has fewer accuracy checkpoints. This system is also more likely to produce errors because information must be posted (copied) separately to each of the bookkeeping forms.

The single-entry system uses several basic records, as well as auxiliary records:

- A daily log (also called a general ledger, day sheet, or daily journal) to record charges, payments, and adjustments (or write-offs)
- Patient ledger cards or an accounts receivable ledger, which shows how much each patient owes
- A checkbook register or cash payment journal, which shows the practice expenses
- Payroll records, which show salaries, wages, and payroll deductions

- Petty cash records, which show disbursements for minor office expenses

The double-entry and pegboard systems, discussed later in this chapter, also use these records.

Daily Log. The daily log is a chronological list of the charges to patients and the payments received from patients each day, as shown in Figure 18-1. In the daily log, you write the name of each patient seen that day. Across from the name, you record the service provided, the fee charged, and the payment received (if any). This process is called **journalizing.** You then post (copy) the charges and payments from the daily log to patient ledger cards (described in the next section). Using a daily or monthly cash control sheet, you record checks and cash received as well as deposits made each day.

There are still a few physicians in individual practices who keep a daily log at their desks for entering information after they see each patient. In such cases, it may be helpful to write the name of each scheduled patient in the log to provide an appointment list. You may be responsible for this task.

In most offices, the medical assistants maintain the daily log. You can obtain the information for the log from charge slips and from checks received from patients or insurance companies. (Note: A charge slip is the original record of the doctor's services and the charge for those services. Some practices use a combination charge slip/receipt, which automatically creates a receipt to tear off for the patient. Typically, a charge slip/receipt includes a duplicate copy underneath to use for bookkeeping purposes. Remember, you need to track charges *and* receipts for payment, regardless of whether the practice uses separate charge slips and receipts or a combination.) There may also be records of outside visits, such as to nursing homes or hospital emergency rooms.

Be sure to record any night calls or other unscheduled visits in the daily log. Simply check with the physician each morning. If the physician has not noted the charge amount on a charge slip/receipt or record of outside visits, remember to apply the correct fee.

Record in the daily log all payments that come in the mail. If a check from an insurance company includes payment for more than one patient (which frequently is the case), post the appropriate amount to each patient ledger card. The information will be found on the EOB (explanation of benefits) attached to the check.

If extra columns are available, you can record additional financial information in the daily log. For example, in addition to showing the total amount charged to the patient, you can show a breakdown of that total into the amounts generated by different physicians in a group practice or by different functions of the office, such as laboratory or x-ray.

At the end of each day, total the charges and receipts in the daily log, and post these totals to the monthly summary of charges and receipts. To double-check your totals, perform the following procedures:

- Ensure that the day's total cash and check receipts are the same as the day's total bank deposit.
- Ensure that the sum of the day's charges for each type of service is the same as the total of the day's charges.

Patient Ledger Cards. Another bookkeeping task is preparing a patient ledger card for each patient. The **patient ledger card** includes the patient's name, address, home and work telephone numbers, and the name of the guarantor, who is the person responsible for payment of the charges (if different from the patient). The ledger card also lists the patient's insurance information, Social Security number, employer's name, and any special billing instructions. Figure 18-2 shows an example of a patient ledger card.

You use the patient ledger card to record charges incurred by the patient, payments received, adjustments made, and the resulting balance owed to the doctor. Because these cards document the financial transactions of the patient account, they are sometimes called account cards. In some practices, they are photocopied for use as monthly statements.

The information for the patient ledger cards comes from the daily log or from charge slips. It is best to complete all the cards at the end of the day. If this is not possible, you may complete them as time permits during the day. To prevent double or omitted postings, put a small check mark next to each entry in the daily log after you post it to the proper ledger card.

Take great care when posting, because errors on ledger cards will be reflected on patient billing statements. To ensure accuracy, add up the total charges and receipts from the ledger cards, and make sure the information matches the total charges and receipts in that day's daily log.

Accounts Receivable. Every day, you must also update the accounts receivable record, which shows the total owed to the practice (the amount able to be received but not yet received). Total up the items on the accounts receivable record, and then total up the outstanding balances on the patient ledger cards. The two numbers should match. If they do not, recheck your work to find the cause of the discrepancy.

Accounts Payable. Accounts payable are the amounts the practice owes to vendors (the amount able to be paid but not yet paid). If your responsibilities include accounts payable, keep careful records of equipment and supplies ordered, and compare orders received against the invoices. In the checkbook register, keep detailed and accurate records of accounts paid.

Record of Office Disbursements. The record of office disbursements is a list of the amounts paid for such items as medical supplies, office rent, office utilities, employee wages, postage, and equipment over a certain period of time. It shows the **payee** (the person who will receive the payment), the date, the check number, the amount paid, and the type of expense. Figure 18-3 is an example of a disbursement record.

A checkbook register may be used to record office disbursements. As an alternative, a disbursement journal or the bottom section of the daily log may be used to record office disbursements. For income tax purposes, this record should include only office expenses. The doctor's personal expenses should not be listed here.

Summary of Charges, Receipts, and Disbursements. Charges, receipts, and disbursements are usually summarized at the end of each month, quarter, or year, as shown in Figure 18-4. The summary is used to compare the income and expenses of the current period with the income and expenses from any previous period.

By analyzing summaries, a physician (or practice) can see which functions of the practice are profitable, the total amount charged for services, the payments received for services, the total cost of running the office, and a breakdown of expenses into various categories. Based on this information, the practice can make vital business decisions. For example, after analyzing monthly summaries, it may decide to budget expenses differently, collect payments more promptly, cut unprofitable services, or expand profitable services.

Although an accountant may prepare these reports, an experienced medical assistant can prepare them. If you are asked to prepare them, follow these guidelines.

- Every business day, post the total charges and receipts from the daily log to the appropriate line and column of the monthly summary.
- Every business day, also post the disbursements from the record of office disbursements to the appropriate lines and columns of the monthly summary.
- At the end of the month, total the columns on the monthly summary.

Patient's Name ___Jonathan Jackson___

Home Phone ___(612) 555-9921___ **Work Phone** ___(612) 555-1000___

Social Security No. ___111-21-4114___

Employer ___Ashton School District___

Insurance ___National Insurance Co.___

Policy # ___123-4-56-788___

Person Responsible for Charges (if Different from Patient) _____

> JONATHAN JACKSON
> 123 Fourth Avenue
> Ashton, MN 70809-1222

Date	Reference	Description	Charge	Credits Payments	Adj.	Current Balance
			Balance Forward ——→			$28 00
4/19/–	J128	OV, Stress test	$125 00	$20 00		$133 00
5/23/–	J236	Insurance payment		$92 00		$41 00

Please Pay Last Amount in This Column ▲

OV—Office Visit   C—Consultation   EX—Examination
X—X-ray   NC—No Charge   INS—Insurance
ROA—Received on Account   MA—Missed Appointment

Figure 18-2. Patient ledger cards are used to show how much each patient owes.

Record of Office Disbursements
April 2012

DATE	PAYEE	CK. NO.	TOTAL AMOUNT	TYPES OF EXPENSES										
				RENT	UTILITIES	POSTAGE	LAB/ X-RAY	MEDICAL SUPPLIES	OFFICE SUPPLIES	WAGES	INSURANCE	TAXES	TRAVEL	MISC.
01	Philips' Med. Suppl.	1778	125.00					125.00						
01	Postage	1779	16.85			16.85								
02	Medi Path	1780	32.50				32.50							
02	Quik Service Co.	1781	82.40						82.40					
02	Philips' Med. Suppl.	1782	92.00					92.00						
02	Jean Medina	1783	77.06							77.06				
05	State Dept. of Rev.	1784	189.16									189.16		
06	General Insurance	1785	165.92								165.92			
07	Postage	(Cash)	5.19			5.19								
07	Micah Smith	(Cash)	15.00										15.00	
08	IRS	1786	419.41									419.41		
12	Quik Service Co.	1787	124.00						124.00					
13	City Laundry	1788	75.00											75.00
13	National Insurance	1789	189.00								189.00			
14	Broyer Assoc.	1790	1500.00	1500.00										
14	Postage	(Cash)	12.11			12.11								
15	City Gas Co.	1791	125.00		125.00									
19	Jean Medina	1792	85.92							85.92				
19	Postage	(Cash)	8.95			8.95								
21	Philips' Med. Suppl.	1793	85.00					85.00						
23	Medi Path	1794	67.90				67.90							
24	Micah Smith	(Cash)	10.00										10.00	
24	Elena Paxson	1795	126.00							126.00				
27	Postage	1796	17.32			17.32								
28	Johnson Assoc.	1797	123.45				123.45							
	Total		3770.14	1500.00	125.00	60.42	223.85	302.00	206.40	288.98	354.92	608.57	25.00	75.00

Figure 18-3. A record of office disbursements lists the amounts paid over a certain period of time.

Quarterly Summary of Charges, Receipts, and Disbursements, 2012

	MONTH	1 CHARGES	2 RECEIPTS	3 DISBURSE-MENTS	4 WAGES	5 RENT & UTILITIES	Types of Disbursements 6 OFFICE EXPENSES	7 GENERAL MEDICAL	8 X-RAY/ LAB.	9 TAXES	10 PERSONAL	11 MISC.
1	Jan.	15400.00	14800.00	6218.14	3349.50	1625.00	129.86	93.45	241.86	589.02	100.00	89.45
2	Feb.	18255.00	18950.00	7050.40	3872.80	1683.08	235.00	118.72	266.00	611.20	186.60	77.00
3	Mar.	13850.00	13250.00	6530.14	3666.10	1702.85	43.85	243.11	187.02	577.00	88.11	22.10
4												
5	Subtotal	47505.00	47000.00	19798.68	10888.40	5010.93	408.71	455.28	694.88	1777.22	374.71	188.55
6												
7	Apr.											
8	May											
9	June											
10												
11	Subtotal											
12												
13	July											
14	Aug.											
15	Sept.											
16												
17	Subtotal											
18												
19	Oct.											
20	Nov.											
21	Dec.											
22												
23	Subtotal											
24												
25	Grand Total											
26												
27												
28												
29												
30												
31												
32												
33												
34												
35												
36												

Figure 18-4. Creating a summary of charges, receipts, and disbursements is a regular bookkeeping task, performed monthly, quarterly, or yearly.

PROCEDURE 18-1

Posting Entries, Adjustments, and Collection Payments

Procedure Goal: To maintain a system that promotes accurate record keeping for the practice

Materials: Daily log sheets, patient ledger cards, and check register, or computerized bookkeeping system; summaries of charges, receipts, and disbursements

Method:

1. Use a new log (day) sheet each day. For each patient seen that day, record the patient name, the relevant charges, and any payments received, calculating any necessary adjustments and new balances. If you're using a computerized system, enter the patient's name or account number, the relevant charges, and any payments received and adjustments made in the appropriate areas. The computer will calculate the new balances.

Rationale
Each day's transactions must be accurately and promptly recorded.

2. Create a ledger card for each new patient, and maintain a ledger card for all existing patients. The ledger card should include the patient's name, address, home and work telephone numbers, and insurance company. It should also contain the name of the guarantor (if different from the patient). Update the ledger card every time the patient incurs a charge or makes a payment. Be sure to adjust the account balance after every transaction. In a computerized system, a patient record is the same as a ledger card. This record must also be maintained and updated.

Rationale
The information on each patient's ledger card must match that of the daily log.

3. Record all deposits accurately in the check register. File the deposit receipt—with a detailed listing of checks, cash, and money orders deposited—for later use in reconciling the bank statement. The deposit amount should match the amount of money collected by the practice for that day.

4. When paying bills for the practice, enter each check in the check register accurately, including the check number, date, payee, and amount before writing the check.

Rationale
Record payments first so the step will not be skipped once the check is written.

5. Prepare and/or print a summary of charges, receipts, and disbursements every month, quarter, or year, as directed. Be sure to double-check all entries and calculations from the monthly summary before posting them to the quarterly summary. Also, double-check the entries and calculations from the quarterly summary before posting them to the yearly summary.

Rationale
Double-checking all entries ensures mistakes are found and corrected as soon as possible.

- At the end of each quarter, post the charges, receipts, and disbursements for each of the previous 3 months to the quarterly summary. Then, total each column.
- At the end of the year, post the charges, receipts, and disbursements for each of the previous 12 months (or 4 quarters) to the annual summary. Then, total each column.

Remember that the total charges and total receipts in any summary should be almost the same. They may not be identical because some bills may not have been fully collected. Procedure 18-1 offers a plan for setting up a medical practice accounting system.

Pegboard System

The **pegboard system** lets you write each transaction once while recording it on four different bookkeeping forms.

Because of the convenience of this system it was commonly called the "write-it-once" system and used to be the most widely used bookkeeping system in medical practices. With the advancement of computerized medical billing and records, this system is seldom used in actual practice. However, understanding the principles of this system will be an essential part of your training as a medical assistant and will help you understand the concepts behind the computerized accounting system.

A pegboard system usually includes a lightweight board with pegs on the left or right edges. The pegs match holes that are punched in daily log sheets, patient ledger cards, charge slips/receipts, and deposit slips. The holes allow the forms to be aligned while stacked on top of each other. Information, entered on only one form, is simultaneously transferred to the form(s) below. Generally these forms are printed on NCR (no-carbon-required) paper. If not, you must place carbon paper between the forms.

Starting the Business Day.   Place a daily log sheet on the pegboard at the beginning of each day. Then, place the stack of charge slips/receipts on the pegs, aligning the top line of the first charge slip/receipt with the daily log top line. Because the charge slips/receipts are shingled, or layered one over the other from top to bottom, alignment of the first aligns all the others. The charge slips/receipts are prenumbered. This numbering promotes good cash control and theoretically prevents embezzlement.

Upon Patient Arrival.   As each patient comes into the office, place the patient's ledger card under the next available charge slip/receipt. Be sure to align the card's first blank line with the carbon strip on the charge slip/receipt. Write the date, the patient's name, and the patient's previous balance on the charge slip section. The information will automatically be recorded in the daily log and on the patient ledger card.

Attaching the Charge Slip/Receipt to the Patient Chart.   Next, remove the charge slip/receipt and attach it to the patient chart so that the doctor will see it. After examining the patient, the doctor fills in the appropriate charges on the charge slip/receipt, indicates when the next appointment is needed, and gives the charge slip/receipt to the patient.

Before the Patient Leaves.   The patient comes to you with the completed charge slip/receipt, and you again place the ledger card between the charge slip/receipt and the daily log. Check to be sure you align it properly. On the charge slip/receipt, write the charge slip/receipt number, date, procedure (or code), charges, payments, new balance, and the date and time of the next appointment (if any). As you write this information, it should be automatically transferred onto the ledger card and daily log. Finally, tear off the receipt, and give it to the patient. You can now return the patient ledger card to the file.

Payments After the Patient Visit.   If you receive payments sometime after the patient visit, either by mail or in person, record them on the patient ledger card and day sheet as you normally would. Record charges for doctor visits to hospitalized patients or other out-of-office visits in the same way. If required, you can use the pegboard system to record bank deposits and petty cash disbursements in the daily log, but you will need the appropriate disbursement journal and overlapping forms.

Returned Checks.   If a patient's check does not clear due to nonsufficient funds (NSF), you must adjust the account accordingly. NSF payments are first deducted from the office checking account. The patient's account is then updated with a negative payment (noted in parentheses in the payment column) for the amount of the check, adding that amount back to the patient balance. An office fee may also be charged for the inconvenience of dealing with the NSF check. In addition if the bank imposes a fee on the office, these bank fees should also be passed to the patient to recoup the loss for the practice, and marked on the patient's ledger. Depending on office policy, the patient may now be seen on a *cash only* basis by the practice. Procedure 18-2 explains the procedure for posting an NSF payment.

End of the Day.   At the end of each day, total and check the arithmetic (addition and subtraction) in all columns. If you find an error, correct it immediately by drawing a line through it and making a new entry on the next available writing line. Remember to make the correction on the patient ledger card also and to issue a new receipt to the patient. To balance a pegboard system (or even check your math on a patient ledger card), after adding the figures in each column, use the following formula for the column totals:

Previous balance + Today's charges − (Payments + Adjustments) = New accounts receivable total

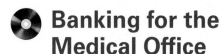

Banking for the Medical Office

Besides bookkeeping, you may be responsible for handling the banking for the practice. Because a practice may use traditional (manual) or electronic (computerized) banking methods, you should be familiar with both. Regardless of which method you use, remember to keep all banking materials secure because they represent the finances of the practice. For example, to prevent theft of checks, always put the checkbook in a securely locked place when it is not in use. Also, file deposit receipts promptly. If they are lost, you have no proof that a deposit was made. Lack of proof could cost the practice thousands of dollars. If you ever suspect checks are stolen from your office, contact the bank and police department as soon as possible.

Banking Tasks

Banking tasks for the medical practice include:

- Writing checks
- Accepting checks
- Endorsing checks
- Making deposits
- Reconciling bank statements

To perform these tasks properly, you must be familiar with several terms and concepts related to banking.

Checks.   A **check** is a bank draft or order for payment. The person who writes the check is called the **payer**. By writing a check, the payer directs the bank to pay a sum of money on demand to the payee. In order to be considered **negotiable** (legally transferable from one person to another), a check must:

- Be written and signed by the payer or maker
- Include the amount of money to be paid, considered a promise to pay a specified sum

PROCEDURE 18-2

Posting a Nonsufficient Funds (NSF) Check

Procedure Goal: To post a nonsufficient funds (NSF) check to patient's account

Materials: Computer, returned check, patient ledger sheet, calculator (optional), daily log sheet (optional)

Method:

1. Locate the patient's account on the computer or pull the patient's ledger card for manual processes.

   Rationale

   To make sure that you have the correct patient (account) for the NSF check.

2. Use your medical facility code for NSF check or charge and create a new billing entry for the patient and then post the returned check using the NSF code. On the daily log sheet, write the NSF check number and the words *check returned by bank* in the *professional services column.* In the adjustment column, place the amount of the check in parentheses to indicate that the amount is debited as an *adjustment.* Add the amount to the old balance and enter it in the *new balance* column as well.

3. Post the fees for the NSF check using the code provided by the medical facility. On the daily log sheet, post the charge for the fee in the *charge* column. Add the new charge to the old balance and record in the new balance column.

4. Use your medical facility's code for an NSF check (if used), and using today's date, create a new charge log for the patient. Using the code and the description *Check returned by bank* in the description column.

5. In the Payment column insert the amount of the NSF check in parentheses

   Rationale

   Parentheses represent a *negative payment* to the patient's account.

6. Add the amount of the NSF check to the previous balance and insert that figure in the *Current Balance* column.

   Rationale

   As a *negative payment* the payment amount is added, not subtracted to the previous balance to obtain the new Current Balance.

7. On the next line, also using today's date, add the description of *NSF Office Fee* with the office charge for NSF checks returned by the bank. Add this charge to the previous balance to obtain the new *Current Balance*

DAILY LOG	Gisele M. Williams, M.D. Will Collins, M.D.						
Date	Code	Patient	Today's Charge	Payment/ Adjustment	Current Balance	Previous Balance	Provider
3/22	Ashley Wilkins	Payment – Ck #102		15.00	0.00	15.00	WC
3/30	Ashley Wilkins	(NSF) Ck returned by Bank		(15.00)	15.00	0.00	WC
3/30	Ashley Wilkins	NSF Office Fee	35.00		50.00	15.00	WC

- Be made payable to the payee or bearer
- Be made payable on demand or on a specific date
- Include the name of the bank that is directed to make payment

Other Negotiable Papers. You may receive other negotiable paper in addition to standard personal and business checks.

- A **cashier's check** is a check issued on bank paper signed by a bank representative. It is usually purchased by individuals who do not have checking accounts.

- A **certified check** is a payer's check written and signed by the payer and stamped "Certified" by the bank. This certification means that the bank has already drawn money from the payer's account to guarantee that the check will be paid when submitted. (The money is set aside to cover this specific check.) Few banks offer certified checks anymore.

- A **money order** is another kind of certificate of guaranteed payment. Money orders may be purchased from banks (bank money orders) or post offices (postal money orders) or from some convenience stores.

Check Codes. The face (front) of every check contains two important items: the American Banking Association (ABA) number and the magnetic ink character recognition (MICR) code. The **ABA number** appears as a fraction, such as 60–117/310, on the upper edge of all printed checks. It identifies the geographic area and specific bank on which the check is drawn.

Found at the bottom of a check, the MICR code consists of numbers and characters printed in magnetic ink, which can be read by MICR equipment at the bank. This code enables checks to be read, sorted, and recorded by computer.

Types of Checking Accounts. A physician is likely to have three different types of checking accounts: a personal account, a business account for office expenses, and an interest-earning account. The interest-earning account will be used for paying special expenses, such as property taxes and insurance premiums. Most of your work will be with the business checking account. You may sometimes, however, make payments from, or transfer money to, the interest-earning account, as directed.

Accepting Checks. Before accepting any check, review it carefully. First be sure the check has the correct date, amount, and signature and that no corrections have been made. Figure 18-5 shows a correctly written and endorsed check. Do not accept a **third-party check** (one made out to the patient rather than to the practice) unless it is from a health insurance company. Also, do not accept a check marked "Payment in Full" unless it actually does pay the

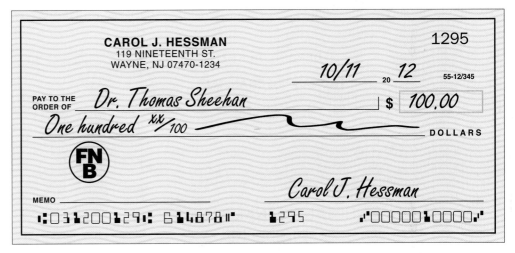

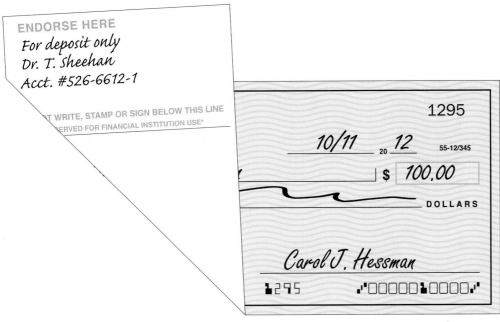

Figure 18-5. After verifying that a patient's check is correct, immediately endorse it with "For Deposit Only," the name of the practice, and the account number.

complete outstanding balance. You may accept a check signed by someone other than the payer if the person who signed the check has power of attorney. **Power of attorney** gives a person the legal right to handle financial matters for another person who is unable to do so. Frequently power of attorney is granted to a patient's spouse, son, or daughter.

Be sure to follow the policy of your practice when accepting a check. For example, if a patient is new or unfamiliar, office policy may require you to request patient identification and to compare the signature on the identification with the signature on the check. Policy may also require that you not accept a check for more than the amount due.

Endorsing Checks. After accepting a check, immediately **endorse** it by writing the name of the doctor or the practice on the back. Include the words "For Deposit Only" and the account number. (For convenience, this statement may be made into a rubber stamp.) This type of endorsement, known as a restrictive endorsement, prevents the check from being cashed if it is lost or stolen because the only way the check can be redeemed is by deposit into the specified account.

Be sure to endorse the check in ink, using a pen or rubber stamp. Place the endorsement in the 1.5-inch area indicated on the back of the check. Most personal and business checks have a number of lines or a shaded area preprinted on the checks for this purpose. Leave the rest of the back of the check blank for the use of the bank.

Completing the Deposit Slip. After endorsing the check, post the payment to the patient ledger card, and put the check with others to be deposited. Then, fill out a deposit slip, as shown in Figure 18-6. The account number is printed on deposit slips in MICR numbers that match those on the checks. As mentioned, these numbers enable checks and deposit slips to be read, sorted, and recorded by computer.

Banks will accept a list of deposited items on something other than the bank-provided deposit slip if the bank's deposit slip is attached. For example, if you are depositing 50 checks, you may create a computer printout listing the payers' names, check numbers, amount of each check, and total. You can then attach the printout to a deposit slip with the total written on the deposit slip. Another

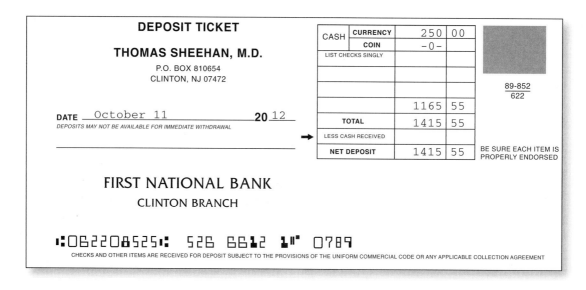

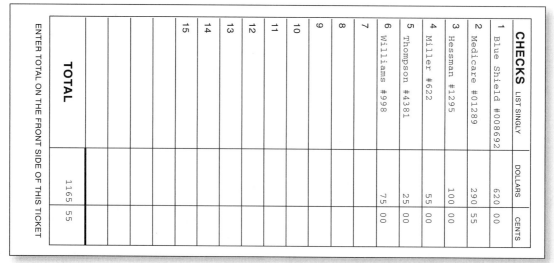

Figure 18-6. List each check on the deposit slip, including the check number and amount.

PROCEDURE 18-3 WORK//PRODUCT

Making a Bank Deposit

Procedure Goal: To prepare cash and checks for deposit and to deposit them properly into a bank account

Materials: Bank deposit slip and items to be deposited, such as checks, cash, and money orders

Method:

1. Divide the bills, coins, checks, and money orders into separate piles.

2. Sort the bills by denomination, from largest to smallest. Then, stack them, portrait side up, in the same direction. Total the amount of the bills, and write this amount on the deposit slip on the line marked "Currency."

   Rationale
   This is the order necessary for the teller to easily verify your totals. The deposit slip separates bill totals from coin totals.

3. If you have enough coins to fill coin wrappers, put them in wrappers of the proper denomination. If not, count the coins, and put them in the deposit bag. Total the amount of coins, and write this amount on the deposit slip on the line marked "Coin."

4. Review all checks and money orders to be sure they are properly endorsed with a restrictive endorsement. List each check on the deposit slip, including the check number and amount.

5. List each money order on the deposit slip. Include the notation "money order" or "MO" and the name of the writer.

6. Calculate the total deposit (total of amounts or currency, coin, checks, and money orders). Write this amount on the deposit slip on the line marked "Total." If you do not use deposit slips that record a copy for the office, photocopy the deposit slip for your office records.

   Rationale
   Doing so provides a legal record for your office.

7. Record the total amount of the deposit in the office checkbook register.

   Rationale
   So that an accurate balance is recorded

8. If you plan to make the deposit in person, place the currency, coins, checks, and money orders in a deposit bag. If you cannot make the deposit in person, put the checks and money orders in a special bank-by-mail envelope, or put all deposit items in an envelope and send it by registered mail.

   Rationale
   If the deposit is not made in person, sending it Registered mail provides proof or receipt and insures the deposit against loss.

9. Make the deposit in person or by mail.

10. Obtain a deposit receipt from the bank. File it with the copy of the deposit slip in the office for later use when reconciling the bank statement.

    Rationale
    For accurate recordkeeping and proof of deposit.

---

method is to attach a calculator or adding machine tape listing the individual check amounts and a total.

Making the Deposit. Plan to deposit checks and cash into the practice's bank account in person at the bank, as described in Procedure 18-3. Make sure you are aware of your surroundings when making deposits because of safety issues. Avoid sending cash through the mail, but if it is absolutely necessary to do so, use registered mail. Always obtain a deposit receipt from the bank.

In a busy physician's office, you may need to make deposits every day. If the physician has a limited practice, you may make deposits less frequently. Keep in mind, however, that making deposits more frequently increases cash flow and reduces the risk of lost or bounced checks.

Reconciling Bank Statements. Another banking task is reconciling the bank statement. **Reconciliation** involves comparing the office's financial records with the bank records to ensure that they are consistent (all numbers agree) and accurate. In most practices this task is performed once a month when the practice receives the monthly checking account statement from the bank. An example of a bank statement is shown in Figure 18-7. The process of reconciliation is explained in Procedure 18-4.

Electronic Banking

Compared with traditional banking methods, electronic banking has several advantages. Electronic banking can improve productivity, cash flow, and accuracy. The use of electronic banking can also speed up many banking tasks.

If your medical office uses electronic banking, your basic tasks will be the same as in an office that uses

First State Bank of Englewood

1st

First State Bank of Englewood
CN 1
Englewood WI 54534-0001

PAGE 1

ACCOUNT NO.   518-833-3

STATEMENT PERIOD
07/19/12 TO 08/20/12

CAROL J CHARLESTON, M.D.
SUITE 49
1013 HUGHES DR
LAWRENCE SQUARE WI 54690-1226

YOUR ACCOUNT SUMMARY

DEPOSIT ACCOUNTS	BALANCE
CHECKING ACCOUNT	2,088.08
SAVINGS ACCOUNT	10,602.54
TOTAL	12,690.62

CHECKING ACCOUNT

CAROL J CHARLESTON, M.D.

SUMMARY OF ACCOUNT   518-833-3

BEGINNING BALANCE ON 07/18/12	3,055.24
DEPOSITS AND CREDITS	+3,819.02
CHECKS & WITHDRAWALS	-4,786.18
ENDING BALANCE ON 08/20/12	2,088.08

CHECKS PAID: 38

CHECK	AMOUNT	DATE PAID	REFERENCE#	CHECK	AMOUNT	DATE PAID	REFERENCE#
CHECK	450.00	07/19/12	81569110	2226	181.00	08/12/12	05105878
2202	146.23	07/31/12	29521570	2227	24.74	08/19/12	06120827
2203	122.03	07/29/12	29141271	2228	140.00	08/12/12	05022086
2210*	43.00	07/29/12	07046380	2229	148.71	08/16/12	27248941
2211	60.09	08/01/12	04597911	2230	53.16	08/13/12	27852752
2214*	123.59	07/24/12	29470425	2231	50.00	08/14/12	01018325
2215	47.70	07/19/12	12357289	2232	50.00	08/13/12	05080148
2216	9.00	07/22/12	05479786	2233	15.00	08/16/12	04709533
2217	30.00	07/26/12	29841864	2234	13.95	08/19/12	06008593
2218	19.00	07/30/12	04330539	2235	123.59	08/14/12	27050650
2219	12.00	07/24/12	04037820	2236	50.00	08/13/12	05099115
2220	35.93	07/24/12	04068844	2237	50.00	08/15/12	03014667
2221	10.00	08/12/12	05091269	2238	20.00	08/16/12	04675854
2222	23.48	07/24/12	29465653	2239	47.70	08/14/12	06172997
2223	242.43	07/26/12	29804419	2240	24.74	08/19/12	06120925
2224	150.00	07/30/12	29405827	2243*	400.00	08/14/12	29652307
2225	830.00	08/07/12	02242873	2344	400.00	08/14/12	29652306

Figure 18-7. Each month you will receive a current bank statement, which you should reconcile with the previous statement and your checkbook register.

traditional banking methods. How these tasks are performed, however, may be quite different. When you use electronic banking, you are still responsible for recording and depositing checks, just as if you were using traditional methods, but you will see these differences.

- Rather than your recording each check in a paper checkbook and determining the new balance, the computer software calculates the new balance for you.
- Rather than your reconciling the office bank statement on paper, the computer software does it automatically.
- Rather than putting the checkbook and banking forms in a securely locked place at the end of the day, you use a computer password for security.

Many medical office software programs are available today. Each one has a different interface, uses different menus, and prompts you for information in different ways. Certain general concepts apply to all. For specific information, consult the user's manual that comes with your practice's computer software. All software will allow you to perform the following tasks:

- Record deposits
- Pay bills
- Display the checkbook
- Balance the checkbook

Record Deposits. If you select "Record Deposits," a message on the computer screen prompts you to enter information about each check to be deposited that day. This information usually includes the check writer's name and the amount of the check. The check's ABA number may also be requested. After you enter this information, the computer gives you a chance to double-check it. If all the information is correct, you continue entering and checking the other deposits, one at a time. You can then select a command to print a deposit slip that contains the information you have just entered. To make the deposit, place the cash and checks in a deposit bag along with the computerized deposit slip and the bank's deposit slip.

Pay Bills. The bill-paying function allows you to log checks that you write into a computerized checkbook register. For each check you want to write, a message on the computer screen should prompt you for information, such as the payee and the amount of the check. The computer should also give you a chance to verify and correct this information before moving on to the next check or printing the actual checks.

Some software programs automatically assign the next available check number to each new check you enter. To double-check that the computer-assigned check numbers match those on the actual checks, print a list of the checks you have entered and compare it with the checks before mailing them.

Display the Checkbook. The checkbook display function allows you to review the electronic checkbook register. Although you cannot change information that appears in the register, you can print it out. Thus, you can be sure the checks have been recorded properly, and you can check your latest balance.

If you select "Display Checkbook" from the "Banking" menu, the computer displays a list of all checks that have been entered into the register. Information includes check number, date, payee, and amount. Scrolling up and down reveals all the checks in the register. (Some banks also allow you to access this information by telephone. The Points on Practice section gives more information about telephone banking.)

Balance Checkbook. The "Balance Checkbook" option electronically reconciles the monthly bank statement. After you enter the appropriate date or dates, the computer screen displays all the checks and deposits that were logged into the register in the order they were posted. Figure 18-8 shows an example of this function.

The next screen highlights each check or deposit that has not been seen on a previous bank statement. You are prompted to indicate whether that item appears on the current statement, usually using Y for yes and N for no. After the computer queries these items, it may ask you to enter any items that appear on the current bank statement but are not in the checkbook, such as service charges.

Finally, a message on the screen prompts you to enter the current account balance from the bank statement. Then, the computer reconciles the bank statement. It will alert you if the system balance does not agree with the balance on the bank statement. If the balance does not agree, recheck the information you entered for possible error. If your work is correct, and the balances still do not agree, call the bank to determine if a bank error has been made.

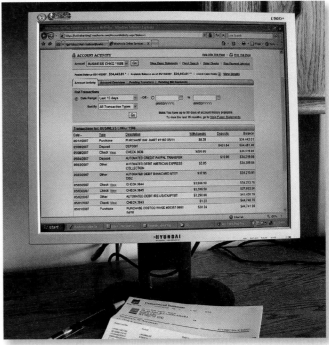

Figure 18-8. Electronic banking will allow you to see the "Balanced Checkbook" on the screen.

PROCEDURE 18-4 WORK//PRODUCT

Reconciling a Bank Statement

Procedure Goal: To ensure that the bank record of deposits, payments, and withdrawals agrees with the practice's record of deposits, payments, and withdrawals

Materials: Previous bank statement, current bank statement, reconciliation worksheet (if not part of current bank statement), deposit receipts, red pencil, check stubs or checkbook register, returned checks

Method:

1. Check the closing balance on the previous statement against the opening balance on the new statement. The balances should match. If they do not, call the bank.

2. Record the closing balance from the new statement on the reconciliation worksheet (Figure 18-9). This worksheet usually appears on the back of the bank statement.

3. Check each deposit receipt against the bank statement. Place a red check mark in the upper right corner of each receipt that is recorded

on the statement. Total the amount of deposits that do *not* appear on the statement. Add this amount to the closing balance on the reconciliation worksheet.

Rationale
Deposits not appearing on the statement have not been recorded by the bank at the time the statement was created.

4. Put the redeemed checks in numerical order. (Your bank may send you several sheets consisting of photocopies of checks instead of the actual checks.)

5. Compare each redeemed check with the bank statement, making sure that the amount on the check agrees with the amount on the statement. Place a red check mark in the upper-right corner of each redeemed check that is recorded on the statement. Also, place a check mark on the check stub or check register entry. Any checks that were written but that do not appear on the

---

HOW TO BALANCE YOUR CHECKING ACCOUNT

1. Subtract any service charges that appear on this statement from your checkbook balance.
2. Add any interest paid on your checking account to your checkbook balance.
3. Check off (✔) in your checkbook register all checks and pre-authorized transactions listed on your statement.
4. Use the worksheet to list checks you have written, ATM withdrawals, and Point of Sale transactions which are not listed on your statement.

5. Enter the closing balance on the statement.	$	.
6. Add any deposits not shown on the statement.	+	.
7. Subtotal	$	.
8. Subtract total transactions outstanding (from worksheet on right).	−	.
9. Account balance (should match balance in your checkbook register).	$	.

IF YOUR ACCOUNT DOES NOT BALANCE
a. Check your addition and subtraction first on this form and then in your checkbook.
b. Be sure the deposit amounts on your statement are the same as those in your checkbook.
c. Be sure all the check amounts on your statement agree with the amounts entered in your checkbook register.
d. Be sure all checks written prior to this reconcilement period but not listed on the statement are listed on the worksheet.
e. Verify that all MAC® ATM, Point of Sale, and other pre-authorized transactions have been recorded in your checkbook register.
f. Review last month's statement to be certain any corrections were entered into your checkbook.

WORKSHEET Transactions Outstanding	
Number or Date	Amount
TOTAL	

Figure 18-9. Use the reconciliation worksheet on the back of the bank statement to reconcile the statement with your checkbook register.

continued ⟶

PROCEDURE 18-4 [WORK // PRODUCT]

Reconciling a Bank Statement (concluded)

statement and were not returned as redeemed are considered "outstanding" checks. You can find these easily on the check stubs or checkbook register because they have no red check mark.

6. List each outstanding check separately on the worksheet, including its check number and amount. Total the outstanding checks, and subtract this total from the bank statement balance.

Rationale

These checks have not cleared yet. The total of these checks will still appear in the medical practice balance.

7. If the statement shows that the checking account earned interest, add this amount to the checkbook balance.

Rationale

You did not know about accrued interest until receiving the statement.

8. If the statement lists such items as a service charge, check printing charge, or automatic payment, subtract them from the checkbook balance.

Rationale

You did not know about these charges until receiving the statement.

9. Compare the new checkbook balance with the new bank statement balance. They should match. If they do not, repeat the process, rechecking all calculations. Double-check the addition and subtraction in the checkbook register. Review the checkbook register to make sure you did not omit any items. Ensure that you carried the correct balance forward from one register page to the next. Double-check that you made the correct additions or subtractions for all interest earned and charges.

10. If your work is correct, and the balances still do not agree, call the bank to determine if a bank error has been made. Contact the bank promptly because the bank may have a time limit for corrections. The bank may consider the bank statement correct if you do not point out an error within 2 weeks (or other period, according to bank policy).

Points on Practice

Telephone Banking

Telephone banking is a form of electronic banking that enables you to access your bank's computer system by phone to obtain account information and perform simple banking tasks. To use telephone banking, you should have a push-button telephone, the telephone personal identification number (TPIN) assigned to your practice by the bank, and the telephone number that accesses the telephone banking system.

The telephone banking system prompts you for information. You use the push-button pad on the telephone to provide the information. For example, an automated voice may ask you to press 1 to inquire about deposits or 2 to inquire about withdrawals. Telephone banking is especially useful for the following banking tasks:

- Checking the current balance of an account
- Determining whether deposited funds are available

- Obtaining the date and amount of the last few deposits and the last few checks paid (usually the last three)
- Finding out if a specific check has been paid
- Transferring funds between accounts (if the practice has more than one account)
- Stopping payment on checks

Although this form of electronic banking is especially useful for some services, you cannot use it to manage all banking tasks. For example, you cannot use it to make deposits or reconcile a bank statement. However, it can be quite convenient for the day-to-day banking tasks just listed. If you have a hearing impairment and have a telecommunications device for the deaf (TDD) installed on the telephone, you can bank by phone.

PROCEDURE 18-5

Setting Up the Accounts Payable System

Procedure Goal: To set up an accounts payable system

Materials: Disbursements journal, petty cash record, payroll register, pen

Method:

Setting Up the Disbursements Journal

1. Write in column headings for the basic information about each check: date, payee's name, check number, and check amount.

2. Write in column headings for each type of business expense, such as rent and utilities.

3. Write in column headings (if space is available) for deposits and the account balance.

4. Record the data from completed checks under the appropriate column headings.

5. Be sure to subtract payments from the balance and add deposits to it.

Rationale

It is important to keep an accurate running total of the disbursements journal.

Setting Up the Petty Cash Record

1. Write in column headings for the date, transaction number, payee, brief description, amount of transaction, and type of expense.

2. Write in a column heading (if space is available) for the petty cash fund balance.

3. Record the data from petty cash vouchers under the appropriate column headings.

4. Subtract payments made from petty cash and when replenishing the fund, add the replenishment amount to the current balance.

Rationale

The petty cash journal must have an accurate accounting of its payments and replenishments.

Setting Up the Payroll Register

1. Write in column headings for check number, employee name, earnings to date, hourly rate, hours worked, regular earnings, overtime hours worked, and overtime earnings.

2. Write in column headings for total gross earnings for the pay period and gross taxable earnings.

3. Write in column headings for each deduction. These may include federal income tax, Federal Insurance Contributions Act (FICA) tax, state income tax, local income tax, and various voluntary deductions.

4. Write in a column heading for net earnings.

5. Each time you write payroll checks, record earning and deduction data under the appropriate column headings on the payroll register.

Managing Accounts Payable

As you learned in Chapter 17, accounts payable are the practice's expenses (money leaving the business), and accounts receivable reflect a practice's income (money coming into the business). This section focuses on accounts payable, including payroll. A basic accounting principle to bear in mind is that when a practice's income exceeds its expenses, it has a profit. When a practice's expenses exceed its income, it has a loss.

Because of this relationship between income and expenses, most practices try to reduce expenses by controlling accounts payable. As a medical assistant, you play an important role in helping control accounts payable and maximize profits.

Accounts payable fall into three main groups:

1. Payments for supplies, equipment, and practice-related products and services
2. Payroll, which may be the largest of the accounts payable
3. Taxes owed to federal, state, and local agencies

A practice's accounting system usually consists of several elements. These elements include the daily log, patient ledger cards, the checkbook, the disbursements journal, the petty cash record, and the payroll register.

The daily log and patient ledger cards are used primarily for accounts receivable. The disbursements journal, petty cash record, and payroll register are used primarily in accounts payable. Procedure 18-5 tells you how to set up and use these accounting tools effectively.

Managing Disbursements

A disbursement is any payment the physician's office makes for goods or services. One of the most common disbursements is payment for office supplies. Other disbursements include payments for equipment, dues, rent, taxes, salary, and utilities. No matter what type of disbursement you make on behalf of the practice, you must keep accurate records of the purchase and the payment.

Managing Supplies

In most practices, the physician authorizes one person to handle the purchasing of supplies and other products. This person is usually the office manager or medical assistant.

Guidelines for purchasing supplies are discussed in detail in Chapter 8. When buying clinical or office supplies, keep these six principles in mind to control expenses.

1. Order only the necessary supplies, and order them only in the proper amounts. Buying too much reduces cash flow. Buying too little may cause you to run out of needed items and you may have to reorder too often.

2. Combine orders when possible. You may save money and time by placing a larger order for several items at once rather than placing a smaller order each time an item is needed.

3. Follow your practice's purchasing guidelines. For example, you may have to get the physician's approval for purchases over a specific dollar amount. Employees may have to submit purchase orders (formal requests for goods or services).

4. Buy from reputable suppliers. They are more likely to provide on-time delivery and satisfactory handling of your order. If your office does not already have a list of reliable suppliers, ask for recommendations from other practices.

5. Get the best-quality supplies for the best price.

6. For clinical supplies, consider the amount for which insurance companies will reimburse the practice. For example, if your office does only a few throat cultures a year, it might make more sense to send those patients elsewhere for the test than to stock the supplies required. The small reimbursement amount for a few throat cultures may not justify purchasing the supplies. Also consider shelf life. Do not buy large amounts of clinical supplies that will expire before use.

Writing Checks

Virtually all disbursements are made by check. Paying by check gives the practice complete, accurate records of all financial transactions.

Before writing a check, make sure the checking account balance is up-to-date and large enough to cover the check you want to write. Enter the date, check number, payee information, and reason for the payment on the check stub, and then subtract the amount of each check from the previous balance, enter the new balance, and carry that balance forward to the next stub. Do this step before writing the check so the payment entry is not accidentally omitted from the disbursement journal.

If you use a pegboard system, you will automatically record the date, check number, payee, and check amount on the check register as you write out the check. You must note the reason for payment and the new balance manually, however. Record that information in the appropriate spaces on the register.

If you make an error when completing a check, write VOID in ink across the front of the check in large letters so that it cannot be used again. Then file the voided check in numerical order with the returned checks.

After filling out the check properly, detach it from the checkbook and give it to the doctor to sign, along with the invoice to be paid. (With experience, you may be trusted to sign checks under a certain amount.) Mark the date, check number, and amount paid on the invoice. Make a copy of the invoice for your records. Keep these copies with supporting documents, such as order forms or packing slips, in a paid-invoice file. Then, mail the check and the original invoice to the payee in a neatly hand-addressed or typewritten envelope. If you use a window envelope, be sure the payee's address shows through the window.

Commonly Used Checks. Most practices use checks from a standard checkbook, or they use **voucher checks,** business checks with stubs attached. Voucher checks come in several styles. A common style is a large, ring-bound checkbook, with three checks to a page. A perforation divides each check from its matching stub, which the practice retains.

Limited checks are sometimes used for payroll. A **limited check** states that it is void after a certain time limit. Many practices use checks that are void after 90 days. Some limited check accounts may also limit the amount for which a limited check may be written.

Other Types of Checks. You or the physician may sometimes need to use other types of checks. The physician may use a cashier's check to pay certain types of taxes. A cashier's check is purchased from a bank, written on the bank's own checking account, and signed by a bank official.

The physician may use a certified check to pay certain taxes or to buy property. A certified check is a standard check that the bank verifies and certifies before it is used. This certification means that funds have been set aside to guarantee payment of the check.

A **counter check** is a special bank check that allows the depositor to withdraw funds from her account only. It states, "Pay to the Order of Myself Only." The physician may use a counter check when she wants to withdraw money but has forgotten her checkbook.

A physician may use **traveler's checks** when attending an out-of-town conference or whenever using a personal check or carrying a lot of cash is not appropriate. Printed in $10, $20, $50, and $100 denominations, these checks must be signed at the location where they are purchased (usually a bank). To use traveler's checks, the physician fills in the payee's name and signs it in a second place. She must sign it in the payee's presence so the payee can ensure that the signatures match.

Recording Disbursements

You may record disbursements in a check register, in a disbursements journal, or on the bottom section of the daily log.

If you use a disbursements journal, follow these steps to record disbursements.

1. When beginning a new journal page, give each column a heading to reflect the type of expense, such as utilities or rent.
2. For each check, fill in the date, payee's name, check number, and check amount in the appropriate columns.
3. Determine the expense category of the check.
4. Record the check amount in the column for that type of business expense.
5. If you must divide a check between two or more expense columns, record the total in the check amount column. Then record the amount that applies to each type of expense in the appropriate column. The total amount must equal the sum of the amounts listed between the columns.

Recording disbursements in columns for each type of expense allows you to total and track expenses by category. **Tracking** (watching for changes) is important because it helps control expenses. Before tracking, check your calculations by performing a trial balance.

1. Total the check amount column.
2. Find the total for each expense column.
3. Add together all the expense column totals. The combined expense column total should match the total in the check amount column.
4. If the amounts do not match, recheck every entry until you find the error. When you find it, draw a line through it, and record the correct information neatly above it or to the side.
5. When the two amounts match (or balance), carry forward all column totals to the disbursements journal for the next month. Remember to prepare summaries and perform balances at the end of every month, quarter, and year.

Managing Petty Cash

Occasionally, you may need to make small (petty) cash disbursements for minor expenses such as postage-due fees or holiday decorations (Figure 18-10). To avoid writing checks for such small amounts, you may pay for them from the **petty cash fund** (also known as the revolving fund), cash kept on hand in the office for small purchases. The doctor should determine the amount of the petty cash account (usually $50) and the minimum amount of cash to be kept on hand (such as $15).

Starting and Maintaining a Petty Cash Fund.
To start the fund with $50, write a check to "Petty Cash" or "Cash" for that amount. Enter the check in the miscellaneous column of the monthly disbursement record. Then, cash the check. Because this money will be used for small disbursements, be sure to get some of it in pennies, nickels, dimes, quarters, and dollar bills. Put this money in a special petty cash box, along with a stack of petty cash vouchers.

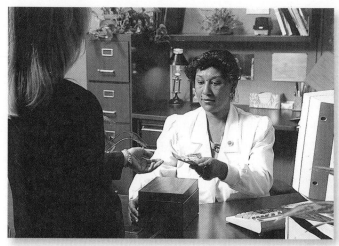

Figure 18-10. You may be in charge of maintaining the practice's petty cash fund. Count cash carefully, and keep accurate records about purchases made.

For each payment from the petty cash fund, obtain a receipt or create a petty cash voucher. The voucher should record the transaction number, date, amount paid, purpose of the expense, your signature (as the person issuing the money), and the signature of the person receiving it. Keep the receipt for any item purchased, along with the completed voucher, in the petty cash box to verify expenses later.

Also, document each petty cash withdrawal on a petty cash record form. Include the transaction number, date, payee, a brief description, amount, and type of expense (such as office expense, auto expense, or miscellaneous expense). If a space is provided, calculate and record the new balance in the petty cash fund.

Replenishing the Petty Cash Fund. At the end of the month (or whenever the fund is low), compare the latest petty cash balance to the money in the petty cash box. If you have not kept a running balance, total the receipts and vouchers, then count the cash on hand. Subtract the total amount on the receipts and vouchers (for example, $35) from the original balance (for example, $50). The difference ($15) should equal the cash on hand in the petty cash box ($15).

To replenish the account, write a check to "Cash" or "Petty Cash" for the amount spent ($35). Cash the check and add the money to the box, bringing the total back up to the original amount of $50. Record the check for $35 on the disbursement record. Also, total the receipts and vouchers by expense category. Record those totals in the appropriate columns on the disbursement record.

Understanding Financial Summaries

The physician may periodically analyze the income and expenses of the practice. Financial summaries provide an easy-to-read report on the business transactions for a given period, such as a month or a year.

An accountant usually prepares financial summaries. Although you will probably not have to create these summaries, you should understand how they are prepared.

Statement of Income and Expense. Also called a profit-and-loss statement, a statement of income and expense highlights the practice's profitability. It shows the physician the practice's total income and then lists and subtracts all expenses.

Cash Flow Statement. A **cash flow statement** shows how much cash is available to cover expenses, to invest, or to take as profits. The cash flow statement begins with the cash on hand at the beginning of the period and shows the income and disbursements made during that period. It concludes with the new amount of cash on hand at the end of the period.

Trial Balance. The doctor may review trial balances periodically to ensure that the books balance. The combined expense column total should match the total in the check amount column. If the amounts do not match, recheck every entry until you find the error.

 Handling Payroll

You may be responsible for handling the office payroll (Table 18-1). If so, your duties may include:

- Obtaining tax identification numbers
- Creating employee payroll information sheets
- Calculating employees' earnings
- Subtracting taxes and other deductions
- Writing paychecks
- Creating employee earnings records
- Preparing a payroll register
- Submitting payroll taxes

Applying for Tax Identification Numbers

Every employer—whether a single physician or a corporate practice—must have an employer identification number (EIN). An EIN is required by law for federal tax accounting purposes. An EIN is obtained by completing Form SS-4

TABLE 18-1 Payroll Duties	
Frequency	**Duties**
Upon assuming payroll responsibilities	Apply for an employer identification number (EIN) with Form SS-4 if the physician does not already have an EIN.
Whenever a new employee is hired	Have the employee complete an Employee's Withholding Allowance Certificate (Form W-4) and Employment Eligibility Verification (Form I-9). Record the employee's name and Social Security number from the employee's Social Security card.
Every payday	Withhold federal income tax as well as state and local income taxes (if any). Withhold the employee's share of FICA taxes (for Social Security and Medicare). Record a matching amount for the employer's share. Calculate how much the practice must pay for each employee's federal and state unemployment tax.
Monthly or biweekly (depending on your deposit schedule)	Deposit withheld income taxes, withheld and employer Social Security taxes, and withheld and employer Medicare taxes.
Quarterly (by April 30, July 31, October 31, and January 31)	File Employer's Quarterly Federal Tax Return (Form 941). With the return, pay any taxes that were not deposited earlier. Deposit federal unemployment tax, if over $100.
At least once a year	Have all employees update their W-4 forms.
On or before January 31	Give employees their Wage and Tax Statements (Form W-2), which show total wages and various withheld taxes. File Employer's Annual Federal Unemployment (FUTA) Tax Return (Form 940) with tax amount due.
On or before February 28	File Transmittal of Wage and Tax Statements (Form W-3) along with the government's copies of the W-2 forms.

(Application for Employer Identification Number) and submitting it to the Internal Revenue Service (IRS). This can be done online at www.irs.gov. Some states also require employer tax reports, for which the practice must have a state identification number, obtained from the proper state agency.

Creating Employee Payroll Information Sheets

The practice must maintain up-to-date, accurate payroll information about each employee. You should prepare a payroll information sheet for each employee. Each sheet should have the following information:

- The employee's name, address, Social Security number, and marital status
- An indication that the employee has completed an Employment Eligibility Verification (Form I-9), verifying that the employee is a U.S. citizen, a legally admitted alien, or an alien authorized to work in the United States
- The employee's pay schedule, number of dependents, payroll type, and voluntary deductions

Pay Schedule. On the payroll information sheet, list the employee's **pay schedule,** showing how often the employee is paid. Common pay schedules are weekly, biweekly, and monthly.

Number of Dependents. Record the number of **dependents** (people who depend on the employee for financial support). Dependents may include a spouse, children, and other family members.

You can find the number of dependents on the Employee's Withholding Allowance Certificate (Form W-4), which should have been completed when the employee was hired (Figure 18-11). Remember to keep the completed W-4 forms in the physician's personnel file, and update them at least annually.

Payroll Type. List the employee's payroll type—hourly wage, salary, or commission—on the payroll information sheet. An hourly wage is a set amount of money per hour of work. A salary is a set amount of money per pay period, regardless of the number of hours worked. A commission is a percentage of the amount an employee earns for the employer. Salespeople, for example, are often paid by commission.

Voluntary Deductions. Finally, document the voluntary deductions to be taken from the employee's check. These may include additional federal withholding taxes, contributions to a 401(k) retirement plan, or payments to a company health insurance plan. Employees who want additional federal taxes taken out of their paycheck will indicate this deduction on their W-4 form.

Gross Earnings

Gross earnings refers to the total amount of income earned before deductions. Gross earnings must be calculated for each employee as a first step in the payroll process.

Calculating Gross Earnings. For every payroll period, use data from the payroll information sheet to compute each employee's gross earnings. For an hourly employee, use this equation:

Hourly Wage × Hours Worked = Gross Earnings

An employee who earns $12.50 per hour and works 35 hours, for example, has gross earnings of $437.50 ($12.50 × 35 hours) per week.

For a salaried employee, use the salary amount as the gross earnings for the pay period, no matter how many hours the employee worked. An employee who earns a weekly salary of $500, for example, receives that amount whether she worked 30, 40, or 50 hours during that week.

Fair Labor Standards Act. The Fair Labor Standards Act primarily affects employees who earn hourly wages. It limits the number of hours they may work, sets their minimum wage, and regulates their overtime pay. It also requires the employer to record the number of hours they work, usually on a time card or in a time book.

For hourly employees, this act mandates payment of:

- Time and a half (1½ times the normal hourly wage) for all hours worked beyond the normal 8 in a regular workday.
- Time and a half for all hours worked on the sixth consecutive day of the work week.
- Twice the normal wage (double time) for all hours worked on the seventh consecutive workday.
- Double time, plus normal holiday pay, for all hours worked on a company-approved holiday.

The Fair Labor Standards Act also requires overtime payments for part-time hourly employees for every hour worked beyond the normal 8 in a day or 40 in a week.

Making Deductions

The law requires all employers to withhold money from employees' gross earnings to pay federal, state, and local (if any) income taxes and certain other taxes. In addition, employees may wish you to make certain voluntary deductions. For example, you might be asked to deduct an amount for child care, if the practice or hospital provides on-site child care. You might also deduct employee contributions to health insurance premiums.

You must deposit all employee deductions and employer payments into separate accounts. Monies from these **tax liability** accounts are used to pay taxes to appropriate government agencies.

Income Taxes. You must withhold enough money to cover the employee's federal income tax for the pay period. You can determine this amount by finding the employee's number of exemptions (from Form W-4) and referring to the tax tables in *Circular E, Employer's Tax Guide,* published by the IRS.

Consult the state and local tax tables for other income taxes. These taxes may be simpler to calculate. For

Form W-4 (2009)

Purpose. Complete Form W-4 so that your employer can withhold the correct federal income tax from your pay. Consider completing a new Form W-4 each year and when your personal or financial situation changes.

Exemption from withholding. If you are exempt, complete **only** lines 1, 2, 3, 4, and 7 and sign the form to validate it. Your exemption for 2009 expires February 16, 2010. See Pub. 505, Tax Withholding and Estimated Tax.

Note. You cannot claim exemption from withholding if (a) your income exceeds $950 and includes more than $300 of unearned income (for example, interest and dividends) and (b) another person can claim you as a dependent on their tax return.

Basic instructions. If you are not exempt, complete the **Personal Allowances Worksheet** below. The worksheets on page 2 further adjust your withholding allowances based on itemized deductions, certain credits, adjustments to income, or two-earner/multiple job situations.

Complete all worksheets that apply. However, you may claim fewer (or zero) allowances. For regular wages, withholding must be based on allowances you claimed and may not be a flat amount or percentage of wages.

Head of household. Generally, you may claim head of household filing status on your tax return only if you are unmarried and pay more than 50% of the costs of keeping up a home for yourself and your dependent(s) or other qualifying individuals. See Pub. 501, Exemptions, Standard Deduction, and Filing Information, for information.

Tax credits. You can take projected tax credits into account in figuring your allowable number of withholding allowances. Credits for child or dependent care expenses and the child tax credit may be claimed using the **Personal Allowances Worksheet** below. See Pub. 919, How Do I Adjust My Tax Withholding, for information on converting your other credits into withholding allowances.

Nonwage income. If you have a large amount of nonwage income, such as interest or dividends, consider making estimated tax payments using Form 1040-ES, Estimated Tax for Individuals. Otherwise, you may owe additional tax. If you have pension or annuity income, see Pub. 919 to find out if you should adjust your withholding on Form W-4 or W-4P.

Two earners or multiple jobs. If you have a working spouse or more than one job, figure the total number of allowances you are entitled to claim on all jobs using worksheets from only one Form W-4. Your withholding usually will be most accurate when all allowances are claimed on the Form W-4 for the highest paying job and zero allowances are claimed on the others. See Pub. 919 for details.

Nonresident alien. If you are a nonresident alien, see the Instructions for Form 8233 before completing this Form W-4.

Check your withholding. After your Form W-4 takes effect, use Pub. 919 to see how the amount you are having withheld compares to your projected total tax for 2009. See Pub. 919, especially if your earnings exceed $130,000 (Single) or $180,000 (Married).

Personal Allowances Worksheet (Keep for your records.)

A   Enter "1" for **yourself** if no one else can claim you as a dependent . . . . **A** _____

B   Enter "1" if: {
- You are single and have only one job; or
- You are married, have only one job, and your spouse does not work; or
- Your wages from a second job or your spouse's wages (or the total of both) are $1,500 or less.
}   **B** _____

C   Enter "1" for your **spouse**. But, you may choose to enter "-0-" if you are married and have either a working spouse or more than one job. (Entering "-0-" may help you avoid having too little tax withheld.) . . . . . . **C** _____

D   Enter number of **dependents** (other than your spouse or yourself) you will claim on your tax return . . . . **D** _____

E   Enter "1" if you will file as **head of household** on your tax return (see conditions under **Head of household** above) . **E** _____

F   Enter "1" if you have at least $1,800 of **child or dependent care expenses** for which you plan to claim a credit . **F** _____
(**Note.** Do **not** include child support payments. See Pub. 503, Child and Dependent Care Expenses, for details.)

G   **Child Tax Credit** (including additional child tax credit). See Pub. 972, Child Tax Credit, for more information.
- If your total income will be less than $61,000 ($90,000 if married), enter "2" for each eligible child; then **less** "1" if you have three or more eligible children.
- If your total income will be between $61,000 and $84,000 ($90,000 and $119,000 if married), enter "1" for each eligible child plus "1" **additional** if you have six or more eligible children.   **G** _____

H   Add lines A through G and enter total here. (**Note.** This may be different from the number of exemptions you claim on your tax return.) ▶ **H** _____

For accuracy, complete all worksheets that apply. {
- If you plan to **itemize or claim adjustments to income** and want to reduce your withholding, see the **Deductions and Adjustments Worksheet** on page 2.
- If you have **more than one job** or are **married and you and your spouse both work** and the combined earnings from all jobs exceed $40,000 ($25,000 if married), see the **Two-Earners/Multiple Jobs Worksheet** on page 2 to avoid having too little tax withheld.
- If **neither** of the above situations applies, **stop here** and enter the number from line H on line 5 of Form W-4 below.
}

- - - - - - - - - - Cut here and give Form W-4 to your employer. Keep the top part for your records. - - - - - - - - - -

Form W-4
Department of the Treasury
Internal Revenue Service

Employee's Withholding Allowance Certificate

OMB No. 1545-0074

2009

▶ Whether you are entitled to claim a certain number of allowances or exemption from withholding is subject to review by the IRS. Your employer may be required to send a copy of this form to the IRS.

1 Type or print your first name and middle initial.	Last name		2 Your social security number

Home address (number and street or rural route)	3 ☐ Single ☐ Married ☐ Married, but withhold at higher Single rate. Note. If married, but legally separated, or spouse is a nonresident alien, check the "Single" box.

City or town, state, and ZIP code	4 If your last name differs from that shown on your social security card, check here. You must call 1-800-772-1213 for a replacement card. ▶ ☐

5	Total number of allowances you are claiming (from line **H** above **or** from the applicable worksheet on page 2)	**5**
6	Additional amount, if any, you want withheld from each paycheck	**6** $

7   I claim exemption from withholding for 2009, and I certify that I meet **both** of the following conditions for exemption.
- Last year I had a right to a refund of **all** federal income tax withheld because I had **no** tax liability **and**
- This year I expect a refund of **all** federal income tax withheld because I expect to have **no** tax liability.

If you meet both conditions, write "Exempt" here . . . . ▶ **7**

Under penalties of perjury, I declare that I have examined this certificate and to the best of my knowledge and belief, it is true, correct, and complete.

Employee's signature
(Form is not valid unless you sign it.) ▶   Date ▶

8 Employer's name and address (Employer: Complete lines 8 and 10 only if sending to the IRS.)	9 Office code (optional)	10 Employer identification number (EIN)

For Privacy Act and Paperwork Reduction Act Notice, see page 2.   Cat. No. 10220Q   Form **W-4** (2009)

Figure 18-11. Update all Employee's Withholding Allowance Certificates (W-4 forms) at least once a year.

example, they may be 4% and 1% of the employee's gross earnings, respectively.

FICA Taxes. For FICA tax, withhold from the employee's check half of the tax owed for the pay period. Pay the other half from the practice's accounts. The amount of FICA tax that funds Social Security differs from the amount that funds Medicare. Report these two amounts separately. Check IRS *Circular E* for the latest FICA tax percentages and level of taxable earnings.

Unemployment Taxes. Federal unemployment tax is not a deduction from employees' paychecks, but it is based on their earnings. It is paid by the practice. The **Federal Unemployment Tax Act (FUTA)** requires employers to pay a percentage of each employee's income, up to a certain dollar amount. The percentage may be reduced if the employer also pays state unemployment taxes.

States calculate unemployment taxes differently. Some states tax employers and employees; others tax only employers. State unemployment tax usually varies with the employer's past employment record. Employers with few layoffs, such as physicians, have lower tax rates than those with many layoffs. To compute state unemployment tax, apply the assigned tax rate to each employee's earnings, up to a maximum for the calendar year. For details, consult your state unemployment insurance department.

Workers' Compensation. Some states require employers to insure their employees against possible loss of income resulting from work-related injury, disability, or disease. Although state laws vary, they typically require doctors to carry this insurance with a state insurance fund or state-authorized private insurer. Usually, a medical practice's insurance agent will audit the payroll books annually and then issue a bill for the workers' compensation premium due.

Calculating Net Earnings

Add each employee's required and voluntary deductions together to determine the total deductions. Then, subtract the total deductions from the gross earnings to get the employee's **net earnings,** or take-home pay. Use the following equation:

$$\text{Gross Earnings} - \text{Total Deductions} = \text{Net Earnings}$$

The exception to this rule may be contributions the employee makes to the employer retirement plan, if available. When sponsored by an employer, as with a 401(k) account, these deductions are often taken before taxes are calculated, reducing the employee's taxable income, which encourages the employee to take part in these plans.

Preparing Paychecks

The way you prepare the practice's payroll will depend on the system the practice uses. In a small practice, you may write paychecks manually. In this case, write the check amount for the employee's net earnings, and deduct the check amount from the office checkbook. Payroll may also be handled through electronic banking; see the Points on Practice section.

If the practice uses a payroll service, you may supply time cards or payroll data to the service by mail or electronically. The service calculates all the deductions, prepares paychecks, and mails them to the practice for distribution.

No matter how paychecks are prepared, they should include information about how the check amount was determined. This information usually appears on the check stub. It should match the information on the employee earnings records and payroll register. Procedure 18-6 explains the process for generating payroll.

Maintaining Employee Earnings Records

You need to keep an employee earnings record for each employee (Figure 18-12). When you create the record, list the employee's name, address, phone number, Social Security number, birth date, spouse's name, number of dependents, job title, employment starting date, pay rate, and voluntary deductions.

Points on Practice

Handling Payroll Through Electronic Banking

An electronic funds transfer system (EFTS) enables you to handle the practice's payroll without writing payroll checks manually. The physician must sign up for EFTS with the bank, and employees must supply their bank account numbers to the employer. Then, the bank electronically deposits employees' paychecks into their bank accounts, as directed.

Most employees like to have their paychecks deposited automatically. The money is available on the day of deposit, and no one has to worry about losing a paycheck, getting to the bank before it closes, or carrying a paycheck around. Also, employees still receive a check stub along with a notification of deposit, so they can track their earnings and deductions.

Contact your bank for more information and specific procedures for setting up EFTS and electronic payroll.

PROCEDURE 18-6

Generating Payroll

Procedure Goal: To handle the practice's payroll as efficiently and accurately as possible for each pay period

Materials: Employees' time cards, employees' earnings records, payroll register, IRS tax tables, check register

Method:

1. Calculate the total regular and overtime hours worked, based on the employee's time card. Enter those totals under the appropriate headings on the payroll register.

   Rationale

   Time calculations and the separation of regular and overtime hours must be accurate in order for the paycheck to be correct.

2. Check the pay rate on the employee earnings record. Then multiply the hours worked (including any paid vacation or paid holidays, if applicable) by the rates for regular time and overtime (time and a half or double time). This yields gross earnings.

   Rationale

   An accurate gross earnings calculation is the basis for taxes and deductions.

3. Enter the gross earnings under the appropriate heading on the payroll register. Subtract any nontaxable benefits, such as health-care or retirement programs.

4. Using IRS tax tables and data on the employee earnings record, determine the amount of federal income tax to withhold based on the employee's marital status and number of exemptions. Also compute the amount of FICA

tax to withhold for Social Security (6.2%) and Medicare (1.45%).

   Rationale

   These tax deductions are required by law.

5. Following state and local procedures, determine the amount of state and local income taxes (if any) to withhold based on the employee's marital status and number of exemptions.

   Rationale

   These tax deductions are required by law.

6. Calculate the employer's contributions to FUTA and to the state unemployment fund, if any. Post these amounts to the employer's account.

7. Enter any other required or voluntary deductions, such as health insurance or contributions to a 401(k) fund.

8. Subtract all deductions from the gross earnings to get the employee's net earnings.

9. Enter the total amount withheld from all employees for FICA under the headings for Social Security and Medicare. Remember that the employer must match these amounts. Enter other employer contributions, such as for federal and state unemployment taxes, under the appropriate headings.

   Rationale

   These deductions are required by law.

10. Fill out the check stub, including the employee's name, date, pay period, gross earnings, all deductions, and net earnings. Make out the paycheck for the net earnings.

11. Deposit each deduction in a tax liability account.

Then, for each pay period, record the employee's gross earnings, individual deductions, net earnings, and related information. Properly completed earnings records show each employee's earning history.

Maintaining a Payroll Register

A payroll register summarizes vital information about all employees and their earnings (Figure 18-13). At the end of each pay period, record each employee's earnings to date, hourly rate, hours worked, overtime hours, overtime earnings, and total gross earnings. Also, list the gross earnings subject to unemployment taxes and FICA, all required

and voluntary deductions, net earnings, and the paycheck number.

Handling Payroll Electronically

Manual payroll preparation and related tasks may take an hour per week for each employee. To save time and to provide the convenience for employees of having their paychecks automatically deposited, some practices handle payroll tasks electronically.

If you work in a relatively small practice, you may handle all payroll tasks in the office, using accounting or payroll software. If you work in a large practice, you may prepare payroll information on the computer and transmit

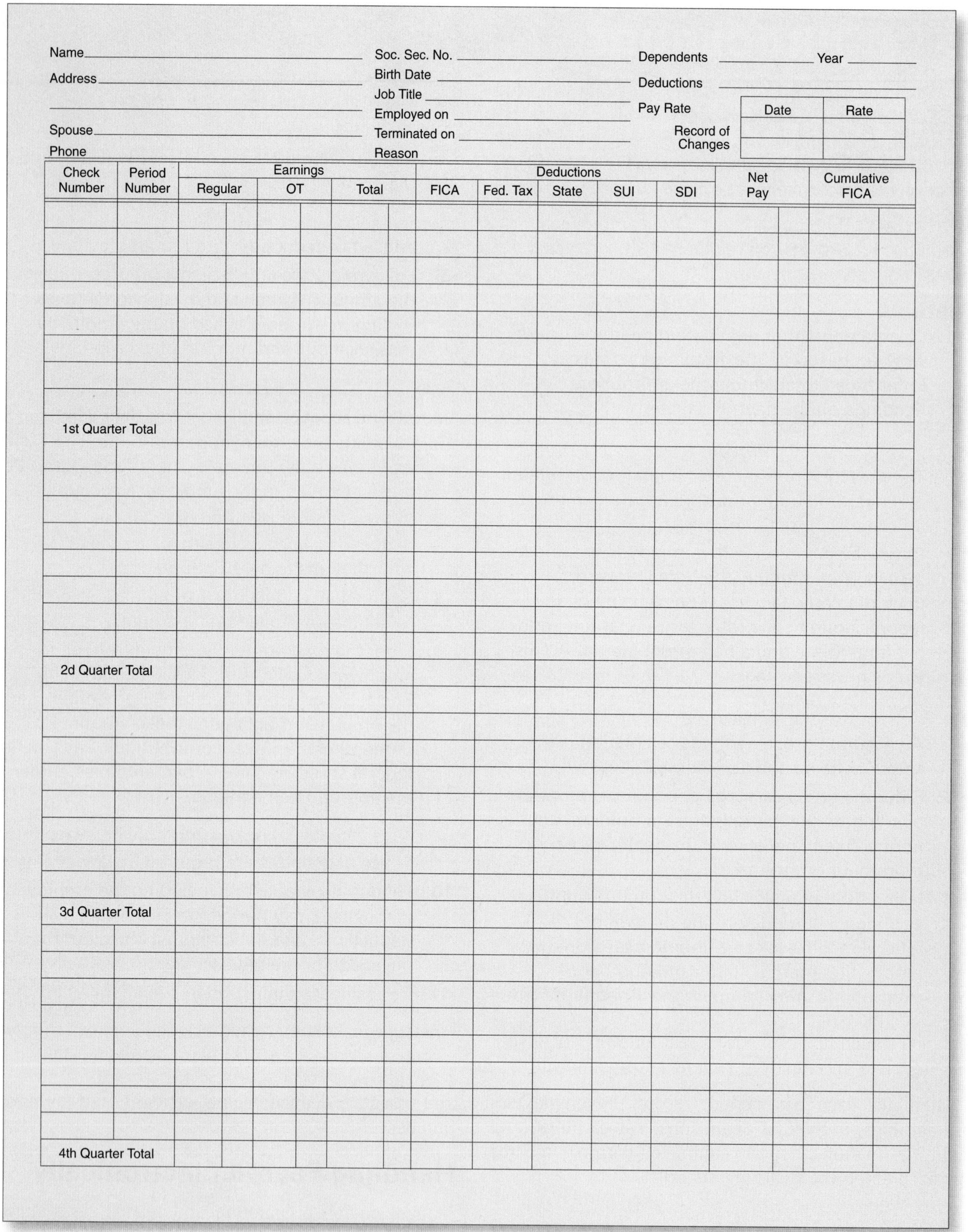

Name _____ Soc. Sec. No. _____ Dependents _____ Year _____

Address _____ Birth Date _____ Deductions _____

_____ Job Title _____

Spouse _____ Employed on _____ Pay Rate

_____ Terminated on _____ Record of Changes

Phone _____ Reason

Check Number	Period Number	Earnings			Deductions					Net Pay	Cumulative FICA
		Regular	OT	Total	FICA	Fed. Tax	State	SUI	SDI		
1st Quarter Total											
2d Quarter Total											
3d Quarter Total											
4th Quarter Total											

Pay Rate:

Date	Rate

Figure 18-12. Earnings records show the earning history of each employee at your practice.

it by modem to an outside payroll service for processing. Depending on which system and software the practice has, you may use the computer to:

- Create, update, and delete employee payroll information files

- Prepare employee paychecks, stubs, and W-2 forms
- Update and print employee earnings records
- Update all appropriate bookkeeping records, such as the payroll ledger and general ledger, with payroll data

Pay Period 6/1–6/14

Emp. No.	Name	Earnings to date	Hrly. Rate	Reg. Hrs.	OT Hrs.	OT Earnings	TOTAL GROSS	Earnings Subject to Unemp.	Earnings Subject to FICA	Social Security (FICA)	Medicare	Federal W/H	State W/H	Health Ins.	Net Pay	Check No.
0010	Scott, B.	9,823.14	14.00	70.00			980.00	980.00	980.00	60.50	14.10	147.92	15.10	25.00	717.38	11747
0020	Wilson, J.	14,290.38	17.00	70.00	6.50	153.00	1343.00	1343.00	1343.00	83.26	19.47	160.45	15.85	67.50	996.47	11748
0030	Diaz, J.	2,750.26	5.50	46.25			254.37	254.37	254.37	15.77	3.68	38.20	3.75		192.97	11749
0040	Ling, W.	2,240.57	6.80	30.00			204.00	204.00	204.00	12.66	2.96	26.02	3.12		159.54	11750
0050	Harris, E.	2,600.98	10.00	23.50			235.00	235.00	235.00	14.57	3.41	33.52	3.36		180.14	11751

Figure 18-13. A payroll register is designed to summarize information about all employees and their earnings.

To perform these payroll functions electronically, follow the specific instructions in the software manual or get instructions from the payroll service. Generally, you would follow these steps.

Select an option from the "Payroll" menu. Wait for the prompt, then select the appropriate employee from a list of employees.

To create an employee payroll information file for a new employee, input the same information that you would record manually on an employee payroll information sheet: name, address, Social Security number, marital status, pay schedule, number of dependents, payroll type, and voluntary deductions. Print two copies of the employee payroll information file—one for the employee and one for the physician's personnel file.

To update an employee payroll information file when an employee moves, marries, has a child, or wants to change deductions, select "Update Employee File." After making the changes, print out two copies of the file. Show one to the employee to confirm that the information is correct. Then have the employee sign and date it. Keep the signed copy for the physician's personnel file, and give the other to the employee. To ensure that payroll information is always correct and current, you should update it once a year for every employee.

To delete an employee payroll information file when an employee leaves the practice, select "Terminate Employee." Remember to print out and file a copy of this information before deleting it, because the physician is required to keep employees' payroll records for 4 years.

To generate paychecks and stubs, select the employee from the list of employees and choose the "Print Paycheck" option. Then, answer each prompt displayed by the computer (for example, hours worked). The computer has the employee's pay rate, payroll type, and deductions on file and automatically calculates the employee's net earnings, generates a paycheck, and prints a pay stub with the appropriate information.

To create an employee earnings record, select this option and follow the prompts for the needed information.

Depending on the software used, each employee's earnings record may be updated automatically every time you generate a paycheck or make changes to other payroll files.

Calculating and Filing Taxes

In many practices, medical assistants set up tax liability accounts for money withheld from paychecks. These accounts are used to submit this money to appropriate agencies. Visit www.irs.gov for further information.

Setting Up Tax Liability Accounts

It is important to hold the money deducted from paychecks until it can be sent to the appropriate government agencies. Deductions from employees' paychecks for federal, state, and local income taxes and FICA taxes, as well as employer payments based on payroll, such as federal and state unemployment taxes, must be deposited until payment is due. For these accounts, choose a bank that is authorized by the IRS to accept federal tax deposits. If the practice makes other paycheck deductions, as for workers' compensation or a 401(k) plan, maintain accurate records for this money as well.

Each time you prepare paychecks, deposit the withheld money into the proper account as dictated by your particular practice. Record the deposited amounts as debits in the practice's checking account.

Understanding Federal Tax Deposit Schedules

You will probably deposit federal income taxes and FICA taxes (which together are known as employment taxes) on a quarterly, monthly, or biweekly (every-other-week) schedule. Every November IRS personnel decide which deposit schedule your office should use for the next year.

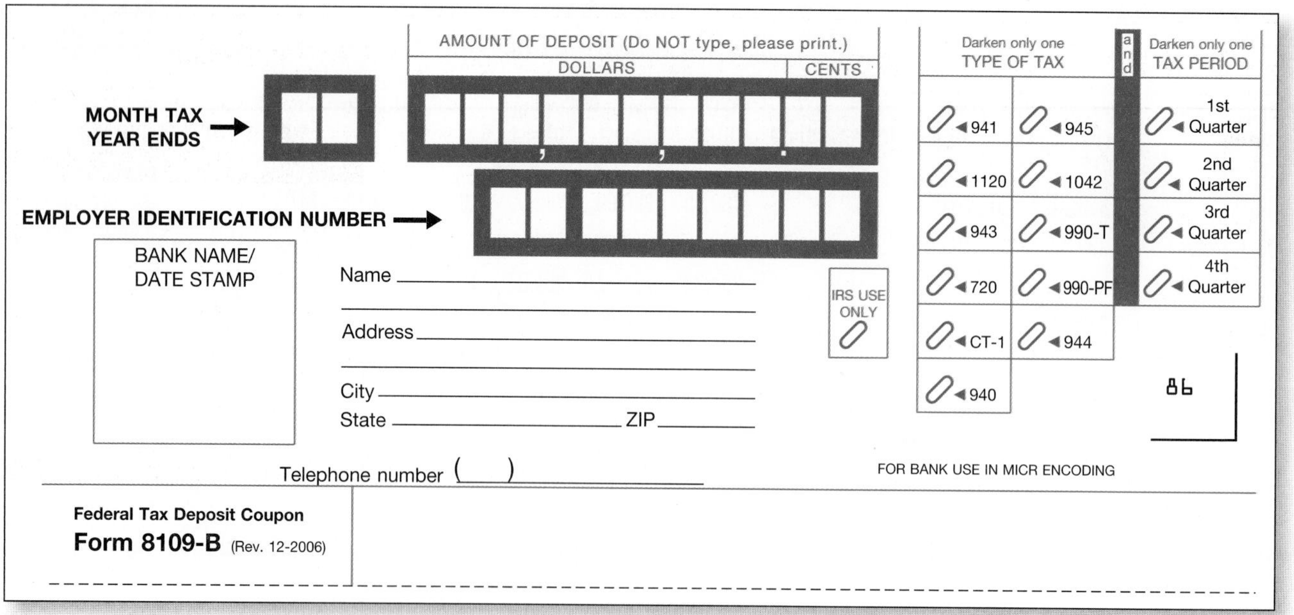
AMOUNT OF DEPOSIT (Do NOT type, please print.)
DOLLARS | CENTS

MONTH TAX YEAR ENDS →

EMPLOYER IDENTIFICATION NUMBER →

BANK NAME/ DATE STAMP

Name
Address
City
State ZIP
Telephone number ( )

IRS USE ONLY

Darken only one TYPE OF TAX: 941, 945, 1120, 1042, 943, 990-T, 720, 990-PF, CT-1, 944, 940

and

Darken only one TAX PERIOD: 1st Quarter, 2nd Quarter, 3rd Quarter, 4th Quarter

86

FOR BANK USE IN MICR ENCODING

Federal Tax Deposit Coupon
Form 8109-B (Rev. 12-2006)

Figure 18-14. Practices that do not use TAXLINK to submit taxes electronically must submit federal income and FICA taxes with a Federal Tax Deposit (FTD) Coupon (Form 8109).

If the IRS does not notify you about this matter, determine your deposit schedule based on the total employment taxes your office reported on the previous year's Employer's Quarterly Federal Tax Returns (Form 941). For example, if your office reported $50,000 or less in employment taxes during the past year, you would make monthly employment tax deposits the present year. If your office reported more than $50,000 during the past year, you would make semimonthly tax deposits.

There are exceptions to the monthly or semimonthly tax deposit schedules: the $500 rule and the $100,000 rule. The $500 rule applies to employers who owe less than $500 in employment taxes during a tax period (such as a quarter). These employers do not have to make a deposit for that period. The $100,000 rule applies to employers who owe $100,000 or more in employment taxes on any one day during a tax period. These employers must deposit the tax by the next banking day after the day that ceiling is reached.

Submitting Federal Income Taxes and FICA Taxes

Some businesses must submit federal income taxes and FICA taxes to the IRS by electronic funds transfer (EFT). The EFT program, known as TAXLINK, began in 1995. Since then, more taxpayers have been required to use it each year. If your practice is not required to use EFT but wishes to do so voluntarily, contact the IRS, Cash Management Site Office, to enroll.

If your practice does not use EFT, you must submit these employment taxes with a Federal Tax Deposit (FTD) Coupon (Form 8109) (see Figure 18-14). FTD Coupons are supplied by the IRS. They are printed with the physician's name, address, and EIN. They have boxes for filling in the type of tax and the tax period for which the deposit is being made.

To make the deposit, write a single check or money order for the total amount of federal income taxes and FICA taxes withheld during the tax period. Make the check payable to the bank where you make the deposit. This must be a Federal Reserve Bank or another bank authorized to make payments to the IRS. Also, complete the FTD Coupon. Then, mail or deliver the check and FTD Coupon to the bank. The bank will give you a deposit receipt.

If you work in a practice with a large payroll, you may need to make deposits every few days. In most practices, however, you will probably make deposits once a month. Then, every 3 months, a more complete accounting is required on a **quarterly return,** called the Employer's Quarterly Federal Tax Return (Form 941).

Submitting Federal Unemployment Tax Act (FUTA) and State Unemployment Tax Act (SUTA) Taxes

FUTA taxes provide money to workers who are unemployed. If the practice owes more than $100 in federal unemployment tax at the end of the quarter, deposit the tax amount with an FTD Coupon (Form 8109). At the end of the year, file an Employer's Annual Federal Unemployment (FUTA) Tax Return (Form 940) with any final taxes owed (Figure 18-15).

Form **940 for 2008:** **Employer's Annual Federal Unemployment (FUTA) Tax Return**   850108

Department of the Treasury — Internal Revenue Service

OMB No. 1545-0028

(EIN)
Employer identification number   ☐☐ – ☐☐☐☐☐☐☐

Name *(not your trade name)*

Trade name *(if any)*

Address
Number   Street   Suite or room number

City   State   ZIP code

Type of Return
(Check all that apply.)

☐ **a.** Amended

☐ **b.** Successor employer

☐ **c.** No payments to employees
   in 2008

☐ **d.** Final: Business closed or
   stopped paying wages

Read the separate instructions before you fill out this form. Please type or print within the boxes.

Part 1: Tell us about your return. If any line does NOT apply, leave it blank.

1   If you were required to pay your state unemployment tax in ...

   1a One state only, write the state abbreviation . . .   **1a** ☐☐
   - OR -
   1b More than one state (You are a multi-state employer) . . . .   **1b** ☐ Check here. Fill out Schedule A.
      Skip line 2 for 2008 and go to line 3.
2   If you paid wages in a state that is subject to CREDIT REDUCTION . . . .   **2** ☐ Check here. Fill out Schedule A (Form 940), Part 2.

Part 2: Determine your FUTA tax before adjustments for 2008. If any line does NOT apply, leave it blank.

3   Total payments to all employees . . . .   **3** ☐☐ .

4   Payments exempt from FUTA tax . . . .   **4** ☐☐ .

   Check all that apply: **4a** ☐ Fringe benefits   **4c** ☐ Retirement/Pension   **4e** ☐ Other
      4b ☐ Group-term life insurance   **4d** ☐ Dependent care

5   Total of payments made to each employee in excess of
   $7,000 . . . .   **5** ☐☐ .

6   **Subtotal** (line 4 + line 5 = line 6) . . . .   **6** ☐☐ .

7   **Total taxable FUTA wages** (line 3 – line 6 = line 7) . . . .   **7** ☐☐ .

8   **FUTA tax before adjustments** (line 7 × .008 = line 8) . . . .   **8** ☐☐ .

Part 3: Determine your adjustments. If any line does NOT apply, leave it blank.

9   If ALL of the taxable FUTA wages you paid were excluded from state unemployment tax,
   multiply line 7 by .054 (line 7 × .054 = line 9). Then go to line 12 . . . .   **9** ☐☐ .

10   If SOME of the taxable FUTA wages you paid were excluded from state unemployment tax,
   OR you paid ANY state unemployment tax late (after the due date for filing Form 940), fill out
   the worksheet in the instructions. Enter the amount from line 7 of the worksheet onto line 10 . . .   **10** ☐☐ .

      Skip line 11 for 2008 and go to line 12.
11   If credit reduction applies, enter the amount from line 3 of Schedule A (Form 940) . . . .   **11** ☐☐ .

Part 4: Determine your FUTA tax and balance due or overpayment for 2008. If any line does NOT apply, leave it blank.

12   Total FUTA tax after adjustments (lines 8 + 9 + 10 + 11 = line 12) . . . .   **12** ☐☐ .

13   FUTA tax deposited for the year, including any payment applied from a prior year . . .   **13** ☐☐ .

14   **Balance due** (If line 12 is more than line 13, enter the difference on line 14.)
   ● If line 14 is more than $500, you must deposit your tax.
   ● If line 14 is $500 or less, you may pay with this return. For more information on how to pay, see
   the separate instructions . . . .   **14** ☐☐ .

15   **Overpayment** (If line 13 is more than line 12, enter the difference on line 15 and check a box
   below.) . . . .   **15** ☐☐ .

Check one: ☐ Apply to next return.
          ☐ Send a refund.

▶ You **MUST** fill out both pages of this form and **SIGN** it.

Next ➡

For Privacy Act and Paperwork Reduction Act Notice, see the back of Form 940-V, Payment Voucher.   Cat. No. 11234O   Form **940** (2008)

Figure 18-15. Tax dollars filed with FUTA tax returns (Form 940) provide money to workers who are unemployed.

Form **941 for 2009:** Employer's QUARTERLY Federal Tax Return

(Rev. April 2009)

Department of the Treasury — Internal Revenue Service

950109

OMB No. 1545-0029

(EIN)
Employer identification number ☐☐ – ☐☐☐☐☐☐☐

Name (not your trade name)

Trade name (if any)

Address

Number   Street   Suite or room number

City   State   ZIP code

Report for this Quarter of 2009
(Check one.)

☐ **1:** January, February, March

☐ **2:** April, May, June

☐ **3:** July, August, September

☐ **4:** October, November, December

Read the separate instructions before you complete Form 941. Type or print within the boxes.

Part 1: Answer these questions for this quarter.

1   Number of employees who received wages, tips, or other compensation for the pay period
     including: *Mar. 12* (Quarter 1), *June 12* (Quarter 2), *Sept. 12* (Quarter 3), *Dec. 12* (Quarter 4)   **1**

2   Wages, tips, and other compensation **2**

3   Income tax withheld from wages, tips, and other compensation **3**

4   If no wages, tips, and other compensation are subject to social security or Medicare tax   ☐ Check and go to line 6.

5   Taxable social security and Medicare wages and tips:

	Column 1		*Column 2*
5a Taxable social security wages		× .124 =	
5b Taxable social security tips		× .124 =	
5c Taxable Medicare wages & tips		× .029 =	

     5d **Total social security and Medicare taxes** (*Column 2,* lines 5a + 5b + 5c = line 5d) . .   **5d**

6   **Total taxes before adjustments** (lines 3 + 5d = line 6) **6**

7   **CURRENT QUARTER'S ADJUSTMENTS,** for example, a fractions of cents adjustment.
     See the instructions.

     7a Current quarter's fractions of cents . . . .

     7b Current quarter's sick pay . . . .

     7c Current quarter's adjustments for tips and group-term life insurance

     7d **TOTAL ADJUSTMENTS.** Combine all amounts on lines 7a through 7c **7d**

8   **Total taxes after adjustments.** Combine lines 6 and 7d **8**

9   **Advance earned income credit (EIC) payments made to employees** **9**

10 **Total taxes after adjustment for advance EIC** (line 8 – line 9 = line 10) **10**

11 Total deposits for this quarter, including overpayment applied from a
     prior quarter and overpayment applied from Form 941-X or
     Form 944-X . . . .

12a COBRA premium assistance payments (see instructions) . . . . .

12b Number of individuals provided COBRA premium
     assistance reported on line 12a . . . . . .

13 Add lines 11 and 12a **13**

14 **Balance due.** If line 10 is more than line 13, write the difference here **14**
     For information on how to pay, see the instructions.   ☐ Apply to next return.

15 **Overpayment.** If line 13 is more than line 10, write the difference here   Check one ☐ Send a refund.

▶ You **MUST** complete both pages of Form 941 and **SIGN** it.   Next ➡

For Privacy Act and Paperwork Reduction Act Notice, see the back of the Payment Voucher.   Cat. No. 17001Z   Form **941** (Rev. 4-2009)

Figure 18-16. Most practices make tax deposits monthly and then make a more complete accounting once every 3 months on the Employer's Quarterly Federal Tax Return (Form 941), the first page of which is shown here.

22222	Void ☐	**a** Employee's social security number	**For Official Use Only ▶** OMB No. 1545-0008		

b Employer identification number (EIN)		**1** Wages, tips, other compensation	**2** Federal income tax withheld
c Employer's name, address, and ZIP code		**3** Social security wages	**4** Social security tax withheld
		5 Medicare wages and tips	**6** Medicare tax withheld
		7 Social security tips	**8** Allocated tips
d Control number		**9** Advance EIC payment	**10** Dependent care benefits

e Employee's first name and initial	Last name	Suff.	**11** Nonqualified plans	**12a** See instructions for box 12
			13 Statutory employee ☐ Retirement plan ☐ Third-party sick pay ☐	**12b**
			14 Other	**12c**
				12d
f Employee's address and ZIP code				

15 State	Employer's state ID number	**16** State wages, tips, etc.	**17** State income tax	**18** Local wages, tips, etc.	**19** Local income tax	**20** Locality name

Form **W-2** Wage and Tax Statement   **2009**   Department of the Treasury—Internal Revenue Service

For Privacy Act and Paperwork Reduction Act Notice, see back of Copy D.

Copy A For Social Security Administration — Send this entire page with Form W-3 to the Social Security Administration; photocopies are **not** acceptable.

Cat. No. 10134D

Do Not Cut, Fold, or Staple Forms on This Page — Do Not Cut, Fold, or Staple Forms on This Page

Figure 18-17. A Wage and Tax Statement (Form W-2) records the total amount of taxes withheld during the previous year for each employee.

Generally, an employer must pay FUTA taxes if employees' wages total more than $1500 in any quarter (3-month period) and if those employees are not seasonal or household workers. The FUTA tax, which is 6.2%, is applied to the first $7000 of income for a year.

Some states are also governed by a **State Unemployment Tax Act (SUTA).** These taxes are filed along with FUTA taxes. Make sure you know the laws governing unemployment taxes in your state.

Filing an Employer's Quarterly Federal Tax Return

Each quarter, file an Employer's Quarterly Federal Tax Return (Form 941) with the IRS (Figure 18-16). This tax return summarizes the federal income and FICA taxes (employment taxes) withheld from employees' paychecks.

As a general rule, you should file Form 941 at the nearest IRS office by the last day of the first month after the quarter ends. If the practice has deposited all taxes on time, you have an additional 10 days after the due date to file.

Handling State and Local Income Taxes

Send withheld state and local income taxes to the proper agencies, using their forms, procedures, and schedules. If required, prepare quarterly or other tax forms for the state and local governments.

Filing Wage and Tax Statements

After the end of each year, file a Wage and Tax Statement (Form W-2) with the appropriate federal, state, and local government agencies for each employee who had federal income and FICA taxes withheld during the previous year (Figure 18-17). Also, supply copies of Form W-2 to each employee.

DO NOT STAPLE

a Control number `33333`	**For Official Use Only ▶** OMB No. 1545-0008	

b Kind of Payer ▶	941 ☐ CT-1 ☐	Military ☐ Hshld. emp. ☐	943 ☐ Medicare govt. emp. ☐	944 ☐ Third-party sick pay ☐	**1** Wages, tips, other compensation	**2** Federal income tax withheld

3 Social security wages	**4** Social security tax withheld

c Total number of Forms W-2   **d** Establishment number   **5** Medicare wages and tips   **6** Medicare tax withheld

e Employer identification number (EIN)   **7** Social security tips   **8** Allocated tips

f Employer's name   **9** Advance EIC payments   **10** Dependent care benefits

11 Nonqualified plans   **12** Deferred compensation

13 For third-party sick pay use only

14 Income tax withheld by payer of third-party sick pay

g Employer's address and ZIP code

h Other EIN used this year

15 State   Employer's state ID number   **16** State wages, tips, etc.   **17** State income tax

18 Local wages, tips, etc.   **19** Local income tax

Contact person   Telephone number ( )   For Official Use Only

Email address   Fax number ( )

Under penalties of perjury, I declare that I have examined this return and accompanying documents, and, to the best of my knowledge and belief, they are true, correct, and complete.

Signature ▶   Title ▶   Date ▶

Form **W-3** Transmittal of Wage and Tax Statements   **2009**   Department of the Treasury Internal Revenue Service

Send this entire page with the entire Copy A page of Form(s) W-2 to the Social Security Administration.

Do not send any payment (cash, checks, money orders, etc.) with Forms W-2 and W-3.

Reminder

Separate instructions. See the 2009 Instructions for Forms W-2 and W-3 for information on completing this form.

Purpose of Form

A Form W-3 Transmittal is completed only when paper Copy A of Form(s) W-2, Wage and Tax Statement, are being filed. Do not file Form W-3 alone. Do not file Form W-3 for Form(s) W-2 that were submitted electronically to the Social Security Administration (see below). All paper forms **must** comply with IRS standards and be machine readable. Photocopies and hand-printed forms are **not** acceptable. Use a Form W-3 even if only one paper Form W-2 is being filed. Make sure both the Form W-3 and Form(s) W-2 show the correct tax year and Employer Identification Number (EIN). Make a copy of this form and keep it with Copy D (For Employer) of Form(s) W-2 for your records.

Electronic Filing

The Social Security Administration strongly suggests employers report Form W-3 and W-2 Copy A electronically instead of on paper. SSA provides two e-file options:

● Free online, fill-in Forms W-2 for employers who file 20 or fewer Form(s) W-2.

● Upload a file for employers who use payroll/tax software to print Form(s) W-2, if the vendor software creates a file that can be uploaded to SSA.

For more information, go to *www.socialsecurity.gov/employer* and select "First Time Filers" or "Returning Filers" under "BEFORE YOU FILE."

When To File

Mail any paper Forms W-2 under cover of this Form W-3 Transmittal by March 1, 2010. Electronic fill-in forms or uploads are filed through SSA's Business Services Online (BSO) Internet site and will be on time if submitted by March 31, 2010.

Where To File Paper Forms

Send this entire page with the entire Copy A page of Form(s) W-2 to:

**Social Security Administration
Data Operations Center
Wilkes-Barre, PA 18769-0001**

Note. If you use "Certified Mail" to file, change the ZIP code to "18769-0002." If you use an IRS-approved private delivery service, add "ATTN: W-2 Process, 1150 E. Mountain Dr." to the address and change the ZIP code to "18702-7997." See Publication 15 (Circular E), Employer's Tax Guide, for a list of IRS-approved private delivery services.

For Privacy Act and Paperwork Reduction Act Notice, see the back of Copy D of Form W-2.

Cat. No. 10159Y

Figure 18-18. Submit a Transmittal of Wages and Tax Statements (Form W-3) with the W-2 forms.

Form W-2 shows the employee's total taxable income for the previous year. It also shows the exact amount of federal income taxes and FICA taxes (for Social Security and Medicare) withheld, along with the amounts of state and local taxes withheld (if any).

Along with the W-2 forms, submit Form W-3, a Transmittal of Wage and Tax Statements (Figure 18-18). This form lists the employer's name, address, and EIN and summarizes the amount of all employees' earnings and the federal income taxes and FICA taxes withheld.

Summary

18.1 Traditional bookkeeping systems in the medical office are also known as patient accounting methods. Many medical offices still use manual systems including single- or double-entry systems or the pegboard system. Most medical practices today use computerized systems. All bookkeeping systems record income (patient charges), disbursements, and other financial information.

18.2 Bookkeeping tasks on the computer save time because you do not have to do repetitive tasks and calculations are done for you.

18.3 Banking tasks include writing checks, accepting checks, endorsing checks, making deposits, and reconciling bank statements.

18.4 Accepting and endorsing checks from patients and insurance companies requires consistency and attentiveness. Endorse all checks with a restrictive endorsement as soon as they are received. Calculate deposits carefully and make deposits promptly, making sure to note the deposit in the disbursements journal or check register.

18.5 In reconciling a bank statement, make sure that the bank record of deposits, payments, and other withdrawals agrees with the medical facility's record of deposits, payments, and withdrawals. When the reconciliation is completed, the practice balance and the bank balance should agree.

18.6 Employee payroll, rent, and utilities payments are examples of medical office disbursements.

18.7 You may record disbursements in a check register, journal, or the bottom section of a daily log. Be consistent in your method and calculate the current checkbook balance after each disbursement.

18.8 A petty cash fund is needed to pay for minor expenses. Treat the petty cash fund like any disbursement journal, recording what the funds were used for, the date, and by whom. Keep all receipts and replenish the fund as needed to maintain the agreed-upon minimum balance.

18.9 In creating an employment payroll information sheet, you must document the employee's pay schedule, number of dependents, payroll type (hourly or salaried), and any voluntary deductions.

18.10 To calculate an employee's gross earnings, multiply the hours worked by the hourly rate. Using state, local, and federal tax guidelines, calculate the employee's tax deductions. Add to these any voluntary deductions and subtract the total deductions to obtain the employee's net earnings.

18.11 Medical offices need to keep an employee earnings record for each employee. When creating the record, obtain the necessary information such as name, social security number, and number of dependents. At the end of each pay period, record earnings for the pay period, adding this amount to the total earnings prior to today's date, to obtain the employee's current earnings to date.

18.12 The practice's liability account, is set up to hold the money deducted from employees' paychecks until the funds can be appropriately disbursed to the government agencies. Record the tax amounts deposited in the lability account as debits in the practice checking account.

18.13 When completing a practice's tax forms, make sure that you submit the appropriate state and federal taxes, file an Employer's Quarterly Federal Tax Return, and, if necessary, prepare state and local quarterly tax returns as well. Additionally, you will have to file Wage and Tax Statements for the practice.

18.14 Federal, state, and local tax returns should be filed quarterly for the medical office practice.

REVIEW

CHAPTER 18

CASE STUDY QUESTIONS

Now that you have completed this chapter, review the case study at the beginning of the chapter and answer the following questions:

1. What should Ben do to properly record the payment?

Multiple-Choice Questions

1. If you make an error when completing a check, you should
   a. use correction fluid to cover up the incorrect amount and write in the correct amount.
   b. tear up the check and throw it away.
   c. write VOID in ink across the front of the check and file it in numerical order with the returned checks.
   d. scratch out the error and fill in the correct amount above it.
2. Business checks with stubs attached are
   a. counter checks.
   b. voucher checks.
   c. limited checks.
   d. traveler's checks.
3. Which of the following checks may a physician use when she wants to withdraw money but forgot her checkbook?
   a. Counter
   b. Voucher
   c. Limited
   d. Certified
4. Money from the petty cash fund should be used for purchases such as
   a. new office furniture.
   b. postage-due fees and holiday decorations.
   c. everyday office supplies, such as tongue blades, cotton swabs, and bandages.
   d. medications that are administered in the office.
5. An employee payroll information sheet should include
   a. a completed I-9 form and verification of U.S. citizenship or legally admitted alien.
   b. the employee's work history, including salary requirements.
   c. all current and previous performance evaluations.
   d. the beneficiary in case of death.

Discussion Questions

1. Name three things that are required in a single-entry accounting system.
2. Discuss the meaning of a payroll deduction.
3. Why is the reconciliation of the bank statement so important?
4. Discuss the advantages and disadvantages of electronic banking.
5. When creating a payroll information sheet, name what it should contain.

Critical Thinking Questions

1. Why is it important for an employer to have an Employer Identification Number?
2. From an employer's perspective, when might a medical assistant contract be advisable?
3. Name some of the banking tasks of the medical practice.
4. Generating payroll is a very important part of a medical assistant's job. What could be the result if the payroll is inaccurate?

Application Activities WORK//PRODUCT

1. Record the following disbursements made on September 9, 2011, in a disbursements journal: Check no. 1234, payee—Tom Jones (electrician), check amount—$125; Check no. 1235, payee—Postmaster (postage), check amount—$32; Check no. 1236, payee—Gateway Property Management (rent), check amount—$900
2. A medical assistant in a medical practice is hired to work 8 hours a day, 4 days a week at an hourly rate of $10.00/hour. Checks are issued every 2 weeks. Her total deductions each week equal 10% of her gross earnings. What are her gross earnings per week? What is her "take home" pay in each check?
3. Prepare your personal federal income tax return, using information from the Wage and Tax Statement (Form W-2) and the Employee's Withholding Allowance Certificate (Form W-4) provided by your employer.

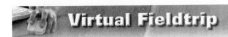

Virtual Fieldtrip

Visit the McGraw-Hill Higher Education Medical Assisting website at www.mhhe.com/medicalassisting4e to complete the following activity:

Imagine that you are a medical assistant in a busy medical practice. You are assisting a new employee with the completion of the W-4 form. Go online and visit the U.S. government website and any other sites that offer information about how to complete the W-4 form. Then answer the following questions for submission to your instructor.

1. What general instruction would you give the employee?
2. Is claiming "exempt" the same thing as claiming "0"?
3. Under what conditions will the employee be exempt from any income tax withholding?

Open the CD and complete this chapter's practice activities, play the games, listen to the key terms, and test yourself with the interactive review. E-mail, print, and/or save your results to document your proficiency.

APPENDIX I

Prefixes, Suffixes, and Word Roots in Commonly Used Medical Terms

Prefixes

a-, an- without, not
ab- from, away
ad-, -ad to, toward
ambi-, amphi- both, on both sides, around
ante- before
antero- in front of
anti- against, opposing
auto- self
bi- twice, double
brachy- short
brady- slow
cata- down, lower, under
centi- hundred
chol-, chole-, cholo- gall
circum- around
co-, com-, con- together, with
contra- against
cryo- cold
de- down, from
deca- ten
deci- tenth
demi- half
dextro- to the right
di- double, twice
dia- through, apart, between
dipla-, diplo- double, twin
dis- apart, away from
dys- difficult, painful, bad, abnormal
e-, ec-, ecto- away, from, without, outside
em-, en- in, into, inside
endo- within, inside
ento- within, inner
epi- on, above
erythro- red
eu- good, true, normal
ex-, exo- outside of, beyond, without
extra- outside of, beyond, in addition
fore- before, in front of
gyn-, gyno-, gyne-, gyneco- woman, female

hemi- half
hetero- other, unlike
homeo, homo- same, like
hyper- above, over, increased, excessive
hypo- below, under, decreased
idio- personal, self-produced
im-, in-, ir- not
in- in, into
infra- beneath
inter- between, among
intra-, intro- into, within, during
juxta- near, nearby
leuco-, leuko- white
macro- large, long
mal- bad
mega-, megalo- large, great
melan-, melano- black
mes-, meso- middle
meta- beyond
micro- small
mono- single, one
multi- many
neo- new
non-, not- no
nuli- none
olig-, oligo- few, less than normal
ortho- straight
oxy- sharp, acid
pachy- thick
pan- all, every
par; para- alongside of, with; woman who has given birth
per- through, excessive
peri- around
pluri- more, several
poly- many, much
post- after, behind
pre-, pro- before, in front of
presby-, presbyo- old age
primi- first
pseudo- false
quadri- four
re- back, again
retro- backward, behind
semi- half

steno- contracted, narrow
stereo- firm, solid, three-dimensional
sub- under
super-, supra- above, upon, excess
sym-, syn- with, together
tachy- fast
tele- distant, far
tetra- four
trans- across
tri- three
ultra- beyond, excess
uni- one

Suffixes

-aesthesia sensation
-al characterized by
-algia pain
-ase enzyme
-asthenia weakness
-cele swelling, tumor
-centesis puncture, tapping
-cidal killing
-cide causing death
-cise cut
-cyst bladder, sac
-cyte, cell, cellular
-derm skin
-dynia- pain
-ectomy cutting out, surgical removal
-emesis vomiting
-emia blood
-esthesia sensation
-gene, -genic, -genetic, -genesis arising from, origin, formation
-gram recorded information
-graph instrument for recording
-graphy the process of recording
-gravida pregnant female
-ia condition
-iasis condition of
-ic, -ical pertaining to
-ism condition, process, theory

-itis   inflammation of

-ium   membrane

-ize   to cause to be, to become, to treat by special method

-kinesis, -kinetic   motion

-lepsis, -lepsy   seizure, convulsion

-logy   science of, study of

-lysis   setting free, disintegration, decomposition

-malacia   abnormal softening

-mania   insanity, abnormal desire

-meter   measure

-metry   process of measuring

-odynia   pain

-oid   resembling

-ole   small, little

-oma   tumor

-opia   vision

-opsy   to view

-osis   disease, condition of

-ostomy   to make a mouth, opening

-otomy   incision, surgical cutting

-ous   having

-pathy   disease, suffering

-penia   too few, lack, decreased

-pexy   surgical fixation

phagia, -phage   eating, consuming, swallowing

-phobia   fear, abnormal fear

-phylaxis   protection

-plasia   formation or development

-plastic   molded

-plasty   operation to reconstruct, surgical repair

-plegia   paralysis

-pnea   breathing

-rrhage, -rrhagia   abnormal or excessive discharge, hemorrhage, flow

-rrhaphy   suture of

-rrhea   flow, discharge

-sclerosis   hardening

-scopy   examining

-sepsis   poisoning, infection

-spasm   cramp or twitching

-stasis   stoppage

-stomy   opening

-therapy   treatment

-thermy   heat

-tome   cutting instrument

-tomy   incision, section

-tripsy   surgical crushing

-trophy   nutrition, growth

-tropy   turning, tendency

-uria   urine

Word Roots

adeno-   gland, glandular

adipo-   fat

aero-   air

andr-, andro-   man, male

angio-   blood vessel

ano-   anus

arterio-   artery

arthro-   joint

bili-   bile

bio-   life

blasto-, blast-   developing stage, bud

bracheo-   arm

broncho-   bronchial (windpipe)

carcino-   cancer

cardio-   heart

cephal-, cephalo-   head

cerebr-, cerebro-   brain

cervico-   neck

chondro-   cartilage

chromo-   color

colo-   colon

colp-, colpo-   vagina

coro-   body

cost-, costo-   rib

crani-, cranio-   skull

cysto-   bladder, bag

cyto-   cell, cellular

dacry-, dacryo-   tears, lacrimal apparatus

dactyl-, dactylo-   finger, toe

dent-, denti-, dento-   teeth

derma-, dermat-, dermato-   skin

dorsi-, dorso-   back

encephalo-   brain

entero-   intestine

esthesio-   sensation

fibro-   connective tissue

galact-, galacto-   milk

gastr-, gastro-   stomach

gingiv-   gums

glosso-   tongue

gluco-, glyco-   sugar, sweet

haemo-, hemato-, hem-, hemo-   blood

hepa-, hepar-, hepato-   liver

herni-   rupture

histo-   tissue

hydra-, hydro-   water

hyster-, hystero-   uterus

ictero-   jaundice

ileo-   ileum

karyo-   nucleus, nut

kera-, kerato-   horn, hardness, cornea

lact-   milk

laparo-   abdomen

latero-   side

linguo-   tongue

lipo-   fat

lith-, -lith   stone

mast-, masto-   breast

med-, medi-   middle

meno-   month

metro-, metra-   uterus

my-, myo-   muscle

myel-, myelo-   marrow

narco-   sleep

nas-, naso-   nose

necro-   dead

nephr-, nephro-   kidney

neu-, neuro-   nerve

niter-, nitro-   nitrogen

nucleo-   nucleus

oculo-   eye

odont-   tooth

omphalo-   navel, umbilicus

onco-   tumor

oo-   ovum, egg

oophor-   ovary

ophthalmo-   eye

orchid-   testicle

os-   mouth, opening

oste-, osteo-   bone

oto-   ear

paedo, pedo-   child

palpebro-   eyelid

path-, patho-   disease, suffering

pepso-   digestion

phag-, phago-   eating, consuming, swallowing

pharyng-   throat, pharynx

phlebo-   vein

pleuro-   side, rib

pneumo-   air, lungs

pod   foot

procto-   rectum

psych-   the mind

pulmon-, pulmono-   lung

pyelo-   pelvis (renal)

pyo-   pus

pyro-   fever, heat

reni-, reno-   kidney
rhino-   nose
sacchar-   sugar
sacro-   sacrum
salpingo-   tube, fallopian tube
sarco-   flesh
sclero-   hard, sclera
septi-, septico-   poison, infection

stomato-   mouth
teno-, tenoto-   tendon
thermo-   heat
thoraco-   chest
thrombo-   blood clot
thyro-   thyroid gland
tricho-   hair

urino-, uro-   urine, urinary organs
utero-   uterus, uterine
vaso-   vessel
ventri-, ventro-   abdomen
vesico-   blister
xantho-   yellow

APPENDIX II
Abbreviations and Symbols Commonly Used in Medical Notations

Abbreviations

a before

aa, AA of each

a.c. before meals

ADD attention deficit disorder

ADL activities of daily living

ad lib as desired

ADT admission, discharge, transfer

AIDS acquired immunodeficiency syndrome

a.m.a. against medical advice

AMA American Medical Association

amp. ampule

amt amount

aq., AQ water; aqueous

ausc. auscultation

ax axis

Bib, bib drink

b.i.d., bid, BID twice a day

BM bowel movement

BP, B/P blood pressure

BPC blood pressure check

BPH benign prostatic hypertrophy

BSA body surface area

c̄ with

Ca calcium; cancer

cap, caps capsules

CBC complete blood (cell) count

C.C., CC chief complaint

CDC Centers for Disease Control and Prevention

CHF congestive heart failure

chr chronic

CNS central nervous system

Comp, comp compound

COPD chronic obstructive pulmonary disease

CP chest pain

CPE complete physical examination

CPR cardiopulmonary resuscitation

CSF cerebrospinal fluid

CT computed tomography

CV cardiovascular

d day

D&C dilation and curettage

DEA Drug Enforcement Administration

Dil, dil dilute

DM diabetes mellitus

DOB date of birth

DTP diptheria-tetanus-pertussis vaccine

Dr. doctor

DTs delirium tremens

D/W dextrose in water

Dx, dx diagnosis

ECG, EKG electrocardiogram

ED emergency department

EEG electroencephalogram

EENT eyes, ears, nose, and throat

EP established patient

ER emergency room

ESR erythrocyte sedimentation rate

FBS fasting blood sugar

FDA Food and Drug Administration

FH family history

Fl, fl, fld fluid

F/u follow-up

Fx fracture

GBS gallbladder series

GI gastrointestinal

Gm, gm gram

gr grain

gt, gtt drop, drops

GTT glucose tolerance test

GU genitourinary

GYN gynecology

HA headache

HB, Hgb hemoglobin

HEENT head, ears, eyes, nose, throat

HIV human immunodeficiency virus

HO history of

h.s., hs, HS hour of sleep/at bedtime

Hx history

ICU intensive care unit

I&D incision and drainage

I&O intake and output

IM intramuscular

inf. infusion; inferior

inj injection

IT inhalation therapy

IUD intrauterine device

IV intravenous

KUB kidneys, ureters, bladder

L1, L2, etc. lumbar vertebrae

lab laboratory

lb pound

liq liquid

LLL left lower lobe

LLQ left lower quadrant

LMP last menstrual period

LUQ left upper quadrant

M mix (Latin *misce*)

m- meta-

MI myocardial infarction

mL milliliter

MM mucous membrane

MRI magnetic resonance imaging

MS multiple sclerosis

NB newborn

NED no evidence of disease

no. number

noc, noct night

npo, NPO nothing by mouth

NPT new patient

NS normal saline

NSAID nonsteroidal anti-inflammatory drug

NTP normal temperature and pressure

N&V nausea and vomiting

NYD not yet diagnosed

o- ortho-

OB obstetrics

OC oral contraceptive

OD overdose

oint ointment

OOB out of bed

OPD outpatient department

OPS outpatient services

OR operating room

OTC over-the-counter

p- para-

p̄ after

P&P Pap smear (Papanicolaou smear) and pelvic examination

PA posteroanterior

Pap Pap smear

Path pathology

p.c., pc after meals

PE physical examination

per   by, with

PH   past history

PID   pelvic inflammatory disease

p/o   postoperative

POMR   problem-oriented medical record

PMFSH   past medical, family, social history

PMS   premenstrual syndrome

p.r.n., prn, PRN   whenever necessary

Pt   patient

PT   physical therapy

PTA   prior to admission

PVC   premature ventricular contraction

pulv   powder

q.   every

q2, q2h   every 2 hours

q.a.m., qam   every morning

q.h., qh   every hour

qhs   every night, at bedtime

q.i.d., QID   four times a day

qns, QNS   quantity not sufficient

qs, QS   quantity sufficient

RA   rheumatoid arthritis; right atrium

RBC   red blood cells; red blood (cell) count

RDA   recommended dietary allowance, recommended daily allowance

REM   rapid eye movement

RF   rheumatoid factor

RLL   right lower lobe

RLQ   right lower quadrant

R/O   rule out

ROM   range of motion

ROS/SR   review of systems/systems review

RUQ   right upper quadrant

RV   right ventricle

Rx   prescription, take

s̄   without

SAD   seasonal affective disorder

SIDS   sudden infant death syndrome

Sig   directions

sig   sigmoidoscopy

SOAP   subjective, objective, assessment, plan

SOB   shortness of breath

sol   solution

S/R   suture removal

ss, s̄s̄   one-half (Latin semis)

Staph   staphylococcus

stat, STAT   immediately

STD   sexually transmitted disease

Strep   streptococcus

subling, SL   sublingual

subq, SubQ   subcutaneously

surg   surgery

S/W   saline in water

SX   symptoms

T1, T2, etc.   thoracic vertebrae

T & A   tonsillectomy and adenoidectomy

tab   tablet

TB   tuberculosis

tbs., tbsp   tablespoon

TIA   transient ischemic attack

t.i.d., tid, TID   three times a day

tinc, tinct, tr   tincture

TMJ   temporomandibular joint

top   topically

TPR   temperature, pulse, and respiration

TSH   thyroid stimulating hormone

tsp   teaspoon

Tx   treatment

UA   urinalysis

UCHD   usual childhood diseases

UGI   upper gastrointestinal

ung, ungt   ointment

URI   upper respiratory infection

US   ultrasound

UTI   urinary tract infection

VA   visual acuity

VD   venereal disease

Vf   visual field

VS   vital signs

WBC   white blood cells; white blood (cell) count

WNL   within normal limits

wt   weight

y/o   year old

Symbols

Weights and Measures

\#   pounds

°   degrees

′   foot; minute

″   inch; second

μm   micrometer

μ   micron (former term for micrometer)

mμ   millimicron; nanometer

mEq   milliequivalent

mL   milliliter

dL   deciliter

mg%   milligrams percent; milligrams per 100 mL

Mathematical Functions and Terms

\#   number

+   plus; positive; acid reaction

−   minus; negative; alkaline reaction

±   plus or minus; either positive or negative; indefinite

×   multiply; magnification; crossed with, hybrid

÷ , /   divided by

=   equal to

≈   approximately equal to

>   greater than; from which is derived

<   less than; derived from

≮   not less than

≯   not greater than

≤   equal to or less than

≥   equal to or greater than

≠   not equal to

√   square root

³√   cube root

∞   infinity

:   ratio; "is to"

∴   therefore

%   percent

π   pi (3.14159)—the ratio of circumference of a circle to its diameter

Chemical Notations

Δ   change; heat

⇌   reversible reaction

↑   increase

↓   decrease

Warnings

Ⓒ   Schedule I controlled substance

Ⓒ   Schedule II controlled substance

Ⓒ   Schedule III controlled substance

Ⓒ   Schedule IV controlled substance

Ⓒ   Schedule V controlled substance

☠   poison

☢   radiation

☣   biohazard

Others

℞   prescription; take

□, ♂   male

○, ♀   female

†   one

††   two

†††   three

GLOSSARY

Note: (†) Pronunciation from *Stedman's Medical Dictionary,* 26th edition; all others from *American Heritage,* 4th edition, in case you need to consult.

10× lens (těn) A magnifying lens in the ocular of a microscope that magnifies an image ten times.

24-hour urine specimen (twĕn′tē fôr our yŏŏr′ in spĕs′ ə-mən) A urine specimen collected over a 24-hour period and used to complete a quantitative and qualitative analysis of one or more substances, such as sodium, chloride, and calcium.

abandonment (ə-bǎn′dən-mənt) A situation in which a health-care professional stops caring for a patient without arranging for care by an equally qualified substitute.

ABA number (nŭm′ber) A fraction appearing in the upper-right corner of all printed checks that identifies the geographic area and specific bank on which the check is drawn.

abduction (ab-dŭk′shuň)(†) Movement away from the body.

abscess (ăb′sĕs′) A collection of pus (white blood cells, bacteria, and dead skin cells) that forms as a result of infection.

absorption (əb-sôrp′shən) The process by which one substance is absorbed, or taken in and in-corporated, into another, as when the body converts food or drugs into a form it can use.

abuse (ə-byōōs′) A practice or be-havior that is not indicative of or in line with sound medical or fiscal activity.

access (ăk′sĕs) The way patients enter and exit a medical office.

accessibility (ăk-sĕs′ə-bĭl′ĭ-tē) The ease with which people can move into and out of a space.

accommodation (ă-kom′ə-dā-shən) The ability of the lens to change shape, allowing the eye to focus images of objects that are near or far away.

accounts payable (ə-kounts′ pā′-ă-bəl) Money owed by a business; the practice's expenses.

accounts receivable (ə-kounts′ rĭ-sē′ və-bəl) Income or money owed to a business.

accreditation (ə-krĕd′ĭ-tā′shən) The documentation of official authorization or approval of a program.

acetabulum (as′ətab′yələm) The hip socket.

acetylcholine (as-e-til-kō′lēn)(†) A neurotransmitter released by the parasympathetic nerves onto organs and glands for resting and digesting.

acetylcholinesterase (as′e-til-kō-lin-es′ter-ās) An enzyme within the nervous system that hydro-lyzes acetylcholine to acetate and choline.

acid-fast stain (ăs′ĭd fǎst stān) A staining procedure for identify-ing bacteria that have a waxy cell wall.

acids (ăs′ĭds) Electrolytes that release hydrogen ions in water.

acinar cells (as′i-nar sĕlz)(†) Cells in the pancreas that produce pan-creatic juice.

acquired immunodeficiency syndrome (AIDS) (ə-kwīrd im′yū-nō-dē-fish′en-sē sĭn′drōm′)(†) The most advanced stage of HIV in-fection; it severely weakens the body's immune system.

acromegaly (ak-rō-meg′ă-lē)(†) A disorder in which too much growth hormone is produced in adults.

acrosome (ak′rō-sōm)(†) An enzyme-filled sac covering the head of a sperm that aids in the penetration of the egg during fertilization.

action potential (ăk′shən pə-tĕn′shəl) The flow of electrical current along the axon membrane.

active file (ăk′tĭv fĭl) A file used on a consistent basis.

active listening (ăk′tĭv lĭs′ənĭng) Part of two-way communication, such as offering feedback or ask-ing questions; contrast with **pas-sive listening.**

active transport (ak′-tiv trans-pórt) The movement of a substance across a cell membrane from an area of low concentration to an area of high concentration.

acupressure (ak-you-presh-er) Pressure applied by hands to various areas of the body to restore balance in the body's energy flow.

acupuncture (ak-you-punk-chūr) The practice of inserting needles into various areas of the body to restore balance in the body's energy flow.

acupuncturist (ăk′yōō-pŭngk′chər-ĭst) A practitioner of acupunc-ture. The acupuncturist uses hollow needles inserted into the patient's skin to treat pain, discomfort, or systemic imbalances.

acute (ə-kyōōt′) Having a rapid onset and progress, as acute appendicitis.

*Parenthetical numbers indicate the chapter in which the entry is a key term or is first defined in context. Entries not followed by a chapter number are important terms related to material covered but not specifically defined in the text.

425

addiction (ă-dĭkˊshun)(†) A physical or psychological dependence on a substance, usually involving a pattern of behavior that includes obsessive or compulsive preoccupation with the substance and the security of its supply, as well as a high rate of relapse after withdrawal.

Addison's disease (ă-dĭsuns dĭzēz) A condition in which the adrenal glands fail to produce enough corticosteroids.

add-on code (ădˊon' kōd) A code indicating procedures that are usually carried out in addition to another procedure. Add-on codes are used together with the primary code.

adduction (ă-dŭkˊshŭn)(†) Movement toward the body.

adenoids (ădˊn-oidzˊ) See **pharyngeal tonsils.**

adjustment (ə-jŭstˊ-ment) Manual treatments given by a chiropractor that move the joints of the spine and other joints into proper alignment.

administer (ăd-mĭnˊĭ-stər) To give a drug directly by injection, by mouth, or by any other route that introduces the drug into the body.

adrenocorticotropic hormone (ACTH) (ă-drēˊnō-kōrˊti-kō-trōˊpik horˊmōn) Hormone that stimulates the adrenal cortex to release its hormones.

advance scheduling (ăd-văns skējˊoolˊĭng) Booking an appointment several weeks or even months in advance.

aerobes (ârˊōbsˊ) Bacteria that grow best in the presence of oxygen.

aerobic respiration (â-rōˊbĭk rĕsˊpə-rāˊshən) A process that requires large amounts of oxygen and uses glucose to make ATP.

afebrile (ā-febˊril)(†) Having a body temperature within one's normal range.

afferent arterioles (ăfˊər-ənt ar-tērˊē-ōlz)(†) Structures that deliver blood to the glomeruli of the kidneys.

afferent nerves (ăfˊər-ənt nûrvs) A type of sensory nerves that are responsible for detecting sensory information from the environment or even from inside the body and bringing it to the CNS for interpretation.

affiliation agreement (ə-fĭlˊē-āˊshən ə-grēˊmənt) An agreement that externship participants must sign that states the expectations of the facility and the expectations of the student.

agar (āˊgärˊ) A gelatin-like substance derived from seaweed that gives a culture medium its semi-solid consistency.

age analysis (āj ə-nălˊĭ-sĭs) The process of clarifying and reviewing past due accounts by age from the first date of billing.

agenda (ə-jĕnˊdə) The list of topics discussed or presented at a meeting, in order of presentation.

agent (āˊ-jənt) (legal) A person who acts on a physician's behalf while performing professional tasks; (clinical) an active principal or entity that produces a certain effect, for example, an infectious agent.

agglutination (ă-glū-ti-nāˊshŭn)(†) The clumping of red blood cells following a blood transfusion.

aggressive (ə-grĕsˊĭv) Imposing one's position on others or trying to manipulate them.

agonist (ăgˊənist) See **antagonist.**

agranular leukocyte (ă-granˊ-yulər lūˊkō-sīt)(†) A type of leukocyte (white blood cell) with a solid nucleus and clear cytoplasm; includes lymphocytes and monocytes.

agranulocyte (ă-granˊyū-lō-sīt)(†) See **agranular leukocyte.**

albumins (ăl-byoōˊmĭns) The smallest of the plasma proteins. Albumins are important for pulling water into the bloodstream to help maintain blood pressure.

aldosterone (al-dosˊter-ōn)(†) A hormone produced in the adrenal glands that acts on the kidney. It causes the body to retain sodium and excrete potassium. Its role is to maintain blood volume and pressure.

alimentary canal (ălˊə-mĕnˊtə-rē kə-nălˊ) The organs of the digestive system that extend from the mouth to the anus.

allele (ə-lēlˊ) Any one of a pair or series of **genes** that occupy a specific position on a specific **chromosome.**

allergen (ălˊər-jən) An antigen that induces an allergic reaction.

allergic rhinitis (alˊərjik rīniˊtis) A hypersensitivity reaction to various airborne allergens.

allergist (ălˊər-jĭst) A specialist who diagnoses and treats physical reactions to substances including mold, dust, fur, pollen, foods, drugs, and chemicals.

allopathy (ə-lōˊpăth-ē) The usual medical practice of physicians and other health professionals; also known as conventional medicine.

allowed charge (ə-loudˊ chärj) The amount that is the most the payer will pay any provider for each procedure or service.

alopecia (ălˊə-pēˊshə) The clinical term for baldness.

alphabetic filing system (ălˊfə-bĕtˊĭk fīˊlĭng sisˊtəm) A filing system in which the files are arranged in alphabetic order, with the patient's last name first, followed by the first name and middle initial.

Alphabetic Index (ălˊfə-bĕtˊĭk ĭnˊdĕksˊ) One of two ways diagnoses are listed in the ICD-9-CM. They appear in alphabetic order with their corresponding diagnosis codes.

alternative medicine (ôl-tûrˊ-nə-tĭv mĕdˊ-ĭ-sĭn) The type of medicine used in place of conventional medicine to promote health and treat disease.

alveolar glands (al-vē´ō-lăr glăndz) (†) Glands that make milk under the influence of the hormone **prolactin.**

alveoli (ăl-vē´ə-lī´) Clusters of air sacs in which the exchange of gases between air and blood takes place; located in the lungs.

American Association of Medical Assistants (AAMA) (ə-mĕr´ĭkən ə-sō´sē-ā´shən mĕd´ĭ-kəl ə-sĭs´tənts) The professional organization that certifies medical assistants and works to maintain professional standards in the medical assisting profession.

Americans with Disabilities Act (ADA) (ə-mĕr´ĭ-kəns dĭs´ə-bĭl´ĭ-tēs ăkt) A U.S. civil rights act forbidding discrimination against people because of a physical or mental handicap.

amblyopia (am-blē-ō´pē-ă) (†) Poor vision in one eye without a detectable cause.

amino acids (ə-mē´nō ăs´ĭds) Natural organic compounds found in plant and animal foods and used by the body to create protein.

amnion (ăm´nē-ən) The innermost membrane enveloping the embryo and containing amniotic fluid.

anabolism (ənab´əlĭz´əm) The stage of metabolism in which substances such as nutrients are changed into more complex substances and used to build body tissues.

anaerobe (ăn´ə-rōb´) A bacterium that grows best in the absence of oxygen.

anal canal (ā´nəl kə-năl´) The last few centimeters of the rectum.

anaphase (an´əfāz) The period of mitosis when the centromeres divide and pull the chromosomes (formerly chromatids) toward the centrioles at opposite sides of the cell.

anaphylaxis (an´ă-fī-lak´sis) A severe allergic reaction with symptoms that include respiratory distress, difficulty in swallowing, pallor, and a drastic drop in blood pressure that can lead to circulatory collapse.

anatomical position (ăn´ə-tŏm´ĭ-kəl pə-zĭsh´ən) When the body is standing upright and facing forward with the arms at the side and the palms of the hands facing forward.

anatomy (ə-năt´ə-mē) The scientific term for the study of body structure.

anemia (ə-nē´mē-ə) A condition characterized by low red blood cell count. This condition decreases the ability to transport oxygen throughout the body.

anergic reaction (an-er´jik rē-ăk´shən) A lack of response to skin testing that indicates the body's inability to mount a normal response to invasion by a pathogen.

anesthesia (ăn´ĭs-thē´zhə) A loss of sensation, particularly the feeling of pain.

anesthetic (ăn´ĭs-thĕt´ik) A medication that causes anesthesia.

anesthetist (ă-nes´thĕ-tist) (†) A specialist who uses medications to cause patients to lose sensation or feeling during surgery.

aneurysm (ăn´yə-rĭz´əm) A serious and potentially life-threatening bulge in the wall of a blood vessel.

angiography (an-jē-og´ră-fē) (†) An x-ray examination of a blood vessel, performed after the injection of a contrast medium, that evaluates the function and structure of one or more arteries or veins.

annotate (ăn´ō-tāt´) To underline or highlight key points of a document or to write reminders, make comments, and suggest actions in the margins.

anorexia nervosa (ăn´ə-rĕk´sē-ə nûr-vō´sə) An eating disorder in which people starve themselves because they fear that if they lose control of eating they will become grossly overweight.

antagonist (ăn-tăg´ə-nĭst) A muscle that produces the opposite movement of the **prime mover.**

antecubital space (an-te-kyū´bi-tăl spās) The inner side or bend of the elbow; the site at which the brachial artery is felt or heard when a pulse or blood pressure is taken.

anterior (ăn-tîr´ē-ər) Anatomical term meaning toward the front of the body; also called ventral.

anthracosis (an´thrə kō´sis) Chronic lung disease caused by the inhalation of coal deposits; also known as Black Lung Disease.

antivirus software (an-tē vī-rəs soft-wer) Software that prevents and removes computer virusus. Such programs may also detect and remove adware and spyware.

antibodies (ăn´tĭ-bod´ēs) Highly specific proteins that attach themselves to foreign substances in an initial step in destroying such substances, as part of the body's defenses.

antidiuretic hormone (ADH) (an´tē-dī-yū-ret´ik hôr´mōn´) (†) A hormone that increases water reabsorption, which decreases urine production and helps to maintain blood pressure.

antigen (an´tĭ-jən) A foreign substance that stimulates white blood cells to create antibodies when it enters the body.

antihistamines (ăn´tē-hĭs´tə-mēnz) Medications used to treat allergies.

antimicrobial (an´tē-mī-krō´bē-ăl) (†) An agent that kills microorganisms or suppresses their growth.

antioxidants (ăn´tē-ŏk´sĭ-dənt) Chemical agents that fight cell-destroying chemical substances called free radicals.

antiseptic (ăn´tĭ-sĕp´tĭk) A cleaning product used on human tissue as an anti-infection agent.

anuria (an-yū´rē-ă) (†) The absence of urine production.

aortic semilunar valve (ā ôr´tĭk sem´ē loonər valv) Heart valve that is a semilunar valve and that is situated between the left ventricle and the aorta.

apex (ā´pĕks) The left lower corner of the heart, where the strongest heart sounds can be heard.

apical (ap´i-kăl) (†) Located at the **apex** of the heart.

apnea (ap´nēə) The absence of respiration.

apocrine gland (ap´ō-krin glănd) (†) A type of sweat gland. It produces a thicker type of sweat than other sweat glands and contains more proteins.

aponeurosis (ap´ō-nū-rō´sis) (†) A tough, sheet-like structure that is made of fibrous connective tissue. It typically attaches muscles to other muscles.

appendicitis (ə-pĕn´dĭ-sī´tĭs) Inflammation of the appendix.

appendicular (ap´en-dik´yū-lăr) The division of the skeletal system that consists of the bones of the arms, legs, pectoral girdle, and pelvic girdle.

approximate (a-prŏk´s i māt) To bring the edges of a wound together so the tissue surfaces are close in order to protect the area from further contamination and to minimize scar and scab formation.

aqueous humor (a´kwē-əs hyōō´mər) A liquid produced by the eye's ciliary body that fills the space between the cornea and the lens.

arbitration (är´bĭ-trā´shən) A process in which opposing sides choose a person or persons outside the court system, often someone with special knowledge in the field, to hear and decide a dispute.

areflexia (ā-rē-flek´sē-ă) (†) The absence of reflexes.

areola (ă-rē´ō-lă) (†) The pigmented area that surrounds the nipple.

aromatherapy (a-rō´-mə-thēr´-ə-pē) The use of essential oil extracts or essences from flowers, herbs, and trees to promote health and well-being.

arrector pili (ă-rek´tōr pī´lī) (†) Muscles attached to most hair follicles and found in the dermis.

arrhythmia (ə-rĭth´mē-ə) Irregularity in heart rhythm.

arterial blood gases (är-tîr´ē-əl blŭd găs´ses) A test that measures the amount of gases, such as oxygen and carbon dioxide, dissolved in arterial blood.

arthritis (arth rīt´is) A general term meaning joint inflammation.

arthrography (ar-throg´ră-fē) (†) A radiologic procedure performed by a radiologist, who uses a contrast medium and fluoroscopy to help diagnose abnormalities or injuries in the cartilage, tendons, or ligaments of the joints—usually the knee or shoulder.

arthroscopy (är-thŏs´kə-pē) A procedure in which an orthopedist examines a joint, usually the knee or shoulder, with a tubular instrument called an arthroscope; also used to guide surgical procedures.

articular cartilage (ar-tik´yu-lăr kär´tl-ĭj) (†) The cartilage that covers the **epiphysis** of long bones.

articulations (ärtik´yəla´shən) The area where bones are joined together; joints.

artifact (är´tə-făkt´) Any irrelevant object or mark observed when examining specimens or graphic records that is not related to the object being examined; for example, a foreign object visible through a microscope or an erroneous mark on an ECG strip.

asbestosis (asbestō´sis) Chronic lung disease caused by the inhalation of asbestos fibers.

ascending colon (ə-sĕnd´ĭng ko´lən) The segment of the large intestine that runs up the right side of the abdominal cavity.

ascending tracts (ə-sĕnd´ĭng trăkts) The tracts of the spinal cord that carry sensory information to the brain.

asepsis (ă-sep´sĭs) (†) The condition in which pathogens are absent or controlled.

assault (ə-sôlt´) The open threat of bodily harm to another.

assertive (ə-sûrt´tĭv) Being firm and standing up for oneself while showing respect for others.

asset (ăs´ĕt´) An item owned by the practice that has a dollar value, such as the medical practice building, office equipment, or accounts receivable.

assignment of benefits (ə-sīn´mənt bĕn´ə-fĭts) An authorization for an insurance carrier to pay a physician or practice directly.

asthma (az´mə) A condition in which the tubes of the bronchial tree become obstructed due to inflammation.

astigmatism (ə-stĭg´mə-tĭz´əm) A condition in which the cornea has an abnormal shape, which causes blurred images during near or distant vision.

astrocytes (ăs´-tro-sīts) Star-shaped cells within the nervous system that anchor blood vessels to the nerve cells.

atelectasis (at´ilek´təsis) The collapse of a lung because of fluid, air, pus, or blood.

atherosclerosis (ăth´ə-rō-sklə-rō´sĭs) The accumulation of fatty deposits along the inner walls of arteries.

atlas (ăt´ləs) The first cervical vertebra.

atoms (ăt´əmz) The simplest units of all matter.

atria (ā´trē-ă) (†) [*Singular:* **atrium**] Chambers of the heart that receive blood from the veins and circulate it to the ventricles.

atrial natriuretic peptide (ā´trē-ăl nā´trēyu-ret´ik pep´tīd) (†) A hormone secreted by the heart that regulates blood pressure.

atrioventricular bundle (ā´trē-ō-ventrik´yū-lar bŭn´dl)(†) A structure that is located between the ventricles of the heart and that sends the electrical impulse to the Purkinje fibers.

atrioventricular node (ā´trē-ō-ventrik´yū-lar nōd) A node that is located between the atria of the heart. After the electrical impulse reaches the atrioventricular node, the atria contract and the impulse is sent to the ventricles.

atrioventricular septum (a´treo-ventrik´yu-lar səp´təm) The wall separating the upper atrial chambers from the lower ventricular chambers of the heart.

audiologist (aw-dē-ol´ōjist)(†) A health-care specialist who focuses on evaluating and correcting hearing problems.

audiometer (aw-dē-om´ē-ter) An electronic device that measures hearing acuity by producing sounds in specific frequencies and intensities.

auricle (ôr´ĭ-kəl) The outside part of the ear, made of cartilage and covered with skin.

auscultated blood pressure (ô´skəl-tāt-ĕd blŭd prĕsh´ər) Blood pressure as measured by listening with a stethoscope.

auscultation (ô´skəl-tā´shən) The process of listening to body sounds.

authorization (ô´thər-ĭ-zā´shən) A form that explains in detail the standards for the use and disclosure of patient information for purposes other than treatment, payment, or health-care operations.

autoclave (aw´tō-klāv)(†) A device that uses pressurized steam to sterilize instruments and equipment.

autoimmune disease (aw´tō-ĭmyoŏn di-zēz´) Any condition in which the body attacks its own antigens, causing illness to the patient.

automated external defibrillator (AED) (ô´tə-mā´tĭd ĭk-stûr´nəl dē-fib´ri-lā-ter) A computerized defibrillator programmed to recognize lethal heart rhythms and deliver an electrical shock to restore a normal rhythm.

autonomic (ô´tə-nŏm´ĭk) A division of the peripheral nervous system that connects the central nervous system to viscera such as the heart, stomach, intestines, glands, blood vessels, and bladder.

autonomic nervous system (ANS) (ô´tə-nŏm´ĭk nūr´vəs sĭs´təm) A system that is in charge of the body's automatic functions, such as the respiratory and gastrointestinal systems.

autopsy (ô-top´-sē) The examination of a cadaver to determine or confirm the cause of death.

autosome (ô´tə-sōm´) A chromosome that is not a sex chromosome.

axial (ăk´sē-əl) The division of the skeletal system that consists of the skull, vertebral column, and rib cage.

axilla (ăk-sĭl´ə) Armpit; one of the four locations for temperature readings.

axis (ak´-səs) The second vertebra of the neck on which the head turns.

axon (ăk´sŏn´) A type of nerve fiber that is typically long and branches far from the cell body. Its function is to send information away from the cell body.

Ayurveda (eye-yer-vay-duh) A form of medicine, originated in India, that uses herbal preparations, dietary changes, exercises, and meditation to restore health and promote well-being.

bacillus (ba-sil´ŭs)(†) A rod-shaped bacterium.

bacterial spore (băk-tîr´ēăl spôr) A primitive, thick-walled reproductive body capable of developing into a new individual; resistant to killing through disinfection.

balance billing (băl´əns bĭl´ĭng) Billing a patient for the difference between a higher usual fee and a lower allowed charge.

balloon angioplasty (buh-loon an´je-o-plas´te-) A procedure using a slender, hollow tube passed through a coronary artery to compress a blockage in the artery.

bandwidth (bānd´wĭdth´) A measurement, calculated in bits or bytes, of how much information can be sent or processed with one single instruction.

barium enema (bâr´ē-əm ĕn´ə-mə) A radiologic procedure performed by a radiologist who administers barium sulfate through the anus, into the rectum, and then into the colon to help diagnose and evaluate obstructions, ulcers, polyps, diverticulosis, tumors, or motility problems of the colon or rectum; also called a lower GI (gastrointestinal) series.

barium swallow (bâr´ē-əm swŏl´ō) A radiologic procedure that involves oral administration of a barium sulfate drink to help diagnose and evaluate obstructions, ulcers, polyps, diverticulosis, tumors, or motility problems of the esophagus, stomach, duodenum, and small intestine; also called an upper GI (gastrointestinal) series.

baroreceptors (bar´ō-rē-sep´ters)(†) Structures, located in the aorta and carotid arteries, that help regulate blood pressure.

Bartholin's glands (bär´ tə linz glăndz) Glands lateral to the vagina that produce mucus for lubrication of the vagina.

bases (bā´sēz´) Electrolytes that release hydroxyl ions in water.

basophil (bā-sō-fil)(†) A type of granular leukocyte that produces the chemical histamine, which aids the body in controlling allergic reactions and other exaggerated immunologic responses.

battery (băt´ə-rē) An action that causes bodily harm to another.

behavior modification (bĭ-hāv´yər mŏd´ə-fī-kā-shən) The altering of personal habits to promote a healthier lifestyle.

benefits (bĕn´ə-fĭts) Payments for medical services.

benign (bē-nīn´) A noncancerous or nonmalignant growth or condition.

benign prostatic hypertrophy (bē nīn´ pros-tat´ik hī pur´trə fē) A noncancerous enlargement of the prostate gland.

bicarbonate ions (bī-kar´bon-āt ī´onz) Elements formed when carbon dioxide gets into the bloodstream and reacts with water. In the alimentary canal, these ions neutralize acidic chyme arriving from the stomach.

bicuspids (bī-kŭs´pĭds) Teeth with two cusps. There are two in front of each set of molars.

bicuspid valve (bī-kŭs´pĭd vălv) Heart valve that has two cusps and that is located between the left atrium and the left ventricle. Also known as the mitral valve.

bile (bīl) A substance created in the liver and stored in the gallbladder. Bile is a bitter yellow-green fluid that is used in the digestion of fats.

bilirubin (bili-rū´bin)(†) A bile pigment formed by the breakdown of hemoglobin in the liver.

bilirubinuria (bil´i-rū-bi-nū´rē-ă)(†) The presence of bilirubin in the urine; one of the first signs of liver disease or conditions that involve the liver.

biliverdin (bil-i-ver´din)(†) A pigment released when a red blood cell is destroyed.

biochemistry (bī´ō-kĕm´ĭ-strē) The study of matter and chemical reactions in the body.

bioelectromagnetic-based therapies (bī´ō-ī-lĕk´tro-mag-ne-tik basĕd thĕr´-ə-pēs) The use of measurable energy fields in such things as magnetic therapy, millimeter wave therapy, sound energy therapy, and light therapy.

bioethics (bī-ō-ĕth´ĭks) Principles of right and wrong in issues that arise from medical advances.

biofeedback (bī-ō-fēd´-bāk) A type of therapy in which an individual learns how to control involuntary body responses in order to promote health and treat disease.

biofield therapies (bī-ō-field thĕr´ -ə-pēs) Treatments that affect the energy fields that surround and penetrate the human body in order to promote health and well-being.

biohazard symbol (bī-ō-hăz´ərd sĭm´bəl) A symbol that must appear on all containers used to store waste products, blood, blood products, or other specimens that may be infectious.

biohazardous materials (bī-ō-hăz´ərd-əs mə-tîr´ə-əls) Biological agents that can spread disease to living things.

biohazardous waste container (bī-ō-hăz´ərd-əs wāst kən-tā´nər) A leakproof, puncture-resistant container, color-coded red or labeled with a special biohazard symbol, that is used to store and dispose of contaminated supplies and equipment.

biopsy (bī-op´-sē) The removal and examination of a sample of tissue from a living body for diagnostic purposes.

biopsy specimen (bī´ŏp´sē spĕs´ə-mən) A small amount of tissue removed from the body for examination under a microscope to diagnose an illness.

bioterrorism (bī-ō´tĕr´ə-rĭz´əm) The intentional release of a biologic agent with the intent to harm individuals.

birthday rule (bûrth´dā´rool) A rule that states that the insurance policy of a policyholder whose birthday comes first in the year is the primary payer for all dependents.

blastocyst (blas´tō-sist) A morula that travels down the uterine tube to the uterus and is invaded with fluid. It then implants into the wall of the uterus.

blood-borne pathogen (blŭd-bôrn păth´ə-jən) A disease-causing microorganism carried in a host's blood and transmitted through contact with infected blood, tissue, or body fluids.

blood-brain barrier (blŭd brăn băr´ē-ər) A structure that is formed from tight capillaries to protect the tissues of the central nervous system from certain substances.

B lymphocyte (bē lĭm´fə-sīt´) A type of nongranular leukocyte that produces antibodies to combat specific pathogens.

body (bod-ee) Single-spaced lines of text that are the content of a business letter.

body language (bŏd´ē lăng´gwĭj) Nonverbal communication, including facial expressions, eye contact, posture, touch, and attention to personal space.

bolus (bō´ləs) The mass created when food is combined with saliva and mucus.

bone conduction (bōn kən-dŭk´shən) The process by which sound waves pass through the bones of the skull directly to the inner ear, bypassing the outer and middle ears.

bookkeeping (book´kē´pĭng) The systematic recording of business transactions.

botulism (bŏch´ə-lĭz´əm) A life-threatening type of food poisoning that results from eating improperly canned or preserved foods that have been contaminated with the bacterium *Clostridium botulinum.*

boundaries (bau n-d(ə-)rēs) A physical or psychological space that indicates the limit of appropriate versus inappropriate behavior.

Bowman's capsule (bō´mənz kap´səl) A capsule that surrounds the **glomerulus** of the kidney.

brachial artery (brāk´ē-ăl är´tə-rē) An artery that provides a palpable pulse and audible vascular sounds in the antecubital space (the bend of the elbow).

brachytherapy (brak-ē-thăr′ă-pē′)(†) A radiation therapy technique in which a radiologist places temporary radioactive implants close to or directly into cancerous tissue; used for treating localized cancers.

bradycardia (braid uh card e uh) A slow heart rate; usually less than 60 beats per minute.

brain stem (brān stēm) A structure that connects the cerebrum to the spinal cord.

breach of contract (brēch kŏn′trăkt′) The violation of or failure to live up to a contract's terms.

bronchi (brŏn-kī) The two branches of the trachea that enter the lungs.

bronchial tree (brŏng′kē-al trē) A series of tubes that begins where the distal end of the trachea branches.

bronchioles (brŏng′kē-ōlz) A part of the respiratory tract that branches from the tertiary bronchi.

buccal (bŭk′ăl)(†) Between the cheek and gum.

buffy coat (buf′ē kōt) The layer between the packed red blood cells and plasma in a centrifuged blood sample; this layer contains the white blood cells and platelets.

bulbourethral glands (bŭl′bō-yū-rē′thrăl glăndz)(†) Glands that lie beneath the prostate and empty their fluid into the urethra. Their fluid aids in sperm movement.

bulimia (boō-lē′mē-ə) An eating disorder in which people eat a large quantity of food in a short period of time (bingeing) and then attempt to counter the effects of bingeing by self-induced vomiting, use of laxatives or diuretics, and/or excessive exercise.

bundle of His (bēn′ dl ov hiss) Also known as the AV bundle, this is the node located between the ventricles of the heart that carries the electrical impulse from the AV node to the bundle branches.

burnout (′bər-naŭt) The end result of prolonged periods of stress without relief. Burnout is an energy-depleting condition that can affect one's health and career. It can be common for those who work in health care.

bursitis (bər-sī′tĭs) Inflammation of a bursa.

calcaneus (kal-kā′nē-ŭs)(†) The largest tarsal bone; also called the heel bone.

calcitonin (kal-si-tō′nin) A hormone produced by the thyroid gland that lowers blood calcium levels by activating osteoblasts.

calibrate (kīal′-brat) To determine the caliber of; to standardize a measuring instrument.

calibration syringe (kăl′ə-brā′shən sə-rĭnj) A standardized measuring instrument used to check and adjust the volume indicator on a spirometer.

calorie (kăl′ə-rē) A unit used to measure the amount of energy food produces; the amount of energy needed to raise the temperature of 1 kg of water by 1°C.

calyces (kă′lĭ-sēz′) Small cavities of the renal pelvis of the kidney.

CAM (kăm) The acronym for complementary and alternative medicine. Complementary medicine is used with conventional medicine. Alternative medicine is used in place of conventional medicine.

canaliculi (kan-ă-lik′yū-lī) Tiny canals that connect lacunae to each other.

cancellous (kan′siləs) Bone also known as spongy bone. It contains spaces within it containing the red bone marrow.

capillary (kăp′ə-lĕr′ē) Branches of arterioles and the smallest type of blood vessel.

capillary puncture (kăp′ə-lĕr′ē pŭngk′chər) A blood-drawing technique that requires a superficial puncture of the skin with a sharp point.

capitation (kăp′ĭ-tā′shən) A payment structure in which a health maintenance organization prepays an annual set fee per patient to a physician.

carboxyhemoglobin (kärbok′sēhē′məglō′bin) The term used when the hemoglobin of red blood cells is carrying carbon dioxide.

carboxypeptidase (kar-bok-sē-pep′ti-dās)(†) A pancreatic enzyme that digests proteins.

carcinogen (kär-sĭn′ə-jən) A factor that is known to cause the formation of cancer.

cardiac catheterization (kär′dē-ăk′ kath′ē-ter-ī-zā′shun)(†) A diagnostic method in which a catheter is inserted into a vein or artery in the arm or leg and passed through blood vessels into the heart.

cardiac cycle (kär′dē-ăk′ sī′kəl) The sequence of contraction and relaxation that makes up a complete heartbeat.

cardiac sphincter (kär′dē-ăk sfingk′tər) The valve-like structure composed of a circular band of muscle at juncture of the esophagus and stomach. Also known as the esophageal sphincter.

cardiologist (kär′dē-ŏl′ə-jĭst) A specialist who diagnoses and treats diseases of the heart and blood vessels (cardiovascular diseases).

carditis (kar-dī′tis)(†) Inflammation of the heart.

carpal (kär′pəl) Bones of the wrist.

carpal tunnel syndrome (kär′pəl tŭn′əl sĭn′drōm′) A painful disorder caused by compression of the median nerve in the carpal tunnel of the wrist.

carrier (kăr′ē-ər) A reservoir host who is unaware of the presence of a pathogen and so spreads the disease while exhibiting no symptoms of infection.

cash flow statement (kăsh flō stā′tmənt) A statement that shows the cash on hand at the beginning of a period, the income and disbursements made during the period, and the new amount of cash on hand at the end of the period.

cashier's check (kă-shîrz′ chĕk) A bank check issued by a bank on bank paper and signed by a bank representative; usually purchased by individuals who do not have checking accounts.

cast (kăst) A rigid, external dressing, usually made of plaster or fiberglass, that is molded to the contours of the body part to which it is applied; used to immobilize a fractured or dislocated bone.

Cylinder-shaped elements with flat or rounded ends, differing in composition and size, that form when protein from the breakdown of cells accumulates and precipitates in the kidney tubules and is washed into the urine.

catabolism (kə tăb′əlĭz′əm) The stage of metabolism in which complex substances, including nutrients and body tissues, are broken down into simpler substances and converted into energy.

cataracts (kăt′ə-răkts′) Cloudy areas that form in the lens of the eye that prevent light from reaching visual receptors.

catheterization (kăth′ē-ter-ĭ-zā′shun)(†) The procedure during which a catheter is inserted into a vessel, an organ, or a body cavity.

caudal (kôd′l) See **inferior.**

CD-ROM (sē′dē′rŏm′) A compact disc that contains software programs; an abbreviation for "compact disc—read-only memory."

cecum (sē′kəm) The first section of the large intestine.

celiac disease (sē′lē-ăk′ dĭ-zēz′) An intolerance to gluten that causes an immune response in the body and reduces the absorption of nutrients in the small intestines.

cell body (sĕl bŏd′ē) The portion of the neuron that contains the nucleus and organelles.

cell membrane (sĕl mĕm′brān′) The outer limit of a cell that is thin and selectively permeable. It controls the movement of substances into and out of the cell.

cells (sĕlz) The smallest living units of structure and function.

cellulitis (sel-yū-lī′tis) Inflammation of cellular or connective tissue.

cellulose (sĕl′yə-lōs′) A type of carbohydrate that is found in vegetables and cannot be digested by humans; commonly called fiber.

Celsius (centigrade) (sĕl′sē-əs) One of two common scales for measuring temperature; measured in degrees Celsius, or °C.

Centers for Medicare and Medicaid Services (CMS) (sĕn′tərs mĕd′ĭ-kâr′ mĕd′ĭ-kād′ sûr′vĭs-əz) A congressional agency designed to handle Medicare and Medicaid insurance claims. It was formerly known as the Health Care Financing Administration.

central nervous system (CNS) (sĕn′trəl nûr′vəs sĭs′təm) A system that consists of the brain and the spinal cord.

central processing unit (CPU) (sĕn′trəl prŏs′es′ĭng yōō′nĭt) A microprocessor, the primary computer chip responsible for interpreting and executing programs.

centrifuge (sĕn′trə-fyōōj′) A device used to spin a specimen at high speed until it separates into its component parts.

centrioles (sen′trē ōlz) Two cylinder-shaped organs near the cell nucleus that are essential for cell division, by equally dividing chromosomes to the daughter cells.

cerebellum (sĕr′ə-bĕl′əm) An area of the brain inferior to the cerebrum that coordinates complex skeletal muscle coordination.

cerebrospinal fluid (CSF) (ser′ē-brō-spī′nəl flōō′ĭd) The fluid in the subarachnoid space of the meninges and the central canal of the spinal cord.

cerebrovascular accident (ser′əbrovas′kyələr ak′sidənt) A stroke. Caused by a hemorrhage in the brain or more often by a clot lodged in a cerebral artery.

cerebrum (sĕr′ə-brəm) The largest part of the brain; it mainly includes the cerebral hemispheres.

Certificate of Waiver tests (sər-tĭf′ĭ-kĭt wā′vər tĕsts) Laboratory tests that pose an insignificant risk to the patient if they are performed or interpreted incorrectly, are simple and accurate to such a degree that the risk of obtaining incorrect results is minimal, and have been approved by the Food and Drug Administration for use by patients at home; laboratories performing only Certificate of Waiver tests must meet less stringent standards than laboratories that perform tests in other categories.

certified check (sûr′tə-fīd′ chĕk) A payer's check written and signed by the payer, which is stamped "certified" by the bank. The bank has already drawn money from the payer's account to guarantee that the check will be paid.

Certified Medical Assistant (CMA) (sûr′tə-fīd′ mĕd′ĭ-kəl ə-sĭs′tənt) A medical assistant whose knowledge about the skills of medical assistants, as summarized by the 2003 AAMA Role Delineation Study areas of competence, has been certified by the Certifying Board of the American Association of Medical Assistants (AAMA).

cerumen (sə-rōō′mən) A wax-like substance produced by glands in the ear canal; also called earwax.

cervical enlargement (sûr′vĭ-kəl in-lärj′-mənt) The thickening of the spinal cord in the neck region.

cervical orifice (sûr′vĭ-kəl ôr′ə-fĭs) The opening of the uterus through the cervix into the vagina.

cervicitis (ser-vi-sī′tis) Inflammation of the cervix.

cervix (sûr´vĭks) The lowest portion of the uterus that extends into the vagina.

cesarean section (si zer´ē ən sak´ shən) A surgical incision of the abdomen and uterus to deliver a baby transabdominally.

chain of custody (chān kŭs´tə-dē) A procedure for ensuring that a specimen is obtained from a specified individual, is correctly identified, is under the uninterrupted control of authorized personnel, and has not been altered or replaced.

CHAMPVA (Civilian Health and Medical Program of the Veterans Administration) (sĭ-vĭl´yən hĕlth mĕd´ĭ-kəl prō´ğram vĕtər-enz ăd-mĭn´ĭ-strā´shən) A type of health insurance that covers the expenses of families (dependent spouses and children) of veterans with total, permanent, and service-connected disabilities. It also covers the surviving families of veterans who die in the line of duty or as a result of service-connected disabilities.

chancre (shang´ker) (†) A painless ulcer that may appear on the tongue, the lips, the genitalia, the rectum, or elsewhere.

charge slip (chärj slĭp) The original record of services performed for a patient and the charges for those services.

check (chĕk) A bank draft or order written by a payer that directs the bank to pay a sum of money on demand to the payee.

chemistry (kĕm´ĭ-strē) The study of the composition of matter and how matter changes.

chemoreceptor (kē´mo-rĭ-sĕp´tôr) Any cell that is activated by a change in chemical concentration and results in a nerve impulse. The olfactory or smell receptors in the nose are an example of a chemoreceptor.

Cheyne-Stokes respirations (chain stokes RES per ra shuns) A pattern of breathing that gradually alternates between deep and shallow breaths with a period of apnea or no breathing that can last from 5 to 40 seconds.

chief cells (chēf sĕlz) Cells in the lining of the stomach that secrete **pepsinogen.**

chief complaint (chēf kəm-plān´t) The patient's main issue of pain or ailment.

chiropractor (kī´rə-prăk´tôr) A physician who uses a system of therapy, including manipulation of the spine, to treat illness or pain. This treatment is done without drugs or surgery.

chlamydia (klə mid´ē ah) A common bacterial STD caused by bacterium *Chlamydia trachomatis* that can lead to PID in women.

cholangiography (kō-lan-jē-og´răfē) (†) A test that evaluates the function of the bile ducts by injection of a contrast medium directly into the common bile duct (during gallbladder surgery) or through a T-tube (after gallbladder surgery or during radiologic testing) and taking an x-ray.

cholecystography (kō-lē-sis-tog´răfē) (†) A gallbladder function test performed by x-ray after the patient ingests an oral contrast agent; used to detect gallstones and bile duct obstruction.

cholesterol (kə-lĕs´tə-rôl) A fat-related substance that the body produces in the liver and obtains from dietary sources; needed in small amounts to carry out several vital functions. High levels of cholesterol in the blood increase the risk of heart and artery disease.

chordae tendineae (kōr´dĕ tendin´ā) (†) Cord-like structures that attach the cusps of the heart valves to the papillary muscles in the ventricles.

choroid (kôr´oid´) The middle layer of the eye, which contains the iris, the ciliary body, and most of the eye's blood vessels.

chromosome (krō´mə-sōm´) Thread-like structures composed of DNA.

chronic (krŏn´ĭk) Lasting a long time or recurring frequently, as in chronic osteoarthritis.

chronic obstructive pulmonary disease (COPD) (krŏn´ĭk obstrŭk´tiv po͞olmə-nĕr´ē dĭ-zēz´) A disease characterized by the presence of airflow obstruction as a result of chronic bronchitis or emphysema. It is typically progressive. Cigarette smoking is the leading cause.

chronological résumé (krŏn´ə-lŏj´ĭ-kəl rĕz´o͞o-mā´) The type of résumé used by individuals who have job experience. Jobs are listed according to date, with the most recent being listed first.

chylomicron (kī-lō-mi´kron) The least dense of the lipoproteins; it functions in lipid transportation.

chyme (kīm) (†) The mixture of food and gastric juice.

chymotrypsin (kī-mō-trip´sin) (†) A pancreatic enzyme that digests proteins.

cilia (sil´ēa) Hair-like projections from the outside of the cell membrane on some cell types.

ciliary body (sĭl´ē-ēr´ē bŏd´ē) A wedge-shaped thickening in the middle layer of the eyeball that contains the muscles that control the shape of the lens.

circumduction (ser-kŭm-dŭk´shŭn) Moving a body part in a circle; for example, tracing a circle with your arm.

cirrhosis (sĭ-rō´sĭs) A long-lasting liver disease in which normal liver tissue is replaced with non-functioning scar tissue.

civil law (sĭv´əl lô) Involves crimes against persons. A person can sue another person, business, or the government. Judgments often require a payment of money.

clarification (klăr´ə-fĭ´kā´shən) Asking questions that provide an increased understanding of a problem.

clarity (klăr´i-tē) Clearness in writing or stating a message.

class action lawsuit (klăs-ăk´shən lô´sōōt) A lawsuit in which one or more people sue a company or other legal entity that allegedly wronged all of them in the same way.

clavicle (klăv´ĭ-kəl) A slender, curved long bone that connects the sternum and the scapula; also called the collar bone.

clean-catch midstream urine specimen (klēn-kăch mĭd´strēm yōōr´ĭn spĕs´əmən) A type of urine specimen that requires special cleansing of the external genitalia to avoid contamination by organisms residing near the external opening of the urethra and is used to identify the number and types of pathogens present in urine; sometimes referred to as midvoid.

clearinghouse (klîr´ĭng-hous´) A group that takes nonstandard medical billing software formats and translates them into the standard EDI formats.

cleavage (klē´vĭj) The rapid rate of mitosis of a zygote immediately following fertilization.

clinical coordinator (klĭn´ĭ-kəlkō-ôr´dn-ā´tor) The person associated with the medical assisting school that procures externship sites and qualifies them to ensure that they provide a thorough educational experience.

clinical diagnosis (klĭn´ĭ-kəl dī´əg-nō´sĭs) A diagnosis based on the signs and symptoms of a disease or condition.

clinical drug trial (klĭn´ĭ-kəl drŭg trī´əl) An internationally recognized research protocol designed to evaluate the efficacy or safety of drugs and to produce scientifically valid results.

Clinical Laboratory Improvement Amendments of 1988 (CLIA '88) (klē´ə) A law enacted by Congress in 1988 that placed all laboratory facilities that conduct tests for diagnosing, preventing, or treating human disease or for assessing human health under federal regulations administered by the Health Care Financing Administration (HCFA) and the Centers for Disease Control and Prevention (CDC).

clitoris (klĭt´ər-ĭs) Located anterior to the urethral opening in females. It contains erectile tissue and is rich in sensory nerves.

clock speed (klŏk spēd) A measurement of how many instructions per second that a CPU can process. Clock speed is measured in megahertz (MHz) or gigahertz (GHz).

closed file (klōzd fīl) A file for a patient who has died, moved away, or for some other reason no longer consults the office for medical expertise.

closed posture (klōzd pŏs´chər) A position that conveys the feeling of not being totally receptive to what is being said; arms are often rigid or folded across the chest.

cluster scheduling (klŭs´tər skĕj´ōō l-ĭng) The scheduling of similar appointments together at a certain time of the day or week.

coagulation (kō-ăg´yə-lā´shən) The process by which a clot forms in blood.

coccus (kŏk´əs) A spherical, round, or ovoid bacterium.

coccyx (kŏk´sĭks) A small, triangular-shaped bone consisting of three to five fused vertebrae.

cochlea (kŏk´lē-ă) A spiral-shaped canal in the inner ear that contains the hearing receptors.

code linkage (kōd lĭng´kĭj) Analysis of the connection between diagnostic and procedural information in order to evaluate the medical necessity of the reported charges. This analysis is performed by insurance company representatives.

coinsurance (kō-ĭn-shōōr´əns) A fixed percentage of covered charges paid by the insured person after a deductible has been met.

colitis (kə-lī´tĭs) Inflammation of the colon.

colonoscopy (kō-lon-os´ kŏ-pē)(†) A procedure used to determine the cause of diarrhea, constipation, bleeding, or lower abdominal pain by inserting a scope through the anus to provide direct visualization of the large intestine.

colony (kōl´ə-nē) A distinct group of microorganisms, visible with the naked eye, on the surface of a culture medium.

color family (kūl´ər făm´ə-lē) A group of colors that share certain characteristics, such as warmth or coolness, allowing them to blend well together.

colposcopy (kol-pos´kŏ-pē)(†) The examination of the vagina and cervix with an instrument called a colposcope to identify abnormal tissue, such as cancerous or precancerous cells.

combining vowel (kəm-bīn-ĭng vou´ əl) A vowel (often and o) that is placed between a word root and suffix to ease pronunciation.

common bile duct (kŏm´ən bīl dŭkt) Duct that carries bile to the duodenum. It is formed from the merger of the cystic and hepatic ducts.

compactible file (kəm-păkt´-əbəl fīl) Files kept on rolling shelves that slide along permanent tracks in the floor and are stored close together or stacked when not in use.

complement (kŏm´plə-mənt) A protein present in serum that is involved in specific defenses.

complementary medicine (kŏm´-plə-mĕn-tə-rē mĕd´-ĭ-sĭn) A type of medicine that is used with conventional medicine.

complete proteins (kəm-plēt´ prō´ten´) Proteins that contain all nine essential amino acids.

complex carbohydrates (kəm-plĕks´ kär´bō-hī´drāt´s) Long chains of sugar units; also known as polysaccharides.

complex inheritance (kəm-plĕks´ ĭn-hĕr´ĭ-təns) The inheritance of traits determined by multiple genes.

compliance plan (kəm-plīˊəns plăn)   A process for finding, correcting, and preventing illegal medical office practices.

complimentary closing (kom-pluh-men-tuh-ree kloh-zing)   The closing remark of a business letter found two spaces below the last line of the body of the letter.

compound (kŏmˊpoundˊ)   A substance that is formed when two or more atoms of more than one element are chemically combined.

compound microscope (kŏmˊpoundˊ mīˊkrə-skōpˊ)   A microscope that uses two lenses to magnify the image created by condensed light focused through the object being examined.

computed tomography (kəm-pyootˊĕd tō-mogra-fē) (†)   A radiographic examination that produces a three-dimensional, cross-sectional view of an area of the body; may be performed with or without a contrast medium.

concise (k n-sīsˊ)   Brevity; the use of no unnecessary words.

concussion (kən-kŭshˊən)   A jarring injury to the brain; the most common type of head injury.

conductive hearing loss (kon-dŭk-tivˊhērˊing lôs) (†)   A type of hearing loss that occurs when sound waves cannot be conducted through the ear. Most types are temporary.

condyle (konˊdīl) (†)   Rounded articular surface on a bone.

cones (kōnz)   Light-sensing nerve cells in the eye, at the posterior of the retina, that are sensitive to color, provide sharp images, and function only in bright light.

conflict (kŏnˊflĭktˊ)   An opposition of opinions or ideas.

conjunctiva (kŏnˊjŭngk-tīˊvə)   The protective membrane that lines the eyelid and covers the anterior of the sclera, or the white of the eye.

conjunctivitis (kən-jŭngkˊtə-vīˊtĭs)   A contagious infection of the conjunctiva caused by bacteria, viruses, and allergies. The symptoms may include discharge, red eyes, itching, and swollen eyelids; also commonly called pinkeye.

connective tissue (kə-nĕkˊtĭv)   A tissue type that is the framework of the body.

consent (kən-ˊsēnt)   A voluntary agreement that a patient gives to allow a medically trained person the permission to touch, examine, and perform a treatment.

constructive criticism (kən-streˊk-tiv krˊi-tə-si-zəm)   A type of critique that is aimed at giving an individual feedback about his or her performance in order to improve that performance.

consumable (kən-sooˊmə-bəl)   Able to be emptied or used up, as with supplies.

consumer education (kən-sooˊmər ĕjˊə-kaˊshən)   The process by which the average person learns to make informed decisions about goods and services, including health care.

contagious (kən-tāˊjəs)   Having a disease that can easily be transmitted to others.

contaminated (kən-tămˊə-nātˊĕd)   Soiled or stained, particularly through contact with potentially infectious substances; no longer clean or sterile.

contract (kŏnˊtrăctˊ)   A voluntary agreement between two parties in which specific promises are made.

contraindication (kŏnˊtrə-ĭnˊdĭ-kāˊ-shən)   A symptom that renders use of a remedy or procedure inadvisable, usually because of risk.

contrast medium (kŏnˊtrastˊ mēˊdē-əm)   A substance that makes internal organs denser and blocks the passage of x-rays to photographic film. Introducing a contrast medium into certain structures or areas of the body can provide a clear image of organs and tissues and highlight indications of how well they are functioning.

controlled substance (kən-trōldˊ sūbˊstəns)   A drug or drug product that is categorized as potentially dangerous and addictive and is strictly regulated by federal laws.

control sample (kən-trolˊ sămˊpəl)   A specimen that has a known value; used as a comparison for test results on a patient sample.

contusion (kon-tŭˊshŭn) (†)   A closed wound, or bruise.

conventional medicine (kən-vĕnˊ-shən-əl mĕdˊ-i-sĭn)   The usual practice of physicians and other allied health professionals, such as physical therapists, psychologists, medical assistants, and registered nurses. Also known as allopathy.

conventions (kən-vĕnˊshənz)   A list of abbreviations, punctuation, symbols, typefaces, and instructional notes appearing in the beginning of the ICD-9. The items provide guidelines for using the code set.

convolutions (kŏnˊvə-looˊshənz)   The ridges of brain matter between the sulci; also called gyri.

coordination of benefits (kō-ôrˊdn-āˊshən bĕnˊə-fĭts)   A legal principle that limits payment by insurance companies to 100% of the cost of covered expenses.

co-payment (kō-pāˊmənt)   A small fee paid by the insured at the time of a medical service rather than by the insurance company.

cornea (kôrˊnē-ə)   A transparent area on the front of the outer layer of the eye that acts as a window to let light into the eye.

coronary artery bypass graft (CABG) (korˊ-uh-ner-ee, ahrˊ-tuh-ree, bahyˊ-pas, grahft)   A surgery performed to bypass a blockage within a coronary artery with a vessel taken from another area.

coronary sinus (kôrˊə-nĕrˊē sīˊnəs)   The large vein that receives oxygen-poor blood from the cardiac veins and empties it into the right atrium of the heart.

corporation (kôr-pə-´rā-shən) A type of business group, such as a medical practice, that is established by law and managed by a board of directors.

corpus callosum (kôr´pəs ka-l´ō-səm) A thick bundle of nerve fibers that connects the cerebral hemispheres.

corpus luteum (kôr´pŭs lū-tē´ŭm) (†) A ruptured follicle cell in the ovary following ovulation.

cortex (kôr´təks´) The outermost layer of the cerebrum.

cortisol (kōr´ti-sol) (†) A steroid hormone that is released when a person is stressed. It decreases protein synthesis.

coryza (côrī´zə) Another name for an upper respiratory tract infection. The common cold.

costal (kos´tăl) (†) Cartilage that attaches true ribs to the sternum.

counter check (koun´tər chěk) A special bank check that allows a depositor to draw funds from his own account only, as when he has forgotten his checkbook.

courtesy title (kûr´tĭ-sē tīt´l) A title used before a person's name, such as Dr., Mr., or Ms.

cover sheet (kŭr´ər shēt) A form sent with a fax that provides details about the transmission.

covered entity (kūv´ərd en-tə-tē) Any organization that transmits health information in an electronic form that is related in any way with a HIPAA-covered business.

Cowper's glands (kou´ pərz glāndz) Bulbourethral glands.

coxal (koks-al´) (†) Pertaining to the bones of the pelvic girdle. The coxa is composed of the ilium, ischium, and pubis.

CPT See *Current Procedural Terminology.*

cranial (krā-´nē-ăl) (†) See **superior.**

cranial nerves (krā´nē-ăl nûrvs) (†) Peripheral nerves that originate from the brain.

crash cart (krăsh kärt) A rolling cart of emergency supplies and equipment.

creatine phosphate (krē´ă-tēn fos´fāt) (†) A protein that stores extra phosphate groups.

credit (krĕd´ĭt) An extension of time to pay for services, which are provided on trust.

credit bureau (kre´-dit byür´-o) A company that provides information about the credit worthiness of a person seeking credit.

cricoid cartilage (krī´koyd kär´tl-ĭj) (†) A cartilage of the larynx that forms most of the posterior wall and a small part of the anterior wall.

crime (krīm) An offense against the state committed or omitted in violation of public law.

criminal law (krĭm´ə-nəl lô) Involves crimes against the state. When a state or federal law is violated, the government brings criminal charges against the alleged offender.

cross-reference (krôs´rĕf´ər-əns) The notation within the ICD-9 of the word *see* after a main term in the index. The *see* reference means that the main term first checked is not correct. Another category must then be used.

cross-referenced (krôs´rĕf´ər-ənsd) Filed in two or more places, with each place noted in each file; the exact contents of the file may be duplicated, or a cross-reference form can be created, listing all the places to find the file.

cross-training (krôs-tr´ā-ning) The acquisition of training in a variety of tasks and skills.

cryosurgery (krī´ō-sûr´jə-rē) The use of extreme cold to destroy unwanted tissue, such as skin lesions.

cryotherapy (krī´ō-thĕr´ə-pē) The application of cold to a patient's body for therapeutic reasons.

cryptorchidism (krĭptôr´kidiz´əm) Congenital failure of the testes to descend into the scrotal sac.

crystals (kr˘ıs´təls) Naturally produced solids of definite form; commonly seen in urine specimens, especially those permitted to cool.

culture (kŭl´chər) In the sociologic sense, a pattern of assumptions, beliefs, and practices that shape the way people think and act.

To place a sample of a specimen in or on a substance that allows microorganisms to grow in order to identify the microorganisms present.

culture and sensitivity (C and S) (kŭl´chər sĕn´sĭ-tĭv´ə-tē) A procedure that involves culturing a specimen and then testing the isolated bacteria's susceptibility (sensitivity) to certain antibiotics to determine which antibiotics would be most effective in treating an infection.

culture medium (kŭlchər mē´de-əm) A substance containing all the nutrients a particular type of microorganism needs to grow.

Current Procedural Terminology **(CPT) (kûr´ənt prə-sē´jər-əl tûr´mə-nŏl´ə-jē)** A book with the most commonly used system of procedure codes. It is the HIPAA-required code set for physicians' procedures.

cursor (kûr´sər) A blinking line or cube on a computer screen that shows where the next character that is keyed will appear.

Cushing's disease (kush´ingz dī-zēz´) A condition in which a person produces too much **cortisol** or has used too many steroid hormones. Some of the signs and symptoms include buffalo hump obesity, a moon face, and abdominal stretch marks; also called hypercortisolism.

cuspids (kūs´pĭdz) The sharpest teeth; they act to tear food.

cyanosis (sī´ə-no´sīs) A bluish color of skin that results when the supply of oxygen is low in the blood.

cycle billing (sī´kəl bĭl´ĭng) A system that sends invoices to groups of patients every few days, spreading the work of billing all patients over the month while billing each patient only once.

cystic duct (sĭsˊtĭk dŭkt) The duct from the gallbladder that merges with the hepatic duct to form the common bile duct.

cystitis (sis-tīˊtis)(†) Inflammation of the urinary bladder caused by infection.

cytokines (sīˊtō-kīnz) A chemical secreted by T lymphocytes in response to an antigen. Cytokines increase T- and B-cell production, kill cells that have antigens, and stimulate red bone marrow to produce more white blood cells.

cytokinesis (sīˊtō-ki-nēˊsis)(†) Splitting of the cytoplasm during cell division.

cytoplasm (sīˊtə-plăzˊəm) The watery intracellular substance that consists mostly of water, proteins, ions, and nutrients.

damages (dămˊĭjz) Money paid as compensation for violating legal rights.

database (dāˊtə-bās) A collection of records created and stored on a computer.

dateline (dātˊlīnˊ) The line at the top of a letter that contains the month, day, and year.

debridement (dā-brēd-montˊ) (†) The removal of debris or dead tissue from a wound to expose healthy tissue.

decibel (dĕsˊə-bəl) A unit for measuring the relative intensity of sounds on a scale from 0 to 130.

deductible (dĭ-dŭkˊtə-bəl) A fixed dollar amount that must be paid by the insured before additional expenses are covered by an insurer.

deep (dēp) Anatomical term meaning closer to the inside of the body.

defamation (dĕfˊə-māˊshən) Damaging a person's reputation by making public statements that are both false and malicious.

defecation reflex (def-ē-kāˊshŭn rēˊflĕksˊ) The relaxation of the anal sphincters so that feces can move through the anus in the process of elimination.

deflection (dĭ-flĕkˊshən) A peak or valley on an electrocardiogram.

dehydration (dē-hīˊdrāˊshən) The condition that results from a lack of adequate water in the body.

dementia (dĭ-mĕnˊshə) The deterioration of mental faculties from organic disease of the brain.

dendrite (dĕnˊdrītˊ) A type of nerve fiber that is short and branches near the cell body. Its function is to receive information from the neuron.

deoxyhemoglobin (dē-oks-ē-hē-mō-glōˊbin)(†) A type of hemoglobin that is not carrying oxygen. It is darker red in color than hemoglobin.

dependent (dĭ-pĕnˊdənt) A person who depends on another person for financial support.

depolarization (dē-pōˊlăr-i-za-shūn)(†) The loss of polarity, or opposite charges inside and outside; the electrical impulse that initiates a chain reaction resulting in contraction.

depolarized (dē-pōˊlăr-īzd)(†) A state in which sodium ions flow to the inside of the cell membrane, making the outside less positive. Depolarization occurs when a neuron responds to stimuli such as heat, pressure, or chemicals.

depression (diˊ-pre-shan) The lowering of a body part.

dermatitis (dûrˊmə-tīˊtĭs) Inflammation of the skin.

dermatologist (der-mă-tolˊō-jist)(†) A specialist who diagnoses and treats diseases of the skin, hair, and nails.

dermatome (durˊmə tōm) An area of skin innervated by a spinal nerve.

dermis (dûrˊmĭs) The middle layer of the skin, which contains connective tissue, nerve endings, hair follicles, sweat glands, and oil glands.

descending colon (dĭ-sĕndˊĭng kōˊlən) The segment of the large intestine after the transverse colon that descends the left side of the abdominal cavity.

descending tracts (dĭ-sĕndˊĭng trăkts) Tracts of the spinal cord that carry motor information from the brain to muscles and glands.

detrusor muscle (dē-trŭsˊor mŭsˊəl) A smooth muscle that contracts to push urine from the bladder into the urethra.

diabetes insipidus (dīˊə bētĭs ĭn sĭpˊĭdəs) The condition of excessive thirst and excessive urination related to hyposecretion of ADH so that water is not retained by the kidney.

diabetes mellitus (dīˊə-bēˊtĭs mə-līˊtəs) Any of several related endocrine disorders characterized by an elevated level of glucose in the blood, caused by a deficiency of insulin or insulin resistance at the cellular level.

diagnosis (Dx) (dīˊəg-nōˊsĭs) The primary condition for which a patient is receiving care.

diagnosis code (dīˊəg-nōˊsĭs kōd) The way a diagnosis is communicated to the third-party payer on the health-care claim.

diagnostic radiology (dīˊəg-nosˊtik rāˊdē-ŏlˊə-jē) The use of x-ray technology to determine the cause of a patient's symptoms.

diapedesis (dīˊă-pĕ-dēˊsis)(†) The squeezing of a cell through a blood vessel wall.

diaphoresis (dīˊəfarēˊsis) Excessive sweating as a result of illness or injury.

diaphragm (dīˊə-frămˊ) A muscle that separates the thoracic and abdominopelvic cavities.

diaphysis (dīˊ-afˊi-sis) The shaft of a long bone.

diastolic pressure (dīˊə-stŏlˊĭk prĕshˊər) The blood pressure measured when the heart relaxes.

diathermy (dīˊə-thŭrˊmē) A type of heat therapy in which a machine produces high-frequency waves that achieve deep heat penetration in muscle tissue.

diencephalon (dī-en-sef´ă-lon)(†) A structure that includes the thalamus and the hypothalamus. It is located between the cerebral hemispheres and is superior to the brain stem.

dietary supplement (dī´-ĭ-tĕr-ē sŭp´-lə-mənt) Vitamins, minerals, herbals, and other substances taken by mouth without a prescription to promote health and well-being.

differential diagnosis (dĭf´ə-rĕn´shəl dī´əg-nō´sĭs) The process of determining the correct diagnosis when two or more diagnoses are possible.

differently abled (dĭf´ər-ənt-lē ā´bəld) Having a condition that limits or changes a person's abilities and may require special accommodations.

diffusion (di-fyū´zhŭn)(†) The movement of a substance from an area of high concentration to an area of low concentration.

digital examination (dĭj´ĭ-tl ĭg-zam´ə-nā´shən) Part of a physical examination in which the physician inserts one or two fingers of one hand into the opening of a body canal such as the vagina or the rectum; used to palpate canal and related structures.

diluent (dĭl´yōō-ənt) A liquid used to dissolve and dilute another substance, such as a drug.

disability insurance (dĭs´ə-bĭlĭ-tē ĭn-shōor´əns) Insurance that provides a monthly, prearranged payment to an individual who cannot work as the result of an injury or disability.

disaccharide (dī-sak´ă-rīd) (†) A type of carbohydrate that is a simple sugar.

disbursement (dĭs-bûrs´mənt) Any payment of funds made by the physician's office for goods and services.

disclaimer (dĭs-klā´mər) A statement of denial of legal liability or that refutes the authenticity of a claim.

disclosure (dĭ-sklō´zhər) The release of, the transfer of, the provision of access to, or the divulgence in any manner of patient information.

disclosure statement (dĭ-sklō´zhər stāt´mənt) A written description of agreed terms of payment; also called a federal Truth in Lending statement.

discrimination (dĭs-´skrĭm-ə-´nā-shən) Unequal and unfair treatment.

disinfectant (dĭs´ĭn-fĕk´tănt) A cleaning product applied to instruments and equipment to reduce or eliminate infectious organisms; not used on human tissue.

disk clean up (dĭsk kleen uph) A computer maintenance untility designed to free up disk space on computer users' hard drive.

disk defragmentation (dĭsk di-fragmen-ta-shun) A computer program designed to increase access speed by rearranging files stored on a disk to occupy contiguous storage locations, a technique commonly known as defragmenting.

dislocation (dĭs´lō-kā´shən) The displacement of a bone end from a joint.

dispense (dĭ-spĕns´) To distribute a drug, in a properly labeled container, to a patient who is to use it.

distal (dĭs´təl) Anatomic term meaning farther away from a point of attachment or farther away from the trunk of the body.

distal convoluted tubule (dĭs´təl kon´vō-lū-ted tū´byūl) The last twisted section of the renal tubule; it is located after the loop of Henle. Several of these tubules merge together to form collecting ducts.

distribution (dĭs´trĭ-byōō´shən) The biochemical process of transporting a drug from its administration site in the body to its site of action.

diverticulitis (dī´ver-tik-yū-li´tis)(†) Inflammation of the diverticuli, which are abnormal dilations in the intestine.

diverticulosis (dī´ver-tik-yū-lō-sis) Abnormal outpouchings or dilations of the intestine.

DNA (dē´ĕn-ā´) A nucleic acid that contains the genetic information of cells.

doctor of osteopathy (dok´tər ŏs´tē-ŏp´ə-thē) A doctor who focuses special attention on the muscu-loskeletal system and uses hands and eyes to identify and adjust structural problems, supporting the body's natural tendency toward health and self-healing.

doctrine of informed consent (dōk-´trĭn of ĭn-fôrmd´ kən-´sēnt) The legal basis for informed consent, usually outlined in a state's medical practice act.

doctrine of professional discretion (dōk-´trĭn of prə-fĕsh´ə-nəl dĭ-skrēsh´ən) A principle under which a physician can exercise judgment as to whether to show patients who are being treated for mental or emotional conditions their records.

documentation (dŏk´yə-mən-tā´shən) The recording of information in a patient's medical record; includes detailed notes about each contact with the patient and about the treatment plan, patient progress, and treatment outcomes.

dorsal (dôr´səl) See **posterior.**

dorsal root (dôr´səl rōōt) A portion of a spinal nerve that contains axons of sensory neurons only.

dorsiflexion (dōr-si-flek´shŭn)(†) Pointing the toes upward.

dosage (dōs´aj) The size, frequency, and number of doses.

dose (dōs) The amount of a drug given or taken at one time.

dot matrix printer (dŏt mā´trĭks prĭn´tər) An impact printer that creates characters by placing a series of tiny dots next to one another.

double-booking system (dŭb´əl bōōk´ing sĭs´təm) A system of scheduling in which two or more patients are booked for the same appointment slot, with the assumption that both patients will be seen by the doctor within the scheduled period.

douche (dōōsh)   Vaginal irrigation, which can be used to administer vaginal medication in liquid form.

drainage catheter (drā´nij kăth´ĭ-tər)   A type of catheter used to withdraw fluids.

dressing (drĕs´ĭng)   A sterile material used to cover a surgical or other wound.

DSL (digital subscriber line) (dĭj´ĭ-tl səb-skrīb´ līn)   A type of modem that operates over telephone lines but uses a different frequency than a telephone, allowing a computer to access the Internet at the same time that a telephone is being used.

ductus arteriosus (dŭk´tŭs ar-tēr´ē-ō´sus)(†)   The connection in the fetus between the pulmonary trunk and the aorta.

ductus venosus (duk´tŭs ven-ō´sus)(†)   A blood vessel that allows most of the blood to bypass the liver in the fetus.

duodenum (dōō´ə-dē´nəm)   The first section of the small intestine.

durable item (dōor´ə-bəl ī´təm)   A piece of equipment that is used repeatedly, such as a telephone, computer, or examination table; contrast with **expendable item.**

durable power of attorney (dōor´ə-bəl poúər ə-tûr´nē)(†)   A document naming the person who will make decisions regarding medical care on behalf of another person if that person becomes unable to do so.

dwarfism (dwôrf´ĭzm)   A condition in which too little growth hormone is produced, resulting in an abnormally small stature.

dysmenorrhea (dis-men-ōr-ē´ă)(†)   Severe menstrual cramps that limit daily activity.

dyspnea (disp-nē´ă)(†)   Difficult or painful breathing.

ear ossicles (îr os´i-kl)(†)   Three tiny bones called the malleus, the incus, and the stapes located in the middle ear cavity. They are the smallest bones of the body.

eccrine gland (ek´rin glănd)(†)   The most numerous type of sweat gland. Eccrine sweat glands produce a watery type of sweat and are activated primarily by heat.

echocardiography (ek´ō-kar-dē-og´ră-fē)(†)   A procedure that tests the structure and function of the heart through the use of reflected sound waves, or echoes.

E code (ē kŏd)   A type of code in the ICD-9. E-codes identify the external causes of injuries and poisoning.

ectoderm (ek´tō-derm)(†)   The primary germ layer that gives rise to nervous tissue and some epithelial tissue.

ectropion (ek-trō´pē-ŭn)   Eversion of the lower eyelid.

eczema (ĕk´sə-mə)   Inflammatory condition of the skin.

edema (ĭ-dē´mə)   An excessive buildup of fluid in body tissue.

editing (ĕd´ĭt-ĭng)   The process of ensuring that a document is accurate, clear, and complete; free of grammatical errors; organized logically; and written in the appropriate style.

effacement (i fās´mənt)   Thinning of the cervix in preparation for childbirth.

effectors (ĭ-fĕk´tərs)   Muscles and glands that are stimulated by motor neurons in the peripheral nervous system.

efferent arterioles (ĕf´ər-ənt ar-tēr´ē-ōlz)(†)   Structures that deliver blood to peritubular capillaries that are wrapped around the renal tubules of the nephron in the kidneys.

efferent nerves (ĕf´ər-ənt nûrvs)   Motor nerves that bring information or impulses from the Central nervous System to the Peripheral nervous System to allow for the movement or action of a muscle or gland.

efficacy (ĕf´ĭ-kə-sē)   The therapeutic value of a procedure or therapy, such as a drug.

efficiency (ĭ-fĭsh´ən-sē)   The ability to produce a desired result with the least effort, expense, and waste.

elective procedure (ĭ-lĕk´tĭv prə-sē´jər)   A medical procedure that is not required to sustain life but is requested for payment to the third-party payer by the patient or physician. Some elective procedures are paid for by third-party payers, whereas others are not.

electrocardiogram (ECG or EKG) (ĭ-lĕk´trō-kär´dē-ə-grăm´)   The tracing made by an **electrocardiograph.**

electrocardiograph (ĭ-lĕk´trō-kär´dē-ə-grăf´)   An instrument that measures and displays the waves of electrical impulses responsible for the cardiac cycle.

electrocardiography (ĭ-lĕk´trō-kär´dē-ŏg´rə-fē)   The process by which a graphic pattern is created to reflect the electrical impulses generated by the heart as it pumps.

electrocauterization (ĭ-lĕk´trō-kô´tər-ĭ-zā´shən)   The use of a needle, probe, or loop heated by electric current to remove growths such as warts, to stop bleeding, and to control nosebleeds that either will not subside or continually recur.

electrodes (ĭ-lĕk´trōds´)   Sensors that detect electrical activity.

electroencephalography (ĭ-lĕk´trō-ĕn-sĕf´ə-lŏ´grə-fē)   A procedure that records the electrical activity of the brain as a tracing called an electroencephalogram, or EEG, on a strip of graph paper.

electrolytes (ĭ-lĕk´trə-līts)   Substances that carry electrical current through the movement of ions.

electromyography (ĭ-lĕk´trō-mī-ŏg´rə-fē)   A procedure in which needle electrodes are inserted into some of the skeletal muscles and a monitor records the nerve impulses and measures conduction time; used to detect neuromuscular disorders or nerve damage.

electronic data interchange (EDI) (ĭ-lĕk-trŏn´ĭk dā´tə ĭn´tər-chānj´) Transmitting electronic medical insurance claims from providers to payers using the necessary information systems.

electronic health records (EHR) (i-lek-tron-ik helth rĭ-kôrd´) Patient health record created and stored on a computer or other electronic storage device. Also known as **electronic medical records.**

electronic mail (ĭ-lĕk´trŏn´ĭks) A method of sending and receiving messages through a computer network; commonly known as e-mail.

electronic media (i-lek-tron´-ik mee´-dee-uh) Any transmissions that are physically moved from one location to another through the use of magnetic tape, disk, compact disk media, or any other form of digital or electronic technology.

electronic medical records (EMR) (i-lek-tron-ik med-i-kuhl rĭ-kôrd´) Patient medical record created and stored on a computer or other electronic storage device. Also known as **electronic health records.**

electronic transaction record (ĭ-lĕk´trŏn´ĭk trăn-săk´shən rĭ-kôrd) The standardized codes and formats used for the exchange of medical data.

elevation (e-lə-v´ā-shən) The raising of a body part.

embolism (ĕm´bə-lĭz´əm) An obstruction in a blood vessel.

embolus (ĕm´bə-ləs) A portion of a thrombus that breaks off and moves through the bloodstream.

embryonic period (em-brē-on´ik pîr´ē-əd)(†) The second through eighth weeks of pregnancy.

E/M code (ē/ĕm kōd) Evaluation and management codes that are often considered the most important of all CPT codes. The E/M section guidelines explain how to code different levels of services.

empathy (ĕm´pə-thē) Identification with or sensitivity to another person's feelings and problems.

emphysema (em´fəsēmə) A chronic lung condition consisting of damage to the alveoli of the lungs. It is heavily associated with smoking, which causes stretching of the spaces between the alveoli and paralyzes the cilia of the respiratory system.

employment contract (ĕm-ploi´mənt kŏn´trăkt´) A written agreement of employment terms between employer and employee that describes the employee's duties and the considerations (money, benefits, and so on) to be given by the employer in exchange.

empyema (em´pīē´mə) A collection of pus in the pleural cavity.

enclosure (ĕn-klō´zhərz) Materials that are included in the same envelope as the primary letter.

encounter form (en-´kaun-tər form) A form that combines the charges for services rendered, an invoice for payment or insurance copayment, and all the information for submitting an insurance claim; also known as a superbill.

endocardium (en-dō-kar´dē-ŭm)(†) The innermost layer of the heart.

endochondral (en-dō-kon´drăl)(†) A type of ossification in which bones start out as cartilage models.

endocrine gland (ĕn´də-kra-n glănd) A gland that secretes its products directly into tissue, fluid, or blood.

endocrinologist (ĕn´də-kra-nŏl´ə-jĭst) A specialist who diagnoses and treats disorders of the endocrine system, which regulates many body functions by circulating hormones that are secreted by glands throughout the body.

endoderm (ĕn´dō-derm)(†) The primary germ layer that gives rise to epithelial tissues only.

endogenous infection (ĕn´-dŏj´ə-nəs ĭn-fĕk´shən) An infection in which an abnormality or malfunction in routine body processes causes normally beneficial or harmless microorganisms to become pathogenic.

endolymph (ĕn´dō-limf)(†) A fluid in the inner ear. When this fluid moves, it activates hearing and equilibrium receptors.

endometriosis (en´dō-mē-trē-ō´sis)(†) A condition in which tissues that make up the lining of the uterus grow outside the uterus.

endometrium (en´dō-mē´trē-ŭm)(†) The innermost layer of the uterus. It undergoes significant changes during the menstrual cycle.

endomysium (en´dō-miz´ē-ŭm)(†) A connective tissue covering that surrounds individual muscle cells.

endoplasmic reticulum (en´doplaz´mik ritik´yəlum) The organelles of the endoplasmic reticulum is composed of both smooth and rough types. The rough type contains ribosomes on its surface. The smooth type has no ribosomes. Both types create a network of passageways throughout the cytoplasm.

endorse (ĕn-dôrs´) To sign or stamp the back of a check with the proper identification of the person or organization to whom the check is made out, to prevent the check from being cashed if it is stolen or lost.

endoscopy (ĕn-dôs´kə-pē) Any procedure in which a scope is used to visually inspect a canal or cavity within the body.

endosteum (en-dos´tē-ŭm)(†) A membrane that lines the medullary cavity and the holes of spongy bone.

entropion (en-trō´pē-ūn) Inversion of the lower eyelid.

enunciation (ĭ-nŭn´sē-ā´shən) Clear and distinct speaking.

enzyme immunoassay (EIA) (ĕn´zīm im´yū-nō-as´ā) (†) The detection of substances by immunologic methods. This method involves an antigen, an antibody specific for the antigen, and a second antibody conjugated to an enzyme.

enzyme-linked immunosorbent assay (ELISA) test (ĕn´zīm-lĭngkt im´yū-nō-sōr´bent ăs´ā tĕst) (†) A blood test that confirms the presence of antibodies developed by the body's immune system in response to an initial HIV infection.

eosinophil (ē-ō-sin´ō-fil) (†) A type of granular leukocyte that captures invading bacteria and antigen-antibody complexes through phagocytosis.

epicardium (ep-i-kar´dē-ŭm) (†) The outermost layer of the wall of the heart. Also known as the **visceral pericardium.**

epidermis (ĕp´ĭ-dûr´mĭs) The most superficial layer of the skin.

epididymis (ep-i-did´i-mis) (†) An elongated structure attached to the back of the testes and in which sperm cells mature.

epididymitis (ep-i-did-i-mī´tis) (†) Inflammation of an **epididymis.** Most cases result from infection.

epiglottic cartilage (ep-i-glot´ik kär´tl-ĭj) (†) A cartilage of the larynx that forms the framework of the epiglottis.

epiglottis (ep-i-glot-ī´tis) (†) The flap-like structure that closes off the larynx during swallowing.

epilepsy (ĕp´ə-lĕp´sē) A condition that occurs when parts of the brain receive a burst of electrical signals that disrupt normal brain function; also called **seizures.**

epimysium (ep-i-mis´-ē-ŭm) (†) A thin covering that is just deep to the fascia of a muscle. It surrounds the entire muscle.

epinephrine (ĕp´ə-nĕf´rĭn) An injectable medication used to treat anaphylaxis by causing vasoconstriction to increase blood pressure.

A hormone secreted from the adrenal glands. It increases heart rate, breathing rate, and blood pressure.

epiphyseal disk (ep-i-fiz´ē-ăl dĭsk) (†) A plate of cartilage between the **epiphysis** and the **diaphysis.**

epiphysis (e-pif´i-sis) (†) The expanded end of a long bone.

episiotomy (epē´zēot´əmē) A surgical incision of the female perineum to enlarge the vaginal opening for delivery.

epistaxis (ĕp´i-stak´sis) Nosebleed.

epithelial tissue (ep-i-thē´lē-ĕl tĭsh´ōō) (†) A tissue type that lines the tubes, hollow organs, and cavities of the body.

erectile tissue (ĭ-rĕk´təl tĭsh´ōō) A highly specialized tissue located in the shaft of the penis. It fills with blood to achieve an erection.

erythema (er-i-thē´mă) Redness of the skin.

erythroblastosis fetalis (ĕ-rith´rō-blas-tō´sis fe´tăl-is) (†) A serious anemia that develops in a fetus with Rh-positive blood as a result of antibodies in an Rh-negative mother's body.

erythrocytes (ĭ-rĭth´rə-sīt´s) Red blood cells.

erythrocyte sedimentation rate (ESR) (ĭ-rĭth´rə-sīt´ sĕd´ə-mən-tā´shən rāt) The rate at which red blood cells, the heaviest blood component, settle to the bottom of a blood sample.

erythropoietin (ĕ-rith-rō-poy´ē-tin) (†) A hormone secreted by the kidney and is responsible for regulating the production of red blood cells.

esophageal hiatus (ĭ-sŏf´ə-jē´əl hi-á-ts) Hole in the diaphragm through which the esophagus passes.

established patient (ĭ-stăb´lĭsht pā´shənt) A patient who has seen the physician within the past 3 years. This determination is important when using E/M codes.

estrogen (ĕs´trə-jən) A female sex hormone; when produced during ovulation, estrogen causes a buildup of the lining of the uterus (womb) to prepare it for a possible pregnancy.

ethics (ĕth´ĭks) General principles of right and wrong, as opposed to requirements of law.

ethmoid (ĕth´moyd) (†) Bones located between the sphenoid and nasal bone that form part of the floor of the cranium.

etiologic agent (ē´tē-ə-lŏj´ĭkā´jənt) A living microorganism or its toxin that may cause human disease.

etiquette (ēt´ĭ-ket´) Good manners.

eustachian tube (yōō-stā´shən tōōb) An opening in the middle ear, leading to the back of the throat, that helps equalize air pressure on both sides of the eardrum.

eversion (ē-ver´zhŭn) (†) Turning the sole of the foot laterally.

exclusion (ĭk-sklōōzh´ən) An expense that is not covered by a particular insurance policy, such as an eye examination or dental care.

excretion (ĭk-skrē´shən) The elimination of waste by a discharge; in drug metabolism, the manner in which a drug is eliminated from the body.

exocrine gland (ĕk´sə-krĭn glănd) A gland that secretes its product into a duct.

exogenous infection (ĕk-sŏj´ə-nəs ĭn-fĕk´shən) An infection that is caused by the introduction of a pathogen from outside the body.

exophthalmos (ak´sä f´tha lm s) Bulging of the eyeballs, often related to hyperthyroidism.

expendable item (ĭk-spĕn´dəbəl ī´təm) An item that is used and must then be restocked; also known collectively as supplies. Contrast with **durable item.**

expiration (ĕk´spə-rā´shən) The process of breathing out; also called exhalation.

explanation of benefits (EOB) (ĕk´splə-nā´shən ŭv bĕn´ə-fits) Information that explains the medical claim in detail; also called **remittance advice (RA)**.

expressed contract (ĭk-sprĕst´ kŏn´trăct) A contract clearly stated in written or spoken words.

extension (ĭk-stĕn´shən) An unbending or straightening movement of the two elements of a jointed body part.

external auditory canal (ĭk-stûr´nəl ô´dĭ-tôr´ē kə-năl´) Canal that carries sound waves to the tympanic membrane; commonly called the ear canal.

externship (ĭk-stûrn´shĭp) A period of practical work experience performed by a medical assisting student in a physician's office, hospital, or other health-care facility.

extrinsic eye muscles (ĭk-strĭn´ sĭk ĭmūs´əlz) The skeletal muscles that move the eyeball.

facsimile machine (făk-sĭm´ə-lēmə-shēn´) A piece of office equipment used to send a facsimile, or fax, over telephone lines from one modem to another; more commonly called a fax machine.

facultative (fak-ŭl-tā´tiv)(†) Able to adapt to different conditions; in microbiology, able to grow in environments either with or without oxygen.

Fahrenheit (făr´ən-hīt) One of two common scales used for measuring temperature; measured in degrees Fahrenheit, or °F.

fallopian tubes (fə-l´ō-pē-ən tübz) Tubes that extend from the uterus on each side and that open near an ovary.

family practitioner (făm´ə-lē prăk-tĭsh´ə-nər)(†) A physician who does not specialize in a branch of medicine but treats all types and ages of patients; also called a general practitioner.

fascia (fash´e-ă)(†) A structure that covers entire skeletal muscles and separates them from each other.

fascicle (făs´ĭ-kəl) Sections of a muscle divided by connective tissue called perimysium.

febrile (fĕb´rəl) Having a body temperature above one's normal range.

feces (fē´sēz) Material found in the large intestine and made from leftover chyme. Feces are eventually eliminated through the anus.

Federal Unemployment Tax Act (FUTA) () This act requires employers to pay a percentage of each employee's income up to a certain dollar amount.

feedback (fēd´băk´) Verbal and nonverbal evidence that a message was received and understood.

feedback loop (fēd´bāk lōōp) A mechanism to control hormone levels. The two types are positive and negative feedback loops.

fee-for-service (fē fôr sûr´vĭs) A major type of health plan. It repays policyholders for the costs of health care that are due to illness and accidents.

fee schedule (fē skĕj´ōol) A list of the costs of common services and procedures performed by a physician.

felony (fĕl´ə-nē) A serious crime, such as murder or rape, that is punishable by imprisonment. In certain crimes, a felony is punishable by death.

femoral (fem´ŏ-răl)(†) Relating to the femur or thigh.

femur (fē´mər) The bone in the upper leg; commonly called the thigh bone.

fenestrated drape (fĕn´ĭ-strāt´ĕd drăp) A drape that has a round or slit-like opening that provides access to the surgical site.

fertilization (fer´til-i-zā´shŭn) The process in which an egg unites with a sperm.

fetal period (fĕt´l pîr´ē-əd) A period that begins at week nine of pregnancy and continues through delivery of the offspring.

fiber (fī´bər) The tough, stringy part of vegetables and grains, which is not absorbed by the body but aids in a variety of bodily functions.

fibrinogen (fī-brin´ō-jen)(†) A protein found in plasma that is important for blood clotting.

fibroid (fī´broid) A benign tumor in the uterus composed of fibrous tissue.

fibromyalgia (fī-brō-mī-al´jē-ă)(†) A condition that exhibits chronic pain primarily in joints, muscles, and tendons.

fibula (fĭb´yə-lə) The lateral bone of the lower leg.

file guide (fīlgīd) A heavy cardboard or plastic insert used to identify a group of file folders in a file drawer.

filtration (fĭl-trā´shən) A process that separates substances into solutions by forcing them across a membrane.

fimbriae (fĭ´m-brē-ə) Fringe-like structures that border the entrances of the **fallopian tubes**.

firewall (fīr´wôl) A system that protects a computer network from unauthorized access by users on its own network or another network such as the Internet.

first morning urine specimen (fûrst môr´nĭng yōōr´ĭn spĕs´ə-mən) A urine specimen that is collected after a night's sleep; contains greater concentrations of substances that collect over time than specimens taken during the day.

fixative (fĭk´sə-tĭv) A solution sprayed on a slide immediately after the specimen is applied. It is used to preserve and hold the cells in place until a microscopic examination is performed.

flaccid (flak´sid) Weak, soft; not erect.

flagellum (flajel´əm) The "tail-like" structure on some cell membranes that provides cell movement.

flexion (flek´shŭn)(†) A bending movement of the two elements of a jointed body part.

floater (flō´tər) A nonsterile assistant who is free to move about the room during surgery and attend to unsterile needs.

fluidotherapy (flōō´ĭd-ōthĕr´ə-pē) A technique for stimulating healing, particularly in the hands and feet, by placing the affected body part in a container of glass beads that are heated and agitated with hot air.

follicle (fŏl´ĭ-kəl) An accessory organ of the skin that is found in the dermis and the sites at which hairs emerge.

follicle-stimulating hormone (FSH) (fŏl´ĭ-kəl stim´yū-lā-ting hôr´mōn) A hormone that in females stimulates the production of estrogen by the ovaries; in males, it stimulates sperm production.

follicular cells (fə-li´-kyə-lər selz) Small cells contained in the primordial follicle along with a large cell called a primary **oocyte.**

folliculitis (fŏ-lik-yū-lī´tis)(†) Inflammation of the hair follicle.

fomite (fō´mīt)(†) An inanimate object, such as clothing, body fluids, water, or food, that may be contaminated with infectious organisms and thus serve to transmit disease.

fontanel (fän-tə-n´el) The soft spot in an infant's skull that consists of tough membranes that connect to incompletely developed bone.

food exchange (fōōd ĭks-chānj´) A unit of food in a particular food category that provides the same amounts of protein, fat, and carbohydrates as all other units of food in that category.

foramen magnum (fə-rā´-mən mag-nəm) The large hole in the occipital bone that allows the brain to connect to the spinal cord.

foramen ovale (fō-rā´men ō-va´lē)(†) A hole in the fetal heart between the right atrium and the left atrium.

forced vital capacity (FVC) (fôrst vīt´l kə-păs´i-tē) The greatest volume of air that a person is able to expel when performing rapid, forced expiration.

formalin (fōr-mă-lin)(†) A dilute solution of formaldehyde used to preserve biological specimens.

formed elements (fôrmd ĕl´ə-mənts) Red blood cells, white blood cells, and platelets; compose 45% of blood volume.

formulary (fōr´myū-lā-rē)(†) An insurance plan's list of approved prescription medications.

fracture (frăk´chər) Any break in a bone.

fraud (frôd) An act of deception that is used to take advantage of another person or entity.

frequency (frē´kwən-sē) The number of complete fluctuations of energy per second in the form of waves.

frontal (frŭn´tl) Anatomic term that refers to the plane that divides the body into anterior and posterior portions. Also called coronal.

fulgurated (ful´gy ə rā təd) The use of heat or laser to burn or destroy tissue.

full-block letter style (fōōl blŏk lĕt´ər stīl) A letter format in which all lines begin flush left; also called block style.

functional résumé (fŭngk´shə-nəl rĕz´ōō-mā´) A résumé that highlights specialty areas of a person's accomplishments and strengths.

fundus (fun´dus) The upper domed portion of an organ.

fungus (fŭng´gəs) A eukaryotic organism that has a rigid cell wall at some stage in the life cycle.

gait (gāt) The way a person walks, consisting of two phases: stance and swing.

ganglia (găng´glē-ə) Collections of neuron cell bodies outside the central nervous system.

gastric juice (găs´trĭk jüs) Secretions from the stomach lining that begin the process of digesting protein.

gastritis (gă-strī´tis) Inflammation of the stomach lining.

gastroenterologist (găs´trō-ĕn-ter-ol´ō-jist)(†) A specialist who diagnoses and treats disorders of the entire gastrointestinal tract, including the stomach, intestines, and associated digestive organs.

gastroesophageal reflux disease (GERD) (gas´trō-ē-sof´ă-jē´ăl rē´flĕks dĭ-zēz´) A condition that occurs when stomach acids are pushed into the esophagus and cause heartburn.

gene (jēn) A segment of DNA that determines a body trait.

general physical examination (jĕn´ər-əl fĭz´ĭ-kəl ĭg-zăm´ə-nā´shən) An examination performed by a physician to confirm a patient's health or to diagnose a medical problem.

generic name (jə-nĕr´ĭk nām) A drug's official name.

gerontologist (jĕr´ən-tŏl´ə-jĭst) A specialist who studies the aging process.

gigantism (jī´gan-tizm)(†) A condition in which too much growth hormone is produced in childhood, resulting in an abnormally increased stature.

glans penis (glanz pē´nĭs) A cone-shaped structure at the end of the penis.

glaucoma (glou-kō´mə) A condition in which too much pressure is created in the eye by excessive aqueous humor. This excess pressure can lead to permanent damage of the optic nerves, resulting in blindness.

global period (glō´bəl pîr´ē-əd) The period of time that is covered for follow-up care of a procedure or surgical service.

globulins (glob´yū-lin)(†) Plasma proteins that transport lipids and some vitamins.

glomerular filtrate (glō-mār´yū-lăr fĭl´trāt´)(†)   The fluid remaining in the **glomerular capsule** after **glomerular filtration.**

glomerular filtration (glō-mār´yū-lăr fĭl-trā´shən)(†)   The process by which urine forms in the kidneys as blood moves through a tight ball of capillaries called the glomerulus.

glomerulonephritis (glō-mār´yū-lō-nef-rī´tis)(†)   An inflammation of the glomeruli of the kidney.

glomerulus (glō-mār´yū-lŭs)(†)   A group of capillaries in the renal corpuscle.

glottis (glot´is)(†)   The opening between the vocal cords.

glucagon (glōō´kə-gŏn´)   A hormone that increases glucose concentrations in the bloodstream and slows down protein synthesis.

glycogen (glī´kə-jən)   An excess of glucose that is stored in the liver and in skeletal muscle.

glycosuria (glī-kō-sū´rē-ă)(†)   The presence of significant levels of glucose in the urine.

goiter (goi´tər)   Enlargement of the thyroid gland, which causes swelling of the neck, often related to iodine insufficiency in the diet.

Golgi apparatus (gôl´jē ap´ərat´es)   The cell's Golgi apparatus synthesizes carbohydrates and also appears to prepare and store secretions for discharge from the cell.

gonadotropin-releasing hormone (GnRH) (gō´na-dō-trō´pin rĭ-lēs´ĭng hôr´mōn´)   Hormone that stimulates the anterior pituitary gland to release **follicle-stimulating hormone (FSH).**

gonads (gō´nădz)   The reproductive organs; namely, in women, the ovaries, and in men, the testes.

goniometer (gō-nē-ă´-me-tər)   A protractor device that measures range of motion.

gout (gowt)(†)   A medical condition characterized by an elevated uric acid level and recurrent acute arthritis.

G-protein (jē-prō´tēn)(†)   A substance that causes enzymes in the cell to activate following the activation of the hormone-receptor complex in the cell membrane.

gram-negative (grăm´nĕg´ə-tĭv)   Referring to bacteria that lose their purple color when a decolorizer has been added during a Gram's stain.

gram-positive (grăm´pŏz´ĭ-tĭv)   Referring to bacteria that retain their purple color after a decolorizer has been added during a Gram's stain.

Gram's stain (grămz stăn)   A method of staining that differentiates bacteria according to the chemical composition of their cell walls.

granular leukocyte (grăn´yə-lər lōō´kəsīt´)   A type of leukocyte (white blood cell) with a segmented nucleus and granulated cytoplasm; also known as a polymorphonuclear leukocyte.

granulocyte (grăn´yū-lō-sīt)(†)   See **granular leukocyte.**

Grave's disease (grāvz dĭ-zēz´)   A disorder in which a person develops antibodies that attack the thyroid gland.

gray matter (grā măt´ər)   The inner tissue of the brain and the spinal cord that is darker in color than **white matter.** It contains all the bodies and dendrites of nerve cells.

gross earnings (grōs ûr´nĭngz)   The total amount an employee earns before deductions.

group practice (grˉoˉop prˇak´tˇıs)   A medical management system in which a group of three of more licensed physicians share their collective income, expenses, facilities, equipment, records, and personnel.

growth hormone (GH) (grōth hôr´mōn´)   A hormone that stimulates an increase in the size of the muscles and bones of the body.

growth plate (grōth plāt)   A shaft of cartilage between the epiphysis and the diaphysis; also knows as the **epiphyseal disk.**

gustatory receptors (gə´s-tə-tör-ē ri-se´p-tər)   Taste receptors that are found on taste buds.

gynecologist (gī´nĭ-kŏi´lə-jĭst)   A specialist who performs routine physical care and examinations of the female reproductive system.

gyri (jī´rī)(†)   The ridges of brain matter between the sulci; also called **convolutions.**

hairy leukoplakia (hâr´ē lū-kō-plā´kē-ă)(†)   A white lesion on the tongue associated with AIDS.

hapten (hap´tĕn)(†)   Foreign substances in the body too small to start an immune response by themselves.

hard copy (härd´ kŏp´ē)   A readable paper copy or printout of information.

hardware (härd´wâr´)   The physical components of a computer system, including the monitor, keyboard, and printer.

hazard label (hăz´ərd lā´bəl)   A shortened version of the Material Safety Data Sheet; permanently affixed to a hazardous substance container.

HCPCS Level II codes (āch sē pē sē ĕs lĕv´əl tōō kōdz)   Codes that cover many supplies such as sterile trays, drugs, and durable medical equipment; also referred to as national codes. They also cover services and procedures not included in the CPT.

Health Care Common Procedure Coding System (HCPCS) (hĕlth kâr kŏm´ən prə-sē´jər kōd´ĭng sĭs´təm)   A coding system developed by the Centers for Medicare and Medicaid Services that is used in coding services for Medicare patients.

health fraud (hĕlth frôd)   A deception or trickery related to health prevention or care for profit.

health maintenance organization (HMO) (hĕlth mān´tə-nəns ôr´gə-nĭ-zā´shən)   A health-care organization that provides specific services to individuals and their dependents who are enrolled in the plan. Doctors who enroll in an HMO agree to provide certain services in exchange for a prepaid fee.

helper T-cells (hĕl′pər tē′ sĕlz) White blood cells that are a key component of the body's immune system and that work in coordination with other white blood cells to combat infection.

hematemesis (hē′-mă-tem′ĕ-sis) The vomiting of blood.

hematocrit (hē′mă-tō-krit)(†) The percentage of the volume of a sample made up of red blood cells after the sample has been spun in a centrifuge.

hematology (hē′mə-tŏl′ə-jē) The study of blood.

hematoma (hē′mə-tō′me) A swelling caused by blood under the skin.

hematopoiesis (hēmətōpōē′sis) The process of new blood cell formation in the red bone marrow of cancellous bone.

hematuria (hē-mă-tu′rē-ă)(†) The presence of blood in the urine.

hemocytoblast (hē′mă-sī′tō-blast)(†) Cells of the red bone marrow that produce most red blood cells.

hemoglobin (hē′mə-glō′bĭn) A protein that contains iron and bonds with and carries oxygen to cells; the main component of erythrocytes.

hemoglobinuria (hē′mō-glō-bi-nū′rē-ă) (†) The presence of free **hemoglobin** in the urine; a rare condition caused by transfusion reactions, malaria, drug reactions, snake bites, or severe burns.

hemolysis (hē-mol′ĭ-sis)(†) The rupturing of red blood cells, which releases hemoglobin.

hemolytic anemias (hē mō lit′ ik ənē′mēə) Types of anemia that cause red blood cells to be destroyed faster than they can be made.

hemoptysis (hi mop′ ti sis) The spitting up of blood from the respiratory tract.

hemorrhoids (hĕm′ə-roidz′) Varicose veins of the rectum or anus.

hemostasis (hē′mō-stā-sis)(†) The stoppage of bleeding.

hemothorax (hē′ mō thôr′ aks) Blood collection in the pleural cavity causing collapse of the lung.

hepatic duct (hĭ-păt′ĭk dŭkt) A duct that leaves the liver carrying bile and merges with the cystic duct to form the common bile duct.

hepatic lobule (he-păt′ĭk lob′yūl)(†) Smaller divisions within the lobes of the liver.

hepatic portal system (he-pat′ik pôr′tl sĭs′təm)(†) The collection of veins carrying blood to the liver.

hepatic portal vein (hˇı-pˇat′ˇık pôr′tl vˉan) A blood vessel that carries blood from the other digestive organs to the **hepatic lobules.**

hepatitis (hĕp′ə-tī′tĭss) Inflammation of the liver usually caused by viruses or toxins.

hepatocytes (hep′ă-tō-sītz)(†) The cells within the lobules of the liver. Hepatocytes process nutrients in the blood and make bile.

hernia (hûr′nē-ə) The protrusion of an organ through the wall that usually contains it, such as a hiatal or inguinal hernia.

herpes simplex (her′pēz sĭm′plĕks)(†) A medical condition characterized by an eruption of one or more groups of vesicles on the lips or genitalia.

herpes zoster (her′pēz zos′ter)(†) A medical condition characterized by an eruption of a group of vesicles on one side of the body following a nerve root.

hierarchy (hī′ə-rär′kē) A term that pertains to Abraham Maslow's hierarchy of needs. This hierarchy states that human beings are motivated by unsatisfied needs and that certain lower needs must be satisfied before higher needs can be met.

hilum (hī′lŭm)(†) The indented side of a lymph node. The entrance of the renal sinus that contains the renal artery, renal vein, and ureter.

HIPAA (Health Insurance Portability and Accountability Act) (hĭp′ə) A set of regulations whose goals include the following: (1) improving the portability and continuity of health-care coverage in group and individual markets; (2) combating waste, fraud, and abuse in health-care insurance and health-care delivery; (3) promoting the use of a medical savings account; (4) improving access to long-term care services and coverage; and (5) simplifying the administration of health insurance.

Holter monitor (hol′tər mŏn′ĭ-tər) An electrocardiography device that includes a small portable cassette recorder worn around a patient's waist or on a shoulder strap to record the heart's electrical activity.

homeopathic medicine (hō-mē-ō-păth′-ĭk mĕd′-ĭ-sĭn) A system of medicine that uses remedies in an attempt to stimulate the body to recover itself.

homeostasis (hō′mē-ō-stā′sĭs) A balanced, stable state within the body.

homologous chromosome (hō-mŏl′ō-gŭs krō′mə-sōm′)(†) Members in each pair of chromosomes.

hormone (hôr′mōn′) A chemical secreted by a cell that affects the functions of other cells.

hospice (hŏs′pĭs) Volunteers who work with terminally ill patients and their families.

human chorionic gonadotropin (HCG) (hyōō′mən kō-rē-on′ik gō′nad-ōtrō′pin) A hormone secreted by cells of the embryo after implantation. It maintains the corpus luteum in the ovary so it will continue to secrete estrogen and progesterone.

human immunodeficiency virus (HIV) (hyōō´mən im´yū-nō-dē-fish´en-sē vī´rəs) A retrovirus that gradually destroys the body's immune system and causes AIDS.

humerus (hyü´-mə-rəs) The bone of the upper arm.

humors (hyōō´mərz) Fluids of the body.

hydrotherapy (hī´drə-thĕr´ə-pē) The therapeutic use of water to treat physical problems.

hydrothorax (hī´ drō thôr´ aks) Fluid collection in the pleural cavity causing collapse of the lung.

hyoid (hī´-ȯid) The bone that anchors the tongue.

hyperextension (hī´per-eks-ten´shŭn)(†) Extension of a body part past the normal anatomic position.

hyperglycemia (hī´pər-glī-sē´mē-ə) High blood sugar.

hyperopia (hī-per-ō´pē-ă) A condition that occurs when light entering the eye is focused behind the retina; commonly called farsightedness.

hyperpnea (hī-per-nē´ă)(†) Abnormally deep, rapid breathing.

hyperpyrexia (hy per py rex´ e a) An exceptionally high fever.

hyperreflexia (hī´per-rē-flek´sē-ă) Reflexes that are stronger than normal reflexes.

hypertension (hī´pər-tĕn´shən) High blood pressure.

hyperventilation (hī´pər-vĕn´tl-ā´shən) The condition of breathing rapidly and deeply. Hyperventilating decreases the amount of carbon dioxide in the blood.

hypnosis (hīp-nō´-sĭs) A trance-like state usually induced by another person to access the subconscious mind and promote healing.

hypodermis (hī´pə-dûr´mĭs) The subcutaneous layer of the skin that is largely made of adipose tissue.

hypoglycemia (hī´pō-glī-sē´mē-ə) Low blood sugar.

hyporeflexia (hī´pō-rē-flek´sē-ă)(†) A condition of decreased reflexes.

hypotension (hī´pō-tĕn´shən) Low blood pressure.

hypothalamus (hī´pō-thăl´ə-məs) A region of the **diencephalon.** It maintains homeostasis by regulating many vital activities such as heart rate, blood pressure, and breathing rate.

hypovolemic shock (hī´per-vō-lē´mik shŏk)(†) A state of shock resulting from insufficient blood volume in the circulatory system.

hypoxia (hī pôk´ sē ə) Inadequate oxygenation of the cells of the body.

hysterectomy (hĭs´tə-rĕk´tə-mē) Surgical removal of the uterus.

ICD-9 See *International Classification of Diseases, Ninth Revision, Clinical Modification.*

icon (ī´kŏn´) A pictorial image; on a computer screen, a graphic symbol that identifies a menu choice.

identification line (ī-dĕn´tə-fĭ-kā´shən līn) A line at the bottom of a letter containing the letter writer's initials and the typist's initials.

idiopathic (ĭd-ē-ō-path´ik) A disease or condition of unknown cause.

ileocecal sphincter (ĭl´ē ō sē´kəl sfĭngk´ ter) A structure that controls the movement of **chime** from the ileum to the **cecum.**

ileum (ĭl´ē-əm) The last portion of the small intestine. It is directly attached to the large intestine.

ilium (i´-lē-əm) The most superior part of the hip bone. It is broad and flaring.

immunity (ĭ-myoōn´ĭ-tē) The condition of being resistant or not susceptible to pathogens and the diseases they cause.

immunization (im´yū-nī-zā-shən) The administration of a vaccine or toxoid to protect susceptible individuals from communicable diseases.

immunocompromised (im´yū-nōkom´pro-mīzd)(†) Having an impaired or weakened immune system.

immunofluorescent antibody (IFFA) test (im´yū-nō-flūr-es´ent ăn´tĭ-bŏd-ē tĕst)(†) A blood test used to confirm enzyme-linked immunosorbent assay (ELISA) test results for HIV infection.

immunoglobulins (im´yū-nō-glob´yū-linz)(†) A class of structurally related proteins that include IgG, IgA, IgM, and IgE; also called **antibodies.**

impetigo (im´pĭ-tī´gō) A contagious skin infection usually caused by germs commonly called staph and strep.

implied consent (im-plahyd kuhn sent) A form of consent which is not expressly granted by a person, but rather inferred from a person's actions and the facts and circumstances of a particular situation (or in some cases by a person's silence or inaction).

implied contract (ĭm-plīd kŏn´trăct´) A contract that is created by the acceptance or conduct of the parties rather than the written word.

impotence (ĭm´pō-tens)(†) A disorder in which a male cannot maintain an erect penis to complete sexual intercourse; also called erectile dysfunction.

inactive file (ĭn-ăk´tĭv fīl) A file used infrequently.

incision (ĭn-sĭzh´ən) A surgical wound made by cutting into body tissue.

incisors (ĭn-sī´zərz) The most medial teeth. They act as chisels to bite off food.

incomplete proteins (ĭn´kəm-plēt´ prō´tēnz´) Proteins that lack one or more of the essential amino acids.

incontinence (in-kon´ti-nens)(†) The involuntary leakage of urine.

incus (ĭng´kəs) A small bone in the middle ear, located between the malleus and the stapes; also called the anvil.

indexing (ĭn´dēks´ ing) The naming of a file.

indexing rules (ĭn´dēks´ ing rōōls) Rules used as guidelines for the sequencing of files based on current business practice.

indication (ĭn´dĭ-kā´shən) The purpose or reason for using a drug, as approved by the FDA.

individual identifiable health information (IIHI) (in-duh-vij-oo-uh ahy-den-tuh-fahy-able hĕlth ĭn´fər-mā´shən) Any part of an individual's health information, including demographic information, collected from an individual that is received by a covered entity (e.g., a health-care provider).

induration (in-də-´rā-shən) The process of hardening or of becoming hard.

infection (ĭn-fĕk´shən) The presence of a pathogen in or on the body.

infectious waste (ĭn-fĕk´shəs wāst) Waste that can be dangerous to those who handle it or to the environment; includes human waste, human tissue, and body fluids as well as potentially hazardous waste, such as used needles, scalpels, and dressings, and cultures of human cells.

inferior (ĭn-fîr´ē-ər) Anatomic term meaning below or closer to the feet; also called caudal.

inflammation (ĭn´flə-mā´shən) The body's reaction when tissue becomes injured or infected. The four cardinal signs are redness, heat, pain, and swelling.

inflammatory phase (in-flam´-a-tor-ee fāz) The initial phase of wound healing in which bleeding is reduced as blood vessels in the affected area constrict.

informed consent (ĭn-fôrmd´ kən-sĕnt) The patient's right to receive all information relative to his or her condition and then make a decision regarding treatment based upon that knowledge.

informed consent form (ĭn-fôrmd´ kən-sĕnt fôrm) A form that verifies that a patient understands the offered treatment and its possible outcomes or side effects.

infundibulum (in-fŭn-dib´yū-lŭm)(†) The funnel-like end of the uterine tube near an ovary. It catches the secondary oocyte as it leaves the ovary.

infusion (in-fyū´zhŭn)(†) A slow drip, as of an intravenous solution into a vein.

ink-jet printer (ĭngk´jĕt´ prĭn´tər) A nonimpact printer that forms characters by using a series of dots created by tiny drops of ink.

innate immunity (ĭn āt ĭmyoōn´ītē) The body's mechanisms to protect itself against pathogens in general; also called nonspecific defenses.

inner cell mass (ĭn´ər sĕl măs) A group of cells in a blastocyte that gives rise to an embryo.

inorganic (ĭn´ôr-găn´ĭk) Matter that generally does not contain carbon and hydrogen.

insertion (ĭn-sûr´shən) An attachment site of a skeletal muscle that moves when a muscle contracts.

inside address (ĭn-sĭd´ ə-drĕs´) The name and address of the person to whom the letter is being sent. It appears on a business letter two to four spaces down from the date. It should be two, three, or four lines in length.

inspection (ĭn-spĕk´shən) The visual examination of the patient's entire body and overall appearance.

inspiration (in-spə-rā´-shən)(†) The act of breathing in; also called inhalation.

instruction set (ĭn-strŭk´shən set) Includes the groups of instructions from installed programming that a CPU can implement.

insulin (ĭn´sə-lĭn) A hormone that regulates the amount of sugar in the blood by facilitating its entry into the cells.

integrative medicine (ĭn´-tĭ-grāt´-tĭv mĕd´-ĭ-sĭn) The combination of components of conventional medicine with complementary and alternative medicine modalities.

interactive pager (ĭn´tər-ăk´tĭv pāj´ər) A pager designed for two-way communication. The pager screen displays a printed message and allows the physician to respond by way of a mini keyboard.

interatrial septum (in´tər ā´trē əl səp´təm) The wall separating the right and left atria from each other.

intercalated disc (in-ter´kă-lā-ted disk)(†) A disk that connects groups of cardiac muscles. This disc allows the fibers in that group to contract and relax together.

interferon (in-ter-fēr´on)(†) A protein that blocks viruses from infecting cells.

interim room (ĭn´tər-ĭm rōōm) A room off the patient reception area and away from the examination rooms for occasions when patients require privacy.

***International Classification of Diseases, Ninth Revision, Clinical Modification*(ICD-9) (ĭn´tər-năsh´ə-nəl klăs´ə-fīkā´shən dĭ-zēz´əz nĭnth rĭ-vĭzh´ən klĭn´ĭ-kəl mŏd´ə-fī-kā´shən)** Code set that is based on a system maintained by the World Health Organization of the United Nations. The use of the ICD-9 codes in the health-care industry is mandated by **HIPAA** for reporting patients' diseases, conditions, and signs and symptoms.

Internet (ĭn´tər-nĕt´) A global network of computers.

interneuron (ĭn´ter-nū´ron)(†) A structure found only in the central nervous system that functions to link sensory and motor neurons together.

internist (ĭn-tûr´nĭst) A doctor who specializes in diagnosing and treating problems related to the internal organs.

interpersonal skills (ĭn´tər-pûr´sə-nəl sk ĭlz) Attitudes, qualities, and abilities that influence the level of success and satisfaction achieved in interacting with other people.

interphalangeal (intərfəlan´jeal) Pertaining to the joints between the phalangeal bones.

interphase (in´ter-fāz)(†) The state of a cell carrying out its normal daily functions and not dividing.

interstitial cell (in-ter-stish´ăl sĕl) A cell located between the seminiferous tubules that is responsible for making testosterone.

interstitial fluid (in-ter-stish´āl flōō´īd) Fluid found between tissue cells that is absorbed by lymph capillaries to become lymph.

interventricular septum (in´tər ventrik´yələr səp´təm) The wall separating the right and left ventricles from each other.

intestinal lipase (in-tĕs´tĭ-n lip´ās) An enzyme that digests fat.

intradermal (ID) (in´tră-der´măl) Within the upper layers of the skin.

intradermal test (in´tră-der´măl tĕst) An allergy test in which dilute solutions of allergens are introduced into the skin of the inner forearm or upper back with a fine-gauge needle.

intramembranous (in-trə-me´m-brə-nəs) A type of ossification in which bones begin as tough fibrous membranes.

intramuscular (IM) (in´tră-mŭs´kyū-lăr) Within muscle; an IM injection allows administration of a larger amount of a drug than a subcutaneous injection allows.

intraoperative (in´tră-ŏp´ər-ə-tĭv) Taking place during surgery.

intravenous (IV) (in´trə-vē´nəs) Injected directly into a vein.

intravenous pyelography (IVP) (in´trə-vē´nəs pī´ĕ-log´ră-fē)(†) A radiologic procedure in which the doctor injects a contrast medium into a vein and takes a series of x-rays of the kidneys, ureters,

and bladder to evaluate urinary system abnormalities or trauma to the urinary system; also known as excretory urography.

intrinsic factor (ĭn-trĭn´zĭk făk´tər) A substance secreted by **parietal cells** in the lining of the stomach. It is necessary for vitamin B$_{12}$ absorption.

invasive (ĭn-vā´sĭv) Referring to a procedure in which a catheter, wire, or other foreign object is introduced into a blood vessel or organ through the skin or a body orifice. Surgical asepsis is required during all invasive tests.

inventory (ĭn´vən-tôrē) A list of supplies used regularly and the quantities in stock.

inversion (ĭn-vûr´zhən) Turning the sole of the foot medially.

invoice (ĭn´vois´) A bill for materials or services received by or services performed by the practice.

ions (ī´ənz) Positively or negatively charged particles.

iris (ī´rĭs) The colored part of the eye, made of muscular tissue that contracts and relaxes, altering the size of the pupil.

ischium (is´-kē-əm) A structure that forms the lower part of the hip bone.

islets of Langerhans (ī´lĭts lan´ger-hans) Structures in the pancreas that secrete insulin and glucagon into the bloodstream.

itinerary (ī-tĭn´ə-rĕr´ē) A detailed travel plan listing dates and times for specific transportation arrangements and events, the location of meetings and lodgings, and phone numbers.

jaundice (jôn´dĭs) A condition characterized by yellowness of the skin, eyes, mucous membranes, and excretions; occurs during the second stage of hepatitis infection.

jejunum (jə-jōō´nəm) The midportion and the majority of the small intestine.

journalizing (jûr´nə-līz´ĭng) The process of logging charges and receipts in a chronological list each day; used in the single-entry system of bookkeeping.

juxtaglomerular apparatus (jŭks´tă-glŏmer´yū-lăr ăp´ə-răt´əs)(†) A structure contained in the nephron and made up of the macula densa and **juxtaglomerular cells**.

juxtaglomerular cells (jŭks´tă-glŏmer´yū-lăr sĕlz) Enlarged smooth muscle cells in the walls of either the afferent or efferent arterioles.

Kaposi's sarcoma (kap´ō-sēz sar-kō´mă) Abnormal tissue occurring in the skin, and sometimes in the lymph nodes and organs, manifested by reddish-purple to dark blue patches or spots on the skin.

keratin (kĕr´ə-tĭn) A tough, hard protein contained in skin, hair, and nails.

keratinocyte (kĕ-rat´i-nō-sīt)(†) The most common cell type in the epidermis of the skin.

key (kē) The act of inputting or entering information into a computer.

KOH mount (kā´ō-āch mount) A type of mount used when a physician suspects a patient has a fungal infection of the skin, nails, or hair and to which potassium hydroxide is added to dissolve the keratin in cell walls.

Krebs cycle (krēbz sī´kəl) Also called the citric acid cycle. This cycle generates ATP for muscle cells.

KUB radiography (kā´yōō-bē rā´dēog´ră-fē)(†) The process of x-raying the abdomen to help assess the size, shape, and position of the urinary organs; evaluate urinary system diseases or disorders; or determine the presence of kidney stones. It can also be helpful in determining the position of an intrauterine device (IUD) or in locating foreign bodies in the digestive tract; also called a flat plate of the abdomen.

kyphosis (kī-fō´sis) A deformity of the spine characterized by a bent-over position; more commonly called humpback.

labeling (lā´bəl-ĭng) Information provided with a drug, including FDA-approved indications and the form of the drug.

labia majora (lā´bē-ă mă´jôr-ă) The rounded folds of adipose tissue and skin that serve to protect the other female reproductive organs.

labia minora (lā´bē-ă mĭ´nôr-ă) The folds of skin between the labia majora.

labyrinth (lăb´ə-rĭnth´) The inner ear.

laceration (lăs´ə-rā´shən) A jagged, open wound in the skin that can extend down into the underlying tissue.

lacrimal apparatus (lăk´rə-məl ăp´ə-răt´əs) A structure that consists of the lacrimal glands and nasolacrimal ducts.

lacrimal gland (lăk´rə-məl glănd) A gland in the eye that produces tears.

lactase (lăk´tās) (†) An enzyme that digests sugars.

lactic acid (lăk´tĭk ăs´ĭd) A waste product that must be released from the cell. It is produced when a cell is low on oxygen and converts pyruvic acid.

lactiferous (lak-tif´ə rus) Pertaining to producing milk.

lactogen (lak´tō-jen) Substance secreted by the placenta that stimulates the enlargement of the mammary glands.

lacunae (l-kü-na) Holes in the matrix of bone that hold osteocytes.

lamella (lə-me´-lə) Layers of bone surrounding the canals of osteons.

LAN (lān) Abbreviation for Local Area Network.

lancet (lăn´sĭt) A small, disposable instrument with a sharp point used to puncture the skin and make a shallow incision; used for capillary puncture.

laryngopharynx (lă-ring´gō-far-ingks) (†) The portion of the pharynx behind the **larynx.**

larynx (lăr´ĭngks) The part of the respiratory tract between the pharynx and the trachea that is responsible for voice production; also called the voice box.

laser printer (lā´zər prĭn´tər) A high-resolution printer that uses a technology similar to that of a photocopier. It is the fastest type of computer printer and produces the highest-quality output.

lateral (lăt´ər-əl) A directional term that means farther away from the midline of the body.

lateral file (lăt´ər-əl fīl) A horizontal filing cabinet that features doors that flip up and a pull-out drawer, where files are arranged with sides facing out.

law (lô) A rule of conduct established and enforced by an authority or governing body, such as the federal government.

law of agency (lô ā´jən-sē) A law stating that an employee is considered to be acting on the physician's behalf while performing professional duties.

lead (lēd) A view of a specific area of the heart on an electrocardiogram.

lease (lēs)) To rent an item or piece of equipment.

legal custody (lēgəl kŭs´tə-dē) The court-decreed right to have control over a child's upbringing and to take responsibility for the child's care, including health care.

lens (lēnz) A clear, circular disc located in the eye, just posterior to the iris, that can change shape to help the eye focus images of objects that are near or far away.

letterhead (lĕt´ər-hĕd´) Formal business stationery, with the doctor's (or office's) name and address printed at the top, used for correspondence with patients, colleagues, and vendors.

leukemia (lōō-kē´mē-ə) A medical condition in which bone marrow produces a large number of white blood cells that are not normal.

leukocyte (lōō-kə-sīt) White blood cells.

leukocytosis (lū´kō-sī-tō´sis) (†) A white blood cell count that is above normal.

leukopenia (lū´kō-pē´nē-ə) (†) A white blood cell count that is below normal.

liability insurance (lī´ə-bĭl´ĭ-tē ĭn-shōōr´əns) A type of insurance that covers injuries caused by the insured or injuries that occurred on the insured's property.

liable (lī´ə-bəl) Legally responsible.

libel (lī´bəl) A false publication, as in writing, print, signs, or pictures, that damages a person's reputation.

lifetime maximum benefit (līf´tīm´ măk´sə-məm bĕn´ə-fĭt) The total sum that a health plan will pay out over the patient's life.

ligament (lĭg´ə-mənt) A tough, fibrous band of tissue that connects bone to bone.

ligature (lĭg´ə-chōōr´) Suture material.

limbus (lĭm bŭs) The corneal-scleral junction, which is the area where the sclera (the white of the eye) gives way to the clear covering of the iris (cornea).

limited check (lĭm´ĭ-tĭd chĕk) A check that is void after a certain time limit; commonly used for payroll.

lingual frenulum (ling´gwăl fren´yūlŭm) (†) A flap of mucosa that holds the body of the tongue to the floor of the oral cavity.

lingual tonsils (ling´gwăl ton´silz) (†) Two lumps of lymphatic tissue on the back of the tongue that act to destroy bacteria and viruses.

linoleic acid (lin-ō-lē′ik as′id)(†) An essential fatty acid found in corn and sunflower oils.

lipoproteins (lip-ō-prō′tēnz) Large molecules that are fat-soluble on the inside and water-soluble on the outside and carry lipids such as cholesterol and triglycerides through the bloodstream.

living will (lĭv′ĭng wĭl) A legal document addressed to a patient's family and health-care providers stating what type of treatment the patient wishes or does not wish to receive if he becomes terminally ill, unconscious, or permanently comatose; sometimes called an advance directive.

lobe (lōb) The frontal, parietal, temporal, or occipital regions of the cerebral hemisphere.

locum tenens (lō′kum tĕn′ens)(†) A substitute physician hired to see patients while the regular physician is away from the office.

loop of Henle (lōōp hen′lē) The portion of the renal tubule that curves back toward the renal corpuscle and twists again to become the distal convoluted tubule.

lubricant (loo-bri-k*uh* nt) A water-soluble gel used during examination of the rectum or vaginal cavity.

lumbar enlargement (lŭm′bər ĕnlärj′mənt) The thickening of the spinal cord in the low back region.

lunula (lū′nū-lă) The white half-moon–shaped area at the base of a nail.

luteinizing hormone (LH) (lū′tē-in-izing hôr′mōn′)(†) Hormone that in females stimulates ovulation and the production of estrogen; in males, it stimulates the production of testosterone.

lymph (limf) The fluid found inside of the lymphatic vessels.

lymphedema (limf′e-dē′mă) The blockage of lymphatic vessels that results in the swelling of tissue from the accumulation of lymphatic fluid.

lymphocyte (lĭm′fō-sīt)(†) An agranular leukocyte formed in lymphatic tissue. Lymphocytes are generally small. See **T lymphocyte** and **B lymphocyte.**

lymphokines (lĭmf′ō kĭnz) A type of cytokine secreted by T cells that increases T-cell production and directly kills cells with antigens.

lysosomes (lī′səsōmz) Structures that are known to perform the digestive function of the cells.

lysozyme (lī′sō-zīm)(†) An enzyme in tears that destroys pathogens on the surface of the eye.

macrophage (măk′rə-fāj′) A type of phagocytic cell found in the liver, spleen, lungs, bone marrow, and connective tissue. Macrophages play several roles in humoral and cell-mediated immunity, including presenting the antigens to the lymphocytes involved in these defenses; also known as monocytes while in the bloodstream.

macula densa (mak′yū-lă den′sa)(†) An area of the distal convoluted tubule that touches afferent and efferent arterioles.

macular degeneration (mak′yū-lăr dējen-er-ā′shŭn)(†) A progressive disease that usually affects people older than the age of 50. It occurs when the retina no longer receives an adequate blood supply.

magnetic resonance imaging (MRI) (măgnĕt′ĭk rĕz′ə-nəns ĭ-măj′ing) A viewing technique that uses a powerful magnetic field to produce an image of internal body structures.

magnetic therapy (măg-nĕt′-ĭk thĕr′-ə-pē) A type of therapy in which magnets are placed on the body to penetrate and correct the body's energy fields.

maintenance contract (mān′tə-nəns kŏn′trăkt′) A contract that specifies when a piece of equipment will be cleaned, checked for worn parts, and repaired.

major histocompatibility complex (MHC) (mā′jər his′tō-kom-pat-ī-bil′i-tē kəm-pleks) A large protein complex that plays a role in T-cell activation.

malignant (mə-lĭg′nənt) A type of tumor or neoplasm that is invasive and destructive and that tends to metastasize; it is commonly known as cancerous.

malleus (măl′ē-əs) A small bone in the middle ear that is attached to the eardrum; also called the hammer.

malpractice claim (măl-prăk′tĭs klăm) A lawsuit brought by a patient against a physician for errors in diagnosis or treatment.

maltase (mawl-tās) An enzyme that digests sugars.

mammary glands (mam′ă-rē glăndz) Accessory organs of the female reproductive system that secrete milk after pregnancy.

mammography (mă-mŏg′rə-fē) X-ray examination of the breasts.

managed care organization (MCO) (măn′ĭjd kâr ôr′gə-nī-zā′shən) A health-care business that, through mergers and buyouts, can deliver health care more cost-effectively.

mandible (man′-də-bəl) A bone that forms the lower portion of the jaw.

manipulation (mə-nĭp′yə-la′shən) The systematic movement of a patient's body parts.

margin (mahr-jin) The space or measurement around the edges of a form or letter that is left blank.

marrow (mer′-ō) A substance that is contained in the medullary cavity. In adults, it consists primarily of fat.

massage (mə-säzh) The use of pressure, kneading, stroking, and the human touch to alleviate pain and promote healing through relaxation.

massage therapist (mə-säzh′thĕr′ ə-pĭst) An individual who is trained to use pressure, kneading, and stroking to promote muscle and full-body relaxation.

mastoid process (mas´-to´id pr¨ä-ses) A large bump on each temporal bone just behind each ear. It resembles a nipple, hence the name mastoid.

Material Safety Data Sheet (MSDS) (mə-tîr´e-əl sāf´tē dā´tə shēt) A form that is required for all hazardous chemicals or other substances used in the laboratory and that contains information about the product's name, ingredients, chemical characteristics, physical and health hazards, guidelines for safe handling, and procedures to be followed in the event of exposure.

matrix (mā´trĭks) The basic format of an appointment book, established by blocking off times on the schedule during which the doctor is able to see patients. The material between the cells of connective tissue.

matter (măt´er) Anything that takes up space and has weight. Liquids, solids, and gases are matter.

maturation phase (măch´ə-rā´shən fāz) The third phase of wound healing, in which scar tissue forms.

maxillae (mak-si´-lə) A bone that forms the upper portion of the jaw.

Mayo stand (mā´ō stănd) A movable stainless steel instrument tray on a stand.

medial (mē´dē-əl) A directional term that describes areas closer to the midline of the body.

Medicaid (měd´ĭ-kād´) A federally funded health cost assistance program for low-income, blind, and disabled patients; families receiving aid to dependent children; foster children; and children with birth defects.

medical asepsis (měd´ĭ-kəl ə-sěp´sĭs) Measures taken to reduce the number of microorganisms, such as hand washing

and wearing examination gloves, that do not necessarily eliminate microorganisms; also called clean technique.

medical practice act (měd´ĭ-kəl prăk´tĭs ăkt) A law that defines the exact duties that physicians and other health-care personnel may perform.

Medicare (měd´ĭ-kâr´) A national health insurance program for Americans aged 65 and older.

Medicare + Choice Plan (měd´ĭ-kâr´ chois plăn) Medicare benefit in which beneficiaries can choose to enroll in one of three major types of plans instead of the **Original Medicare Plan.**

Medigap (měd´ĭ-găp´) Private insurance that Medicare recipients can purchase to reduce the gap in coverage—the amount they would have to pay from their own pockets after receiving Medicare benefits.

meditation (měd´-ĭ-tā-shən) A state in which the body is consciously relaxed and the mind becomes calm and focused.

medullary cavity (me´-de-ler-ē ka´-və-tē) The canal that runs through the center of the **diaphysis.**

megakaryocytes (meg-ă-kar´ē-ō-sīts)(†) Cells within red blood marrow that give rise to platelets.

meiosis (mī-ō´sis)(†) A type of cell division in which each new cell contains only one member of each chromosome pair.

melanin (měl´ə-nĭn) A pigment that is deposited throughout the layers of the epidermis.

melanocyte (měl´ă-nō-sīt)(†) A cell type within the epidermis that makes the pigment **melanin.**

melanocyte-stimulating hormone (MSH) (məl´ən ō sīt stim´ yū lāting hôr mōn´) A hormone released from the anterior pituitary to stimulate melanin production in the skin's epidermal cells.

melatonin (měl´ə-tō´nĭn) A hormone that helps to regulate circadian rhythms.

membrane potential (měm´brān´ pə-těn´shəl) The potential inside a cell relative to the fluid outside the cell.

menarche (me-nar´ke) The first menstrual period.

Meniere's disease (Mən´yerz dĭzēz) An inner-ear disease characterized by attacks of vertigo, tinnitus, and nausea. Permanent hearing loss may result.

meninges (mě-nin´jēz)(†) Membranes that protect the brain and spinal cord.

meningitis (měn´ĭn-jī´tĭs) An inflammation of the **meninges.**

meniscus (mə-nĭs´kəs) The curve in the air-to-liquid surface of a liquid specimen in a container.

menopause (měn´ə-pôz´) The termination of the menstrual cycle due to the normal aging of the ovaries.

menses (měn´sēz) The clinical term for menstrual flow.

menstrual cycle (měn´strōō-əl sī´kəl) The female reproductive cycle. It consists of regular changes in the uterine lining that lead to monthly bleeding.

mensuration (měn´sə-rā´-shən) The process of measuring.

meridian (mə-rĭd´-ē-ən) Pathways of energetic flow that are distributed symmetrically throughout the body. These pathways are used in acupuncture, traditional Chinese medicine, and Ayurveda.

mesentery (me´sen´tərē) The fan-like tissue that attaches the jejunum and ileum to the posterior abdominal wall.

mesoderm (mez´ō-derm)(†) The primary germ layer that gives rise to connective tissue and some epithelial tissue.

metabolism (mĭ-tăb´ə-lĭz´əm) The overall chemical functioning of the body, including all body processes that build small molecules into large ones (anabolism) and break down large molecules into small ones (catabolism).

metacarpals (me-tə-kär′-pəl) The bones that form the palms of the hand.

metacarpophalangeal (met′əkar′pōfəlan′jēəl) Pertaining to the joints that join the phalanges to the metacarpals.

metaphase (met′əfāz) Period of mitosis when the chromosomes line up on the spindle fibers created by the centrioles during prophase.

metastasis (mĕ-tăs′tə-sĭs) The transfer of abnormal cells to body sites far removed from the original tumor; the spread of tumor cells.

metatarsals (mĕt′ə-tär′salz) The bones that form the front of the foot.

metatarsophalangeal (met′ətar′sōfəlan′jēəl) Pertaining to the joints that join the phalanges to the metatarsals.

microbiology (mī′krō-bī-ŏl′ə-jē) The study of microorganisms.

microfiche (mī′krō-fēsh′) Microfilm in rectangular sheets.

microfilm (mī′krə-fĭlm′) A roll of film stored on a reel and imprinted with information on a reduced scale to minimize storage space requirements.

microglia (mī-krŏg′lĕa) Small cells within the nervous system that act as phagocytes, watching for and engulfing invaders.

microorganism (mī′krō-ôr′gə-nĭz′əm) A simple form of life, commonly made up of a single cell and so small that it can be seen only with a microscope.

micropipette (mī′krō-pĭ-pet′) A small pipette that holds a small, precise volume of fluid; used to collect capillary blood.

microvilli (mī′krō-vil′-ī) (†) Structures found in the lining of the small intestine. They greatly increase the surface area of the small intestine so it can absorb many nutrients.

micturition (mik-chū-rish′ŭn) (†) The process of urination.

middle digit (′mi-dəl ′di-jət) A small group of two to three numbers in the middle of a patient number that is used as an identifying unit in a filing system.

midsagittal (mid′saj′i-tăl) (†) Anatomical term that refers to the plane that runs lengthwise down the midline of the body, dividing it into equal left and right halves.

minerals (mĭn′ər-əlz) Natural, inorganic substances the body needs to help build and maintain body tissues and carry on life functions.

minors (mī-nərs) Anyone under the age of majority—18 in most states, 21 in some jurisdictions.

minutes (mi-nətz′) A report of what happened and what was discussed and decided at a meeting.

mirroring (mĭr′ər-ĭng) Restating in your own words what a person is saying.

misdemeanor (mĭs′dĭ-mē′nər) A less serious crime such as theft under a certain dollar amount or disturbing the peace. A misdemeanor is punishable by fines or imprisonment.

mitochondria (mīto′kon′drēə) Structures that provide energy for cells and are the respiratory centers for the cell.

mitosis (mī-tō′sĭs) A type of cell division that produces ordinary body, or somatic, cells; each new cell receives a complete set of paired chromosomes.

mitral valve (mī′trăl vălv) (†) See **bicuspid valve.**

mobility aid (mō′bəl-ə-tē ād) Device that improves one's ability to move from one place to another; also called mobility assistive device.

modeling (mŏd′l-ĭng) The process of teaching the patient a new skill by having the patient observe and imitate it.

modem (mō′dəm) A device used to transfer information from one computer to another through telephone lines.

modified-block letter style (mŏd′ə-fīd blŏk lĕt′ər stīl) A letter format similar to full-block style, except that the dateline, complimentary closing, signature block, and notations are aligned and begin at the center of the page or slightly to the right of center.

modified-wave schedule (mŏd′ə-fīd wāv skĕj′ool) A scheduling system similar to the wave system, with patients arriving at planned intervals during the hour, allowing time to catch up before the next hour begins.

modifier (mŏd′ə-fī′ər) One or more two-digit codes assigned to the five-digit main code to show that some special circumstance applied to the service or procedure that the physician performed.

molars (mō′lərz) Back teeth that are flat and are designed to grind food.

mold (mōld) Fungi that grow into large, fuzzy, multicelled organisms that produce spores.

molecule (mŏl′ĭ-kyool′) The smallest unit into which an element can be divided and still retain its properties; it is formed when atoms bond together.

money order (mŭn′ē ôr′dər) A certificate of guaranteed payment, which may be purchased from a bank, a post office, or some convenience stores.

monocyte (mon′-o-s-īt) (†) A type of phagocyte that is formed in bone marrow and circulates throughout the blood for a very short period of time. It then migrates to specific tissues and is called a macrophage.

monokines (mon′ō kīnz) A type of cytokine secreted by lymphocytes and macrophages that assists in regulating the immune response by increasing B-cell production and stimulating red bone marrow to produce more white blood cells.

mononucleosis (mon´ō nōō klē ō´sis)
A highly contagious viral infection caused by the Epstein-Barr virus (EBV).

monosaccharide (mon-ō-sak´ă-rīd)(†)
A type of carbohydrate that is a simple sugar.

mons pubis (m´änz py´ü-bəs) A fatty area that overlies the public bone.

moral values (môr´əl văl´yōōz) Values or types of behavior that serve as a basis for ethical conduct and are formed through the influence of the family, culture, or society.

mordant (môr´dnt) A substance, such as iodine, that can intensify or deepen the response a specimen has to a stain.

morphology (môr-fŏl´ə-jē) The study of the shape or form of objects.

morula (mōr´ū-lă)(†) A zygote that has undergone cleavage and results in a ball of cells.

motherboard (mŭth´ər-bôrd´) The main circuit board of a computer that controls the other components in the system.

motility (mō´ti li tē) To be capable of movement.

motor (mō´tər) Efferent neurons that carry information from the central nervous system to the effectors.

mouse (mous) A pointing device that can be added to a computer that directs activity on the computer screen by positioning a pointer or cursor on the screen. It can be directly attached to the computer or can be wireless.

moxibustion (mŏk-ĭ-bŭs´-chən)
The application of heat at the points where the needles are inserted during acupuncture.

mucocutaneous exposure (myü-kō-kyü´-tā-nē-əs ik-spō´-zhər)
Exposure to a pathogen through mucous membranes.

mucosa (myōō-kō´sə) The innermost layer of the wall of the alimentary canal.

mucous cells (myōō´-kəs sĕlz)
Cells that are found in the salivary glands and the lining of the stomach and that secrete mucous.

MUGA scan (mŭg´ə skăn) A radiologic procedure that evaluates the condition of the heart's myocardium; it involves injection of radioisotopes that concentrate in the myocardium, followed by the use of a gamma camera to measure ventricular contractions to evaluate the patient's heart wall.

multimedia (mŭl´tē-mē´dē-ə)
More than one medium, such as in graphics, sound, and text, used to convey information.

multitasking (mŭl´tē-tăs´kĭng)
Running two or more computer software programs simultaneously.

multi-unit smooth muscle (mŭl´tə-yōō´nĭt smōōth mŭs´əl) A type of smooth muscle that is found in the iris of the eye and in the walls of blood vessels.

murmur (mûr´mər) An abnormal heart sound heard when the ventricles contract and blood leaks back into the atria.

muscle fatigue (mŭs´əl fa-tēg´) A condition caused by a buildup of lactic acid.

muscle fiber (mŭs´əl fī´bər)
Muscle cells that are called fibers because of their long lengths.

muscle tissue (mŭs´əl tĭsh´ōō) A tissue type that is specialized to shorten and elongate.

muscular dystrophy (mŭs´kyə-lər dis´trō-fē)(†) A group of inherited disorders characterized by a loss of muscle tissue and by muscle weakness.

mutation (myōō-ta´shən) An error that sometimes occurs when DNA is duplicated. When it occurs, it is passed to descendent cells and may or may not affect them in harmful ways.

myasthenia gravis (mī-as-thē´nē-ă grav´is) An autoimmune disorder that is characterized by muscle weakness.

myelin (mī´ə-lĭn) A fatty substance that insulates the axon and allows it to send nerve impulses quickly.

myelography (mī´ĕ-log´ră-fē) An x-ray visualization of the spinal cord after the injection of a radioactive contrast medium or air into the spinal subarachnoid space (between the second and innermost of three membranes that cover the spinal cord). This test can reveal tumors, cysts, spinal stenosis, or herniated disks.

myocardial infarction (mī´ō-kär´dē-ăl ĭn-fark´shən) A heart attack that occurs when the blood flow to the heart is reduced as a result of blockage in the coronary arteries or their branches.

myocardium (mī´ō-kär´dē-əm)
The middle and thickest layer of the heart. It is made primarily of cardiac muscle.

myocytes (mī´ō sīts) Muscle cells; also called muscle fibers.

myofibrils (mī-ō-fī´brils)(†) Long structures that fill the sarcoplasm of a muscle fiber.

myoglobin (mī-ō-glō´bin)(†) A pigment contained in muscle cells that stores extra oxygen.

myoglobinuria (mī´ō-glō-bi-nūrē-ă)
The presence of myoglobin in the urine; can be caused by injured or damaged muscle tissue.

myometrium (mī´ō-mē´trē-ŭm)(†)
The middle, thick muscular layer of the uterus.

myopia (mī-ō´pē-ə) A condition that occurs when light entering the eye is focused in front of the retina; commonly called nearsightedness.

myxedema (mik-se-dē´mă)(†) A severe type of hypothyroidism that is most common in women older than the age of 50.

nail bed (nāl bĕd) The layer beneath each nail.

narcotic (när-kŏt´ĭk) A popular term for an opioid and term of choice in government agencies; see **opioid.**

nares (ner´ēz) The openings of the nose or nostrils.

nasal (nā′zəl) Relating to the nose. The nasal bones fuse to form the bridge of the nose.

nasal conchae (nā′zəl kon′kē)(†) Structures that extend from the lateral walls of the nasal cavity.

nasal mucosa (nā′zəl myōō-kō′sə) The lining of the nose.

nasal septum (nā′zəl sĕp′tə m) A structure that divides the nasal cavity into a left and right portion.

nasolacrimal duct (nā-zō-lăk′rə-məl dŭkt) A structure located on the medial aspect of each eyeball. These ducts drain tears into the nose.

nasopharynx (nā′zō-far′ingks)(†) The portion of the pharynx behind the nasal cavity.

National Center for Complementary and Alternative Medicine (NCCAM) (năsh′ə-nəl sĕn′tər for kŏm′-plə-mĕn-tə-rē and ôl-tûr′-nə-tĭv mĕd′-ĭ-sĭn) National organization that conducts and supports CAM research and provides CAM information to health-care providers and the public.

natural killer (NK) cells (năch′ ər-el kĭl′ər selz) Non-B and non-T lymphocytes. NK cells kill cancer cells and virus-infected cells without previous exposure to the antigen.

naturopathic medicine (nă′-chə-rŏp′-ə-thĭk mĕd′-ĭ-sĭn) A system of medicine that relies on the healing power of the body and supports that power through various health-care practices, such as nutritional counseling, lifestyle counseling, and exercise.

needle biopsy (nēd′l bī′ŏp′sē) A procedure in which a needle and syringe are used to aspirate (withdraw by suction) fluid or tissue cells.

negligence (nĕg′lĭ-jəns) A medical professional's failure to perform an essential action or performance of an improper action that directly results in the harm of a patient.

negotiable (nĭ-gō′shē-ə-bəl) Legally transferable from one person to another.

neonatal period (nē-ō-nā′tăl pîr′ē-əd)(†) The first 4 weeks of the postnatal period of an offspring.

neonate (nē′ə-nāt′) An infant during the first 4 weeks of life.

nephrologist (ne-frol′ō-jĭst)(†) A specialist who studies, diagnoses, and manages diseases of the kidney.

nephrons (nef′ronz)(†) Microscopic structures in the kidneys that filter blood and form urine.

nerve fiber (nûrv fī′bər) A structure that extends from the cell body. It consists of two types: axons and dendrites.

nerve impulse (nûrv ĭm′pŭls′) Electrochemical messages transmitted from neurons to other neurons and effectors.

nervous tissue (nûr′vəs tĭsh′ōō) A tissue type located in the brain, spinal cord, and peripheral nerves.

netbook (′net bŭk) A small portable laptop computer designed for wireless communication and access to the Internet.

net earnings (nĕt ûr′nĭngz) Take-home pay, calculated by subtracting total deductions from gross earnings.

network (nĕt′wûrk′) A system that links several computers together.

networking (nĕt′wûrk′ĭng) Making contacts with relatives, friends, and acquaintances that may have information about how to find a job in your field.

neuralgia (nōō-răl′jə) A medical condition characterized by severe pain along the distribution of a nerve.

neuroglia (n˄ur-˘og′l̄ea) Structures that function as support cells for other neurons, including astrocytes, microglia, and oligodendrocytes. See also **neuroglial cells.**

neuroglial cell (nū-rog′lē-ăl sĕl)(†) Non-neuronal type of nervous tissue that is smaller and more abundant than neurons. Neuroglial cells support neurons.

neurologist (nōō-rəl′ə-jēst) A specialist who diagnoses and treats disorders and diseases of the nervous system, including the brain, spinal cord, and nerves.

neuron (nōōr′ŏn′) A nerve cell; it carries nerve impulses between the brain or spinal cord and other parts of the body.

neurotransmitter (nōōr′ō-trăns′ mĭt-ər) A chemical within the vesicles of the synaptic knob that is released into the postsynaptic structures when a nerve impulse reaches the synaptic knob.

neutrophil (nū′trō-fil)(†) A type of granular leukocyte that aids in phagocytosis by attacking bacterial invaders; also responsible for the release of pyrogens.

new patient (nōō pā′shənt) Patient that, for CPT reporting purposes, has not received professional services from the physician within the past 3 years.

nocturia (nok-tū′rē-ă)(†) Excessive nighttime urination.

noncompliant (nŏn′kəm-plī′ent) The term used to describe a patient who does not follow the medical advice given.

noninvasive (non-in-vā′siv)(†) Referring to procedures that do not require inserting devices, breaking the skin, or monitoring to the degree needed with invasive procedures.

nonsteroidal hormone (non-stēr′oyd-al hôr′mōn′)(†) A type of hormone made of amino acids and proteins.

norepinephrine (nōr′ep-i-nef′rin)(†) A neurotransmitter released by sympathetic neurons onto organs and glands for fight-or-flight (stressful) situations.

no-show (nō shō) A patient who does not call to cancel and does not come to an appointment.

nosocomial infection (nos-ō-kō´mē-ăl ĭn-fĕk-shən) An infection contracted in a hospital.

notations (nō-tā´shən) Information found at the end of a business letter indicating enclosures included with the letter and the names of other people who will be receiving copies of the letter.

Notice of Privacy Practices (NPP) (nō´tĭs prī´və-sē prăk´tis-əs) A document that informs patients of their rights as outlined under **HIPAA**.

nuclear medicine (noo´klē-ər mĕd´ĭ-sĭn) The use of radionuclides, or radioisotopes (radioactive elements or their compounds), to evaluate the bone, brain, lungs, kidneys, liver, pancreas, thyroid, and spleen; also known as radionuclide imaging.

nucleases (nū´klē-ās-ez) Pancreatic enzymes that digest nucleic acids.

nucleus (noo´klē-əs)(†) The control center of a cell; contains the chromosomes that direct cellular processes.

numeric filing system (noo-mĕr´ĭk fīl´ĭng sĭs´təm) A filing system that organizes files by numbers instead of names. Each patient is assigned a number in the order in which she joins the practice.

nystagmus (nis-tag´mŭs) Rapid involuntary eye movements that may be the result of drug or alcohol use, brain injury or lesion, or cerebrovascular accident (CVA).

O&P specimen (ō ənd pē spĕs´ə-mən) An ova and parasites specimen, or a stool sample, that is examined for the presence of certain forms of protozoans or parasites, including their eggs (ova).

objective (əb-jĕk´tĭv) Pertaining to data that is readily apparent and measurable, such as vital signs, test results, or physical examination findings.

objective data (əb-jĕk´tĭv dā´tə) Information about the patient's condition that is readily apparent or measureable.

objectives (ob-jek´tĭvs) The set of magnifying lenses contained in the nosepiece of a compound microscope.

occipital (ŏk-sĭp´ĭ-tl) Relating to the back of the head. The occipital bone forms the back of the skull.

occult blood (ə-kŭlt blŭd) Blood contained in some other substance, not visible to the naked eye.

ocular (ŏk´yə-lər) An eyepiece of a microscope.

oil-immersion objective (oil ĭ-mûr´zhən əb-jĕk´tĭv) A microscope objective that is designed to be lowered into a drop of immersion oil placed directly above the prepared specimen under examination, eliminating the air space between the microscope slide and the objective and producing a much sharper, brighter image.

ointment (oint´mənt) A form of topical drug; also known as a salve.

Older Americans Act of 1965 (ōl´dər ə-mĕr´ĭ-kəns ăkt) A U.S. law that guarantees certain benefits to elderly citizens, including health care, retirement income, and protection against abuse.

olfactory (ŏl-făk´tə-rē) Relating to the sense of smell.

oligodendrocytes (ōl´igōden´drəsit) Specialized neuroglial cells that assist in the production of the myelin sheath.

oliguria (ol´i-gu´re-ah) Insufficient production (or volume) of urine.

oncologist (ŏn-kŏl´ə-jĭst) A specialist who identifies tumors and treats patients who have cancer.

onychectomy (ŏn-i-kek´tō-mē) The removal of a fingernail or toenail.

oocyte (ō´ō-sīt)(†) The immature egg.

oogenesis (ō-ō-jen´ĕ-sis)(†) The process of egg cell formation.

open-book account (ō´pən bŏŏk ə-kount´) An account that is open to charges made occasionally as needed.

open-hours scheduling (ō´pən ourz skĕj´ool-ĭng) A system of scheduling in which patients arrive at the doctor's office at their convenience and are seen on a first-come, first-served basis.

open posture (ōpən pŏs´chər) A position that conveys a feeling of receptiveness and friendliness; facing another person with arms comfortably at the sides or in the lap.

ophthalmologist (ŏf-thəl-mŏl´ə-jĭst) A medical doctor who is an eye specialist.

ophthalmoscope (of-thal´mōskōp)(†) A hand-held instrument with a light; used to view inner eye structures.

opioid (ō´-pē-ȯid) A natural or synthetic drug that produces opium-like effects.

opportunistic infection (ŏp´ər-toon ĭs´tĭk ĭn-fĕk-shən) Infection by microorganisms that can cause disease only when a host's resistance is low.

optical character reader (OCR) (ŏp´tĭ-kəl kār´ək-tər-rek-tər rēdər) An electronic scanner that can "read" typed letters.

optical character recognition (OCR) (ŏp´tĭ-kəl kār´ək-tər rek-uhg-nish-uhn) The process or technology of reading data in printed form by a device that scans and identifies characters.

optical microscope (op´ti-kăl mī´krə-skōp´) A microscope that uses light, concentrated through a condenser and focused through the object being examined, to project an image.

optic chiasm (ŏp´tĭk kī´azm)(†) A structure located at the base of the brain where parts of the optic nerves cross. It carries visual information to the brain.

optician (ōp-tĭ´shən) An eye professional who fills prescriptions for eyeglasses and contact lenses.

optometrist (ŏp-tŏm´ĭ-trĭst) A trained and licensed vision specialist who is not a physician.

orbicularis oculi (ōr-bik´yū-lā´ris ok´yū-lī) The muscle in the eyelid responsible for blinking.

orbit (ôr´bĭt) The eye socket, which forms a protective shell around the eye.

organ (ôr´gan) Structure formed by the organization of two or more different tissue types that carries out specific functions.

organ of Corti (ôr´gən əv kôr´tē) The organ of hearing, located within the cochlea of the inner ear.

organelle (ôr´gə-nəl´) A structure within a cell that performs a specific function.

organic (ôr-găn´ĭk) Pertaining to matter that contains carbon and hydrogen.

organism (ôr´gə-nĭz´əm) A whole living being that is formed from organ systems.

organ system (ôr´gən sĭs´təm) A system that consists of organs that join together to carry out vital functions.

orifice (ôr´ĭ fĭs) An opening.

origin (ôr´ə-jĭn) An attachment site of a skeletal muscle that does not move when a muscle contracts.

Original Medicare Plan (ə-rĭj´ə-nəl mĕd´ĭ-kâr´ plăn) The Medicare fee-for-service plan that allows the beneficiary to choose any licensed physician certified by Medicare.

oropharynx (ôr´ō-far´ingks)(†) The portion of the pharynx behind the oral cavity.

orthopedist (ôr´thə-pēd´ĭst) A specialist who diagnoses and treats diseases and disorders of the muscles and bones.

orthopnea (ôr thop´nē a) Condition of difficulty breathing except while in an upright position.

orthostatic hypotension (ôr´-thə-stăt´-ĭk hi´po-tĕn´ shən) A situation in which blood pressure becomes low and the pulse increases when a patient is moved from a lying to standing position; also known as postural hypotension.

OSHA (Occupational Safety and Health Act) (ō´shə) A set of regulations designed to save lives, prevent injuries, and protect the health of workers in the United States.

osmosis (ŏz-mō´sĭs) The diffusion of water across a semipermeable membrane such as a cell membrane.

ossification (ä-sə-fə-kā´-shən) The process of bone growth.

osteoblast (os´tē-ō-blast)(†) Bone-forming cells that turn membrane into bone. They use excess blood calcium to build new bone.

osteoclast (os´tē-ō-klast)(†) Bone-dissolving cells. When bone is dissolved, calcium is released into the bloodstream.

osteocyte (äs´-tē-ə-sīt) A cell of osseous tissue; also called a bone cell.

osteon (äs´-tē-ən) Elongated cylinders that run up and down the long axis of bone.

osteopathic manipulative medicine (OMM) (ŏs´tē-ō-păth´ĭk mə-nĭp´ū-lă´tĭv mĕd´ĭ-sĭn) A system of hands-on techniques that help relieve pain, restore motion, support the body's natural functions, and influence the body's structure. Osteopathic physicians study OMM in addition to medical courses.

osteoporosis (ŏs´tē-ō-pə-rō´sĭs) An endocrine and metabolic disorder of the musculoskeletal system, more common in women than in men, characterized by hunched-over posture.

osteosarcoma (os´tē-ō-sar-kō´mă) A type of bone cancer that originates from osteoblasts, the cells that make bony tissue.

otologist (ō-tol´ŏ-jist)(†) A medical doctor who specializes in the health of the ear.

otorhinolaryngologist (ō-tō-rī´nōlar-ing-gol´ŏ-jist) A specialist who diagnoses and treats diseases of the ear, nose, and throat.

otosclerosis (ō-tō-sklŭ rōsis) Hardening or immobilization of the stapes within the inner ear.

out guide (out gīd) A marker made of stiff material and used as a placeholder when a file is taken out of a filing system.

ova (ō va) Eggs.

oval window (ō´vəl wĭn´dō) The beginning of the inner ear.

overbooking (ō´vər-bŏŏk´ĭng) Scheduling appointments for more patients than can reasonably be seen in the time allowed.

oviduct (ō´və´duct) A Fallopian tube.

ovulation (ō´vyə-lā´shən) The process by which the ovaries release one ovum (egg) approximately every 28 days.

ovum (ō vəm) One egg. The female "egg" that unites with the male sperm to begin reproduction.

oxygenated (ok´səjənātəd) Oxygenated blood refers to blood that has been to the lungs and is carrying oxygen in the hemoglobin.

oxygen debt (ok´sĭ-jən det) A condition that develops when skeletal muscles are used strenuously for a minute or two.

oxyhemoglobin (oks-ē-hē-mō-glō´bin)(†) Hemoglobin that is bound to oxygen. It is bright red in color.

oxytocin (OT) (ok-sē-tō´sin)(†) A hormone that causes contraction of the uterus during childbirth and the ejection of milk from mammary glands during breast-feeding.

packed red blood cells (păkt rĕd blud sĕlz) Red blood cells that collect at the bottom of a centrifuged blood sample.

palate (pal´ăt)(†) The roof of the mouth.

palatine (pa´-lə-tĭn) Bones that form the anterior potion of the roof of the mouth and the **palate.**

palatine tonsils (pal´ă-tīn tŏn´ sils)(†) Two masses of lymphatic tissue located at the back of the throat.

palpation (păl-pā´shən) A type of touch used by health-care providers to determine characteristics such as texture, temperature, shape, and the presence of movement.

palpatory method (pal-pa´tôr´ē mĕth´əd) Systolic blood pressure measured by using the sense of touch. This measurement provides a necessary preliminary approximation of the systolic blood pressure to ensure an adequate level of inflation when the actual auscultatory measurement is made.

palpitations (păl´pĭ-tā´shənz) Unusually rapid, strong, or irregular pulsations of the heart.

pancreatic amylase (pan-krē-at´ik am´il-ās)(†) An enzyme that digests carbohydrates.

pancreatic lipase (pan-krē-at´ik lip´ās) (†) An enzyme that digests lipids.

panel (păn´əl) Tests frequently ordered together that are organ or disease oriented.

papillae (pə-pĭl´ē) The "bumps" of the tongue in which the taste buds are found.

paranasal sinuses (par-ă-nā´zəl sī´nŭs-ĕz) Air-filled spaces within skull bones that open into the nasal cavity.

parasite (păr´ə-sīt´) An organism that lives on or in another organism and relies on it for nourishment or some other advantage to the detriment of the host organism.

parasympathetic (păr´ə-sĭm´pə-thĕt´ĭk) (†) A division of the autonomic nervous system that prepares the body for rest and digestion.

parathyroid glands (para-ă-thī royd glăndz) Four small glands embedded in the posterior thyroid gland that secrete parathyroid hormone (PTH); also known as parathormone.

parathyroid hormone (PH) (par-ă-thī´royd hôr´mōn´)(†) A hormone that helps regulate calcium levels in the bloodstream. It increases blood calcium by decreasing bone calcium.

parenteral nutrition (pă-ren´ter-ăl nōo-trĭsh´ən) Nutrition obtained when specially prepared nutrients are injected directly into patients' veins rather than taken by mouth.

paresthesias (par-es-thē´zē-ăs)(†) Abnormal sensations ranging from burning to tingling.

parietal (pă-rī´ĕ-tăl) Bones that form most of the top and sides of the skull.

parietal cells (pă-rī´ĕ-tăl sĕlz) Stomach cells that secrete hydrochloric acid, which is necessary to convert **pepsinogen** to **pepsin.** Parietal cells also secrete **intrinsic factor,** which is necessary for vitamin B_{12} absorption.

parietal pericardium (pă-rī´ĕ-tăl per-i-kar´dē-ŭm)(†) The layer on top of the visceral pericardium.

parietal peritoneum (pă-rī´ĕ-tăl per-ə-tŏnē´əm) The lining of the abdominal cavity.

parotid glands (pă-rot´id glăndz)(†) The largest of the salivary glands. The parotid glands are located beneath the skin just in front of the ears.

participating physicians (pär-tĭs´ə-pāt´ĭng fĭ-zĭsh´ənz) Physicians who enroll in managed care plans. They have contracts with MCOs that stipulate their fees.

partnership (pärt´n r shĭp) A form of medical practice management in which two or more parties practice together under a written agreement, specifying the rights, obligations, and responsibilities of each partner.

parturition (pär´ tur ish´ ən) The act of giving birth.

passive listening (păs´ĭv lĭs´ən-ĭng) Hearing what a person has to say without responding in any way; contrast with **active listening.**

patch test (păch tĕst) An allergy test in which a gauze patch soaked with a suspected allergen is taped onto the skin with nonallergenic tape; used to discover the cause of contact dermatitis.

patella (pə-té-lə) The bone commonly referred to as the kneecap.

pathogen (păth´ə-jən) A microorganism capable of causing disease.

pathologist (pă-thŏl´ə-jĭst) A medical doctor who studies the changes a disease produces in the cells, fluids, and processes of the entire body.

patient compliance (pā´shənt kəmplī´əns) Obedience in terms of following a physician's orders.

patient ledger card (pā´shənt lĕj´ər kärd) A card containing information needed for insurance purposes, including the patient's name, address, telephone number, Social Security number, insurance information, employer's name, and any special billing instructions. It also includes the name of the person who is responsible for charges if this is anyone other than the patient.

patient record/chart (pā´shənt rĕk´ərd/chärt) A compilation of important information about a patient's medical history and present condition.

pay schedule (pā skĭej´ool) A list showing how often an employee is paid, such as weekly, biweekly, or monthly.

payee (pā-ē´) A person who receives a payment.

payer (pā´ər) A person who pays a bill or writes a check.

pectoral girdle (pĕk´ tər əl gr-dl) The structure that attaches the arms to the axial skeleton.

pediatrician (pē´dē-ə-trĭshən) A specialist who diagnoses and treats childhood diseases and teaches parents skills for keeping their children healthy.

pediculosis (pədik´yoolō´sis) The medical term for lice.

pegboard system (pĕg´bôrd sĭs´təm) A bookkeeping system that uses a lightweight board with pegs on which forms can be stacked, allowing each transaction to be entered and recorded on four different bookkeeping forms at once; also called the one-write system.

pelvic girdle (pĕl´vik gr-dl) The structure that attaches the legs to the axial skeleton.

pepsin (pep´sin)(†) An enzyme that allows the body to digest proteins.

pepsinogen (pep-sin´ō-jen)(†) Substance that is secreted by the chief cells in the lining of the stomach and becomes **pepsin** in the presence of acid.

peptidases (pep´ti-dās-ez)(†) Enzymes that digest proteins.

percussion (pər-kŭsh´ən) Tapping or striking the body to hear sounds or feel vibration.

percutaneous exposure (per-kyūtā´nē-ŭs ĭk-spō´zhər)(†) Exposure to a pathogen through a puncture wound or needlestick.

pericardium (per-i-kar´dē-ŭm)(†) A membrane that covers the heart and large blood vessels attached to it.

perilymph (per´i-limf)(†) A fluid in the inner ear. When this fluid moves, it activates hearing and equilibrium receptors.

perimetrium (peri-mē´trēum) The thin layer that covers the myometrium of the uterus.

perimysium (per-i-mis´ē-ŭm)(†) The connective tissue that divides a muscle into sections called fascicles.

perineum (per i nē´üm) In the male, the area between the scrotum and anus; in the female, the area between the vagina and rectum.

periosteum (pĕr´ē ŏs´tē əm) The membrane that surrounds the **diaphysis** of a bone.

peripheral nervous system (PNS) (pə-rĭf´ər-əl nûr´vəs sĭs´təm) A system that consists of nerves that branch off the central nervous system.

peristalsis (pĕr´ĭ-stôl´sĭs) The rhythmic muscular contractions that move a substance through a tract, such as food through the digestive tract and the ovum through the fallopian tube.

personal protective equipment (PPE) (pur-suh-nl pruh-tek-tiv i-kwip-muh nt) Any type of protective gear worn to guard against physical hazards.

personal space (pûr´sə-nəl spās) A certain area that surrounds an individual and within which another person's physical presence is felt as an intrusion.

petty cash fund (pĕt´ē kăsh fŭnd) Cash kept on hand in the office for small purchases.

phagocyte (făg´ə-sīt´) A specialized white blood cell that engulfs and digests pathogens.

phagocytosis (fag´ō-sī-tō´sis)(†) The process by which white blood cells defend the body against infection by engulfing invading pathogens.

phalanges (f-lan´-jez) The bones of the fingers.

pharmaceutical (fär´mə-soo´tĭ-kəl) Pertaining to medicinal drugs.

pharmacodynamics (far´m̆-a-k̄o-d̄nam´iks)(†) The study of what drugs do to the body: the mechanism of action, or how they work to produce a therapeutic effect.

pharmacognosy (far-mă-kog´nō-sē)(†) The study of characteristics of natural drugs and their sources.

pharmacokinetics (far´mă-kō-kinet´iks) (†) The study of what the body does to drugs: how the body absorbs, metabolizes, distributes, and excretes the drugs.

pharmacology (fär´ma-kŏl´ə-jē)(†) The study of drugs.

pharmacotherapeutics (far´mă-kō-thĕr´ə-pyoo´tĭks) The study of how drugs are used to treat disease; also called clinical **pharmacology.**

pharyngeal tonsils (fă-rin´jē-ăl tŏn´səls)(†) Two masses of lymphatic tissue located above the palatine tonsils; also called adenoids.

pharynx (făr´ĭngks) Structure below the mouth and nasal cavities that is an organ of the respiratory system as well as the digestive system.

phenylketonuria (PKU) (fen´il-kē´tō-nū´rē-ă)(†) A genetically inherited disorder in which the body cannot properly metabolize the nutrient phenylalanine, resulting in the buildup of phenylketones in the blood and their presence in the urine. The accumulation of phenylketones results in mental retardation.

philosophy (fĭ-lŏs´ə-fē) The system of values and principles an office has adopted in its everyday practice.

phlebotomy (flĭ-bŏt´ə-mē) The insertion of a needle or cannula (small tube) into a vein for the purpose of withdrawing blood.

photometer (fō-tŏm´ĭ-tər) An instrument that measures light intensity.

physiatrist (fiz-ī´ă-trist)(†) A physical medicine specialist, who diagnoses and treats diseases and disorders with physical therapy.

physical therapy (fĭz´ĭ-kəl thĕr´ə-pē) A medical specialty that uses cold, heat, water, exercise, massage, traction, and other physical means to treat musculoskeletal, nervous, and cardiopulmonary disorders.

physician assistant (PA) (fĭ-zĭsh´ən ə-sĭs´tənt) A health-care provider who practices medicine under the supervision of a physician.

physician's office laboratory (POL) (fĭ-zĭsh´ənz ô´fĭs lăb´rə-tôr´ē) A laboratory contained in a physician's office; processing tests in the POL produces quick turnaround and eliminates the need for patients to travel to other test locations.

physiology (fĭz´ē-ŏl´ə-jē) The science of the study of the body's functions.

pineal body (pĭn´ē-ăl bŏd´ē) A small gland located between the cerebral hemispheres that secretes melatonin.

pitch (pĭch) The high or low quality in the sound of a person's speaking voice.

placebo effect (plə´-sē-bō ĭ-fěkt´) The belief that a medication or treatment works even though it is not scientifically substantiated. In research, a placebo is an inactive substance or preparation used as a control to determine the effectiveness of a medicinal drug.

placenta (plə-sěn´tə) An organ located between the mother and the fetus. It permits the absorption of nutrients and oxygen. In some cases, harmful substances such as viruses are absorbed through the placenta.

plantar flexion (plan´tăr flek´shŭn)(†) Pointing the toes downward.

plasma (plăz´mə) The fluid component of blood, in which formed elements are suspended; makes up 55% of blood volume.

plastic surgeon (plăs´tĭk sûr´jən) A specialist who reconstructs, corrects, or improves body structures.

platelets (plāt´lĭts) Fragments of cytoplasm in the blood that are crucial to clot formation; also called thrombocytes.

pleura (plūr´ă)(†) The membranes that surround the lungs.

pleural effusion (plŏŏr´ əl if yōō´ zhən) A buildup of fluid within the pleural cavity.

pleurisy (plŏōr´əsē) Also known as pleuritis; this is an inflammation of the parietal pleura of the lungs.

pleuritis (ploor-í-tis) A condition in which the **pleura** become inflamed, which causes them to stick together. It can also cause an excess amount of fluid to form between the membranes.

plexus (plěk´səs) A structure that is formed when spinal nerves fuse together. It includes the cervical, brachial, and lumbosacral nerves.

pneumoconiosis (nŏŏ mŏ kō´nē ō´sis) This is the name given to lung diseases that result from years of exposure to different environmental or occupational types of dust.

pneumothorax (nū-mō-thōr´aks)(†) The presence of air or gas in the pleural cavity. The lung typically collapses with pneumothorax.

podiatrist (pə-dī´-ə-trist) Physician who specializes in the study and treatment of the foot and ankle.

polar body (pō´lər bŏd´ē) A nonfunctional cell that is one of two small cells formed during the division of an oocyte.

polarity (pō-lăr´ĭ-tē) The condition of having two separate poles, one of which is positive and the other, negative.

polarized (pō´lə-rīzd´) The state in which the outside of a cell membrane is positively charged and the inside is negatively charged. Polarization occurs when a neuron is at rest.

polysaccharide (pol-ē-sak´ă-rīd)(†) A type of carbohydrate that is a starch.

POMR (pē´ō-ěm-är) The problem-oriented medical record system for keeping patients' charts. Information in a POMR includes the database of information about the patient and the patient's condition, the problem list, the diagnostic and treatment plan, and progress notes.

portfolio (pôrt-fō´lē-ō´) A collection of an applicant's résumé, reference letters, and other documents of interest to a potential employer.

positive tilt test (pŏz´-ĭ-tĭv tĭlt těst) When the pulse rate increases more than 10 beats per minute (bpm) and the blood pressure drops more than 20 points while taking vital signs in the lying, sitting, and standing positions.

positron emission tomography (PET) (pah´-zih-tron ee-mih´-shun toh-mah´-gruh-fee) A radiologic procedure that entails injecting isotopes combined with other substances involved in metabolic activity, such as glucose. These special isotopes emit positrons, which a computer processes and displays on a screen.

posterior (pŏ-stîr´ē-ar) Anatomic term meaning toward the back of the body. Also called dorsal.

postnatal period (pōst-nā´tăl pîr´ē-əd)(†) The period following childbirth.

postoperative (pōst-ŏp´ər-ə-tĭv) Taking place after a surgical procedure.

postural hypotension (pŏs-chěr-ăl hī-pō-těn-shŭn) A situation in which blood pressure becomes low and the pulse increases increases when a patient is moved from a lying to a standing position; also known as orthostatic hypotension.

posture (pŏs´chər) Body position and alignment.

power of attorney (pou´ər ə-tûr´nē) The legal right to act as the attorney or agent of another person, including handling that person's financial matters.

practitioner (prăk-tĭsh´ə-nər) One who practices a profession.

pre-authorization (prē ô´thər-ĭ-zā´shən) Authorization or approval for payment from a third-party payer requested in advance of a specific procedure.

pre-certification (prē sûr´tə-fĭ-kā´shən) A determination of the amount of money that will be paid by a third-party payer for a specific procedure before the procedure is conducted.

preferred provider organization (PPO) (prĭ-fûrd´ prə-vīd´ər or´gə-nĭ-zā´shən) A managed care plan that establishes a network of providers to perform services for plan members.

prefix (prē-fĭks) A word part that comes at the beginning of a medical term that alters the meaning of the term.

premenstrual syndrome (PMS) (prē-mĕ′n-strə-wal sin′-drōm)(†) A syndrome that is a collection of symptoms that occur just before the menstrual period.

premium (prē′mē-əm) The basic annual cost of health-care insurance.

prenatal period (prē-nā′tăl pîr′ē-əd)(†) The period that includes the embryonic and fetal periods until the delivery of the offspring.

preoperative (prē-ŏp′ər-ə-tĭv) Taking place prior to surgery.

prepuce (prē′pūs)(†) A piece of skin in the uncircumcized male that covers the glans penis.

presbyopia (prez-bē-ō′pē-ă) A common eye disorder that results in the loss of lens elasticity. Presbyopia develops with age and causes a person to have difficulty seeing objects close up.

prescribe (prĭ-skrīb′) To give a patient a prescription to be filled by a pharmacy.

prescription (prĭ-skrĭp′shən) A physician's written order for medication.

prescription drug (prĭ-skrĭp′shən drŭg) A drug that can be legally used only by order of a physician and must be administered or dispensed by a licensed health-care professional.

primary care physician (prī′mĕr′ē kâr fĭ-zĭsh′ən) A physician who provides routine medical care and referrals to specialists.

primary germ layer (prī′mĕr′ē jûrm lā′ər) An inner cell mass that organizes into layers: the ectoderm, mesoderm, and endoderm.

prime mover (prīm mōō′vər) The muscle responsible for most of the movement when a body

movement is produced by a group of muscles.

primordial follicle (prī-mōr′dĕl-ăl fŏl′ĭ-kəl)(†) A structure that develops in the ovarian cortex of a female infant before she is born.

Privacy Rule (prī′və-sē rōōl) Common name for the **HIPAA** Standard for Privacy of Individually Identifiable Health Information, which provides the first comprehensive federal protection for the privacy of health information. The Privacy Rule creates national standards to protect individuals' medical records and other personal health information.

procedure code (prə-sē′jər kōd) Codes that represent medical procedures, such as surgery and diagnostic tests, and medical services, such as an examination to evaluate a patient's condition.

proctologist (prok-tŏl′ə-jĭst) Physician who diagnoses and treats disorders of the anus, rectum, and intestines.

proctoscopy (prok-tos′kō-pē) An examination of the lower rectum and anal canal with a 3-inch instrument called a proctoscope to detect hemorrhoids, polyps, fissures, fistulas, and abscesses.

proficiency testing program (prə-fĭ′shən-cē tĕst′ĭng prō′grăm′) A required set of tests for clinical laboratories; the tests measure the accuracy of the laboratory's test results and adherence to standard operating procedures.

progesterone (prō-jĕs′tə-rōn′) A female steroid hormone primarily produced by the ovary.

prognosis (prŏg-nō′sĭs) A prediction of the probable course of a disease in an individual and the chances of recovery.

prolactin (PRL) (prō-lak′tin)(†) A hormone that stimulates milk production in the mammary glands.

proliferation phase (prə-lĭf′ər-ā′shən fāz) The second phase of wound healing, in which new tissue forms, closing off the wound.

pronation (prō-nā′shŭn)(†) Turning the palms of the hand downward.

pronunciation (prə-nun′cē-ā′shən) The sounding out of words.

proofreading (prōōf′rēd′ĭng) Checking a document for formatting, data, and mechanical errors.

prophase (prō′faz) Movement of the replicated centrioles to the opposite ends of the cell, creating spindle-like fibers during mitosis.

prostaglandin (pros-tă-glan′din)(†) A local hormone derived from lipid molecules. Prostaglandins typically do not travel in the bloodstream to find their target cells because their targets are close by. This hormone has numerous effects, including uterine stimulation during childbirth.

prostate gland (prŏs′tāt′ glănd) A chestnut-shaped gland that surrounds the beginning of the urethra in the male.

prostatitis (pros-tă-tī′tis) Inflammation of the prostate gland, which can be acute or chronic.

protected health information (PHI) (prə-tĕkt-əd hĕlth ĭn′fər-mă′shən) Individually identifiable health information that is transmitted or maintained by electronic or other media, such as computer storage devices. The core of the **HIPAA Privacy Rule** is the protection, use, and disclosure of protected health information.

proteinuria (prō-tē-nū′rē-ă) An excess of protein in the urine.

protozoan (prō′-tə-zō′ən) A single-celled eukaryotic organism much larger than a bacterium; some protozoans can cause disease in humans.

protraction (prō-trăk′shən) Moving a body part anteriorly.

proximal (prok′si-măl)(†) Anatomic term meaning closer to a point of attachment or closer to the trunk of the body.

proximal convoluted tubule (prok´sĭmăl kon´vō-lū-ted tū´byūl)(†) The portion of the renal tubule that is directly attached to the glomerular capsule and becomes the loop of Henle.

psoriasis (sə-rī´ə-sĭs) A common skin condition characterized by reddish-silver scaly lesions most often found on the elbows, knees, scalp, and trunk.

puberty (pyo͞o´bər-tē) The period of adolescence when a person begins to develop secondary sexual traits and reproductive functions.

pubis (pyü´-bəs) The area that forms the front of a hip bone.

pulmonary circuit (po͞ol´mə-nĕr´ē sûr´kĭt) The route that blood takes from the heart to the lungs and back to the heart again.

pulmonary semilunar valve (p ŭl´mənerē sem´ē loonər valv) A heart valve that is a semilunar valve. It is situated between the right ventricle and the pulmonary trunk.

pulmonary trunk (po͞ol´mə-nĕr´ē trŭngk) A large artery that branches into the pulmonary arteries and carries blood to the lungs.

pulmonary function test (po͞ol´mə-nĕr´ē fŭngk´shən tĕst) A test that evaluates a patient's lung volume and capacity; used to detect and diagnose pulmonary problems or to monitor certain respiratory disorders and evaluate the effectiveness of treatment.

puncture wound (pŭngk´chər wound) A deep wound caused by a sharp, pointed object.

punitive damages (pyo͞o´nĭ-tĭv dăm´ĭjz) Money paid as punishment for intentionally breaking the law.

pupil (pyo͞o´pəl) The opening at the center of the iris, which grows smaller or larger as the iris contracts or relaxes, respectively; it

regulates the amount of light that enters the eye.

purchase order (pûr´chĭs ôr´dər) A form that authorizes a purchase for the practice.

purchasing groups (pur´chĭs-ĭng gro͞ops) Groups of medical offices associated with a nearby hospital that order supplies through the hospital to obtain a quantity discount.

Purkinje fibers (per´kin-jē fī´bərz) Cardiac fibers that are located in the lateral walls of the ventricles.

pyelonephritis (pī´ĕ-lō-ne-frī-tis)(†) A urinary tract infection that involves one or both of the kidneys.

pyloric sphincter (pī-lôrĭk sfingk´tər) The valve-like structure composed of a circular band of muscle at the juncture of the stomach and small intestine.

pyothorax (pī ō thôr´ aks) Pus or infected fluid in the pleural cavity causing collapse of the lung.

pyrogens (pī´rō-jenz)(†) Fever-producing substances released by neutrophils.

qi (chē) According to traditional Chinese medicine, a vital energy that flows throughout the body.

quadrants (kwŏd´rəntz) Four equal sections, such as those into which the abdomen is figuratively divided during an examination.

qualitative analysis (kwŏl´ĭ-tā´tĭv-ənăl´ĭ-sĭs) In microbiology, identification of bacteria present in a specimen by the appearance of colonies grown on a culture plate.

qualitative test response (kwŏl´ĭ-tā´tĭv tĕst rĭ-spŏns´) A test result that indicates the substance tested for is either present or absent.

quality assurance program (kwŏl´ĭ-tē ə-sho͞or´əns prō´gram´) A required program for clinical laboratories designed to monitor the quality of patient care, including quality control,

instrument and equipment maintenance, proficiency testing, training and continuing education, and standard operating procedures documentation.

quality control (QC) (kwŏl´ĭ-tē kən-trol´) An ongoing system, required in every physican's office, to evaluate the quality of medical care provided.

quality control program (kwŏl´ĭ-tē kəntrōl´ prō´grăm´) A component of a quality assurance program that focuses on ensuring accuracy in laboratory test results through careful monitoring of test procedures.

quantitative analysis (kwŏn´tĭ-tā´tĭv ə-năl´ĭ-sĭs) In microbiology, a determination of the number of bacteria present in a specimen by direct count of colonies grown on a culture plate.

quantitative test results (kwŏn´tĭ-tā´tĭv tĕst rĭ-zŭlt´) The concentration of a test substance in a specimen.

quarterly return (kwŏr´tar-lē rĭ-tûrn´) The Employer's Quarterly Federal Tax Return, a form submitted to the IRS every 3 months that summarizes the federal income and employment taxes withheld from employees' paychecks.

qui tam **(k -´t m)** Latin, meaning "to bring action for the king and for one's self."

radial artery (rā´dē-əl är´tə-rē) An artery located in the groove on the thumb side of the inner wrist, where the pulse is taken on adults.

radiation therapy (rā´dē-ā´shən thĕr´ə-pē) The use of x-rays and radioactive substances to treat cancer.

radiologist (rā´dē-ŏl´ə-jĭst) A physician who specializes in taking and reading x-rays.

radius (rā-dā-əs) The lateral bone of the forearm.

rales (ralz) Noisy respirations usually due to blockage of the bronchial tubes.

random access memory (RAM) (răn´dəm ăk´sĕs mĕm´ə-rē) The temporary, or programmable, memory in a computer.

random urine specimen (răn´dəm yŏŏr´ĭn spĕs´ə-mən) A single urine specimen taken at any time of the day; the most common type of sample collected.

range of motion (ROM) (rānj mō´shən) The degree to which a joint is able to move.

rapport (ră-pôr´) A harmonious, positive relationship.

read only memory (ROM) (rĕd ōn´lē mĕm´ə-rē) A computer's permanent memory, which can be read by the computer but not changed. It provides the computer with the basic operating instructions it needs to function.

reagent (rē-ā´jənt) A chemical or chemically treated substance used in test procedures and formulated to react in specific ways when exposed under specific conditions.

reconciliation (rĕk´ən-sĭl´ē-ā´shən) A comparison of the office's financial records with bank records to ensure that they are consistent and accurate; usually done when the monthly checking account statement is received from the bank.

records management system (rĭ-kôrdz măn´ĭj-mənt sĭs´təm) How patient records are created, filed, and maintained.

recovery position (rĭ-kŭv´ər-ē pə-zĭsh´ən) The position a person is placed in after receiving first aid for choking or cardiopulmonary resuscitation.

rectum (rĕk´təm) The last section of the sigmoid colon that straightens out and becomes the anal canal.

reference (rĕf´ər-əns) A recommendation for employment from a facility or a preceptor.

reference laboratory (rĕf´ər-əns lăb´rə-tôr´ē) A laboratory owned and operated by an organization outside the physician's practice.

referral (rĭ-fûr´əl) An authorization from a medical practice for a patient to have specialized services performed by another practice; often required for insurance purposes.

reflection (rĭ-flĕk´shən) When a thought, idea or opinion is formed as a result of deeper thought.

reflex (rē´flĕks´) A predictable automatic response to stimuli.

reflexology (rē -flĕk-sŏl´-ə-jē) Manual therapy to the foot and/or hand in which pressure is applied to "reflex" points mapped out on the feet or hands.

refraction (rĭ-frăk´shən) The bending of light by the cornea, lens, and eye fluids to focus light onto the retina.

refraction examination (rĭ-frăk´shən ĭg-zăm´ə-nā´shən) An eye examination in which the patient looks through a succession of different lenses to find out which ones create the clearest image.

refractometer (rē-frak-tom´ē-ter) (†) An optical instrument that measures the refraction, or bending, of light as it passes through a liquid.

Registered Medical Assistant (RMA) (rĕj´ĭ-stərd mĕd´ĭ-kəl ə-sĭs´tənt) A medical assistant who has met the educational requirements and taken and passed the certification examination for medical assisting given by the American Medical Technologists (AMT).

Reiki (ray-key) The use of visualization and touch to balance energy flow and bring healthy energy to affected body parts.

relaxin (rē-lak´sin) (†) A hormone that comes from the corpus luteum. It inhibits uterine contractions and relaxes the ligaments of the pelvis in preparation for childbirth.

remedy (rĕm´-ĭ-dē) A treatment prescribed by a homeopath in small amounts that in large doses would produce the same symptoms seen in the patient.

remittance advice (RA) (rĭ-mĭt´ns ad-vīz´) A form that the patient and the practice receive for each encounter that outlines the amount billed by the practice, the amount allowed, the amount of subscriber liability, the amount paid, and notations of any service not covered, including an explanation of why that service is not covered; also called an explanation of benefits.

renal calculi (rē´nəl kăl´ kyə-lī´) Kidney stones.

renal column (rē´nəl kŏl´əm) The portion of the **renal cortex** between the **renal pyramids**.

renal corpuscle (rē´nəl kôr´pə-səl) Corpuscle that is composed of the glomerulus and the glomerular capsule. The filtration of blood occurs here.

renal cortex (rē´nəl kôr´tĕks´) The outermost layer of the kidney.

renal medulla (rē´nəl mĭ-dŭl´ə) The middle portion of the kidney.

renal pelvis (rē´nəl pĕl´vĭs) The internal structure of the kidney. Urine flows from the renal pelvis down the ureter.

renal pyramids (rē´nəl pĭr´ə -mĭdz) Triangular-shaped areas in the medulla of the kidney.

renal sinus (rē´nəl sī´nəs) The medial depression of a kidney.

renal tubule (rē´nəl tū´byūl) Structure that extends from the glomerular capsule of a nephron and is composed of the proximal convoluted tubule, the loop of Henle, and the distal convoluted tubule.

renin (ren´in) (†) A hormone secreted by the kidney that helps to regulate blood pressure.

repolarization (rē´pō-lăr-i-zā´shŭn) (†) The process of returning to the original polar (resting) state.

reputable (rĕpyə-tə-bəl) Having a good reputation.

requisition (rĕk´wĭ-zĭsh´ən) A formal request from a staff member or doctor for the purchase of equipment or supplies.

res ipsa loquitur (reez ip-suh loh-kwi-ter) Latin, meaning "the thing speaks for itself," which is also known as the doctrine of common knowledge.

reservoir host (rĕz´ər-vwär´ hōst) An animal, insect, or human whose body is susceptible to growth of a pathogen.

resident normal flora (´re-zə-dənt, ´nōr-məl, ´flōr-ə) Bacteria, fungi, and protozoa that have taken up residence either in or on the human body. Some of these organisms neither help nor harm the host and some are beneficial, creating a barrier against pathogens.

resource-based relative value scale (RBRVS) (rē´sôrs´ bāst rĕl´ə-tĭvvăl´yōō skāl) The payment system used by Medicare. It establishes the relative value units for services, replacing the providers' consensus on usual fees.

respiratory distress syndrome (res´pərətôr´ə distres sin´drəm) Condition found usually in premature babies, who lack the substance surfactant in their lungs, causing the lungs to collapse on expiration.

respiratory hygiene/cough etiquette (rĕs´pər-ə-tôr´ēhī´jēn´ kôfĕt´ī-kĭt) Infection control guideline that includes teaching the patient to cover their mouth/nose when coughing and dispose of tissues in the proper receptacle.

respiratory volume (rĕs´pər-ə-tôr´ē vŏl´yōōm) The different volumes of air that move in and out of the lungs during different intensities of breathing. These volumes can be measured to assess the healthiness of the respiratory system.

respondeat superior (rehs-pond-dee-at soo-peer-e-or) Latin, meaning "let the master answer," a doctrine under which an employer is legally liable for the acts of his or her employees, if such acts were performed within the scope of the employee's duties.

restatement (rē-stāt´ment) Repeating what a patient says in your own words back to the patient.

résumé (rĕz´ŏŏ-mā´) A typewritten document summarizing one's employment and educational history.

retention schedule (rĭ-tĕn´shən skĕj´ōōl) A schedule that details how long to keep different types of patient records in the office after they have become inactive or closed and how long the records should be stored.

retina (rĕt´n-ə) The inner layer of the eye; contains light-sensing nerve cells.

retraction (rĭ-trăk´shən) Moving a body part posteriorly.

retrograde pyelography (rĕt´rə-grād´pī´ē-log´ră-fē)(†) A radiologic procedure in which the doctor injects a contrast medium through a urethral catheter and takes a series of x-rays to evaluate function of the ureters, bladder, and urethra.

retroperitoneal (re-trō-per-ə-tə-nē´əl) An anatomic term that means behind the peritoneal cavity. It is where the kidneys lie.

return demonstation (rĭ-tûrn´ dĕm´ən-strā´shən) Participatory teaching method in which the technique is first described to the patient and then demonstrated to the patient; the patient is then asked to repeat the demonstration.

rhabdomyolysis (rab´dō-mī-ol´i-sis)(†) A condition in which the kidneys have been damaged due to toxins released from muscle cells.

Rh antigen (är´ach an´tĭ-jən) A protein first discovered on the red

blood cells of rhesus monkeys, hence the name Rh.

RhoGAM (rō´găm) A medication that prevents an Rh-negative mother from making antibodies against the Rh antigen.

ribosomes ((rībəsomz) The organelle within the cytoplasm responsible for protein synthesis.

RNA (är´ĕn-ā´) A nucleic acid used to make protein.

rods (rŏdz) Light-sensing nerve cells in the eye, at the posterior of the retina, that function in dim light but do not provide sharp images or detect color.

rosacea (rō-zā´shē-ă)(†) A condition characterized by chronic redness and acne over the nose and cheeks.

rotation (rō-tā´shən) Twisting a body part.

route (rōōt) The way a drug is introduced into the body.

rugae (rōō´gā) The expandable folds of an organ. The folds of the stomach lining.

sacrum (sa´-krəm) A triangular-shaped bone that consists of five fused vertebra.

sagittal (saj´i-tăl)(†) An anatomic term that refers to the plane that divides the body into left and right portions.

salutation (săl´yə-tā´shən) A written greeting, such as "Dear," used at the beginning of a letter.

sanitization (săn´ĭ-tĭ-zā´shən)(†) A reduction of the number of microorganisms on an object or a surface to a fairly safe level.

sarcolemma (sar´kō-lem´ă) The cell membrane of a muscle fiber.

sarcoplasm (sar´-kō-pla-zim) The cytoplasm of a muscle fiber.

sarcoplasmic reticulum (sar-kō-plaz´mik re-tik´yū-lŭm) The endoplasmic reticulum of a muscle fiber.

SARS (severe acute respiratory syndrome) (särz; sivĕr əkyōōt res´pərətôr´ē sin´drəm) A severe and acute respiratory illness characterized by fever and a nonproductive cough that progresses to the point at which insufficient oxygen is present in the blood.

saturated fat (săch´ə-rā´tĭd făt) Fats, derived primarily from animal sources, that are usually solid at room temperature and that tend to raise blood cholesterol levels.

scabies (skā´bēz) Skin lesions that are very itchy and caused by a burrowing mite. Scabies is most commonly found between the fingers and on the genitalia.

scanner (skăn´ər) An optical device that converts printed matter into a format that can be read by the computer and inputs the converted information.

scapula (sk´a-pyə-la) Thin, triangular-shaped, flat bones located on the dorsal surface of the rib cage; also called shoulder blades.

Schwann cell (shwahn sĕl)(†) A neuroglial cell whose cell membrane coats the axons.

sciatica (sī-ăt´ĭ-kə) Pain in the low back and hip radiating down the back of the leg along the sciatic nerve.

sclera (sklîr´ə) The tough, outermost layer, or "white," of the eye, through which light cannot pass; covers all except the front of the eye.

scoliosis (skō´lē-ō´sĭs) A lateral curvature of the spine, which is normally straight when viewed from behind.

scratch test (skrăch tĕst) An allergy test in which extracts of suspected allergens are applied to the patient's skin and the skin is then scratched to allow the extracts to penetrate.

screening (skrēn´ĭng) Performing a diagnostic test on a person who is typically free of symptoms.

screen saver (skrēn săv´ər) A program that automatically changes the monitor display at short intervals or constantly shows moving images to prevent burn-in of images on the computer screen.

scrotum (skrō´təm) In a male, the sac of skin below the pelvic cavity that contains the testes.

sebaceous (sĭ-bā´shəs) A type of oil gland found in the dermis.

sebum (sē´bŭm)(†) An oily substance produced by sebaceous glands.

Security Rule (sĭ-kyŏor´ĭ-tē rōol) The technical safeguards that protect the confidentiality, integrity, and availability of health information covered by **HIPAA.** The Security Rule specifies how patient information is protected on computer networks, the Internet, disks, and other storage media.

seizure (sē´zhər) A series of violent and involuntary contractions of the muscles; also called a convulsion.

sella turcica (sel´ă tŭr´sē-kă)(†) A deep depression in the sphenoid bone where the pituitary gland sits.

semen (sē´mən) Sperm and the various substances that nourish and transport them.

semicircular canals (sĕm´ē-sûr´kyə-lər kə-nălz´) Structures in the inner ear that help a person maintain balance; each of the three canals is positioned at right angles to the other two.

seminal vesicles (sem´-năl ves´ĭ-klz)(†) A pair of convoluted tubes that lie behind the bladder. These tubes secrete a fluid that provides nutrition for the sperm.

seminiferous tubules (sem´ĭ-nif´er-ŭs tū´byūlz)(†) These tubes contain spermatogenic cells and are located in the lobules of the testes.

sensorineural hearing loss (sen´sōr-i-nūr´ăl hîr´ĭng lôs) This type of hearing loss occurs when neural structures associated with the ear are damaged. Neural structures include hearing receptors and the auditory nerve.

sensory (sĕn´sə-rē) Afferent neurons that carry sensory information from the periphery to the central nervous system.

sensory adaptation (sĕn´sə-rē ăd´ăp-tā´shən) A process in which the same chemical can stimulate receptors only for a limited amount of time until the receptors eventually no longer respond to the chemical.

septic shock (sĕp´tĭk shŏk) A state of shock resulting from massive, widespread infection that affects the blood vessels' ability to circulate blood.

sequential order (sĭ´kwĕn´shəl ôr´dər) One after another in a predictable pattern or sequence.

serosa (se-rō´să)(†) The outermost layer of the alimentary canal; also known as the visceral peritoneum.

serous cells (sēr´ŭs sĕlz)(†) One of two types of cells that make up the salivary glands. These cells secrete a watery fluid that contains amylase.

serum (sēr´ŭm)(†) The liquid portion of blood (plasma) when all of the clotting factors have been removed.

service contract (sûr´vĭs kŏn´trăkt´) A contract that covers services for equipment that are not included in a standard maintenance contract.

sex chromosome (sĕks krō´mə-sōm´) Chromosome of the 23rd pair.

sex-linked trait (sĕks lĭngk trāt) Traits that are carried on the sex chromosomes, or X and Y chromosomes.

sigmoid colon (sig-mȯid ko-lən) An S-shaped tube that lies between the **descending colon** and the **rectum.**

sigmoidoscopy (sig´moy-dos´kŏ-pē) A procedure in which the interior of the sigmoid area of the large intestine, between the descending colon and the rectum, is examined with a sigmoidoscope, a lighted instrument with a magnifying lens.

sign (sīn) An objective or external factor, such as blood pressure, rash, or swelling, that can be seen or felt by the physician or measured by an instrument.

signature block (sig´-nuh-cher blok´) The writer's name and business title found four lines below the complimentary closing in a business letter.

silicosis (sil´ i kō´ sis) Chronic lung disease caused by the inhalation of silica dust.

simplified letter style (sĭm´plə-fīd´ lĕt´ər stīl) A modification of the full-block style in which the salutation and complimentary closing are omitted and a subject line typed in all capital letters is placed between the address and the body of the letter.

single-entry account (sĭng´gəl-ĕn´trē ə-kount´) An account that has only one charge, usually for a small amount, for a patient who does not come in regularly.

sinoatrial node (sī´nō-ā´trē-ăl nōd)(†) A small bundle of heart muscle tissue in the superior wall of the right atrium that sets the rhythm (or pattern) of the heart's contractions; also called sinus node or pacemaker.

sinusitis (sī´nə-sī´tĭs) Inflammation of the lining of a sinus.

skinfold test (skĭn´ fōld tĕst) A method of measuring fat as a percentage of body weight by measuring the thickness of a fold of skin with a caliper.

slander (slăn´ dər) The speaking of defamatory words intended to prejudice others against an individual in a manner that jeopardizes his or her reputation or means of livelihood.

sleep apnea (slēp ap-ne´ah) A condition characterized by pauses in breathing during sleep.

slitlamp (slĭt lămp) An instrument composed of a magnifying lens combined with a light source; used to provide a minute examination of the eye's anatomy.

smear (smîr) A specimen spread thinly and unevenly across a slide.

SOAP (sōp) An approach to medical records documentation that documents information in the following order: S (**subjective** data), O (**objective** data), A (assessment), P (plan of action).

software (sôft´wâr´) A program, or set of instructions, that tells a computer what to do.

sole proprietorship (sōl prə -prī´-tər shĭp) A form of medical practice management in which a physician practices alone, assuming all benefits, and liabilities for the business.

solution (sə-lōō´shən) A homogeneous mixture of a solid, liquid, or gaseous substance in a liquid, such as a dissolved drug in liquid form.

somatic (sō-măt´ĭk) A division of the peripheral nervous system that connects the central nervous system to skin and skeletal muscle.

somatic nervous system (SNS) (sō-măt´ĭk nûr´vəs sĭs´təm) A system that governs the body's skeletal or voluntary muscles.

SPECT (spĕkt) Single photon emission computed tomography; a radiologic procedure in which a gamma camera detects signals induced by gamma radiation and a computer converts these signals into two- or three-dimensional images that are displayed on a screen.

speculum (spĕk´yə-ləm) An instrument that expands the vaginal opening to permit viewing of the vagina and cervix.

spermatids (sper´mă-tidz)(†) Immature sperm before they develop their flagella (tails).

spermatocytes (sper´mă-tō-sīts)(†) The cells that result

when spermatogonia undergo mitosis.

spermatogenesis (sper´mă-tō-jen´ĕ-sis)(†) The process of sperm cell formation.

spermatogenic cells (sper´mă-tō-jen´ik sĕlz)(†) The cells that give rise to sperm cells.

spermatogonia (sper´mă-tō-gō´nē-ă)(†) The earliest cell in the process of **spermatogenesis.**

sphenoid A bone that forms part of the floor of the cranium.

sphincter (sfĭngk´tər) A valve-like structure formed from circular bands of muscle. Sphincters are located around various body openings and passages.

sphygmomanometer (sfĭg´mō-mănom´ĕter)(†) An instrument for measuring blood pressure; consists of an inflatable cuff, a pressure bulb used to inflate the cuff, and a device to read the pressure.

spinal nerves (spī´năl nûrvs)(†) Peripheral nerves that originate from the spinal cord.

spirillum (spī-ril´ŭm)(†) A spiral-shaped bacterium.

spirometer (spī-rom´ĕ-ter)(†) An instrument that measures the air taken in and expelled from the lungs.

spirometry (spī-rom´ĕ-trē)(†) A test used to measure breathing capacity.

splenectomy (splən ek´ tō me) Surgical removal of the spleen.

splint (splĭnt) A device used to immobilize and protect a body part.

splinting catheter (splĭnt´ĭng kăth´ĭ-tər) A type of catheter inserted after plastic repair of the ureter; it must remain in place for at least a week after surgery.

sprain (sprān) An injury characterized by partial tearing of a ligament that supports a joint, such as the ankle. A sprain may also involve injuries to tendons, muscles, and local blood vessels and contusions of the surrounding soft tissue.

stain (stān) In microbiology, a solution of a dye or group of dyes that impart a color to microorganisms.

standard (stăn´dərd) A specimen for which test values are already known; used to calibrate test equipment.

standardization (stăn-dər-dĭ -zā´-shən) The consistency of the active ingredient(s) in a supplement from batch to batch and from manufacturer to manufacturer.

Standard Precautions (stăn´dərd prĭ-kô´shənz) A combination of Universal Precautions and Body Substance Isolation guidelines; used in hospitals for the care of all patients.

stapes (stā´pēz) A small bone in the middle ear that is attached to the inner ear; also called the stirrup.

statement (stāt´mənt) A form similar to an invoice; contains a courteous reminder to the patient that payment is due.

State Unemployment Tax Act (SUTA) Some states are also governed by this act; these taxes are filed along with FUTA taxes.

statute of limitations (stăch´oot lĭm´ĭ-tā´shənz) A state law that sets a time limit on when a collection suit on a past-due account can legally be filed.

stent (stĕnt-) A metal mesh tube used to hold a vessel open.

stereoscopy (ster-¯e--os´k˘o-p¯e)(†) An x-ray procedure that uses a specially designed microscope (stereoscopic, or Greenough, microscope) with double eye-pieces and objectives to take films at different angles and produce three-dimensional images; used primarily to study the skull.

sterile field (stĕr´əl fēld) An area free of microorganisms used as a work area during a surgical procedure.

sterile scrub assistant (stĕr´əl skrŭb ə-sĭs´tənt) An assistant who handles sterile equipment during a surgical procedure.

sterilization (stĕr´ə-lĭ-zā´shən) The destruction of all microorganisms, including bacterial spores, by specific means.

sterilization indicator (stĕr´ə-lĭ-zā´shən in´dĭ-kā´tor) A tag, insert, tape, tube, or strip that confirms that the items in an autoclave have been exposed to the correct volume of steam at the correct temperature for the correct amount of time.

sternum (st´ər-nəm) A bone that forms the front and middle portion of the rib cage; also called the breastbone or breast plate.

steroidal hormone (stîr´oid´əl hôr´mōn´) A hormone derived from steroids that are soluble in lipids and can cross cell membranes very easily.

stethoscope (stĕth´ə-skōp´) An instrument that amplifies body sounds.

strabismus (strə-bĭz´məs) A condition that results in a lack of parallel visual axes of the eyes; commonly called crossed eyes.

strain (strān) A muscle injury that results from overexertion or overstretching.

stratum basale (strat´ŭm bā-sā´le)(†) The deepest layer of the epidermis of the skin.

stratum corneum (strat´um kōr´nē ŭm)(†) The most superficial layer of the epidermis of the skin.

stratum germinativum (strat´ŭm jur´minə tē´vūm) The deepest layer of the epidermis; also known as staratum basale.

stressor (stres´or)(†) Any stimulus that produces stress.

stress test (strĕs tĕst) A procedure that involves recording an electrocardiogram while the patient is exercising on a stationary bicycle, treadmill, or stair-stepping ergometer, which measures work performed.

striations (strī-ā´shŭns)(†) Bands produced from the arrangement of filaments in myofibrils in skeletal and cardiac muscle cells.

stroke (strōk) A condition that occurs when the blood supply to the brain is impaired. It may cause temporary or permanent damage.

stylus (stī´ləs) A pen-like instrument that records electrical impulses on ECG paper.

subarachnoid space (sŭb-ă-rak´noyd spās)(†) An area between the arachnoid mater and the pia mater.

subclinical case (sŭb-klin´i-kăl kās)(†) An infection in which the host experiences only some of the symptoms of the infection or milder symptoms than in a full case.

subcutaneous (sub-Q) (sŭb´kyoo-tā´nē-əs) Under the skin.

subject line (sŭb´jĭkt līn) Optional line of two to three words that appears three lines below the inside address of a business letter.

subjective (səb-jĕk´tĭv) Pertaining to data that is obtained from conversation with a person or patient.

subjective data (səb-jĕk´tĭv dā´tə) Information about the patient's condition that includes thoughts feelings and perceptions.

sublingual (sŭb-ling´gwăl) (†) Under the tongue.

sublingual gland (sŭb-ling´gwăl glănd)(†) The smallest of the salivary glands.

submandibular gland (sŭb-man-dib´yu-lăr glănd)(†) The gland that is located in the floor of the mouth.

submucosa (sŭb-mū-kō´s ă)(†) The layer of the alimentary canal located between the mucosa and the muscular layer.

subpoena (sə-pē´nə) A written court order that is addressed to a specific person and requires that person's presence in court on a specific date at a specific time.

subpoena duces tecum (suh-pee-nuh doo-seez tee-kum) Latin; a legal document that requires the recipient to bring certain written records to court to be used as evidence in a lawsuit.

substance abuse (sŭb´stəns ə-byōoz´) The use of a substance in a way that is not medically approved, such as using diet pills to stay awake or consuming large quantities of cough syrup that contains codeine. Substance abusers are not necessarily addicts.

sucrase (sū´krās)(†) An enzyme that digests sugars.

sudoriferous (sōo´dərif´ərəs) The sweat glands.

suffix (sŭ-fĭks) A word part that comes at the end of medical term that alters the meaning of the term.

sulci (sŭl´si)(†) The grooves on the surface of the cerebrum.

superbill (sōo´pər-bĭl´) A form that combines the charges for services rendered, an invoice for payment or insurance copayment, and all the information for submitting an insurance claim; also known as an encounter form.

superficial (sōo´pər-fĭsh´əl) Anatomic term meaning closer to the surface of the body.

superior (sōo´-pîr´-ē-ər) Anatomic term meaning above or closer to the head; also called cranial.

supernatant (sū-per-nā´tănt)(†) The liquid portion of a substance from which solids have settled to the bottom, as with a urine specimen after centrifugation.

supination (sū´pi-nā´shŭn)(†) Turning the palm of the hand upward.

surfactant (sər fak´ tənt) Fatty substance secreted by some alveolar cells that helps maintain the inflation of the alveoli so that they do not collapse in on themselves between inspirations.

surgeon (sûr´jən) A physician who uses hands and medical instruments to diagnose and correct deformities and treat external and internal injuries or disease.

surgical asepsis (sûr´jə-kəl ă-sep´sis)(†) The elimination of all microorganisms from objects or working areas; also called sterile technique.

susceptible host (sə-sĕp´təbal hōst) An individual who has little or no immunity to infection by a particular organism.

suture (sōo´chər) Fibrous joints in the skull.
A surgical stitch made to close a wound.

symmetry (sĭm´ĭ-trē) The degree to which one side of the body is the same as the other.

sympathetic (sĭm´pə-thĕt´ĭk) A division of the autonomic nervous system that prepares organs for fight-or-flight (stressful) situations.

symptom (sĭm´təm) A subjective, or internal, condition felt by a patient, such as pain, headache, or nausea, or another indication that generally cannot be seen or felt by the doctor or measured by instruments.

synaptic knob (si-nap´tik nŏb)(†) The end of the axon branch.

synaptic space (si-nap-tik spās) The space between the axon of one neuron and the dendrite of the next.

synergist (sĭn´ər-jist´) Muscles that help the **prime mover** by stabilizing joints.

synovial (sin-ō-vā-əl) A type of joint, such as the elbow or knee, that is freely moveable.

systemic circuit (sĭ-stĕm´ĭk sûr´kĭt) The route that blood takes from the heart through the body and back to the heart.

systemic lupus erythematosus (SLE) (si-stĕm´ĭk loo´p s er the m´to´s s) An autoimmune disorder in which a person produces antibodies that target the person's own cells and tissues.

systolic pressure (sĭ-stŏl´ĭk prĕsh´ər) The blood pressure measured when the left ventricle of the heart contracts.

tab (tăb) A tapered rectangular or rounded extension at the top of a file folder.

tablet PC (´ta-blət pē sē) A laptop or slate-shaped mobile computer, equipped with a touchscreen or graphics tablet to operate the computer with a digital pen, or a fingertip instead of a keyboard or mouse.

Tabular List (tăb´yə-lər lĭst) One of two ways that diagnoses are listed in the **ICD-9**. In the Tabular List, the diagnosis codes are listed in numerical order with additional instructions.

tachycardia (tak´i-kar´dē-ă)(†) Rapid heart rate, generally in excess of 100 beats per minute.

tachypnea Abnormally rapid breathing.

targeted résumé (tär´gĭt-əd rĕz´ōo-mā´) A résumé that is focused on a specific job target.

tarsals (tär´-səlz) Bones of the ankle.

taste bud (tāst bŭd) A structure that is made of taste cells (a type of chemoreceptor) and supporting cells.

tax liability (tăks lī´ə-bĭl´ĭ-tē) Money withheld from employees' paychecks and held in a separate account that must be used to pay taxes to appropriate government agencies.

telephone triage (tĕl´ə-fōn´ trē-äzh´) A process of determining the level of urgency of each incoming telephone call and how it should be handled.

teletherapy (tel-ĕ-thār´əpē)(†) A radiation therapy technique that allows deeper penetration than brachytherapy; used primarily for deep tumors.

teletype (TTY) device (tĕl´ə-tīp) A specially designed telephone that looks very much like a laptop computer with a cradle for the receiver of a traditional telephone. It is used by the hearing impaired to type communications onto a keyboard.

telophase (tel´əfāz) The final stage of mitosis; chromosomes reach the centrioles and the division creating two cells, each with a complete set of chromosomes is completed.

template (tĕm´plĭt) A guide that ensures consistency and accuracy.

temporal (tem´-p(a)-rəl) Bones that form the lower sides of the skull.

temporal scanner (temp´-or-al skăn-ĕr) An instrument used to measure the body temperature by scanning the temporal artery in the forehead.

tendon (tĕn´dən) A cord-like fibrous tissue that connects muscle to bone.

tendonitis (ten dŭn ĭ tis) Inflammation of a tendon.

terminal (tûr´mə-nəl) Fatal.

terminal digit (tûrmə-nəl dĭjĭt) A small group of two to three numbers at the end of a patient number that is used as an identifying unit in a filing system.

testes (tĕs´tēz) The primary organs of the male reproductive system. Testes produce the hormone **testosterone**.

testosterone (tĕs-tŏs´tə-rōn´) A hormone produced by the testes that maintains the male reproductive structures and male characteristics such as deep voice, body hair, and muscle mass.

tetanus (tĕt´n-əs) A disease caused by *Clostridium tetani* living in the soil and water; more commonly called lockjaw.

thalamus (th˘al´ə-məs) Structure that acts as a relay station for sensory information heading to the cerebral cortex for interpretation; a subdivision of the **diencephalon**.

thalassemia (thal´ə sē´mēaə) An inherited form of anemia with a defective hemoglobin chain causing micocytic (small), hypochromic (pale), and short-lived red blood cells.

therapeutic team (thĕr´ə-pyōō´tĭk tēm) A group of physicians, nurses, medical assistants, and other specialists who work with patients dealing with chronic illness or recovery from major injuries.

therapeutic touch (thĕr´ -ə-pyōō-tĭk tŭch) The use of touch to detect and correct an person's energy fields, thus promoting healing and health.

thermography (ther-mog´ră-fē)(†) A radiologic procedure in which an infrared camera is used to take photographs that record variations in skin temperature as dark (cool areas), light (warm areas), or shades of gray (areas with temperatures between cool and warm); used to diagnose breast tumors, breast abscesses, and fibrocystic breast disease.

thermometer (ther-mom´ə-ter) An instrument, either electronic or disposable, that is used to measure body temperature.

thermotherapy (ther´mō-thār´ă-pē) (†) The application of heat to the body to treat a disorder or injury.

third-party check (thûrd pär´tē chĕk) A check made out to one recipient and given in payment to another, as with one made out to a patient rather than the medical practice.

third-party payer (thûrd pär´tē pā´ər) A health plan that agrees to carry the risk of paying for patient services.

thoracocentesis (thôr´ə kō´sen tē´ sis) Medical procedure where a sterile needle is introduced into the chest to remove fluid and pus.

thoracostomy (thor´ə kos´ tə mē) The surgical insertion of a chest tube to provide continuous drainage of the thoracic (chest) cavity.

thorax (thôr´aks) The chest cavity.

thrombocytes (throm´bō-sīts) See **platelets**.

thrombophlebitis (thrŏm´bō-flĕ-bī´tis) (†) A medical condition that most commonly occurs in leg veins when a blood clot and inflammation develop.

thrombus (thrŏm´bəs) A blood clot that forms on the inside of an injured blood vessel wall.

thymosin (thī´mō-sin)(†) A hormone that promotes the production of certain lymphocytes.

thymus gland (thī´məs glănd) A gland that lies between the lungs. It secretes a hormone called **thymosin**.

thyroid cartilage (thī´roid´ kär´tl-ĭj) The largest cartilage in the larynx. It forms the anterior wall of the larynx.

thyroid hormone (thī´roid´ hôr´mōn´) A hormone produced by the thyroid gland that increases energy production, stimulates protein synthesis, and speeds up the repair of damaged tissue.

thyroid-stimulating hormone (TSH) (thī´roid´stim´yū-lā-ting hôr´mōn´) A hormone that stimulates the thyroid gland to release its hormone.

tibia (ti-bē-ə) The medial bone of the lower leg; commonly called the shin bone.

tickler file (tĭk´lər fīl) A reminder file for keeping track of time-sensitive obligations.

timed urine specimen (tīmd yōōr´ĭn spĕs´ə-mən) A specimen of a patient's urine collected over a specific time period.

time-specified scheduling (tīm spĕs´ə-fīd skĕj´ōol-ĭng) A system of scheduling where patients arrive at regular, specified intervals, assuring the practice a steady stream of patients throughout the day.

tinea (tin ē´ă) A fungal infection.

tinnitus (ti-nī´tus)(†) An abnormal ringing in the ear.

tissue (tĭsh´o͞o) A structure that is formed when cells of the same type organize together.

T lymphocyte (tē lĭm´fə-sīt) A type of nongranular leukocyte that regulates immunologic response; includes helper T cells and suppressor T cells.

topical (tŏp´ĭ-kəl) Applied to the skin.

tort (tôrt) In civil law, a breach of some obligation that causes harm or injury to someone.

torticollis (tôr´tikol´is) A muscular disease causing a cervical deformity in which the head bends toward the affected side while the chin rotates to the opposite side.

touchpad (tūch pād) A type of pointing device common to laptop and notebook computers that directs activity on the computer screen by positioning a pointer or cursor on the screen. It is a small, flat device or surface that is highly sensitive to touch.

touch screen (tūch skrēn) A type of computer monitor that acts as an intake device, receiving information thought the touch of a pen, wand, or hand directly to the screen.

tower case (tou´ər kās) A vertical housing for the system unit of a personal computer.

toxicology (tŏk´sĭ-kŏl´ə-jē) The study of poisons or poisonous effects of drugs.

trachea (trā´kē-ə) The part of the respiratory tract between the larynx and the bronchial tree that is tubular and made of rings of cartilage and smooth muscle; also called the windpipe.

trackball (trāk bôl) A pointing device with a ball that is rolled to position a pointer or cursor on a computer screen. It can be directly attached to the computer or can be wireless.

tracking (trăk´ĭng) (financial) Watching for changes in spending so as to help control expenses.

traction (trăk´shən) The pulling or stretching of the musculoskeletal system to treat dislocated joints, joints afflicted by arthritis or other diseases, and fractured bones.

trade name (trād nām) A drug's brand or proprietary name.

traditional Chinese medicine (TCM) (trə-dĭsh´-ə-nəl chĭ-nĕz mĕd´-ĭ-sĭn) An ancient system of medicine originating in China that involves herbal and animal source preparations to treat illness. TCM includes various treatments such as acupuncture and acupressure.

transcription (trăn-skrĭp´shən) The transforming of spoken notes into accurate written form.

transcutaneous absorption (trans-kyū-tā´nē-ŭs əb-sorp´shən)(†) Entry (as of a pathogen) through a cut or crack in the skin.

transdermal (trans-der´mel) A type of topical drug administration that slowly and evenly releases a systemic drug through the skin directly into the bloodstream; a transdermal unit is also called a patch.

transfer (trăns-fûr´) To give something, such as information, to another party outside the doctor's office.

transurethral resection of prostate (trans´yŏo rĕ thrəl rĕ-sək´ shən) Removal of the prostate through the urethra.

transverse (trăns-vŭrs´) Anatomic term that refers to the plane that divides the body into superior and inferior portions.

transverse colon (trăns-vûrs´ kō´lən) The segment of the large intestine that crosses the upper abdominal cavity between the ascending and descending colon.

traveler's check (trăv´əl-rz chĕk) A check purchased and signed at a bank and later signed over to a payee.

treatment, payments, and operations (TPO) (trēt´mənt pā´mənts ŏp´ə-rā´shəns) The portion of HIPAA that allows the provider to use and share patient healthcare information for treatment, payment, and operations (such as quality improvement).

triage (trē-äzh´) To assess the urgency and types of conditions patients present as well as their immediate medical needs.

TRICARE (trī´kâr) A program that provides health-care benefits for families of military personnel and military retirees.

trichinosis (trik-i-nō´sis)(†) A disease caused by a worm that is usually ingested from undercooked meat.

tricuspid valve (trī-kŭs´pid vălv)(†) A heart valve that has three cusps and is situated between the right atrium and the right ventricle.

triglycerides (trī-glĭs´ə-rīd´z) Simple lipids consisting of glycerol (an alcohol) and three fatty acids.

trigone (trī´gōn)(†) The triangle formed by the openings of the two ureters and the urethra in the internal floor of the bladder.

troubleshooting (trŭb´əl-sho͞o´tĭng) Trying to determine and correct a problem without having to call a service supplier.

trypsin (trip´sin)(†) A pancreatic enzyme that digests proteins.

tubular reabsorption (tū´byū-lăr re-ab-sôrp´sh n)(†) The second process of urine formation in which the glomerular filtrate flows into the proximal convoluted tubule.

tubular secretion (tū´byū-lăr sĭ-krē´shən)(†) The third process of urine formation in which substances move out of the blood in the peritubular capillaries into renal tubules.

tutorial (too-tôr´ē-əl) A small program included in a software package designed to give users an overall picture of the product and its functions.

tympanic membrane (tĭm-păn´ĭk mĕm´brān´) A fibrous partition located at the inner end of the ear canal and separating the outer ear from the middle ear; also called the eardrum.

tympanic thermometer (tim-pan´ik ther-mom´ĕ-ter) A type of electronic thermometer that measures infrared energy emitted from the tympanic membrane.

ulna (əl´-nə) The medial bone of the lower arm.

ultrasonic cleaning (ŭl´trə-sŏn´ĭk klēn´ĭng) A method of sanitization that involves placing instruments in a cleaning solution in a special receptacle that generates sound waves through the cleaning solution, loosening contaminants. Ultrasonic cleaning is safe for even very fragile instruments.

ultrasound The noninvasive theraputic or diagnostic use of ultrasound for examination of internal body structures.

umami (oo-mom´ē) Savory taste produced by glutamic acid (monosodium glutamate), recognized as the fifth taste sensation.

umbilical cord (ŭm-bĭl´ĭ-kəl kôrd) The rope-like connection between the fetus and the placenta. It contains the umbilical blood vessels.

underbooking (ŭn´dər-bŏŏkĭng) Leaving large, unused gaps in the doctor's schedule; this approach does not make the best use of the doctor's time.

uniform donor card (yoo´nə-fôrm´ dō´nər kärd) A legal document that states a person's wish to make a gift upon death of one or more organs for medical research, organ transplants, or placement in a tissue bank.

unit (yoo´nĭt) A part of an individual's name or title, described in indexing rules.

unit price (yoo´nĭt prīs) The total price of a package divided by the number of items that comprise the package.

Universal Precautions (yoo´nə-vur´səl prĭ-kô´shənz) Specific precautions required by the Department of Health and Human Services' Centers for Disease Control and Prevention (CDC) to prevent health-care workers from exposing themselves and others to infection by blood-borne pathogens.

unsaturated fats (ŭn-săch´ə-rā´tĭd făts) Fats, including most vegetable oils, that are usually liquid at room temperature and tend to lower blood cholesterol.

upper respiratory (tract) infection (upper res´pərətôr´ē tract infek´shən) The common cold.

urea (yoo-rē´ə) Waste product formed by the breakdown of proteins and nucleic acids.

ureters (yoo-rē´tərz) Long, slender, muscular tubes that carry urine from the kidneys to the urinary bladder.

urethra (yoo-rē´thrə) The tube that conveys urine from the bladder during urination.

uric acid (yoor´ĭk as´id) Waste product formed by the breakdown of proteins and nucleic acids.

urinalysis (yoor´ə-năl´ĭ-sĭs) The physical, chemical, and microscopic evaluation of urine to obtain information about body health and disease.

urinary catheter (yoor´ə-nĕr´ē kăth´ĭ-tər) A sterile plastic tube inserted to provide urinary drainage.

urinary pH (yoor´ə-nĕr´ē pē´ăch) A measure of the degree of acidity or alkalinity of urine.

urine specific gravity (yoor´ĭn spĭ-sĭf´ĭk grăv´ĭ-tē) A measure of the concentration or amount (total weight) of substances dissolved in urine.

urobilinogen (yūr-ō-bī-lin´ō-jen)(†) A colorless compound formed by the breakdown of hemoglobin in the intestines. Elevated levels in urine may indicate increased red blood cell destruction or liver disease, whereas lack of urobilinogen in the urine may suggest total bile duct obstruction.

urologist (yoo-rŏl´ə-jĭst) A specialist who diagnoses and treats diseases of the kidney, bladder, and urinary system.

use (yooz) The sharing, employing, applying, utilizing, examining, or analyzing of individually identifiable health information by employees or other members of an organization's workforce.

uterus (yoo´tər-əs) A hollow, muscular organ that functions to receive an embryo and sustain its development; also called the womb.

uvula (yoo´vyə-lə) The part of the soft palate that hangs down in the back of the throat.

uvulotomy (yoo´vyəlot´əmē) Surgical procedure removing all or part of the uvula of the soft palate.

vaccine (văk-sēn´) A special preparation made from microorganisms and administered to a person to produce reduced sensitivity to, or increased immunity to, an infectious disease.

vagina (və-jī´nə) A tubular organ that extends from the uterus to the labia.

vaginal introitus (vaj´ i-nəl in trō´i təs) The vaginal os or orifice. The opening of the vagina to the outside of the body.

vaginitis (vaj-i-nī´tis)(†) Inflammation of the vagina characterized by an abnormal vaginal discharge.

varicose veins (vār´i-kōs vānz)(†) Distended veins that result when vein valves are destroyed and blood pools in the veins, causing these veins to dilate.

vas deferens (văs´ dĕf´ər-ənz) A tube that connects the epididymis with the urethra and that carries sperm.

vasectomy (və-sĕk´tə-mē) A male sterilization procedure in which a section of each vas deferens is removed.

vasoconstriction (vā´sō-kon-strik´shŭn)(†) The constriction of the muscular wall of an artery to increase blood pressure.

vasodilation (vā-sō-dī-lā´shŭn)(†) The widening of the muscular wall of an artery to decrease blood pressure.

V code (vē kōd) A code used to identify encounters for reasons other than illness or injury, such as annual checkups, immunizations, and normal childbirth.

vector (vĕk´tər) A living organism, such as an insect, that carries microorganisms from an infected person to another person.

venipuncture (ven´i-pŭnk-chŭr)(†) The puncture of a vein, usually with a needle, for the purpose of drawing blood.

ventilation (vĕn´tə-lā´shən) Moving air in and out of the lungs; also called breathing.

ventral (vĕn´trəl) See **anterior.**

ventral root (vĕn´trəl rōot) A portion of the spinal nerve that contains axons of motor neurons only.

ventricle (vĕn´trĭ-kəl) Interconnected cavities in the brain filled with cerebrospinal fluid.

ventricular fibrillation (VF) (ven-trik´yū-lăr fĭ-bri-lā´shŭn) An abnormal heart rhythm that is the most common cause of cardiac arrest.

verbalizing (vûr´bə-līz´-ĭng) Stating what you believe the patient is suggesting or implying.

vermiform appendix (ver´mi-fōrm ə-pĕn´dĭks)(†) A structure made mostly of lymphoid tissue and projecting off the cecum. It is commonly referred to as simply the appendix.

vertical file (vûr´tĭ-kəl fīl) A filing cabinet featuring pull-out drawers that usually contain a metal frame or bar equipped to handle letter- or legal-sized documents in hanging file folders.

vertigo (vûr´tĭ g ō) Dizziness.

vesicles (vĕs´ĭ-kəlz) Small sacs within the synaptic knobs that contain chemicals called neurotransmitters.

vestibule (ves ti b´yule) The space enclosed by the labia minora.

vestibule (vĕs´tə-byōōl´) The area in the inner ear between the semicircular canals and the cochlea.

vial (vī´əl) A small glass bottle with a self-sealing rubber stopper.

vibrio (vib´rē-ō) (†) A comma-shaped bacterium.

Virtual Private Network (VPN) (vur - choo-ul prahy-vit net-wurk) These are used to connect two or more computer systems.

virulence (vîr´yə-ləns) A microorganism's disease-producing power.

virus (vī´rəs) One of the smallest known infectious agents, consisting only of nucleic acid surrounded by a protein coat; can live and grow only within the living cells of other organisms.

visceral pericardium (vis´er-ăl per-i-kar´dē-ŭm)(†) The innermost layer of the pericardium that lies directly on top of the heart; also known as the epicardium.

visceral peritoneum (vīs´er-āl per-ə-tōnē´əl) Also known as the serosa, the outermost layer of the abdominal organs that secretes serous fluid to keep the organs from sticking to each other

visceral smooth muscle (vĭs´ər-əl smōōth mŭs´əl) A type of smooth muscle containing sheets of muscle that closely contact each other. It is found in the walls of hollow organs such as the stomach, intestines, bladder, and uterus.

vitamins (vī´tə-mĭnz) Organic substances that are essential for normal body growth and maintenance and resistance to infection.

vitreous humor (vĭt´rē-əs hyōō´mər) A jelly-like substance that fills the part of the eye behind the lens and helps the eye keep its shape.

voice mail (vois māl) An advanced form of answering machine that allows a caller to leave a message when the phone line is busy.

void (void) (legal) A term used to describe something that is not legally enforceable.

volume (vŏl´yōōm) The amount of space an object, such as a drug, occupies.

vomer (vō´-mər) A thin bone that divides the nasal cavity.

voucher check (vou´chər chĕk) A business check with an attached stub, which is kept as a receipt.

vulva (vul´ vah) External female genitalia.

vulvovaginitis (vul vō vaj´i-nī´tis) Inflammation of the external female genitalia and vagina.

walk-in (wôk´ĭn) A patient who arrives without an appointment.

WAN (wŏn) Abbreviation for Wide Area Network.

warranty (wôr´ən-tē) A contract that specifies free service and replacement of parts for a piece of equipment during a certain period, usually a year.

warts (wôrts) Flesh-colored skin lesions with distinct round borders that are raised and often have small finger-like projections; also called verruca.

wave scheduling (wāv skĕj´ōol-ĭng) A system of scheduling in which the number of patients seen each hour is determined by dividing the hour by the length of the average visit and then giving that number of patients appointments with the doctor at the beginning of each hour.

Western blot test (wĕs´tərn blŏt tĕst) A blood test used to confirm enzyme-linked immunosorbent assay (ELISA) test results for HIV infection.

wet mount (wĕt mount) A preparation of a specimen in a liquid that allows the organisms to remain alive and mobile while they are being identified.

white matter (hwīt măt´ər) The outer tissue of the spinal cord that is lighter in color than **gray matter.** It contains myelinated axons.

whole blood (hōl blŭd) The total volume of plasma and formed elements, or blood in which the elements have not been separated by coagulation or centrifugation.

whole-body skin examination (hōl bŏd´ē skĭn ĭg-zăm´ə-nā´shən) An examination of the visible top layer of the entire surface of the skin, including the scalp, genital area, and areas between the toes, to look for lesions, especially suspicious moles or precancerous growths.

Wood's light examination (wŏŏdz līt ĭg-zăm´ə-nā´shən) A type of dermatologic examination in which a physician inspects the patient's skin under an ultraviolet lamp in a darkened room.

word root (wûrd rōōt) The base meaning of a medical term.

written-contract account (rĭt´n kŏn´trăkt´ ə-kount´) An agreement between the physician and patient stating that the patient will pay a bill in more than four installments.

X12 837 Health Care Claim (hĕlth kâr klām) An electronic claim transaction that is the **HIPAA** Health Care Claim or Equivalent Encounter Information ("HIPAA claim").

xeroradiography (zē´rō-rā´dē-og´ră-fē)(†) A radiologic procedure in which x-rays are developed with a powder toner, similar to the toner in photocopiers, and the x-ray image is processed on specially treated xerographic paper; used to diagnose breast cancer, abscesses, lesions, or calcifications.

xiphoid process (zif´oyd prŏs´ĕs)(†) The lower extension of the breastbone; the cartilaginous tip of the sternum.

yeast (yēst) A fungus that grows mainly as a single-celled organism and reproduces by budding.

yoga (yō´-gə) A series of poses and breathing exercises that provide awareness of the unity of the whole being. The practice of yoga also increases flexibility and strength.

yolk sac (yōk săk) The sac that holds the materials for the nutrition of the embryo.

zip drive (zˇĭp drˉĭv) A Zip drive is a high-capacity floppy disk drive developed by Iomega®. Zip disks are slightly larger and about twice as thick as a conventional floppy disk. Zip drives can hold 100 to 750 MB of data. They are durable and relatively inexpensive. They may be used for backing up hard disks and transporting large files.

zona pellucida (zō´nă pe-lū´sid-ă)(†) A layer that surrounds the cell membrane of an egg.

Z-track method (zē´trăk mĕth´əd) A technique used when injecting an intramuscular (IM) drug that can irritate subcutaneous tissue; involves pulling the skin and subcutaneous tissue to the side before inserting the needle at the site, creating a zigzag path in the tissue layers that prevents the drug from leaking into the subcutaneous tissue and causing irritation.

zygomatic (zī-gə-m´a-tik) The bones that form the prominence of the cheeks.

zygote (zī´gōt) The cell that is formed from the union of the egg and sperm.

CREDITS

Photo Credits

CHAPTER 1
Fig. 1.1(a-b): © Total Care Programming, Inc.; Fig. 1.2: © Royalty-Free/Corbis; Page 16: © David Kelly Crow; Fig. 1.4: © Somos/Veer/Getty Images RF.

CHAPTER 2
Fig. 2.1: © Donn Thompson/Getty Images; Fig. 2.2: © Royalty-Free/Corbis; Fig. 2.3: © Lester Lefkowitz/Getty Images; Page 32: © John Cole, Photo Researchers, Inc.; Fig. 2.4: © Time & Life Pictures/Getty Images; Fig. 2.5: © David Kelly Crow; Fig. 2.6: © Creatas/Punchstock RF; Fig. 2.7: © Will and Deni McIntrye.

CHAPTER 4
Fig. 4.3: © Sean Justice/Getty Images; Fig. 4.4: © Cliff Moore; Fig. 4.5: © Richard Shock/Getty Images; Fig. 4.6: © Cliff Moore.

CHAPTER 5
Fig. 5.1: © Duncan Smith/Getty Images RF; Fig. 5.3: © Comstock Images/Alamy RF; Fig. 5.5: © Terry Wild Studio; Fig. 5.6: © David Kelly Crow; Fig. 5.7: © Total Care Programming, Inc.; Fig. 5.8: © Terry Wild Studio; Fig. 5.9: © PNC/Digital Vision/Getty Images RF.

CHAPTER 6
Fig. 6.2, Fig. 6.4, Fig. 6.7, Fig. 6.8: Courtesy of Total Care Programming, Inc.; Fig. 6.10: © Photodisc Collection/Getty Images RF; Fig. 6.11: Courtesy of Total Care Programming, Inc.; Fig. 6.12: Tim Flach/Getty Images.

CHAPTER 7
Fig. 7.1: Courtesy of Total Care Programming, Inc.; Fig. 7.12-Fig. 7.13: © Cliff Moore.

CHAPTER 8
Fig. 8.1, Fig. 8.5: © David Kelly Crow.

CHAPTER 9
Fig. 9.1: © Hank Morgan/Photo Researchers, Inc.; Fig. 9.6: © UpperCut Images/Getty Images; Fig. 9.7: Courtesy of Total Care Programming, Inc.; Fig. 9.9: © David Kelly Crow; Page 208: © Kathy Sloan; Fig. 9.10: © David Kelly Crow.

CHAPTER 10
Fig. 10.1: © Image Source/Jupiter Images RF; Fig. 10.2, Fig. 10.4: Courtesy Bibbero Systems, Inc. Petaluma, CA (800) 242.2376, www.bibbero.com; Fig. 10.5: © Image Source/Jupiter Images; Fig. 10.7: © Jon Feingersh/Getty Images; Page 235: © Stewart Cohen/Pam Ostrow/Getty Images RF.

CHAPTER 11
Fig. 11.2: Courtesy of Total Care Programming, Inc.; Fig. 11.4: © Terry Wild Studio.

CHAPTER 12
Fig. 12.8: © Terry Wild Studio.

CHAPTER 13
Page 281: Courtesy of Total Care Programming, Inc.; Fig. 13.2: © Keith Brofsky/Getty Images RF; Fig. 13.3: © Royalty-Free/Corbis; Fig. 13.4: © Cliff Moore; Fig. 13.5: © Terry Wild Studio; Fig. 13.6: Rob Melnychuk/Digital Vision/Getty Images RF; Fig. 13.7: © Stockbyte/Getty Images RF.

CHAPTER 14
Fig. 14.1: © Terry Wild Studio; Fig. 14.2: © Image Source/Getty Images RF; Fig. 14.5: © Terry Wild Studio; Page 311: © Ken Lax.

CHAPTER 15
Fig. 15.3: © David Kelly Crow.

CHAPTER 17
Fig. 17.4: © Stockbyte RF.

CHAPTER 18
Fig. 18.8: Courtesy of Total Care Programming, Inc.; Fig. 18.10: © Terry Wild Studio.

Text and Line Art Credits

FRONTMATTER
Correlation of Text to ABHES Competencies–Reprinted with permission from the Medical Assistant Education Review Board. All rights reserved.

Correlation of Text to AMT Task List-© 2009 AMT. All rights reserved.; Reprinted with permission from the Medical Assistant Education Review Board. All rights reserved

Correlation of Text to CAAHEP Core Curriculum for Medical Assistants- Reprinted with permission from the Medical Assistant Education Review Board. All rights reserved.

Correlation of Text to Occupational Analysis of the CMA (AAMA)- Reprinted with permission from the Medical Assistant Education Review Board. All rights reserved.

Certified Medical Administrative Specialists (CMAS)–Reprinted with permission from the Medical Assistant Education Review Board. All rights reserved.

Correlation of Text to National Healthcareer Association (NHA) Medical Assisting Duty/Task List-© 2003-2009 National Healthcareer Association. All rights Reserved.

CHAPTER 3
Pages 41–42: *Law & Ethics for Medical Careers*, 4th ed. Judson/Hicks/Harrison, McGraw-Hill, 2006, ISBN 0-07-302263-2.; Page 44: *Law & Ethics for Medical Careers*, 4th ed. Judson/Hicks/Harrison, McGraw-Hill, 2006, ISBN 007-302263-2.: Page 56: *Law & Ethics for Medical Careers*, 4th ed. Judson/Hicks/Harrison, McGraw-Hill, 2006, ISBN 007-302263-2.; Pages 61–62: *Law & Ethics for Medical Careers*, 4th ed. Judson/Hicks/Harrison, McGraw-Hill, 2006, ISBN 007-302263-2.; Pages 62–63: *Law & Ethics for Medical Careers*, 4th ed. Judson/Hicks/Harrison, McGraw-Hill, 2006, ISBN 007-302263-2.

CHAPTER 4
Fig. 4-2: Maslow's Pyramid.; Page 85-Adapted with permission of Atria Books, a Division of Simon & Schuster, Inc. from THE STRESS SOLUTION: An Action Plan to Manage the Stress in Your Life by Lyle H. Miller, Ph.D. and Alma Dell Smith, Ph.D. with Larry R. Rothstein, Ed.D. Copyright © 1993 by Lyle H. Miller, Alma Dell Smith, and Larry Rothstein

CHAPTER 5
Fig. 5-4: Reprinted with permission of Heavenly Office. www.heavenlyoffice.com.

CHAPTER 6
Fig. 6-6: Corel, permissions@corel.com, Fig. 6-9: Manage Bytes Software. support@managebytes.com

CHAPTER 7
Fig. 7-8: Reprinted with permission from English Plus. Copyright © English Plus. All rights reserved.

CHAPTER 8
Fig. 8-6: Reprinted with permission from Bibbero Systems, Inc., Petaloma, CA (800)242-2376, www.bibbero.com

CHAPTER 9
Fig. 9-11: The Medical Record Audit form was provided by the American Medical Association/Specialty Society Medical Liability Project.

CHAPTER 10
Table 10-1: Source: Adapted from William A. Sabin, The Gregg Reference Manual, 10th ed. (Columbus, OH: Glencoe/McGraw-Hill, 2005)

CHAPTER 12
Fig. 12-4: Screen capture of Office Hours Professional courtesy of McKesson Corporation.

CHAPTER 15
Fig. 15-1: Copyright 2007. The Managed Care Information Center., Fig. 15-7: NUCC www.nucc.org.

CHAPTER 16
Fig. 16-2: CPT copyright 2008 American Medical Association. All rights reserved. CPT is a registered trademark of the American Medical Association.

CHAPTER 17
Fig. 17-6: Reprinted with permission from Bibbero Systems, Inc., Petaloma, CA (800)242-2376, www.bibbero.com

INDEX

Page numbers in **boldface** indicate figures. Page numbers followed by b indicate box features, p procedures, and t tables, respectively.

A

AAMA. *See* American Association of Medical Assistants
Abandonment, 49
ABA number, 395
Abbreviations
    appointment book, 262
    claims form processing, 325t
    mailing, 150t, 162, 162t
    medical, in patient records, 201, 201t
ABHES. *See* Accrediting Bureau of Health Education Schools
ABMS. *See* American Board of Medical Specialties
ABN. *See* Advance Beneficiary Notice of Noncoverage
Acceptance, in stages of dying/grief, 86–87
Access
    to files, limiting, 229, **229**
    to patient records, for minors, 211
Accessibility, of office, 286, **286,** 290–291, **291,** 292p
Accessories, in reception area decor, 282–283
Account(s)
    open-book, 370
    past-due
        age-analysis of, **374,** 374, 375p
        collection of, 370–378
    single-entry, 370
    tax liability, 411
    written-contract, 370
Accounting, 384–419
    accuracy of, importance of, 386
    basic, 363
    computerized, 386–387
    establishing procedures for, 386
    patient, methods of, 386–393
    pegboard system of, 392–393
    setting up system of, 392p
    single-entry system of, 387–392
    software for, 134
Accounts payable (A/P), 363, 388
    categories of, 402
    management of, 402
    setting up system of, 402p
Accounts receivable (A/R), 363, 378, 388
Accreditation, 10, 12–13
    AAMA standards for, 12–13
    definition of, 12
    topics covered in programs with, 12
Accredited Records Technician (ART), 31
Accrediting Bureau of Health Education Schools (ABHES), 10, 12
Accuracy
    of bookkeeping and banking, 386
    of patient records, 204
ACP. *See* American College of Physicians
Acquired immune deficiency syndrome. *See* HIV/AIDS
Active files, *vs.* inactive or closed, 230–231
Active listening, 78–79, **79**
Active voice, in writing, 152–154
Activity-monitoring systems, 139

Acupuncturists, 30
ADA. *See* Americans with Disabilities Act of 1990
Adding machines, 110
Add-on codes, of CPT, 351
Address(es)
    change, and payment collection, 382
    delivery, 161, **161**
    format on envelope, 162
    inside, **149,** 149–150
    placement on envelope, 161, **161**
    USPS abbreviations for, 162, 162t
Address labels, 148
ADEA. *See* Age Discrimination in Employment Act of 1967
Administrative assistant, medical, 31
Administrative duties
    advanced, 16
    daily, of medical assistants, 15–17
    entry-level, 15
    importance of, 98
    and law, 52
    simplification of, HIPAA and, 62
Administrative supplies, 173, 174t, 175
ADNs. *See* Associate degrees in nursing
Adolescent(s), minor status of, 47, 211
    emancipated, 367
    mature, 211
    payment responsibility in, 367
Adolescent medicine, 29
Advance Beneficiary Notice of Noncoverage (ABN), 331, **332**
Advanced duties
    administrative, 16
    clinical, 17
    laboratory, 17
Advance directive, 56
Advance scheduling, 263
Advice, telephone requests for, 247
Age analysis, of past-due accounts, **374,** 374, 375p
Age Discrimination in Employment Act of 1967 (ADEA), 67
Agency, law of, 50
Agenda, for meeting, 274
Agent, 50
Aggressive behavior, in communication, 81, 81t
Aging. *See* Elderly patients
Agreement
    in contracts, 46
    externship, 13, **14**
AHA. *See* American Hospital Association
AHDI. *See* Association for Healthcare Documentation Integrity
AHIMA. *See* American Health Information Management Association
Airmail supplies, 163
Alcohol dependence, patient education resources on, 310t
Allergies
    medical specialty in, 27
    patient education resources on, 310t
Allergist, 27

Allied health profession(s)
    medical assisting as, 9
    working with others, 30
All-in-one printer, 132, **132**
Allowable benefits, 328
Allowed charges, 330
Allscripts, 205
Alphabetic filing system, **222,** 222–223
    color coding in, 225–226
    indexing rules in, 222–223, 224b
    personal names in, 223t, 224b
Alphabetic Index, of ICD-9-CM, 344–346, **345**
Alzheimer's disease, 86
    patient education on, 306, 310t
Alzheimer's Disease Education and Referral Center, 310t
AMA. *See* American Medical Association
American Academy of Medical Administrators, 32b
American Academy of Otolaryngology, 29
American Academy of Pediatrics, 310t
American Academy of Professional Coders, 358b
American Association of Medical Assistants (AAMA), 38, 39t
    accreditation standards of, 12–13
    certification by, 10–11
        for office administrator or manager, 32b
        pins designating, 9, **9**
    code of ethics, 9–10, 21, 65b, 66
    creation of, 9–10
    creed of, 9
    definition of medical assisting, 15
    malpractice insurance from, 50
    networking in, 12
    Occupational Analysis of CMA, 10, 21
    professional support from, 11–12, **12**
    purpose of, 9
American Association of Nurse Anesthetists, 27
American Banking Association (ABA) number, 395
American Board of Medical Specialties (ABMS), 26, 29
American Board of Physical Medicine and Rehabilitation, 29
American Cancer Society, 310t
American Collectors Association International, 377b
American College of Physicians (ACP), 38, 39t
American Diabetes Association, 310t
American Dietetic Association, 310t
American Health Information Management Association (AHIMA), 230, 358b
American Heart Association, 310t
American Hospital Association (AHA), 38, 39t, 66, 233
American Medical Association (AMA), 39t, 40
    and authorization of disclosure, 64
    code of ethics, 65–66
    CPT coding of, 351–356
    Internet resources of, 136t
    and retention of files/records, 233
American Medical Informatics Association and Health Email, 134

American Medical Technologists (AMT), 39t, 40
  certification by, 9, 11, 40
    for office administrator or manager, 32b
    pins designating, 9, **9**
  professional support from, 12
American Pharmacists Association (APhA), 39t, 40
American Red Cross, 13–15
American Registry of Radiologic Technologists, 33
American Society of Clinical Pathology (ASCP), 33, 39t
American Society of Phlebotomy Technicians (ASPT), 39t
Americans with Disabilities Act of 1990 (ADA), 67, 286, 290–291
AMT. *See* American Medical Technologists
Anatomical models, for patient education, 309, **309**
Anatomic pathologist, 29
Anesthesiology, 27
Anesthetist(s), 27
Anesthetist's assistant, 36
Anger, in stages of dying/grief, 86
Angry patient, communication with, 82
Annotating mail, 166
Answering machine, 105
Answering service, 105, 252, 253p
Antivirus software, 140
Anxiety. *See* Anxious patient
Anxious patient
  communication with, 82, **83**, 83p
  preoperative, patient education for, 309
A/P. *See* Accounts payable
APhA. *See* American Pharmacists Association
Appearance
  neat, of medical assistants, 19–20
  of patient records, 203–204
Application software, 132–138
Appointment(s)
  advance, 263
  arranging, 266–268
  cancellations of, 270
  missed, 270
    charging for, 270
    documentation of, 53, 270
    reminders for patients with history of, 268
  new patient, 266–267
  reminders of, 267–268, **268**
  return, 267
  scheduling of, 258–277
    cluster, 263, 266p
    combination, 266
    computerized, 266, **267**
    for diabetic patients, 269
    double-booking, 263
    for emergencies, 268, 269p
    for fasting patients, 269
    for late arrivals, 270
    modified-wave, 263, **265**
    online, 266
    open-hours, 262–263
    outside appointments, 271
    patient information on, 302
    patient situations and, 268–270
    physician situations and, 270
    for referrals, 268–269
    for repeat visits, 269
    software for, 134
    special situations and, 268–270
    standard procedure times and, 262
    for surgery, 271, 271p, **272**

systems of, 262–266
  telephone calls for, 245
  time-specific, 263, **264**
  wave, 263
  walk-ins and, 270
  wrong-day, 270
Appointment book, 260–262
  abbreviations used in, 262
  as legal record, 52, 262
  matrix for, 260, **261**
  obtaining patient information for, 260–262
  preparation of, 260
Appointment cards, 267, **268**
A/R. *See* Accounts receivable
Arbitration, 49–50
Area codes, 253
ART. *See* Accredited Records Technician
Arthritis, patient education resources on, 310t
Arthritis Foundation, 310t
ASCP. *See* American Society of Clinical Pathology
Assault, 45
Assertiveness skills, 81, 81t
Assessment, in patient record, 203
Assignment, Medicaid, 322
Assignment of benefits, 331
Associate degrees in nursing (ADNs), 35
Association(s), 38–40, 39t
  membership in, 11–12
  networking in, 12
  patient education resources of, 309, 310t
  professional support from, 11–12, **12**
Association for Healthcare Documentation Integrity (AHDI), 38, 39t
Asthma, patient education resources on, 310t
Asthma and Allergy Foundation of America, 310t
Attention
  to detail, 18
  physician's, telephone calls requiring, 244
  to telephone caller, 250
Attention line, in business letter, 150
Attitude
  positive, 20
  professional, in medical records, 204
Attorneys, telephone calls from, 248
Audit of patient records, 211, **212–213**
  external, 211
  internal, 211
  prospective, 211
  retrospective, 211
Authorization
  AMA forms for, 64
  HIPAA and, 60
Automated menu, for telephone calls, 106b
Automated telephone triage, 254
Automation equipment, 110–116
  adding machines and calculators, 110
  check writers, 114, 115p
  dictation-transcription, 113–114, **114**, 115p
  folding and inserting machines, 111, **112**
  microfiche readers, 116, **117**
  microfilm readers, 116, **117**
  paper shredders, 114–116, **116**, 116b
  photocopiers, 110, 111p
Autopsies, 29
Awakening Phase, 93–94

B

Baccalaureate nurse, 35
Bachelor of science in nursing (BSN), 35

Backup systems, 120, **139**, 139–140
Bait and switch, 187
Balance billing, 330
Balance checkbook, electronic option for, 399, **399**
Bandwidth, 130
Banking, 394–399
  accuracy in, importance of, 386
  deposits, **396**, 396–397, 397p, 399
  electronic, 397–399
    advantages of, 397
    balance checkbook, 399, **399**
    bill-paying, 399
    checkbook display, 399
    payroll handing through, 408b, 409–411
    recording deposits in, 399
  establishing procedures for, 386
  tasks of, 394
  telephone, 401b
Bank statements
  example of, **398**
  reconciliation of, 397, 400p–401p
Bargaining, in stages of dying/grief, 86
Bariatrics, 27
Basic needs, 75–77
Battery (crime), 45
Battery power backup, 120
Beepers. *See* Pagers
Benefits, insurance
  allowable, 328
  assignment of, 331
  explanation of, 328
  lifetime maximum, 317
Better Business Bureau, 187
Billing, 31, 361–383
  balance, 330
  coding for, 31, 342–360
  collection, 370–378. *See also* Collection
  cycle, 370
  electronic, 370
  ethics of, 66
  false claims in, 57
  health insurance, 315–341. *See also* Insurance claims
  independent service for, 370
  invoices for, 148, 368–370, **369**
  software for, 134
  standard procedures for, 367–370
  statements for, 148, 372–374
  superbills, 148, 353, 354, **354**, 370, **371**, 372p
  telephone inquiries about, patient, 245
Billing cycles, managing, 370
Billing provider, 339b
Bill of Rights, Patient's, 66
Bill-paying, electronic, 399
Binders, for files, 222, 227
Bioethics, 65–66
Biopsy, 29
Birthday rule, in insurance coverage, 326
Blindness. *See also* Visual impairments
  ICD-9-CM coding for, 345–346
Bloodborne pathogens. *See also* HIV/AIDS
  OSHA protection standards against, 57
  Standard Precautions against, 57
Bloodborne Pathogens Protection Standards of 1991, 57
Blue Cross and Blue Shield, 323
Board of Primary Care and Orthopedics, 29
Body, of business letter, **149**, 151
Body language, 78
Bone infection, CPT coding for, 354

Bookkeeping, 386–393
  accounts payable, 363, 388
  accounts receivable, 363, 378, 388
  accuracy in, importance of, 386
  on computer, 386–387
  daily log, **387**, 387–388
  disbursement record, 388
  establishing procedures for, 386
  patient ledger card, 387, 388, **389**
  pegboard system of, 392–393
  setting up system of, 392p
  single-entry system of, 387–392
  summary of charges, receipts, and
    disbursements, 388–392, **391**
Booklets, for patient education, 297–298
Books, in reception area, 287
Boundaries, setting, 90
Bound printed matter, mailing, 163
Boxes, for filing, 219–220
Brace, in ICD-9-CM coding, 347
Brackets, in ICD-9-CM, 347
Breach of contract, 46
Brochures, for patient education, 297–298
Brownout Phase, 94
BSN. *See* Bachelor of science in nursing
Budget, for office supplies, 180
Bulletin board, 288–289, **289**
Burnout
  definition of, 93
  prevention of, 93–94
  stages leading to, 93–94
Business letter
  folding and inserting, 156, **160**
  parts of, **149**, 149–151
  procedure for creating, 159p–160p
Business side of practice, 386
  accounting, 384–419
  banking, 386, 394–399
  billing, 367–370
  bookkeeping, 386–393
  collection, 370–378
  payment, 363–367

C

CAAHEP. *See* Commission on Accreditation of
  Allied Health Education Programs
Cabinets
  filing, 219
  storage, 175
Cable modem, 128
Calculators, 110
Calm in crisis, 20
Cancellations, of appointments, 270
Cancer
  care and treatment in (oncology), 28
  patient education resources on, 310t
*Candidate's Guide to the Certification
  Examination*, 11
Capitation, 318, 330–331
Cardboard tubs or boxes, for filing, 219–220
Cardiologists, 27
Cardiology, 27
Caring, and malpractice prevention, 51
Carpal tunnel syndrome, computer use and,
  129, 129b
Carpeting, in reception area, 282
Cartridge(s), for file storage, 232
Cash flow statement, 405
Cashier's check, 394
Cash-only basis, 365
Cash payment, 365, **365**

Cash payment journal, 387
Category II codes, 351
Category III codes, 351
Cause of illnesses, multicultural attitudes
  and, 84b
Caution
  cleanliness in reception area, 285b
  warning signs of disease, 301
CC. *See* Chief complaints
CCA. *See* Certified Coding Assistant
CCS-P. *See* Certified Coding
  Specialist–Physician-based
CD burner or recorder (CD-R), 130, 142
CDC. *See* Centers for Disease Control and
  Prevention
CD-ROM, 130, **131**
  care and maintenance of, 141, **141**
  file storage on, 232
  patient education via, 309
  research via, 136
CD-ROM drive, 130
CEJA. *See* Council of Ethical and Judicial
  Affairs
Cellular (cell) phones, 104, 120, 248, 255
Centers for Disease Control and Prevention
  (CDC), 310t
  Internet resources of, 134
  Standard Precautions, 57
Centers for Medicare and Medicaid Services
  (CMS), 318, 319, 347, 353
Central processing unit (CPU), 130
Certification, 10–11
  AAMA, 9, **9**, 10–11, 32b
  AMT, 9, **9**, 11, 40
  benefits of, 13
  examinations for
    eligibility for, 11
    major areas of, 11
  pins designating, 9, **9**
  recertification requirements, 11
  state and federal regulations on, 10
Certified check, 394
Certified Coding Assistant (CCA), 358b
Certified Coding Specialist–Physician-based
  (CCS-P), 358b
Certified laboratory assistant, 36
Certified mail, 164, **165**, 168
Certified Medical Assistant (CMA), 10–11, 16b
  duties and skills of, 16b
  educational requirements for, 16b
  examination for, major areas of, 11
  nature of job, 16b
  Occupational Analysis of, 10, 21
  as office administrator or manager, 32b
  pins worn by, 9, **9**
  professional support for, 11–12, **12**
  workplace settings for, 16b
Certified Office Laboratory Technician
  (COLT), 10
Certified pharmacy technician (CPhT), 33, 37
Certified Professional Coder (CPC), 358b
Certified Professional Coder-Apprentice
  (CPC-A), 358b
Certified registered nurse anesthetist
  (CRNA), 27
CF. *See* Conversion factor
CHAMPVA, 323
Charge(s), 328–332
  allowed, 330
  appropriate, determining, 363
  communication with patients about, 331
  fee schedule, 328–332, 363, **364**
  patient, calculation of, 331

  summary of, 388–392, **391**
  usual and customary fees, 363
Charge slips, **364**, 364–365
Charts. *See* Patient records
Check(s), 394–397
  accepting, 395–396
  cashier's, 394
  certified, 394
  correctly written, 395, **395**
  counter, 403
  depositing, **396**, 396–397, 397p
  endorsing, **395**, 396
  limited, 403
  negotiable, 393
  paychecks, preparation of, 408
  returned (NSF), 393, 394p
  third-party, 395
  traveler's, 403
  voided, 144, 403
  voucher, 403
  writing, for disbursement, 403
Checkbook balancing, electronic, 399, **399**
Checkbook display, electronic, 399
Checkbook register, 387, 388
Check codes, 395
Checking accounts, types of, 395
Check payment, 365
Checkup. *See* General physical exam
Check writers, 114
  operating, 115p
  voiding check, 114
CHEDDAR format, 203
Chief complaints (CC), 344, 354
Children
  access to medical records, 211
  anxious, communication with, 82,
    83, 83p
  care and treatment of (pediatrics), 29
  communicating with, 87–88
  health plan for, 323
  in reception area
    accommodation for, 284
    items for, 289, **289**, 290p
Chiropractors, 30
Chronological filing, 225
Chronological order, in patient records, 202
Civil law, 45, 49
Civil penalties, HIPAA, 62
Civil Rights Act of 1964, Title VII of, 66
Civil Rights Act of 1991, 67
Claim(s), insurance. *See* Insurance claims
Claim scrubber, 338
Clarifying, in therapeutic communication, 80
Clarity
  in patient record, 201
  in writing, 154
Classes, for patient education, 299
Clean insurance claims, 338
Cleanliness, of reception area, 284–286, 285b
Clearinghouse, for electronic claims, 338
CLIA '88. *See* Clinical Laboratory
  Improvement Amendments of 1988
  (CLIA '88)
Client's words, in patient record, 200–201
Clinical duties
  advanced, 17
  entry-level, 16–17
Clinical Laboratory Improvement
  Amendments of 1988 (CLIA '88), 10
Clinical laboratory technician (CLT), 31
Clinical supplies, 173, 174t, 175–176
Clinics, 68
Clock speed, 130

Closed files
    active *vs.*, 230–231
    storage of, 231–233
Closed posture, 78
CLT. *See* Clinical laboratory technician
Cluster scheduling, 263, 266p
CMA Today, 11
CMS. *See* Centers for Medicare and Medicaid
        Services
CMS-1500 claim, 333–338, **334,**
        335p–337p, 351
Code first underlying disease, in ICD-9-CM
        coding, 348
Code linkage, 356–357
Code of ethics, 60–66
    AAMA, 9–10, 21, 65b, 66
    AMA, 65–66
*Code of Medical Ethics: Current Opinions with
        Annotations* (AMA), 65–66
Codes for Laterality, 349
Coding
    filing, 225–226, **226,** 229
    medical, 31, 62, 326, 342–360
        compliance with, 356–358
        CPT, **350,** 351–356
        diagnosis, 344–349
        HCPCS, 62, 353–354, 355p
        HIPAA and, 344, 351
        ICD-9-CM, 62, 344–349
        ICD-10-CM, 348–349
        ICD-10-PCS, 348–349
        on invoices, 369–370
Coding, billing, and insurance specialist, 381b
Coding specialists, 358b
Coinsurance, 317
Collection
    address change/relocation and, 382
    age analysis and, **374,** 374, 375p
    common problems in, 380–382
    hardship cases and, 381–382
    laws governing, 374–377, 376t
    letters for, 372, **373**
    standard procedures of, 370–378
    statute of limitations and, 370
    techniques for, 372–374
    telephone calls for, 372
Collection agencies, 377–378, 377b
Colon, in ICD-9-CM coding, 347
Color(s), in reception area decor, 282
Color coding, in filing, 225–226, **226**
Color family, 282
COLT. *See* Certified Office Laboratory
        Technician
Combination codes, 348–349
Combination scheduling, 266
Commercial records centers, 232, **232**
Commission on Accreditation of Allied Health
        Education Programs (CAAHEP), 10, 12
Communication, 71–97
    about charges, 331
    with AIDS/HIV patient, 88
    with angry patient, 82
    with anxious patient, 82, **83,** 83p
    community resources for, 90–91, 92p
    with coworkers, 88–90
    with elderly patient, 86, 87b
    electronic, 134–136
    with families and friends, 88
    humanizing, in medical office, 75
    interview. *See* Interview, patient
    and malpractice prevention, 51
    with management, 89
    negative verbal, 77

    nonverbal, 78
    with parents, 88
    with patients, 73–88
    with patients of other cultures, 82–85
    with patient who is mentally or
        emotionally disturbed, 86
    with patient with hearing impairment, **85,**
        85–86
    with patient with visual impairment, 85
    positive verbal, 77
    in special circumstances, 82–88
    with terminally ill patients, 86–87
    types of, 77–78
    via telephone. *See* Telephone calls
    written, 90–92, 146. *See also*
        Correspondence; Letter(s)
    with young patient, 87–88
Communication circle, **74,** 74–75
Communication equipment, 103–110, **104**
    fax machine, 107, 108p–109p, **110**
    pagers (beepers), 105–107, 255
    telephones, 103–105. *See also*
        Telephone calls
    typewriters, 107–110
Communication skills
    improving, 78–81
    as personal qualification of medical
        assistants, 20
    for telephone calls, 242
    therapeutic, 79–81
Community-assistance directory, 298–299
Community resources, 90–91, 92p, 309
Compactible files, 219
Compensation, as defense mechanism, 80
Competence
    and accreditation, 10
    areas of, 21
    and malpractice prevention, 51
Competitive prices, for office supplies,
        180–182
Complaints
    chief, in coding, 344, 354
    patient, via telephone, 247
Completeness, of patient record, 201
Compliance
    coding, 356–358
    patient, 192
Compliance plan, 357–358
Complimentary closing, in business letter,
        149, 151
Comprehensive Drug Abuse Prevention and
        Control Act of 1970, 53
Computer(s), 123–144
    activity-monitoring systems for, 139
    antivirus software and firewalls, 140
    backup systems for, 120, **139,** 139–140
    banking on, 397–399
    bookkeeping on, 386–387
    care and maintenance of, 140–142
    carpal tunnel syndrome with use,
        129, 129b
    choosing vendor for, 139
    components of, 126–133, **128**
    contamination, preventing, 140
    disaster recovery plan, 142
    file storage on, 232
    of future, 142
    hardware, 126–132
    HIPAA and, 60–61, 117, 140b
    input devices, 127–130
    invoice generation by, 370
    network, 126, 138–139
    output devices, 130–132

    passwords, 139, 339–340
    patient education resources on, 309, 310t
    patient records on, 204–205, **205,** 218
    payroll handling on, 408b, 409–411
    processing devices, 130
    safeguarding confidential files on, 139
    security of, 60–61, 139–140, 140b,
        338–340
    selecting, 138–139
    software, 127, 132–138
    storage devices, 130
    tickler files on, 227
    types of, 125–126
    upgrading system, 138
Computer-generated invoices and
        statements, 148
Computerized scheduling, 266, **267**
Computer Revolution, 125
Conciseness
    in patient record, 201
    in writing, 152
Concurrent care, in CPT coding, 354
Conference calls, 248, 254
Confidentiality
    computer, 139
    ethical issues of, 63–64
    HIPAA and, 58–60, 198b
    legal issues of, 56, 63–64
    mandatory disclosure *vs.*, 63–64, 63b–64b
    in numeric filing system, 225
    patient information on, 302–303
    of patient records, 58–60, 202, 211
Conflict, dealing with, 89–90
Confusion, in elderly patients, 86
Consent, 47
    implied, 47
    informed, 47, 193, **197**
Consent for Surgery form, **307**
Consent for Treatment form, 303, **304**
Consideration
    in contracts, 46
    as interpersonal skill, 79
Consumer Credit Protection Act, 378
Consumer education, 299
Consumer rights, 44
Contagious patients, 284, 292–293
Contaminated supplies, 17
Content, editing for, 156
Continuing education, 11
Contract(s), 46–48
    breach of, 46
    expressed, 46
    implied, 46
    legal elements of, 46
    medical assistant, 46
    patient-physician, 46–48
    types of, 46
    void, 46
Contracted fee schedule, 330
Controlled substances, 53
    disposal of, 53, **54–55**
    storage of, 175
Controlled Substances Act of 1970 (CSA), 53
Conventional medical records, 202
Conventions, ICD-9-CM, 347–348
Conversion factor (CF), 330
Coordination of benefits, 326
Copayment, 317
    forgiveness or waiver of, 357
Copiers. *See* Photocopiers
Coping strategies, 80
Copy machine. *See* Photocopiers
Corporations, 68

Corrections, in medical record, 53, 204, 208, 209p
Correspondence, 145–170. *See also* Mail
  basic rules for, 156, 157t
  business letter, **149**, 149–151, 159p–160p
  editing and proofreading of, 154–156
  effective writing in, 152–154
  inclusion in patient records, 197
  interoffice memorandums, 154, **155**
  letter format, 151
  letter styles, 151–152, **152, 153, 154**
  misspellings in, common, 156, 158t–159t
  and professionalism, 147, **147**
  punctuation style in, 151
  signing, 161
  supplies for, choosing, 147–148
  types in medical office, 148–149
  written, 148–156
Cost controls, 182
Council of Ethical and Judicial Affairs (CEJA), 40
Counseling, in CPT coding, 354
Counter checks, 403
Couriers, 166
Courtesy
  professional, in payment, 367
  in telephone calls, 250
Courtesy phone, patient, 104
Courtesy title, 149
Courtroom conduct, 50
Covered entity, 116b
Coworkers
  boundaries with, setting, 90
  communicating with, 88–90
  conflict with, dealing with, 89–90
  rapport with, 88, **88**
CPC. *See* Certified Professional Coder
CPC-A. *See* Certified Professional Coder-Apprentice
CPhT. *See* Certified pharmacy technician
CPT, 62, 351–356
  add-on codes of, 351
  Category II codes of, 351
  Category III codes of, 351
  evaluation and management services in, 351–353
  for immunizations, 353
  for laboratory procedures, 353
  locating code, 354, 356p
  modifiers in, 351, 352t, 355
  new *vs.* established patient in, 352, 354
  organization of manual, **350**, 351
  panels of, 353
  for superbills, 353, **354**
  for surgical procedures, **350**, 353
  symbols in, 351, **352**
  unlisted procedure codes of, 351
  updates of, 351
  using, 354–356
CPT 4, 62
CPU. *See* Central processing unit
Cramming, telephone, 255
Credentials, 10–11
  AAMA, 10–11
  state and federal regulations on, 10
Credit
  arrangements for, 378–380
  extension of, 379–380
    laws governing, 378–379
    mutual agreement on, 379–380
    unilateral decision on, 379
Credit balance, 367, 368p
Credit bureau, 378

Credit card payment, 365–366, **366**
Credit check, 378
Credit report, 378, **379**
Creed, AAMA, 9
Crime, 45
Criminal law, 45
Criminal penalties, HIPAA, 62
Crisis, remaining calm in, 20
Critical thinking skills, 17
CRNA. *See* Certified registered nurse anesthetist
Cross-references
  in filing system, 228–229
  in ICD-9-CM coding, 346
Cross-training, 15, 92
CSA. *See* Controlled Substances Act of 1970
Culture (ethnic)
  and attitudes about modern medicine, 84b
  beliefs in, respecting, 305b
  and communication, 82–85
  and patient information packet, 303
  and reception area, 291–292
Current Procedural Terminology. See CPT
Custodial parents, and payment responsibility, 367
Customary fees, 363
Customer service, 74
Cycle billing, 370

D

Daily duties, of medical assistants, 15–17
Daily journal. *See* Daily log
Daily log, in bookkeeping, **387**, 387–388, 403
Damages, in negligence, 49
Data, direct entry of, 338
Database, 132, 202
Database management, 134
Data elements, of HIPAA claim, 333, 339b
Data errors, proofreading for, 156
Data mailers, 148
Dateline, in business letter, 149, **149**
Dates, tickler files and, 226–227, 227p
Dating, of patient records, 197–199
Day sheet. *See* Daily log
DDE. *See* Direct data entry
DEA. *See* Drug Enforcement Administration
Deaf. *See* Hearing loss
Death, 86–87
Debit card payment, 365
Debt collection. *See* Collection
Decor, of reception area, **282**, 282–283
Deductible, in insurance, 317
  forgiveness or waiver of, 357
Deductions, from pay, 406
Defamation of character, 45
Defense mechanisms, 80–81
Delayed treatment, 49
Delivery addresses, 161, **161**
Delivery confirmation, 164
Delivery services
  express, 164
  messengers and couriers, 166
  overnight, 163
  regular mail, 163–164
  special, 164
  United Parcel Service, 164
  U.S. Postal Service, 163–164
Dementia. *See also* Alzheimer's disease
  patient education for patients with, 306

Denial
  in elderly patients, 86
  in stages of dying/grief, 86
Denial, as defense mechanism, 80
Dental assistant, 36
Dependents, number of, 406, **407**
Deposits, bank, **396**, 396–397, 397p, 399
Depression (mood)
  in elderly patients, 86
  in stages of dying/grief, 86
Dereliction, in negligence, 49
Dermatologists, 27
Dermatology, 27
Desktop computers, 126, **126**
Detail, attention to, 18
Developmental stages, of life cycle, 75, **76**
DHL, 164
Diabetes mellitus
  ICD-9-CM coding for, 348
  patient education on, 310t
  scheduling appointments for patients with, 269
Diabetic retinopathy, ICD-9-CM coding for, 348
Diagnosis, 344
  locating, for ICD-9-CM, 348, 349p
  in patient records, 193, **196**, 202, 348, 349p
Diagnosis codes, 344–349
Diagnosis-related group (DRG), 236b
Dictation, direct, 205–208
Dictation-transcription, 33, 199, 205–208
Dictation-transcription equipment, 113–114, **114**, 115p
Dictionary, 155
Dietitian, registered, 34, **34**
Digestive system, care and treatment of (gastroenterology), 27
Digital subscriber line modem, 128
Diplomacy, 20
Diploma graduate nurses, 35
Direct cause, in negligence, 49
Direct data entry (DDE), 338
Direct dictation, 206–208
Disabilities, patients with, accessibility for, to office, 286, **286**, 290–291, **291**, 292p
Disaster recovery plan, computer, 142
Disbursements
  definition of, 402
  financial summaries of, understanding, 404–405
  management of, 402–405
  for ordered supplies, 186, 402–403
  petty cash, 404, **404**
  record of, 388, 403–404
  summary of, 388–392, **391**
  tracking of, 404
  writing checks for, 403
Discharge summary form, 197
Disclosure
  authorization for, 60, 64
  HIPAA and, 59–60, 198b
  mandatory, 63, 63b–64b
Disclosure statement, on credit/lending, 378–379, **380**
Discretion, professional, 53
Discrimination, 66–67, 290
Disease prevention, 299–301
Disk cleanup, 140
Disk defragmentation, 140
Diskette backup, 139–140, **140**
Diskette care and maintenance, 142
Diskette drive, 130
Dismissals, documentation of, 53

Displacement, as defense mechanism, 80
Disposal, of controlled substances, 53, **54–55**
Dissociation, as defense mechanism, 81
Distributing mail, 166
DNR (do not resuscitate) order, 56
DO. *See* Doctor of osteopathy
Doctor(s). *See* Physician(s)
Doctor of osteopathy, 27
Doctor of pharmacy (PharmD), 33
Doctrine of informed consent, 47
Doctrine of professional discretion, 53
Documentation. *See also* Patient records
    legal issues in, 53
    and malpractice prevention, 51
    of noncompliance, 192
    SOAP, 202–203, **203**
    of software, 138
Donor card, uniform, 56
Dot matrix printer, 132
Double-booking system, 263
Dressing change, CPT coding for, 355
DRG. *See* Diagnosis-related group
Drug(s), patient questions about, via telephone, 245–247
Drug and product samples, handling of, 166–167
Drug dependence, patient education resources on, 310t
Drug Enforcement Administration (DEA), 53
    disposal guidelines, 53, **54–55**
DSL modem, 128
Durable items, 173
Durable power of attorney, 56
Duties
    advanced administrative, 16
    advanced clinical, 17
    advanced laboratory, 17
    certified medical assistant, 16b
    coding, billing, and insurance specialist, 381b
    daily, of medical assistants, 15–17
    entry-level administrative, 15
    entry-level clinical, 16–17
    entry-level laboratory, 17
    medical office administrator or manager, 32b
    medical receptionist, 281b
    medical transcriptionist, 207b
    occupational therapist assistant, 311b
    payroll, 405, 405t
    registered health information technologist, 235b–236b
Duty, and negligence, 49
DVD, 130, 232
    for patient education, 299, **299**
DVD-R, 142
Dx. *See* Diagnosis
Dying, 86–87

E

Ear, nose, and throat (ENT) specialist, 29
Earnings
    gross, 406
    net, 408
Earnings records, employee, 408, **410**
ECG. *See* Electrocardiography
ECOA. *See* Equal Credit Opportunity Act
E codes, in ICD-9-CM, 346, 347
EDI. *See* Electronic data interchange

Editing, 154–156
    for content, 156
    for language usage, 156
    for style, 156
    tools for, 154–156
Education
    certified medical assistant, 16b
    coding, billing, and insurance specialist, 381b
    consumer, 299
    continuing, 11
    medical office administrator or manager, 32b
    medical receptionist, 281b
    medical transcriptionist, 208b
    occupational therapist assistant, 311b
    patient. *See* Patient education
    physician, 26
    registered health information technologist, 236b
Educational newsletters, 298
Educational summary, in patient record, 202
EEG. *See* Electroencephalogram
EEO. *See* Equal Employment Opportunity
Effective writing, 152–154
Efficiency, 173
EFT. *See* Electronic funds transfer
EFTS. *See* Electronic funds transfer system
E-health, 134–136
EHR. *See* Electronic health records
EIN. *See* Employer Identification Number
EKG. *See* Electrocardiography
Elderly patients
    communicating with, 86, 87b
    depression in, 86
    with hearing loss, 305b
    importance of touch to, 86
    office accommodations for, 291
    patient education for, 304–305
    payment responsibility for, 367
Elective procedure, 317
Electricity, backup system for, 120
Electrocardiograph technician, 30, **31**
Electrocardiography (ECG/EKG), 30, **31**
Electroencephalogram (EEG), 30
Electroencephalographic technologist, 30
Electronic banking, 397–399
    advantages of, 397
    balance checkbook, 399, **399**
    bill-paying, 399
    checkbook display, 399
    payroll handing through, 408b, 409–411
    recording deposits in, 399
Electronic claims, 134, 338, 370
    clearinghouse for, 338
    direct data entry for, 338
    direct transmission of, 338
    HIPAA, 333, 339b
Electronic communication, 134–136
Electronic data interchange (EDI), 326, 338
Electronic funds transfer (EFT), 412
Electronic funds transfer system (EFTS), 408b
Electronic health records (EHRs), 204–205, 206b, 218
Electronic mail. *See* E-mail
Electronic media, HIPAA and, 117
Electronic media claims (EMCs), 338
Electronic medical records (EMRs), 204–205, **205**, 206b, 218
Electronic signatures, 218
Electronic telephone log, 252
Electronic transaction(s), 134–136

Electronic transaction records, 62
E-mail, 134
    HIPAA and, 135b
    managing, 134
    sending and receiving, 137b
Emancipated minor, 367
E/M codes, 351–353
EMCs. *See* Electronic media claims
eMedicineHealth, 136t
Emergencies. *See* Medical emergencies
Emergency appointments, 268, 269p
Emergency medical technician (EMT), 36
Emergency medicine, 27
Emergency telephone calls, 247, 248t, 249p, 268
Emotionally disturbed patient, communicating with, 86
Empathy, 18, 79
Employee(s)
    laws protecting, 57
    payment to. *See* Payroll
Employee records, retention of, 233
Employee's Withholding Allowance Certificate (Form W-4), 406, **407**
Employer identification number (EIN), 339b, 405
Employer's Annual Federal Unemployment Tax Return (Form 940), 412, **413**
Employer's Quarterly Federal Tax Return (Form 941), 412, **414**, 415
Employment laws, 66–67
Employment taxes, 406–408, 411–412
Employment verification, in credit check, 378
EMRs. *See* Electronic medical records
EMT. *See* Emergency medical technician
Enclosures, in business letter, **149**, 151
Encounter forms, **364**, 365, 370
Endocrinologists, 27
Endocrinology, 27
Endorsement, check, **395**, 396
English grammar and usage manuals, 155
Entrances, office, 286
Entry-level duties
    administrative, 15
    clinical, 16–17
    laboratory, 17
Enunciation, in telephone calls, 250
Envelopes, 148
    address format on, 162, 162t
    address placement on, 161, **161**
    for overnight delivery services, 163
    preparation of, 161–162
EOB. *See* Explanation of benefits
Eponym, in CPT coding, 354
Equal Credit Opportunity Act (ECOA), 376t, 378, 381–382
Equal Employment Opportunity (EEO), 358
Equal Pay Act of 1963, 67
Equifax Inc., 378
Equipment
    filing, 218–221
    housekeeping, 284
    inventory of, 120, **120**
    mailing, 111–113, **112**, 163
    office, 101–122
Ergonomics, of filing equipment, 220
Erikson, Erik, 75
Errors, written, proofreading for, 156
Established patient, in CPT coding, 352, 354
Esteem needs, **76**, 77
Ethical behavior, 21

Ethics
  code of, 64–66
    AAMA, 9–10, 21, 65b, 66
    AMA, 65–66
  definition of, 21, 45
  issues of, 42–70
  of mandatory disclosure, 63–64, 63b–64b
  reasons for studying, 44
  social issues (bioethics), 65–66
Etiquette, for telephone calls, 248–251
Evaluation and management services, in CPT, 351–353
Examination(s). *See* Physical examination
Excludes, in ICD-9-CM coding, 347
Exclusions, in insurance, 317
Exits, office, 287
Expendable item, 173
Expense statement, 404
Explanation of benefits (EOB), 328
Exploring, in therapeutic communication, 80
Express delivery services, 164
Expressed contract, 46
Express Mail, 163–164
External audit, 211
Externships, 12–13
  agreement for, 13, **14**
  duties in, 13
  requirements for, 13
Eye(s), care and treatment of (ophthalmology), 28
Eye contact, 78

F

Fabrics, in reception area decor, 282
Facial expression, 78
Facsimile machine. *See* Fax machine
Fact sheets, 297–298
Factual preoperative education, 306–308
Fair Credit Reporting Act (FCRA), 376t, 378
Fair Debt Collection Practices Act of 1977 (FDCPA), 375–376, 376t
Fair Labor Standards Act of 1938, 67, 406
Fair pay regulations, 67
False billing claims, 57
False claims, federal legislation on, 56–57, 230
False imprisonment, 45
Families
  communication with, 73–88, 88
  telephone calls from, 247–248
Family Leave Act of 1991, 67
Family practice, 26–27
Fasting patients, scheduling appointments for, 269
Fax machine, 107, **110**, 255
  in all-in-one printer, 132, **132**
  benefits of, 107
  HIPAA and, 61, 107b, 255
  information received via, in patient records, 197
  messages on, 105
  ordering supplies via, 180, 183b
  receiving fax, 107
  sending fax, 107p–108p
  thermal *vs.* plain paper for, 107
Fax modem, 128
FCRA. *See* Fair Credit Reporting Act
FDCPA. *See* Fair Debt Collection Practices Act of 1977
Fears. *See also* Anxious patient
  preoperative, 309
Federal Express, 164

Federal False Claims Act, 56–57, 230
Federal legislation, affecting health care, 56–62
Federal Tax Deposit Coupon (Form 8109), 412, **412**
Federal tax deposit schedules, 411–412
Federal Unemployment Tax Act (FUTA), 408, 412–415, **413**
Fee(s)
  appropriate, determining, 363
  usual and customary, 363
Feedback, in communication circle, **74**, 75
Fee-for-service plans, 318
  Medicare, 320, 322
Feelings, communicating in telephone calls, 251
Fee schedules, 328–332, 363, **364**
  contracted, 330
  Medicare, 328, 330, 363–364
Fee slips, **364**, 364–365
Felony, 45
Female reproductive system, care and treatment of (OB/GYN), 28, **28**
Femoral fracture, ICD-10-CM coding for, 349
Fetal tissue transplant, ethics of, 65
FICA tax, 408, 411–412
File(s)
  active *vs.* inactive or closed, 230–231
  compactible, 219
  lateral, 219
  limiting access to, 229, **229**
  misplaced, locating, 230
  retention of, 53, 233–234, 234p–235p
  rotary circular, 219
  storage of, 219–220, 229, 231–233
    basic options for, 231–232
    computer, 232
    facilities for, 232, **232**
    paper, 231–232
    safety of, 232–233
  supplemental, 227–228
  tickler, 226–227, 227p, 268, 274
  vertical, 219
File folders, 221
File guides, 222
File jackets, 221
File sorters, 222
File storage, 219–220, 229
Filing cabinets, 219
Filing equipment, 218–221
  ergonomics of, 220
  HIPAA and, 220b
  labeling, 220
  purchasing, 221
  safety of, 220–221
  security of, 220
Filing process, **228**, 228–231
  guidelines for, 229–230
  indexing in, 228–229
  inspecting in, 228
  limiting access in, 229, **229**
Filing shelves, 219, **219**
Filing supplies, **221**, 221–222
Filing systems, 222–228
  alphabetic, **222**, 222–223, 223t, 224b
  chronological, 225
  color coding in, 225–226, **226**
  creation for patient records, 226p
  evaluation of, 231b
  numeric, 225, 226
  for office supply inventory, 176–178, 176p–177p, 186, **186**
  tickler, 226–227, 227p

Financial records, retention of, 233
Financial summaries, understanding, 404–405
Fire extinguishers, 120
Firewalls, 140
First-class mail, 163
First impressions, in reception area, 280–284
First party, in health insurance, 317
Flash drive, 232
Flatbed scanner, 129–130
Flexibility, 19
Focusing, in therapeutic communication, 80
Folding and inserting machines, 111, **112**
Folding letters, 156, **160**, 162–163
Follow-up, in patient records, 193, 199–200
Forensic pathologist, 29
Form 41 (Registrants Inventory of Drug Surrender), 53, **54–55**
Formatting errors, proofreading for, 156
Form letter, word processing for creating, 135p
Formulary, 317
Four Ds of negligence, 49
Fourth-class mail, 163
Fraud, 45
  coding compliance and avoiding, 356–358
  insurance, 357
Friendliness, 79
Friends
  communication with, 88
  telephone calls from, 247–248
FTD. *See* Federal Tax Deposit Coupon (Form 8109)
Full-block letter style, 152, **152**
Full-Scale Burnout Phase, 94
Furnishings (furniture), in reception area, 280, **283**, 283–284
FUTA. *See* Federal Unemployment Tax Act

G

GAF. *See* Geographic adjustment factor
Gastroenterologists, 27
Gastroenterology, 27
Generalists, 7, 7b–8b
Generalizations, 84
General ledger. *See* Daily log
General physical exam, preparing patient for, 199
General practitioners, 26–27
General supplies, 173, 174t
Genuineness, 79
Geographic adjustment factor (GAF), 330
Geriatric patients. *See* Elderly patients
Gerontologists, 27
Gerontology, 27
Goal-setting, 8, 8t
Government health plans, 319–324. *See also* Medicaid; Medicare
Grammar, 154, 155, 156
Graphical user interface (GUI), 132, **133**
Grief, stages of, 86–87
Gross earnings, 406
Group buying pools, 182, **182**
Group practice, 68
GUI. *See* Graphical user interface
Gynecologists, 27–28
Gynecology, 27–28

H

Haines, Sue, 2
Handheld scanner, 129

Handicapped access, 286, **286,** 290–291, **291,** 292p
Hard copy, 131, **131**
Hard disk drive, 130
Hardship cases, 381–382
Hardware, computer, 126–132
    functions of, 127
    input devices, 127–130
HBV. *See* Hepatitis B/hepatitis B virus (HBV)
HCPCS. *See* Health Care Common Procedure Coding System
HCQIA. *See* Health Care Quality Improvement Act of 1986
Health care, managed care, 318
Health Care Common Procedure Coding System (HCPCS), 62, 353–354
    Level I codes, 353
    Level II codes, 353
    locating, 355p
Health-care portability, 58
Health Care Quality Improvement Act of 1986 (HCQIA), 56
Health-care workers. *See specific occupations*
Health information. *See also* Patient records
    disclosure of, HIPAA and, 59
    improper release of, preventing, 63–64
    individually identifiable, 58–59, 198b
    managing/storing, HIPAA and, 59
    protected, 58–59, 198b
    security of, HIPAA and, 60–61
    sharing, HIPAA and, 59
    use of, HIPAA and, 59
Health information technologist, registered, **235,** 235b–236b
Health insurance, 317
    billing claims under. *See* Insurance claims
    fee-for-service, 318
    fraud in, 357
    government plans, 319–324
    patient information about policies on, 302
    portability of, 58
    terminology of, 317
    third-party liability in, 366–367
    types of, 318–319, **319**
Health Insurance Portability and Accountability Act (HIPAA), 11, 44, 56, 57–62, 198b
    and administrative simplification, 62
    authorization under, 60
    and computer, 60–61, 117, 140b
    and disclosure of health information, 59, 198b
    and electronic media, 60–61, 117
    and e-mail, 135b
    and faxing, 61, 107b, 255
    and filing equipment, 220b
    frequently asked questions about, 62
    goals and purposes of, 57–58
    and identifiers, 318
    and insurance claims, 333, 339–340, 339b
    and insurance fraud, 357
    and management of patient records, 218
    and managing/storing patient information, 59
    and medical coding, 344, 351
    Notice of Privacy Practices under, 60, 198b, 303
    and original documentation, 204
    and ownership of patient records, 53
    and paper shredding, 116
    patient information on, 302–303
    Privacy Rule of, 58–60, 302–303
    and retention of files/records, 233

Security Rule of, 60–61
    and sharing health information, 59–60
    and telephone calls, 243, 248
    Title I, 58
    Title II of, 58–62
    and use of health information, 59, 198b
    violations and penalties of, 61–62
Health maintenance organization (HMO), 66, 319
Health-promoting behaviors, 301
Health promotion, 299–301
Healthy habits, 299
Hearing aids, patients wearing, 305b
Hearing loss, patients with
    communicating with, **85,** 85–86
    office accommodations for, 291
    patient education for, 305b, 306
    telephone banking for, 401b
Heart, care and treatment of (cardiology), 27
Hepatitis B/hepatitis B virus (HBV), 57
Hierarchy of human needs, 75–77, **76**
HIPAA. *See* Health Insurance Portability and Accountability Act
Hippocrates, 65
Hippocratic oath, 65
Hiring, successful, 92
History, patient. *See* Medical history, patient
HIV/AIDS
    communicating with patients with, 88
    contagious patients and, 292–293
    numeric filing system in, 225
    OSHA regulations on, 57
    patient education on, 310t
HMO. *See* Health maintenance organization
Hold, telephone call on, 250
Honesty, 20
Honeymoon Phase, 93
Hospice, Medicare coverage for, 320
Hospital(s)
    Medicare coverage for, 319
    reserving operating rooms in, 273
    scheduling surgery in, 271, 271p, **272**
Hospital discharge summary forms, 197
Hospital records, in patient records, 193
Housekeeping, reception area, 284–286, 285b
Human behavior, and provider-patient relationship, 75–77
Human immunodeficiency virus (HIV). *See* HIV/AIDS
Human resources, 92

I

IBM Roadrunner, 126
ICD-9-CM, 62, 344–349
    Alphabetic Index (Volume 2) of, 344–346, **345**
    code structure in, 347
    conventions of, 347–348
    E codes in, 346, 347
    locating diagnosis for, 348, 349p
    new revision of, 348–349
    Tabular List (Volume 1) of, 344, **345,** 346–347, 346t
    using, 344–345
    V codes in, 346, 347
ICD-10-CM, 348–349
ICD-10-PCS, 348–349
Identification, as defense mechanism, 81
Identification line, in business letter, **149,** 151

Identifiers
    national, HIPAA, 339b
    provider, 318, 318t
Illiteracy, among patients, 85
Immunization(s)
    CPT coding for, 353
    retention of records, 233
Implied consent, 47
Implied contracts, 46
Inactive files
    active *vs.*, 230–231
    storage of, 231–233
Incidental supplies, 174
Includes, in ICD-9-CM coding, 347
Income statement, 404
Income taxes, 406, 411–412
Incoming mail, processing, 166–167
Incoming telephone calls
    guidelines for, 243
    HIPAA and, 243
    managing, 242–244
    screening of, 243, 245b, 246p
    types of, 244–248
Independent billing service, 370
Indexing, and filing, 228–229
Indexing rules, 222–223, 224b
Individually identifiable health information, 58–59
Infection control, Bloodborne Pathogens Standard for, 57
Infectious waste, 285–286
Information packet, patient, 288, 301–304
    benefits of, 301
    Consent for Treatment form in, 303, **304**
    contents of, 301–303
    culture and, 303
    distribution of, 303, **303**
    special concerns and, 303
Informed consent, 47
Informed consent forms, 193, **197**
Initialing, of patient records, 197–199
Initial interview, patient, 199, **199**
Injuries, prevention of, 299–300, 300t
Ink-jet printer, 132
Input devices, computer, 127–130
Inside address, **149,** 149–150
Inspecting, in filing process, 228
Instructions, medical, in patient record, 200
Instruction set, computer, 130
Insurance
    basic terminology of, 317
    disability, 318
    health, 317
        billing claims under. *See* Insurance claims
        fee-for-service, 318
        fraud in, 357
        government plans, 319–324
        managed care, 318
        patient information about policies on, 302
        portability of, 58
        third-party liability in, 366–367
        types of, 318–319, **319**
    liability, 317
Insurance claims
    abbreviations used in, 325t
    allowable benefits, 328
    clean, generating, 338
    coding for, 342–360
    coordination of benefits, 326
    delivery of services in, 326–327
    electronic filing of, 134, 333, 338, 339b, 370

Insurance claims—*Cont.*
  errors in, common, 338, 338t
  filing of, 327, **327**
  HIPAA, 333, 339b
  insurer's processing and payment, 328
  medical coding in, 326
  medical necessity review, 328
  obtaining patient information for, 326
  paper, 333–338, **334**, 335p–337p
  patient eligibility for services, 326
  payment of
    Medicare system of, 328, 330
    methods of, 330
  physician services in, 326
  preparation of, 327, 333–340
  primary coverage guidelines, 326, 327t
  process of, overview of, 325–328
  referrals to other services, 327
  remittance advice on, 328, **329**
  security of, 338–340
  time limits for, 328
  transmission of, 333–340
Insurance fraud, 357
Integrity, 20
Intentional torts, 45–46
Interactive pagers (I-Pagers), 106–107
Interim room, 284
Internal audit, 211
Internal medicine, 28
Internal Revenue Service, 233, 405
  Federal Tax Deposit (FTD) Coupon (Form 8109), 412, **412**
  Form W-4, 406, **407**
  FUTA tax return (Form 940), 412, **413**
  quarterly return (Form 941), 412, **414,** 415
  Transmittal of Wages and Tax Statements (Form W-3), **416,** 417
  Wage and Tax Statement (Form W-2), **415,** 415–417
International Classification of Diseases, Ninth Revision, Clinical Modification. See ICD-9-CM
International mail, 164
Internet, 134–136, 136t
  medical practice websites on, 139
  ordering supplies via, 180, 183b, **184**
  patient education resources on, 309, 310t
  research via, 137b
Internet service providers (ISPs), 137b
Internists, 28
Interoffice memorandums, 154, **155**
Interpersonal skills, 79
Interview, patient, 199, **199**
Introjection, as defense mechanism, 81
Invasion of privacy, 45–46
Inventory
  of office equipment, 120, **120**
  of office supplies, 176–179
    filing system for, 176–178, 176p–177p, 186, **186**
    reorder reminder cards for, 178–179, **179**
    scheduling, 179
    understanding responsibilities for, 176
Inventory card or record page, 178, **178**
Inventory reminder kits, 179
Invoices, 148
  computer generation of, 370
  filing system for, 178
  for office supplies, 186
  patient ledger card as, 370
  preparation of, 368–370, **369**
  using codes on, 369–370
I-Pagers, 106–107

ISPs. *See* Internet service providers
Itinerary, travel, 273, **274**

J

JCAHO. *See* The Joint Commission (TJC)
Joint Commission on Accreditation of Healthcare Organizations (JCAHO). *See* The Joint Commission (TJC)
Journalizing, 387
Judgment, proper, 20
Jump drive, 130, 141, **141,** 232

K

Kansas Medical Assistants Society, 9
Key, 149
Keyboard, computer, 126–127
Kickbacks, 57
Knowledge base, 9
Kübler-Ross, Elisabeth, 86

L

Labels
  correspondence (address), 148
  filing, 220, 221
Laboratory duties
  advanced, 17
  entry-level, 17
Laboratory procedures/tests
  CPT coding for, 353
  results of
    in patient records, 193, **195,** 199
    telephone calls requesting, patient, 245
Laboratory technician, clinical, 31
Labor laws, 66–67
Labor Standards Act, 233
Language barriers, 85, 303
Language usage, editing for, 156
LANs. *See* Local-area networks
Laptop computer, 126
Laser printer, 131–132
Late arrivals, 270
Lateral file, 219
Laterality, codes for, 349
Law. *See also* Legal issues
  of agency, 50
  civil, 45, 49
  classifications of, 45–46
  criminal, 45
  definition of, 45
  reasons for studying, 44
Lawsuits, 45–46
  malpractice, 10, 49–51
  patient reasons for, 50–51
  preventing, 49–56
  prevention of, four Cs of, 51
Lawyers, telephone calls from, 248
LCD monitors, 126, 130
LCME. *See* Liaison Committee on Medical Education
Learning, willingness for, 18–19, **19**
Lease agreement, 118, **118**
Leasing
  advantages of, 118–119
  vs. buying, 118–119
  negotiating for, 119
Ledger, general. *See* Daily log
Ledger card, patient, 365, 370, 387, 388, **389**

Legal custody, 367
Legal document(s)
  appointment book as, 52, 262
  for/by patient, 56
Legal issues
  administration duties and law, 52
  confidentiality, 56, 63–64
  contracts, 46–48
  controlled substances, 53
  credit, 378–379
  debt collection, 375–377, 376t
  documentation, 53
  employee protection, 57
  labor and employment, 66–67
  legal documents and patient, 56
  malpractice, 10, 49–51
  malpractice prevention, four Cs of, 51
  mandatory disclosure, 63–64, 63b–64b
  medical practice models, 67–68
  patient reasons for lawsuits, 50
  patient rights and responsibilities, 47–48
  physician rights and responsibilities, 47
  preventing lawsuits, 49–56
  special circumstances for physician practices, 48–49
  standard of care, 51–52
  statute of limitations, 50–51
  termination of care, 51, **52**
  termination of services, **48,** 48–49
Legal subject matter, in contracts, 46
Legibility, of patient records, 203–204
Letter(s), 148–152. *See also* Mail
  automation equipment for, 111–113, **112**
  business
    parts of, **149,** 149–151
    procedure for creating, 159p–160p
  collection, 372, **373**
  editing and proofreading of, 154–156
  effective writing in, 152–154
  folding and inserting, 111, **112,** 156, **160,** 162–163
  form, word processing for creating, 135p
  format of, 151
  full-block, 152, **152**
  modified-block, 152, **153**
  modified-block with indented paragraphs, 152, **153**
  punctuation style in, 151
  signing, 161
  simplified style, 152, **154**
  styles of, 151–152
  transcription of, 207p
Letterhead, 147–148, 149, **149**
Letterhead paper, 147–148
Liability, 47, 50
  third-party, for payment, 366–367
Liability coverage, professional, 50
Liaison Committee on Medical Education (LCME), 26
Libel, 45
Licensed practical nurses (LPNs), 34–35
Licensed vocational nurses (LVNs), 34–35
Licensure, physician, 26
Life cycle, developmental stages of, 75, **76**
Lifespan Development, 75, **76**
Lifetime maximum benefit, 317
Lighting, in reception area, 281–282
Limited check, 403
Listening
  active, 78–79, **79**
  passive, 78
Listening skills, 78–79
Living wills, 56

Local-area networks (LANs), 139, 339
Local taxes, 415
Local vendors, benefits of using, 182
Locum tenens, 273
Love/belonging needs, **76**, 77
LPNs. *See* Licensed practical nurses
Lustig, Kaye H., 98
LVNs. *See* Licensed vocational nurses

M

MAERB. *See* Medical Assisting Educational
    Review Board
Magazines, in reception area, 287, **287**, 288b
Magnetic ink character recognition (MICR)
    code, 395
Magnetic tapes, care and maintenance of, 142
Mail, 145–170
    annotating, 166
    automation equipment for, 111–113, **112,** 163
    delivery services for
        express, 164
        overnight, 163, 168
        regular, 163–164
        special, 164
        United Parcel Service, 164
        U.S. Postal Service, 163–164
    distributing, 166
    drug and product samples in, handling,
        166–167
    equipment and supplies, 163
    folding and inserting, 111, **112,** 156, **160,**
        162–163
    incoming, processing, 166–167
    international, 164
    outgoing, preparation of, 156–163
    recording, 166
    reminder, 267–268, **268**
    sorting and opening, 166, 167p
    tracing, 164, **166**
    urgent incoming, how to spot, **168,** 168b
    voice, 104
Mail-order companies, 180, 183b, **184**
Mainframe computers, 125–126
Maintenance
    of computer systems, 140–142
    of office equipment, 119–121
    of patient records, 199–200, 210p
Maintenance contract, 119
Malfeasance, 49
Malpractice, 10, 49–51
    and civil law, 49
    prevention of, four Cs of, 51
    settling suits in, 49–50
Malpractice claims, 49
Malpractice insurance, 50
Managed care organizations (MCOs), 10, 318
Managed care plans, 318, 321–322
Management, communication with, 89
Mandatory disclosure, 63–64, 63b–64b
Manuals
    CPT, organization of, **350,** 351
    English grammar and usage, 155
    equipment, 119, 119b
    policy and procedures, 90, **91**
    software, 138
Maslow, Abraham, 75
Maslow's hierarchy of human needs,
    75–77, **76**
Massage therapist, 30–31
Material data safety sheet (MDSS), 185–186
Matrix, for appointment book, 260, **261**

Mature minor, 211
MCOs. *See* Managed care organizations
MDSS. *See* Material data safety sheet
Mechanical errors, proofreading for, 156
Medasis, 133
Media mail, 163
Medicaid, 322–323
    accepting assignment from, 322
    state guidelines for, 322–323
    time limits for claims, 328
Medical administrative assistant, 31
Medical assistant(s)
    certification of, 10–11
    contracts for, 46
    daily duties of, 15–17
    as generalists, 7, 7b–8b
    pediatric, 37, **37**
    personal qualifications of, 17–21
    role in preoperative patient education, 306
Medical assistant clinical station security, 61
Medical assisting. *See also specific entries*
    AAMA definition of, 15
    growth of profession, 8–9
    history of profession, 9
Medical Assisting Educational Review Board
    (MAERB), 12
Medicalcharting.com, 205
Medical coding. *See* Coding, medical
Medical dictionary, 155
Medical emergencies, telephone, 247, 248t,
    249p, 268
Medical Group Management Association, 32b
Medical history, patient, 193, **195,** 199
Medical information, in reading material, 288
Medical Manager (software), 133
Medical necessity, insurer's review for, 328
Medical office administrator or manager,
    32, 32b
Medical practice models, legal, 67–68
Medical practice websites, 139
Medical receptionist, **281,** 281b
Medical records. *See* Patient records
Medical records technologists, 31
Medical specialties, 26–30
Medical supplies. *See* Supplies, medical
Medical technologists (MTs), 31–33
Medical technology, 31–33
Medical transcription, 33, 113–114, **114,** 115p,
    199, 205–208
    aids for, 208
    of direct dictation, 206–208
    of letters, reports, and notes, 207p
Medical transcriptionist, 33, 207b–208b, **208**
Medicare, 319–322
    Advance Beneficiary Notice of
        Noncoverage, 331, **332**
    coding for, 353–354
    fee-for-service (original), 320
    fee schedule of, 328, 330, 363–364
    fraud, 357
    Medigap, 320
    Part A, 319–320
    Part B, 320
    Part C, 320
    Part D, 320, **321**
    participating and nonparticipating
        providers, 331
    payment system of, 328, 330
    Recovery Audit Contractor program, 322
    time limits for claims, 328
    types of plans, 320–322
Medicare Advantage plans, 320–322
Medicare fee schedule (MFS), 330

Medicare Managed Care Plans, 321–322
Medicare medical savings plans (MSAs), 320
Medicare-participating provider (PAR), 331
Medicare Preferred Provider Organization
    Plan, 322
Medicare Private Fee-for-Service Plan, 322
Medicare Remittance Notice, 328, **329**
Medication(s). *See* Drug(s)
Medicware.com, 205
Medigap, 320
Medi/Medi coverage, 322
MediSoft, 133
MEDLINE, 134
MedlinePlus, 136t
Medware, 133
Meeting planning, 273–274
Memory, computer, 130
Memos, 154, **155**
Mental health technician, 33
Mental impairments, patients with
    communicating with, 86
    patient education for, 306
Message(s), telephone, 105, **251,** 251–252
    ensuring correct information in, 252
    retrieving from answering service,
        252, 253p
    tips for taking, 252
Message pads, telephone, 251–252, **252, 253**
Messengers, 166
MFS. *See* Medicare fee schedule
MICR code. *See* Magnetic ink character
    recognition code
Microfiche readers, 116, **117**
Microfiche storage, 232
Microfilm readers, 116, **117**
Microfilm storage, 232
Microprocessor, 130
Microsoft Office, 133
Middle digit filing, 225
Military dependents and retirees, health plan
    for, 323, **323**
Minicomputers, 125–126
Minor(s), 47, 211
    emancipated, 367
    mature, 211
    payment responsibility for, 367
Minutes, of meeting, 274
Mirroring, in therapeutic communication, 80
Misdemeanors, 45
Misfeasance, 49
Misplaced files, locating, 230
Missed appointments, 270
    charging for, 270
    documentation of, 53, 270
    reminders for patients with history of, 268
Mixed punctuation, 151
Modem, 127–128
    cable, 128
    DSL, 128
    fax, 128
    speed of, 127–128
Modified-block letter style, 152, **153**
Modified-block letter style with indented
    paragraphs, 152, **153**
Modified-wave scheduling, 263, **265**
Modifiers, in CPT coding, 351, 352t, 355
Modulator-demodulator. *See* Modem
Money order, 395
Monitors, computer, 126, 130–131
    care and maintenance of, 141
    LCD, 126, 130
    resolution of, 131
Moral values, 45

Motherboard, 130
Mouse, computer, 127, **128**
MSAs. *See* Medicare medical savings plans
MSHP. *See* Multiskilled health-care professional
MTs. *See* Medical technologists
Multicultural attitudes, about modern medicine, 84b
Multimedia, 130
Multiple lines, in telephone, 104
Multiskilled health-care professional (MSHP), 7, 7b–8b, 15
Multiskill training, 15
  and career opportunities, 15
  and health-care cost reduction, 15
Multitasking system, computer, 132
Muscular system, care and treatment of (orthopedics), 29
Musculoskeletal system, care and treatment of (orthopedics), 29
Music, in reception area, 282
Mutual agreement, on credit, 379–380

N

Names
  alphabetic filing of, 223t
  indexing rules for, 223, 224b
  remembering patient's, in telephone calls, 250–251
Narcotics, storage of, 175
National AIDS Hotline, 310t
National Association of Medical Staff Services, 32b
National Board of Medical Examiners (NBME), 10, 26
National Cancer Institute, 310t
National Certified Medical Assistant (NCMA), 13
National Certified Medical Office Assistant (NCMOA), 13
National Childhood Vaccine Injury Act of 1986, 233
National Clearinghouse for Alcohol and Drug Information, 310t
National Healthcare Association (NHA), 13
National Health Information Center, 310t
National identifiers, HIPAA, 339b
National Institutes of Health (NIH), 134, 136t
National Kidney Foundation, 310t
National Library of Medicine, 134, 136t
National Organization for Rare Disorders, 310t
National Organization of Competency Assurance (NOCA), 13
National Phlebotomy Association, 33
National Practitioner Data Bank, 56
National Provider Identifier (NPI), 318
National Safety Council, 300
National Uniform Claim Committee (NUCC), 318t
NBME. *See* National Board of Medical Examiners
NCMA. *See* National Certified Medical Assistant
NCMOA. *See* National Certified Medical Office Assistant
Neat appearance, 19–20
Neatness, of patient records, 203–204
NEC (not elsewhere classified), 347
Needs
  basic, 75–77
  esteem, **76**, 77
  hierarchy of, 75–77, **76**

  love/belonging, **76**, 77
  physiological, **76**, 77
  safety, **76**, 77
Negative verbal communication, 77
Negligence, 46, 49
  classification of, 49
  four Ds of, 49
Negotiable checks, 393
Negotiable papers, 394–395
Negotiation, for lease or purchase, 119
Nephrologists, 28
Nephrology, 28
Nervous system, care and treatment of (neurology), 28
Netbook, 126
Net earnings, 408
Network, computer, 126, 138–139
Networking, 12
Neurologists, 28
Neurology, 28
New England Journal of Medicine, 136t
New patient
  appointment for, 266–267
  in CPT coding, 352, 354
Newsletters, educational, 298
NHA. *See* National Healthcare Association
NIH. *See* National Institutes of Health
NOCA. *See* National Organization of Competency Assurance
Noise, in communication circle, **74**, 75
Nonassertive behavior, in communication, 81, 81t
Noncompliant patient, 192
Nonessential terms, in ICD-9-CM coding, 346
Nonfeasance, 49
Non-NPI qualifiers, 318t
Nonparticipating provider (nonPAR), 331
Nonsufficient funds (NSF), 393, 394p
Nonverbal communication, 78
NOS (not otherwise specified), 347
No-shows, 53, 268, 270
Notations, in business letter, **149**, 151
Notebook computer, 126
Notice of Privacy Practices (NPP), 60, 198b, 303
Notification, of sexually transmitted disease risk, 63, 63b–64b
NPI. *See* National Provider Identifier
NPP. *See* Notice of Privacy Practices
NSF. *See* Nonsufficient funds
NUCC. *See* National Uniform Claim Committee
Nuclear medicine/imaging, 28
Nuclear medicine technologist, 33
Numeric filing system, 225
  color coding in, 226
  middle digit, 225
  terminal digit, 225
Nurse(s)
  associate degree, 35
  baccalaureate, 35
  diploma degree, 35
  practical/vocational, 34–35
  registered, 35
Nurse anesthetists, 27
Nurse practitioner, 35, **35**
Nursing aide/assistant, 34

O

Obesity, 27
Objective data, in patient record, 203

Obstetrics, 28, **28**
Occupational Analysis of CMA, 10, 21
  areas of competence in, 21
  uses of, 21
Occupational Safety and Health Act, 10
Occupational Safety and Health Administration (OSHA), 56–57
  Bloodborne Pathogens Protection Standards, 57
  compliance with, 358
  on credentials, 10
  Standard Precautions, 57
  on workplace safety, 286
Occupational therapist, 33
Occupational therapist assistant, 36, **311**, 311b
OCR. *See* Optical character recognition
OCRs. *See* Optical character readers
Odor removal, 285
Office administrator or manager, **32**, 32b
Office equipment, 101–122
  adding machines and calculators, 110
  automation, 110–116
  backup systems, 120
  check writers, 114, 115p
  communication, 103–110, **104**
  computers, 123–144
  dictation-transcription, 113–114, **114**, 115p
  fax machine, 61, 105, 107, 108p–109p, **110**
  folding and inserting machines, 111, **112**
  inventory of, 120, **120**
  leasing *vs.* buying, 118–119
  maintenance and service contracts for, 119
  maintenance of, 119–121
  manuals for, 119, 119b
  microfiche readers, 116, **117**
  microfilm readers, 116, **117**
  negotiating for, 119
  pagers (beepers), 105–107
  paper shredders, 114–116, **116**, 116b
  photocopiers, 61, 110
  postage meters, 111–112, **112**
  purchasing of, 116–119
  telephones, 103–105
  troubleshooting for, 119–120
  typewriters, 107–110
Office hours, 302
Office introduction, in information packet, 301
Office staff, introduction to, 302
Office supplies, 171–188
  administrative, 173, 174t, 175
  budget for, 180
  categorization of, 173–175, 174t
  clinical, 173, 174t, 175–176
  competitive prices and quality of, 180–182
  disbursement for, 186, 402–403
  errors in shipment, correcting, 186
  general, 173, 174t
  incidental, 174
  inventory of, 176–179
    filing system for, 176–178, 176p–177p, 186, **186**
    inventory card or record page for, 178, **178**
    reminder kits for, 179
    reorder reminder cards for, 178–179, **179**
    scheduling, 179
    understanding responsibilities for, 176
  invoices for, 186
  list of, 173–174
  location of, 175
  material data safety sheets for, 185–186
  mistakes in purchasing, avoiding, 186–187
  ordering of, 179–187

ahead of schedule, 179
establishing times for, 179
group buying pools for, 182, **182**
procedures for, 182–186
purchase orders for, 185, **185**
purchasing groups for, 182
scheduling, 179
via mail, telephone, fax, or online, 180,
183b, **184**
orders received, checking, 185
organization of, **173,** 173–176
efficiency in, 173
responsibility for, 173
payment schedules for, 182
periodic, 175
shortage of, unanticipated, 179
storage of, 175–176
vendors for
comparison of, 180, **181**
local, benefits of using, 182
locating and evaluating, 180
reputable, 180
vital, 174
Older Americans Act of 1965, 291
Old prescriptions, telephone calls about, 247
OMM. *See* Osteopathic manipulative medicine
Oncologists, 26, 28
Oncology, 28
One-write system. *See* Pegboard system
Online health information, 134–136, 136t, 299
Online help, **133,** 138
Online ordering, 180, 183b, **184**
Online postage, 164
Online scheduling, 266
Online services, 134, 137b
Open-book account, 370
Open-hours scheduling, 262–263
Opening mail, 166, 167p
Openness, 79
Open posture, 78
Open punctuation, 151
Operating rooms, reserving, 273
Operating system, software, 132
Operative reports, in patient records, 193
Ophthalmic assistant, 36
Ophthalmologists, 28
Ophthalmology, 28
Optical character readers (OCRs), 161
Optical character recognition (OCR), 133
Optometrists, 28
Order forms, 182–184
Ordering, of office supplies, 179–187
ahead of schedule, 179
comparing vendors for, 180, **181**
competitive prices and quality in, 180–182
cost controls in, 182
establishing times for, 179
group buying pools for, 182, **182**
local vendors for, benefits of using, 182
locating and evaluating vendors for, 180
procedures for, 182–186
purchase orders for, 185, **185**
purchasing groups for, 182
scheduling, 179
via mail, telephone, fax, or online, 180,
183b, **184**
Orders received, checking, 185
Organizational skills, 8
Organization of office supplies, **173,** 173–176
efficiency in, 173
responsibility for, 173
Original Medicare Plan, 320
Orthopedics, 29

Orthopedist, 29
OSHA. *See* Occupational Safety and Health
Administration
Osteomyelitis, CPT coding for, 354
Osteopathic manipulative medicine
(OMM), 27
Osteopathy, doctor of, 27
Otolaryngology, 29
Otorhinolaryngology, 29
Outgoing mail, preparation of, 156–163
Outgoing telephone calls
applying telephone skills in, 253–254
placing, 252–254
Out guides, 222
Outpatient services, Medicare coverage
of, 320
Output devices, computer, 130–132
Overbooking, 273
Overnight delivery services, 163, 168
Overpayment, 367
Ownership, of patient records, 53

P

PA. *See* Physician assistant
Pagers, 105–107, 255
interactive, 106–107
paging physician, 106
technology of, 103–104
Panels, in CPT coding, 353
Paper
letterhead, 147–148
thermal *vs.* plain, for fax, 107
Paper-based medical records, management
of, 218
Paper claims, 333–338, **334,** 335p–337p
Paper shredders, 114–116, **116**
HIPAA and, 116
how to shred materials, 116
when to shred materials, 116
Paper storage, of files, 231–232
PAR. *See* Medicare-participating provider
Paramedic, 36
Parcel post, 163
Parentheses, in ICD-9-CM coding, 347
Parents
communication with, 88
custodial, and payment responsibility, 367
Parking arrangements, 286, **286**
Parkinson's disease, fetal tissue transplant in,
ethics of, 65
Part A, Medicare, 319–320
Part B, Medicare, 320
Part C, Medicare, 320
Part D, Medicare, 320, **321**
Participating physicians, in managed care
plans, 318
Participatory preoperative patient education,
308–309
Partnership, 67
Passive listening, 78
Passive voice, in writing, 154
Passwords, computer, 139, 339–340
Past-due accounts
age-analysis of, **374,** 374, 375p
collection of, 370–378
Pathogen(s), bloodborne. *See also* Hepatitis B/
hepatitis B virus; HIV/AIDS
OSHA protection standards against, 57
Standard Precautions against, 57
Pathologist, 29
Pathologist's assistant, 36–37

Pathology, 29
Patient(s)
communication with, 73–88
contact with, documentation of, 53
educated, 297. *See also* Patient education
legal documents for, 56
provider relationship with, human behavior
and, 75–77
responsibilities of, 47–48
rights of, 44, 47–48, 66
telephone calls from, 245–247
Patient Care Partnership: Understanding
Expectations, Rights, and
Responsibilities, 66
Patient compliance, 192
Patient education, 295–313
developing plan for, 298p
diabetes mellitus, 310t
for elderly patients, 304–305
HIV/AIDS, 310t
information packet for, 288, 301–304
injury prevention, 299–300, 300t
online resources for, 299
patient records and, 192
for patients with hearing impairment,
305b, 306
for patients with mental impairments, 306
for patients with special needs, 304–309
for patients with visual impairments, 306
preoperative, 306–309
anatomical models for, 309, **309**
benefits of, 306
factual, 306–308
informing patient of guidelines for
surgery, **308**
participatory, 308–309
relieving anxiety in, 309
role of medical assistant in, 306
sensory, 307
types of, 306–308
verifying understanding in, 309
preventive health care, 300–301
printed materials for, 297–299
promoting health and wellness through,
299–301
resources for, 309, 310t
in telephone triage, 254
types of, 297–299
visual materials for, 299
Patient information packet, 288, 301–304
benefits of, 301
Consent for Treatment form in, 303, **304**
contents of, 301–303
culture and, 303
distribution of, 303, **303**
special concerns and, 303
Patient interview. *See* Interview, patient
Patient ledger card, 365, 370, 387, 388, **389**
Patient medical history. *See* Medical history,
patient
Patient notification, under HIPAA, 60
Patient-physician contract, 46–48
Patient reception. *See* Reception area
Patient records, 189–215
abbreviations in, 201, 201t
accuracy of, 204
appearance of, 203–204
audit of, 211, **212–213**
CHEDDAR format of, 203
confidentiality of, 58–60, 202, 211
contents of, 192–199
conventional, 202
corrections to, 53, 204, 208, 209p

Patient records—*Cont.*
  dating and initialing of, 197–199
  diagnosis in, 193, **196**, 202, 348
  dictation-transcription for, 205–208
  electronic, 204–205, **205**, 206b, 218
  for evaluating quality of treatment, 192
  filing equipment for, 218–221
  filing process for, **228**, 228–231
  filing supplies for, **221**, 221–222
  filing systems for, 222–228
  HIPAA and, 53, 58–62, 198b, 204, 218, 220b
  importance of, 191–192
  information received via fax in, 197
  initiation of, 199–200
  laboratory results in, 193, **195**, 199
  legal guidelines for, 192
  maintenance of, 199–200, 210p
  and malpractice prevention, 51
  management of, 216–238
  neatness and legibility of, 203–204
  noncompliance documented in, 192
  ownership of, 53
  paper-based, 218
  for patient education, 192
  preparation of new, 200p
  Privacy Rule and, 58–60
  problem-oriented, 202
  professional attitude and tone in, 204
  progress notes in, 193, **196**, 202
  release of, 209–211, **211**
    procedures for, 209–211
    special cases for, 211
  for research, 192, **193**
  retention of, 53, 233–234, 234p–235p
  security of, 205
  Security Rule and, 60–61
  six Cs of, 200–202
  SOAP documentation in, 202–203, **203**
  source-oriented, 202
  standard information in, 192–197
  standards for, 192
  storage of, 53, 59, 219, 229, 231–233
  telephone calls documented in, 193,
    199–200, **200**, 251
  timeliness of, 204
  transfer of, 209–211, **211**
  treatment plan in, 193, 202, **206**
  types of, 202
  updating of, 208
Patient registration form, 193, **194**
Patient's Bill of Rights, 66
Patient statements, documenting, 199,
    200–201
Paychecks, preparation of, 408
Payee, 388
Payer, 393
Payment
  accepting, 365–366
  cash, 365, **365**
  check, 365
  collection of, 370–378. *See also* Collection
  credit balance in, 367, 368p
  credit card, 365–366, **366**
  debit card, 365
  to employees. *See* Payroll
  of insurance claims, 328–332
    allowed charges and, 330
    capitation, 318, 330–331
    contracted fee schedule and, 330
    Medicare system of, 328, 330
    methods of, 330
  from office. *See* Disbursements
  pegboard system for posting, 366

  policies on, patient information on, 302
  professional courtesy in, 367
  refunds of, 367, 368p
  responsibility for, determining, 366–367
  standard procedures for, 363–367
  third-party liability for, 366–367
Payment schedules, for supplies, 182
Payroll, 405–411
  deductions and, 406–408
  duties for, 405, 405t
  electronic handling of, 408b, 409–411
  generation of, 409p
  gross earnings and, 406
  net earnings and, 408
  number of dependents and, 406, **407**
  records of, 387
  type of, 406
  withholding and, 406–408
Payroll information sheets, 406
Payroll register, 409, **411**
Pay schedule, 406
Pay-to provider, 339b
PDAs. *See* Personal digital assistants
PDR. *See* Physicians' Desk Reference
Pediatrician, 29
Pediatric medical assistant, 37, **37**
Pediatric playroom, 289, **289**, 290p
Pediatrics, 29
Pegboard system, 366, 392–393
Penalties, HIPAA, 61–62
Peptic ulcer, 348
Periodic supplies, 175
Personal computers, 125–126
Personal digital assistants (PDAs), 126, **127**
Personal names, alphabetic filing of, 223t
Personal space, 78
Personal telephone calls, 248
Personnel management, 92
Petty cash
  management of, 404, **404**
  records of, 387
Petty cash fund
  replenishing, 404
  starting and maintaining, 404
Pharmaceutical sales representatives,
    scheduling of, 273, **273**
Pharmacist(s), 33
  professional association of, 39t, 40
Pharmacy technician, 37
Pharmacy technician, certified (CPhT), 33, 37
PharmD. *See* Doctor of pharmacy
Philosophy, office, 301
Phlebotomist, 33
Phoenix Phenomenon, 94
Photocopiers, 110
  HIPAA and, 61
  special features of, 110
  use of, 110, 111p
Physiatrists, 29
Physical examination
  general, preparing patient for, 199
  results in patient records, 193, **195**
Physical medicine, 29
Physical therapist (PT), 33–34
Physical therapist assistant (PTA), 37, **37**
Physician(s)
  contract with patient, 46–48
  education and licensure of, 26
  Hippocratic oath of, 65
  legal practice models for, 67–68
  liability of, 47, 50
  paging, 106
  qualifications, in information packet, 301

  records from others, in patient records, 193
  rights and responsibilities of, 47
  schedule of
    common items on, 275t
    maintaining, 273–274
  scheduling time with, 274
  substitute (*locum tenens*), 273
  telephone calls from other, 248
  telephone calls requiring attention of, 244
  termination of services by, **48**, 48–49
Physician assistant (PA), 34
Physician practices, special circumstances
    for, 48
Physicians' Desk Reference (PDR), 155
Physician services, in insurance claims, 326
Physician's office. *See specific aspects of*
Physiological needs, **76**, 77
Pins, designating certification, 9, **9**
Plan of action, in patient record, 203
Plastic surgeon, 29
Plastic surgery, 29
Plastic tubs or boxes, for filing, 219–220
Playroom, pediatric, 289, **289**, 290p
Podiatrist, 29
Podiatry, 29
Pointing device, computer, 127
Policy and procedure manual, 90
POMR. *See* Problem-oriented medical records
Portability, of health care, 58
Positive attitude, 20
Positive verbal communication, 77
Postage
  online, 164
  prepaying, 112
Postage meters, 111–112, **112**, 113p, 163
Postal rates, 163
Postal scales, 113, 163
Postal Service. *See* U.S. Postal Service
Posture
  closed, 78
  for computer use, **129**, 129b
  as nonverbal communication, 78
  open, 78
Powermed.com, 205
Power of attorney, 395
  durable, 56
PPOs. *See* Preferred provider organizations
Practical/vocational nurse, 34–35
Practice, scope of, 21
Practice description, in information
    packet, 302
Practice models, legal, 67–68
Practitioners, 9
Preauthorization, insurance, 317
Precertification, insurance, 317
Preferred provider organizations (PPOs),
    319, 322
Pregnancy Discrimination Act of 1976, 67
Premium, insurance, 317
Preoperative patient education, 306–309
  anatomical models for, 309, **309**
  benefits of, 306
  factual, 306–308
  informing patient of guidelines for
    surgery, **308**
  participatory, 308–309
  relieving anxiety in, 309
  role of medical assistant in, 306
  sensory, 307
  types of, 306–308
  verifying understanding in, 309
Prepaid postage, 112, 164
Preprinted invoices, 148

Preprinted statements, 148
Prescription(s), renewals, telephone, 246–247
Prescription drug benefit, Medicare, 320, **321**
President's Council on Physical Fitness and
    Sports, 310t
Preventive health care, 300–301
Pricing
    competitive, 180–182
    unit, 180
Primary care physicians, 26
Primary coverage, insurance, 326, 327t
Printed materials, for patient education,
    297–299
Printer, 131–132
    all-in-one, 132, **132**
    dot matrix, 132
    hard copy from, 131, **131**
    HIPAA and, 61
    ink-jet, 132
    laser, 131–132
    maintenance of, 141
Priority Mail, 163
Privacy
    invasion of, 45–46
    in reception area, 283–284
Privacy practices, notice of, 60
Privacy Rule, HIPAA, 58–60, 302–303
Problem list, in patient record, 202
Problem-oriented medical records
    (PROM), 202
Procedure codes, 351–356. See also CPT
Procedure manual, 90, **91**
Procedure times, standard, and
    scheduling, 262
Processing devices, computer, 130
Proctologists, 29
Proctology, 29
Product samples, handling of, 166–167
Professional associations. See Association(s)
Professional corporations, 68
Professional courtesy, 367
Professional discretion, doctrine of, 53
Professionalism, 19
    correspondence and, 147, **147**
Professional liability coverage, 50
Professional support, from associations,
    11–12, **12**
Profit-and-loss statement, 404
Progress notes, 193, **196,** 202
Progress reports, patient, via telephone, 247
Projection, as defense mechanism, 81
Pronunciation, in telephone calls, 250
Proofreading, 154–156
    for data errors, 156
    for formatting errors, 156
    for mechanical errors, 156
    tools for, 154–156
Proper judgment, 20
Prospective audit, 211
Protected health information (PHI), 58–59,
    198b, 220b
Provider(s)
    billing, 339b
    identifiers for, 318, 318t, 339b
    Medicare participating and
        nonparticipating, 331
    pay-to, 339b
Provider-patient relationship, human behavior
    and, 75–77
Psychiatric treatment, Medicare coverage
    for, 320
PT. See Physical therapist
PTA. See Physical therapist assistant

Purchase orders, 185, **185**
Purchase requisitions, 184–185
Purchasing
    computer, 138–139
    contacting suppliers about, 117
    decisions on, 116–119
    evaluating office needs for, 117
    evaluating warranty options in, 117
    filing equipment, 221
    filing supplies, 222
    leasing vs., 118–119
    mistakes in, avoiding, 186–187
    negotiating for, 119
    ordering office supplies, 179–187
    preparing recommendation for, 118
Purchasing groups, 182

Q

Qi, 30
Quality, of office supplies, 180–182
Quality of treatment, patient records for
    evaluating, 192
Quarterly return, 412, **414,** 415
Qui tam, 56–57

R

RAC. See Recovery Audit Contractor program
Radiation therapy technologist, 37
Radiographer, 34
Radiologic technologist, 34
Radiologists, 29
Radiology, 28, 29
RAM. See Random-access memory
Random-access memory (RAM), 130
Rapport, 88, **88**
Rationalization, as defense mechanism, 81
RBRVS. See Resource-based relative value
    scale
Reading material, in reception area, **287,**
    287–289, 288b
Reading problems, patients with, 85
Read-only memory (ROM), 130
Recall notices, 268
Receipts
    return requested (mail), 164
    summary of, 388–392, **391**
Receiver, in communication circle, 74, **74**
Reception area, 278–294
    access to, 286, **286,** 290–291, **291,** 292p
    children in
        accommodation for, 284
        items for, 289, **289,** 290p
    cleanliness of, 284–286, 285b
    contagious patients in, 284, 292–293
    cultural issues and, 291–292
    decor of, **282,** 282–283
    elderly patients in, 291
    first impressions in, 280–284
    furniture in, 280, **283,** 283–284
    keeping patients occupied and informed in,
        287–289
    lighting in, 281–282
    medical office information in, 281
    music in, 282
    patients with special needs in, 290–291,
        291, 292p
    physical components of, 286–287
    privacy in, 283–284
    reading materials in, **287,** 287–289, 288b

room temperature in, 282
    safety of, 286–287
    security of, 61, 286–287
    special situations in, 291–292
    television and videotapes in, 289
Reception desk, 280, **280**
Receptionist, medical, **281,** 281b
Reception window, 280, **280**
Recertification, 11
Reconciliation, of bank statements, 397,
    401p–402p
Recording mail, 166
Record page (inventory card), 178, **178**
Records. See Documentation; Patient
    records
Records management system, 218
Recovery Audit Contractor program
    (RAC), 322
Recycling, 18b
Referrals
    documentation of, 53
    and insurance claims, 327
    scheduling appointments for, 268–269
    self-referrals, 57
Reflecting, in therapeutic communication, 80
Refrigerator, 175–176
Refunds, 367, 368p
Registered dietitian, 34, **34**
Registered health information technologist
    (RHIT), **235,** 235b–236b
Registered mail, 164, 168
Registered medical assistants (RMAs), 11, 40
    examination for, major areas of, 11
    as office administrator or manager, 32b
    pins worn by, 9, **9**
    professional support for, 12
    requirements for, 11
Registered nurse (RN), 35
Registered pharmacist (RPh), 33
Registered Records Administrator (RRA), 31
Registrants Inventory of Drug Surrender, 53,
    54–55
Registration. See Certification
Registration form, patient, 193, **194**
Regression, as defense mechanism, 81
Regular mail service, 163–164
Rehabilitation, 301
Relative value unit (RVU), 330, 363–364
Release of medical records, 209–211, **211**
    procedures for, 209–211
    special cases for, 211
Relocation, patient, and payment
    collection, 382
Reminder calls, 268
Reminder cards, reorder, 178–179, **179**
Reminder kits, inventory, 179
Reminder mailings, 267–268, **268**
Reminders of appointment, 267–268, **268**
Remittance advice (RA), 328, **329**
Renewal, of prescription, by telephone,
    246–247
Reorder reminder cards, 178–179, **179**
Repeat visits, scheduling of, 269
Repression, as defense mechanism, 81
Reputable vendors, 180
Requisition, purchase, for office supplies,
    184–185
Research
    online, 137b
    patient records and, 192, **193**
    software and, 136
Res ipsa loquitur, 49
Resolution, of computer monitor, 131

Resource(s)
   community, 90–91, 92b, 309
   Internet, 134–136, 136t, 299
   patient education, 309, 310t
Resource-based relative value scale (RBRVS),
   328, 330
Resource rooms, 309
Respect, 79
   for cultural beliefs, 305b
Respiratory therapist, 34
Respiratory therapist technician, 38
Respite care, Medicare coverage for, 320
Respondeat superior, 50
Responsibilities
   patient, 47–48
   physician, 47
Résumé, 15
Retention, of patient records/files, 53,
   233–234, 234p–235p
Retention schedule, 233
Retrospective audit, 211
Return appointments, 267
Return demonstration, 308
Returned checks, 393, 394p
Return receipt requested (mail), 164
RHIT. *See* Registered health information
   technologist
Rights
   of patients, 44, 47–48, 66
   of physicians, 47
Risk management, 62
RMAs. *See* Registered medical assistants
RN. *See* Registered nurse
ROM. *See* Read-only memory
Room temperature, for reception area, 282
Rotary circular files, 219
Routing list, 244, **244**
Routing telephone calls, 243–244
   automated menu for, 106b
   calls handled by medical assistant, 243–244
   calls requiring doctor's attention, 244
RPh. *See* Registered pharmacist
RRA. *See* Registered Records Administrator
Rush orders, 180
RVU. *See* Relative value unit

S

Safety
   file storage, 232–233
   filing equipment, 220–221
   office (reception area), 286–287
Safety needs, **76,** 77
Salespeople, telephone calls from, 248
Salutation, in business letter, **149,** 150–151
Sample(s), drug and product, handling of,
   166–167
Scales, postal, 113, 163
Scanner, 129–130, 132
   flatbed, 129–130
   handheld, 129
   single-sheet, 129
Schedule/scheduling
   appointment, 258–277
     cluster, 263, 266p
     combination, 266
     computerized, 266, **267**
     for diabetic patients, 269
     double-booking, 263
     for emergencies, 268, 269p
     for fasting patients, 269
     for late arrivals, 270

modified-wave, 263, **265**
   online, 266
   open-hours, 262–263
   outside appointments, 271
   patient information on, 302
   patient situations and, 268–270
   physician situations and, 270
   for referrals, 268–269
   for repeat visits, 269
   software for, 134
   special situations and, 268–270
   standard procedure times and, 262
   for surgery, 271, 271p, **272**
   systems of, 262–266
   telephone calls for, 245
   time-specific, 263, **264**
   wave, 263
  federal tax deposit, 411–412
  fee, 328–332
  ordering of supplies, 179
  pay, 406
  payment, for supplies, 182
  pharmaceutical sales representatives,
   273, **273**
  physician, common items on, 275t
  physician, maintaining, 273–274
  retention of files, 233
  time with physician, 274
SCHIP. *See* State Children's Health Plan
Scope of practice, 21, 94
Screening
   disease prevention, 301
   telephone calls, 243, 245b, 246p
Screen saver, 141
Search, Internet, 136, 137b
Search engines, 136
Secondary coverage, insurance, 326
Second-class mail, 163
Second party, in health insurance, 317
Section mark symbol, in ICD-9-CM, 347
Security
   activity-monitoring systems, 139
   antivirus software and firewalls, 140
   backup systems, 120, **139,** 139–140
   claims, 338–340
   computer, 60–61, 139–140, 140b, 338–340
   file storage, 232–233
   filing equipment, 220
   office (reception area), 61, 286–287
   patient record, 205
Security Rule, HIPAA, 60–61
Security systems, 287
See reference, in ICD-9-CM coding, 346
Self-actualization, **76,** 77
Self-motivation, 19
Self-referrals, 57
Seminars, for patient education, 299
Sensitivity, 79
Sensory preoperative education, 308
Servers, 134
Service contract, 119
Sexual harassment, 66–67
Sexually transmitted diseases (STDs), risk of,
   notification of, 63, 63b–64b
Sharing health information, HIPAA and,
   59–60
Shelves, filing, 219, **219**
Shortage of supplies, unanticipated, 179
Shredders. *See* Paper shredders
Sign(s), 202
Signature(s), electronic, 218
Signature block, in business letter, **149,** 151
Signing letters, 161

Simplified letter style, 152, **154**
Single-entry account, 370
Single-entry system, 387–392
Single-sheet scanner, 129
Six Cs of charting, 200–202
Skeletal system, care and treatment of
   (orthopedics), 29
Skill(s)
   assertiveness, 81, 81t
   certified medical assistant, 16b
   coding, billing, and insurance
     specialist, 381b
   critical thinking, 17
   interpersonal, 79
   medical office administrator or
     manager, 32b
   medical receptionist, 281b
   medical transcriptionist, 207b
   occupational therapist assistant, 311b
   registered health information technologist,
     235b–236b
   therapeutic communication skills, 79–81
Skilled nursing facility (SNF), Medicare
   coverage for, 319
Skin, care and treatment of (dermatology), 27
Slamming, telephone, 255
Slander, 45
Smoke detectors, 287
SNF. *See* Skilled nursing facility
SOAP documentation, 202–203, **203**
Social issues, ethics of, 65–66
Social Security Act Amendments of 1994, 363
Social Security tax, 408, 411–412
Software, 127, 132–138
   accounting and billing, 134
   antivirus, 140
   application, 132–138
   appointment scheduling, 134
   database management, 134
   documentation with, 138
   electronic medical record, vendors for, 205
   electronic transactions, 134–136
   manuals, 138
   online help with, **133,** 138
   operating system, 132
   optical character recognition, 133
   research, 136
   selection of, 138
   technical support for, 138
   training for, 136–138
   tutorials, 138
   voice (speech) recognition, 114, 142
   word processing, 133, 135p
Sole proprietorship, 67
SOMR. *See* Source-oriented medical records
Sorting files, 229
Sorting mail, 166, 167p
Source, in communication circle, 74, **74**
Source-oriented medical records (SOMR), 202
Special delivery, 164, 168
Special fourth-class mail, 163
Specialization, 17
Special needs, patients with
   office accommodations for, 290–291,
     291, 292p
   patient education for, 304–309
   payment responsibility for, 367
Specialties, medical, 26–30
Specialty career options, 35–38
Specialty items, in reception area, **282,**
   282–283
Speech/language pathologist, 38
Speech recognition software, 114, 142

Spelling checkers, 155–156
Sports medicine, 29
Stages of dying/stages of grief, 86–87
Stain cleaning, 284–285
Standardized code sets, 62
Standard of care, 51–52
Standard Precautions, 57
Standard procedure times, and
    scheduling, 262
State abbreviations, USPS, 150t
State Children's Health Plan (SCHIP), 323
Statements (billing), 148, 372–374
State taxes, 415
State Unemployment Tax Act (SUTA), 412–415
Statute of limitations, 50–51, 233, 370
Stereotyping, 84
Storage
    of controlled substances, 175
    of files, 219–220, 229, 231–233
    of health information, HIPAA and, 59
    of office supplies, 175–176
    of patient records, 53, 59, 219, 229,
        231–233
Storage cabinets, 175
Storage devices, computer, 130
Storage facilities, 232, **232**
Stress
    good *vs.* bad, 93
    managing, 92–93
    potential causes of, 93b
    reducing, 93, 94b
Student(s)
    externships for, 12–13
    success as, 8
Study habits, 8
Style, editing for, 156
Subjective data, in patient record, 203
Subject line, in business letter, **149,** 151
Subluxations, 30
Subnotebook computer, 126
Subpoena, 50
Subpoena duces tecum, 50
Substitute physician, 273
Substitution, as defense mechanism, 81
Subterms, in ICD-9-CM coding, 346
Success as student, 8
Summarizing, in therapeutic
    communication, 80
Superbills, 148, 370, **371**
    CPT coding for, 353, 354, **354**
    use of, 370, 372p
Supercomputers, 125–126
Supervisors, communication with, 89
Supplemental files, 227–228
Supplies
    correspondences, choosing, 147–148
    filing, **221,** 221–222
    mailing, 163
    medical, contaminated, 17
    office, managing, 171–188. *See also* Office
        supplies
Supply list, 173–174
Surgeons, 29, **30**
Surgery, 29
    consent form for, **307**
    CPT coding for, **350,** 353
    guidelines for, informing patient of, 308p
    patient education prior to, 306–309
        anatomical models for, 309, **309**
        benefits of, 306
        factual, 306–308
        informing patient of guidelines for
            surgery, **308**

participatory, 308–309
    relieving anxiety in, 309
    role of medical assistant in, 306
    sensory, 307
    types of, 306–308
    verifying understanding in, 309
reserving operating rooms for, 273
scheduling appointments for, 271,
    271p, **272**
Surgery flow sheet, 271, **272**
Surgical Board of Certification, 29
Surgical reports, in patient records, 193
Surgical room, reserving, 273
Surgical technician, 38
Surrogate mother, ethics of using, 65
Symbols, in CPT coding, 351, **352**
Symptoms
    definition of, 202
    multicultural attitudes and, 84b
    patient education about, 301
    in patient record, 202
    reports on, via telephone, 247

T

Tablet PC, 126
Tabs, filing, 221
Tabular List, of ICD-9-CM, 344, **345,**
    346–347, 346t
Tape backup, 139–140
Tape care and maintenance, 142
Tape drive, 130
Tax(es)
    calculating and filing, 411–417
    employment, 406–408, 411–412
    federal deposit schedules for, 411–412
    FICA, 408, 411–412
    filing wage and tax statements, **415,** 415–417
    income, 406, 411–412
    state and local, 415
    unemployment, 408, 412–415, **413**
Tax identification numbers, 405
Tax liability, 406
Tax liability accounts, 411
Taxonomy code, 339b
TCPA. *See* Telephone Consumer Protection Act
    of 1991
TDD. *See* Telecommunications device for
    the deaf
Team member, willingness to work with,
    20–21
Technical support, software, 138
Teenagers
    adolescent medicine for, 29
    minor status of, 47, 211
        emancipated, 367
        mature, 211
        payment responsibility in, 367
Telecommunications, 254
Telecommunications device for the deaf
    (TDD), 291, 401b
Telemedicine, 142
Telephone(s), 103–105
    backup systems for, 120
    cellular (cell), 104, 120, 248, 255
    effective use of, 242
    multiple lines on, 104
    patient courtesy, 104
Telephone banking, 401b
Telephone calls, 240–257
    answering machine for, 105, 252
    answering service for, 105, 252, 253p

checking for understanding in, 251
collection, 372
communicating feelings in, 251
communication skills for, 242
conference, 248, 254
difficult situations in, handling, 250
dishonest solicitations via, 186–187
documenting in patient records, 193,
    199–200, **200,** 251
emergency, 247, 248t, 249p, 268
ending conversation in, 251
etiquette for, 248–251
good impression in, 250–251
handling of, 103–105
HIPAA and, 243, 248
on hold, 250
incoming
    guidelines for, 243
    managing, 242–244
    types of, 244–248
legal issues in, 52
ordering supplies via, 180, 183b
outgoing
    applying telephone skills in, 253–254
    placing, 252–254
from patients, 245–247
personal, 248
policy on, patient information on, 302
prescription renewal via, 246–247
remembering patient's name in, 250–251
reminder, 268
routing of, 243–244
    calls handled by medical assistant,
        243–244
    calls requiring doctor's attention, 244
    routing list for, 244, **244**
    through automated menu, 106b
screening of, 243, 245b, 246p
taking messages from, 105, **251,** 251–252
    ensuring correct information in, 252
    tips for, 252
voice qualities in, 250
Telephone Consumer Protection Act of 1991
    (TCPA), 376–377
Telephone cramming, 255
Telephone log
    electronic, 252
    manual, 252
Telephone numbers, locating, 252–253
Telephone personal identification number
    (TPIN), 401b
Telephone slamming, 255
Telephone triage, 254
    automated, 254
    categorizing patient problems in, 254
    learning process of, 254
    providing patient education in, 254
    taking action in, 254
Teletype (TTY) device, 291
Television, in reception area, 289
Temperature, room, for reception area, 282
Templates, 148
Terminal digit filing, 225
Terminally ill patients
    communication with, 86–87
    Medicare coverage for, 320
Termination of care, 51, **52,** 53
Termination of services, **48,** 48–49
Terminology, insurance, 317
The Joint Commission (TJC), 38–40
    filing guidelines of, 219–220
    quality review by, 192
    storage guidelines of, 175

Therapeutic communication skills, 79–81
    defense mechanisms and, 80–81
    ineffective, 80
Thermal paper, for fax machine, 107
Thesaurus, 155
Third-class mail, 163
Third party, in health insurance, 317
Third-party check, 395
Third-party liability, 366–367
Third-party payer, 317
Tickler files, 226–227, 227p, 268, 274
Time limits, for insurance claims, 328
Timeliness, of patient records, 204
Time management, 18
Time-specified scheduling, 263, **264**
Title I, of Americans with Disabilities Act of
    1990, 67
Title III, of Americans with Disabilities Act of
    1990, 67
Title II of HIPAA, 58–62
Title I of HIPAA, 58
Title VII of Civil Rights Act of 1964, 66
TJC. *See* The Joint Commission
TLA. *See* Truth in Lending Act
Tone
    professional, in medical records, 204
    voice, in telephone calls, 250
Tort(s), 45
    intentional, 45–46
    unintentional, 46
Touch
    importance to elderly patients, 86
    as nonverbal communication, 78
Touch pad, 127
Touch screen, 127
Tower case, 126, **126**
Toys and games, in reception area, 289,
    289, 290p
TPIN. *See* Telephone personal identification
    number
TPO. *See* Treatment, payment, and
    operations
Tracing mail, 164, **166**
Trackball, 127
Tracking, of disbursements, 404
Training. *See* Education
Training, software, 136–138
Transaction slips, **364,** 365
Transcription, 33, 113–114, **114,** 115p, 199,
    205–208
    aids for, 208
    of direct dictation, 206–208
    of letters, reports, and notes, 207p
Transcriptionist, medical, 33, 207b–208b, **208**
Transfer, of medical records, 209–211, **211**
Transformation Plan in 2002, USPS, 163
Translation services, 85
Transmittal of Wages and Tax Statements
    (Form W-3), **416,** 417
Transplantation, ethics of, 65
Trans Union Credit Information Company, 378
Travel arrangements, 273, **274**
Traveler's checks, 403
Treatment
    consent form for, 303, **304**
    expectations, culture and, 84b
    quality of, patient records for
        evaluating, 192
Treatment, payment, and operations (TPO),
    sharing health information for,
    59–60
Treatment plan, in patient records, 193,
    196, 202

Triage
    definition of, 36
    by EMT/paramedic, 36
    telephone, 254
Trial balance, 405
TRICARE, 323, **323,** 357, 367
Troubleshooting, for office equipment,
    119–120
Truth in Lending Act (TLA), 376t,
    378–379, **380**
TRW Inc., 378
TTY. *See* Teletype device
Tubs, for filing, 219–220
Tutorials, software, 138
Type A personality, 93
Type B personality, 93
Typewriters, 107–110

U

Ulcer(s), peptic, 348
Underbooking, 273
Unemployment taxes, 408, 412–415, **413**
Uniform Anatomical Gift Act of 1968, 56
Uniform donor card, 56
Unilateral decision, on credit, 379
Unintentional torts, 46
Unit, in indexing rules, 223
United Parcel Service, 164
U.S. Medical Licensing Examination
    (USMLE), 26
U.S. Postal Service
    address abbreviations, 162, 162t
    delivery services of, 163–164
    optical character readers of, 161
    preparing outgoing mail for, 156–163
    regular mail service of, 163–164
    special services of, 164
    state abbreviations, 150t
    tracing mail, 164, **166**
    Transformation Plan in 2002, 163
Unit pricing, 180
Universal claim, 333
Unlisted procedure codes, 351
Updating patient records, 208
Urgent incoming mail, how to spot,
    168, 168b
Urologist, 30
Urology, 30
Use additional code, in ICD-9-CM coding, 348
USMLE. *See* U.S. Medical Licensing
    Examination
USPS. *See* U.S. Postal Service
Usual fees, 363

V

Vaccine(s)
    CPT coding for, 353
    retention of records, 233
Vaginal cyst, excision of, CPT coding
    for, 355
V codes, in ICD-9-CM, 346, 347
Vendor(s)
    comparison of, 180, **181**
    computer, choosing, 139
    disbursement to, 186
    for electronic medical record software, 205
    local, benefits of using, 182
    office supply, locating and evaluating, 180
    reputable, 180

Verbal communication
    negative, 77
    positive, 77
Vertical file, 219
Veterans, health plan for, 323
Videotapes
    for patient education, 299, **299**
    in reception area, 289
Violations, HIPAA, 61–62
Virtual Hospital, 136t
Virtual private networks (VPNs), 139
Viruses, computer, 140
Visual impairments
    ICD-9-CM coding for, 345–346
    patients with
        communicating with, 85
        office accommodations for, 291
        patient education for, 306
Visual materials, for patient education, 299
Vital signs, 199
Vital supplies, 174
Vocational nurse, 34–35
Voice, telephone, 250
Voice mail, 104
Voice recognition software, 114, 142
Void contract, 46
Voided check, 114, 403
Voluntary deductions, from pay, 406
Volunteer programs, 13–15
Voucher checks, 403
VPNs. *See* Virtual private networks

W

W-2 (IRS Form), **415,** 415–417
W-3 (IRS Form), **416,** 417
W-4 (IRS form), 406, **407**
Wage and Tax Statement (Form W-2), **415,**
    415–417
Waiting room. *See also* Reception area
    negative connotation of, 281
Walk-ins, 270
WANs. *See* Wide-area networks
Warmth, as interpersonal skill, 79
Warning signs, of disease, 301
Warranty, 117
Waste, infectious, 285–286
Wave scheduling, 263
WebMD Health, 136t
Wellness promotion, 299–301
White coat syndrome, 82
WHO. *See* World Health Organization
Wide-area networks (WANs), 139
Willingness
    to learn, 18–19, **19**
    to work with team member, 20–21
Windows (operating system), 132
Windows Vista, 132
Windows XP, 132
Withdrawal from case, 51, **52,** 53
Withholding, payroll, 406–408
Word processing, 133
    spelling checkers, 155–156
    use of, 135p
Worker's compensation, 324, 324p, 408
Workplace settings
    certified medical assistant, 16b
    coding, billing, and insurance
        specialist, 381b
    medical office administrator or
        manager, 32b
    medical receptionist, 281b

medical transcriptionist, 207b
occupational therapist assistant, 311b
registered health information technologist, 236b
World Health Organization (WHO), 344
Wrist fracture, ICD-9-CM coding for, 345
Writing, effective, 152–154
Written communication, 90–92, 146. *See also* Letter(s); Written correspondence
community resources, 90–91, 92p
interoffice memorandums, 154, **155**
policy and procedures manual, 90, **91**
Written-contract account, 370
Written correspondence, 148–156
basic rules for, 156, 157t
business letter, **149,** 149–151, 159p–160p
editing and proofreading of, 154–156
effective writing in, 152–154
folding and inserting, 111, **112,** 156, **160,** 162–163
full-block letter, 152, **152**
inclusion in patient records, 197
interoffice memorandums, 154, **155**
letter format, 151
letter styles, 151–152, **152, 153, 154**
misspellings in, common, 156, 158t–159t
modified-block letter, 152, **153**
modified-block letter with indented paragraphs, 152, **153**
punctuation style in, 151
signing, 161
simplified letter style, 152, **154**
Wrong-day appointments, 270

X

X12 837 Health Care Claim, 333, 339b

Y

Young patient. *See* Children

Z

Zip drive, 130